# WRITTEN REGISTRY EXAM REVIEW FOR RESPIRATORY CARE: GUIDELINES FOR SUCCESS

## SECOND EDITION

•

## WILLIAM V. WOJCIECHOWSKI

**DELMAR** ™
**THOMSON LEARNING**

Australia Canada Mexico Singapore Spain United Kingdom United States

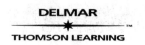

**DELMAR**

**THOMSON LEARNING** ™

## Written Registry Exam Review for Respiratory Care: Guidelines for Success
### by William V. Wojciechowski

**Business Unit Director:**
William Brottmiller

**Executive Editor:**
Cathy L. Esperti

**Acquisitions Editor:**
Candice Janco

**Development Editor:**
Patricia A. Gaworecki

**Editorial Assistant:**
Maria D'Angelico

**Executive Marketing Manager:**
Dawn F. Gerrain

**Channel Manager:**
Tara Carter

**Project Editor:**
Maureen M. E. Grealish

**Production Coordinator:**
John Mickelbank

**Art/Design Coordinator:**
Mary Colleen Liburdi

**Cover Design:**
TDB Publishing Service

Library of Congress Cataloging-in-Publication Data
Written registry exam review for respiratory care: guidelines for success/William V. Wojciechowski, [editor].—2nd ed.
   p. cm.
   Includes bibliographical references.
   ISBN 0-7668-0781-9 (alk. paper)
   1. Respiratory therapy—Examinations, questions, etc.   I. Wojciechowski, William V.
RC735.I5 W75  2001
615.8'36'076—dc21          2001017478

### NOTICE TO THE READER

# Contents

PREFACE                                                                        v

ACKNOWLEDGMENTS                                                              vii

CONTRIBUTORS                                                                  ix

CONTRIBUTORS TO THE ELECTRONIC PRACTICE TEST                                  xi

REVIEWERS                                                                   xiii

INTRODUCTION                                                                   1

TEST OBJECTIVES                                                               1

ORGANIZATION OF BOOK CONTENT                                                  1

HOW TO USE EACH CHAPTER                                                       1

WRITTEN REGISTRY EXAMINATION STRUCTURE                                        3

WRITTEN REGISTRY EXAMINATION MATRIX                                           3

NBRC WRITTEN REGISTRY EXAMINATION FOR ADVANCED
  RESPIRATORY THERAPISTS (RRTs) CONTENT OUTLINE                      4

ANSWERS                                                                      13

WRITTEN EXAMINATION ITEM FORMAT                                              13

WRITTEN REGISTRY EXAMINATION INFORMATION                                     14

WRITTEN EXAMINATION PREPARATION                                              15

CHAPTER 1 • TEST PREPARATION                                                 17

ACADMIC PREPARATION                                                          17

PHYSICAL PREPARATION                                                         19

TESTWISENESS                                                                 19

ATTITUDINAL PREPARATION                                                      20

CHAPTER 2 • PRETEST                                                          22

PRETEST ANSWER SHEET                                                         23

PRETEST ASSESSMENT                                                           25

PRETEST MATRIX CATEGORIES                                                    41

CHAPTER 2 PRETEST WRITTEN REGISTRY EXAMINATION
  MATRIX SCORING FORM                                                42

NBRC WRITTEN REGISTRY EXAMINATION FOR ADVANCED
  RESPIRATORY THERAPISTS (RRTs) CONTENT OUTLINE                       43

PRETEST ANSWERS AND ANALYSES                                                 52

REFERENCES                                                                   80

CHAPTER 3 • CLINICAL DATA                                                    81

CLINICAL DATA ANSWER SHEET                                                   82

CLINICAL DATA ASSESSMENT                                                     86

CLINICAL DATA MATRIX CATEGORIES                                             119

CHAPTER 3 CLININCAL DATA: WRITTEN REGISTRY
    EXAMINATION MATRIX SCORING FORM ..... 121

NBRC WRITTEN REGISTRY EXAMINATION FOR ADVANCED
    RESPIRATORY THERAPISTS (RRTs) CONTENT OUTLINE ..... 123

CLINICAL DATA ANSWERS AND ANALYSES ..... 126

REFERENCES ..... 181

CHAPTER 4 • EQUIPMENT ..... 182

EQUIPMENT ANSWER SHEET ..... 183

EQUIPMENT ASSESSMENT ..... 186

EQUIPMENT MATRIX CATEGORIES ..... 204

CHAPTER 4 EQUIPMENT: WRITTEN REGISTRY
    EXAMINATION MATRIX SCORING FORM ..... 205

NBRC WRITTEN REGISTRY EXAMINATION FOR ADVANCED
    RESPIRATORY THERAPISTS (RRTs) CONTENT OUTLINE ..... 206

EQUIPMENT ANSWERS AND ANALYSES ..... 209

REFERENCES ..... 240

CHAPTER 5 • THERAPEUTIC PROCEDURES ..... 241

THERAPEUTIC PROCEDURES ANSWER SHEET ..... 242

THERAPEUTIC PROCEDURES ASSESSMENT ..... 246

THERAPEUTIC PROCEDURES MATRIX CATEGORIES ..... 280

CHAPTER 5 THERAPEUTIC PROCEDURES: WRITTEN
    REGISTRY EXAMINATION MATRIX SCORING FORM ..... 282

NBRC WRITTEN REGISTRY EXAMINATION FOR ADVANCED
    RESPIRATORY THERAPISTS (RRTs) CONTENT OUTLINE ..... 284

THERAPEUTIC PROCEDURES ANSWERS AND ANALYSES ..... 287

REFERENCES ..... 345

CHAPTER 6 • POSTTEST ..... 346

POSTTEST ANSWER SHEET ..... 347

POSTTEST ASSESSMENT ..... 349

POSTTEST: MATRIX CATEGORIES ..... 366

CHAPTER 6 POSTTEST: ENTRY-LEVEL EXAMINATION
    MATRIX SCORING FORM ..... 367

NBRC WRITTEN REGISTRY EXAMINATION FOR ADVANCED
    RESPIRATORY THERAPISTS (RRTs) CONTENT OUTLINE ..... 368

POSTTEST ANSWERS AND ANALYSES ..... 377

REFERENCES ..... 401

APPENDIX 1 • QUICK REFERENCE MATERIAL—CLINICAL DATA ..... 403

APPENDIX 2 • QUICK REFERENCE MATERIAL—WAVEFORMS
    AND TRACINGS ..... 409

APPENDIX 3 • QUICK REFERENCE MATERIAL—PHYSICAL
    ASSESSMENT OF THE CHEST ..... 425

# Preface

Every five years, the National Board for Respiratory Care (NBRC) conducts job analysis surveys to determine changes in the clinical practice of respiratory therapy. These surveys are the foundation upon which the matrices for all the credentialing examinations are based. The questions appearing on the NBRC examinations are directly related to the matrix of each examination.

The second edition of the *Written Registry* (formerly titled Advanced Practitioner) *Exam Review for Respiratory Care: Guidelines for Success* has undergone a few modifications in this edition in response to changes in the following:

(1) the Written Registry Examination Matrix,
(2) the NBRC's computerized examination policy, and
(3) the inclusion of more application-type questions on the Written Registry Examination.

Therefore, the second edition reflects the most recent NBRC examination specifications.

A special feature included in the second edition is a computerized simulation of the Written Registry Examination on CD-ROM. The computerized examination offers candidates an opportunity to familiarize themselves with the new computerized NBRC testing format, which began in January 2000. Located on the inside back cover, it parallels the NBRC credentialing examination in style and content, including a timing feature.

The authors of this simulated credentialing examination are 27 of the foremost educators, managers, and practitioners in the profession today. These renowned contributors are listed alphabetically on page ix of this text.

Furthermore, the second edition contains close to 900 questions and analyses providing Written Registry Examination candidates with a comprehensive exposure to the Written Registry Examination Matrix. Many people have remarked, "This book contains a gold mine of questions."

Despite the expansion of this book, candidates will be happy to know that the text retains the features and characteristics that made the first edition so successful.

In addition to the computerized Written Registry Examination, the second edition boasts an expanded appendix now containing ventilator waveforms. More graphics have been added to complement those that already enhance understanding.

Candidates who used the *Entry-Level Examination Review for Respiratory Care: Guidelines for Success 2/e* to prepare for the Entry-Level Examination will encounter a smooth transition from entry-level material to subject matter pertaining to the advanced practitioner. Nonetheless, the organization of this text is user-friendly and is designed to produce an organized, systematic, and thorough review process.

Remember, the most efficient method to prepare for an examination is to practice answering questions based on the content covered on the examination for which the candidate is preparing. Merely reading outlines or text amounts to the shotgun approach. This book, with its exhaustive number of questions and analyses, provides the candidate with an empirical and systematic method for identifying areas of strength and weakness. This approach enables the candidate to focus time and effort on specific content. This time is not wasted.

I am gratified and motivated by remarks from numerous respiratory care practitioners who approach me at AARC meetings to express how helpful the first edition of this book was toward their preparation for the NBRC Written Registry Examination. My intention is for the second edition to be even better.

Good luck to you on the Written Registry Examination and throughout your professional career.

—*William V. Wojciechowski, MS, RRT*

# Acknowledgments

This book has evolved from input by colleagues, anonymous practitioners, and NBRC matrix updates. I, therefore, wish to thank the 27 professionals who wrote the electronic Practice Written Registry Examination accompanying this book. The inclusion of this practice test on CD-ROM is sure to have a tremendous positive impact on those who use this review book.

First and probably most important, I wish to thank Deanna Winn for keeping me organized and on track as this project overlapped with other writing commitments. Her diligence, vigilance, and attention to detail were instrumental in retaining the positive qualities of the first edition and in adding beneficial new features to the second.

My friend and colleague, Fred Hill, MA, RRT deserves special recognition for his painstaking review of the manuscript. His input has improved the quality of this text.

Special thanks are also extended to the reviewers for their meticulous review of this manuscript. Their suggestions were illuminating.

The dedicated personnel at Delmar Thomson Learning deserve praise for their professional assistance (Dawn Gerrain, Patty Gaworecki, and Tara Carter).

*—William V. Wojciechowski, MS, RRT*

# Contributors

Bruce S. Brown, BS, RRT
Director Clinical Education
Respiratory Care Program
Brevard Community College
Cocoa, FL

Walter C. Chop, MS, RRT
Program Director
Respiratory Therapy
Southern Maine Technical College
South Portland, ME

Joseph DiPietro, MS, RRT
Professor and Director
Respiratory Care Programs
Southwest Virginia Community College
Richlands, VA

Bill Galvin, MSED, RRT, CPFT
Assistant Professor, Division of Allied Health
Program Director, Respiratory Care Program
Gwynedd-Mercy College
Gwynedd Valley, PA

Paul Mathews, Jr., MPA, EdS, RRT
Tarilyn Dobey, MEd, RRT
Bethene L. Gregg, MS, RRT
L. "Mickey" Mathews, RN, BA
College of Health Sciences
University of Kansas
Kansas City, KS

Paula E. Neff, Esq.
Attorney with Burke, Murphy, Costanza & Cuppy
Merrillville, IN

Donald O'Donohue, MEd, RRT
Ruth S. Dever, BA, RRT
Martha C. Huddleson, AAS, RRT
Kathryn J. Massino, BGS, RRT
J. Sargeant Reynolds Community College
Richmond, VA

David S. Shelledy, PhD, RRT, RPFT
Chairman, Department of Respiratory Care
University of Texas Health Science Center
San Antonio, TX

Debra A. Szymanski, MA, RRT
Director of Clinical Education/Faculty
Respiratory Therapist Program
Henry Ford Community College
Dearborn, MI

David N. Yonutas, MS, RRT
Program Coordinator
Santa Fe Community College
Health Sciences
Gainesville, FL

# Contributors to the Electronic Practice Test

Wesley M. Granger, PhD, RRT
Program Director Respiratory Therapy Program
University of Alabama at Birmingham
Birmingham, Alabama

Kerry E. George, RRT, RCP
Program Director
Des Moines Area Community College
Ankeny, Iowa

Linda Van Scoder, EdD, RRT
Associate Professor
Respiratory Therapy Program
Indiana University School of Medicine
Indianapolis, Indiana

Karen A. Milikowski, MS, RRT
Director of Health Careers
Manchester Community College
Manchester, Connecticut

Fred Hill, MA, RRT
Assistant Professor
Department of Cardiorespiratory Care
University of South Alabama
Mobile, Alabama

William C. Pruitt, MBA, RRT
Instructor
Department of Cardiorespiratory Care
University of South Alabama
Mobile, Alabama

Robert L. Wilkins, PhD, RRT, FAARC
Chairman and Professor
Department of Cardiopulmonary Sciences
Loma Linda University
Loma Linda, California

Georgine W. Bills, MBA/HSA, RRT
Program Director, Respiratory Therapy Education
Weber State University
Ogden, Utah

Leyda Torres de Marin, MA, RRT
Program Director
Sistema Universitario Ana G. Mendez
Universidad Metropolitano
San Juan, Puerto Rico

F. Herbert Douce, MS, RRT, RPFT
Associate Professor and Director
Respiratory Therapy
The Ohio State University
Columbus, Ohio

Bill Galvin, MSEd, RRT, CPFT
Assistant Professor
School of Allied Health Professions
Program Director
Respiratory Care Program
Teaching and Administrative Faculty
TIPS Program
Gwynedd Mercy College
Gwynedd Valley, Pennsylvania

Shelley C. Mishoe, PhD, RRT, FAARC
Professor,
School of Allied Health Sciences and
School of Graduate Studies
Chairperson,
Department of Respiratory Therapy
Medical College of Georgia
Augusta, Georgia

Robert M. Kacmarek, PhD, RRT
Associate Professor of Anesthesiology
Harvard Medical School
Director, Respiratory Care
Massachusetts General Hospital
Boston, Massachusetts

Robert R. Fluck, Jr., MS, RRT
Director of Clinical Education
Department of Cardiorespiratory Sciences
SUNY Upstate Medical University
Syracuse, New York

Dr. Deborah Cullen, RRT, FAARC
Professor and Director
Respiratory Therapy Program
Indiana University
Indianapolis, Indiana

Susan P. Pilbeam, MS, RRT
Program Director
Respiratory Care
Edison Community College
Fort Myers, Florida

Wayne Lawson, MS, RRT
Assistant Professor
Department of Respiratory Care
University of Texas Health Science Center
at San Antonio
San Antonio, Texas

David N. Yonutas, MS, RRT,
Program Director, Respiratory Care and
Surgical Technology
Santa Fe Community College
Gainesville, Florida

Vijay M. Deshpande, MS, RRT, FAARC
Assistant Professor
Georgia State University
Atlanta, Georgia

Vincent C. Madama, MEd, RRT
Director of Clinical Education
Rock Valley College
Rockford, Illinois

Richard D. Branson, BA, RRT
Associate Professor of Surgery
University of Cincinnati
Cincinnati, Ohio

Thomas A. Barnes, EdD, RRT, FAARC
Professor of Cardiopulmonary Sciences
Director, Respiratory Therapy and Cardiovascular
Technology Programs
Bouvé College of Pharmacy & Health Sciences
Northeastern University
Boston, Massachusetts

Patrick L. Johnson, Jr., Phd, RRT
Associate Professor
Division of Cardiopulmonary Science
Florida A & M University
Tallahassee, FL

# Reviewers

Gregory Allred, RRT
Director, Respiratory Care
Marshall Medical Center North
Guntersville, Alabama

Sharon Baer, MBA, RRT, CPFT
Assistant Professor, Program Director
Respiratory Care
Naugatuck Valley Community Technical College
Waterbury, Connecticut

Kathy Beney
SUNY Health Science Center at Syracuse
Department of Cardiorespiratory Sciences
Syracuse, New York

Jim Bierl, MS, RRT
Professor, Director Clinical Education
Respiratory Care Program
Erie Community College
Williamsville, New York

Bruce A. Carr, RRT
Director of Cardiology and Respiratory
Care Services
Fanny Allen Hospital
Colchester, Vermont

Erin Davis, MS, MEd, RRT, CPFT
Our Lady of Holy Cross College
Clinical Education Department
New Orleans, Louisiana

Beverly Edwards, BHS, RRT
Department Chair
Florida Community College at Jacksonville
Jacksonville, FL

Marie Fenske, EdD, RRT
Program Director
Respiratory Care
Gateway Community College
Phoenix, Arizona

Fred Hill, MA, RRT
University of South Alabama
Cardiorespiratory Care
Mobile, Alabama

Gerald E. Hunt, MS, RRT, RPFT
Director of Clinical Education
Respiratory Care Program
Butte Community College
Oroville, California

Arthur Jones, EdD, RRT
Assistant Professor and
Director of Clinical Education
Respiratory Care Department
University of Texas Medical Branch
Galveston, Texas

Paul LaMere, MS, RRT
College of Saint Catherine
Respiratory Care Department
Minneapolis, Minnesota

Gayle Peterson
Director of Clinical Education
Respiratory Care Program
Illinois Central College
Peoria, Illinois

Kathy Jones-Boggs Rye, M.Ed., RRT
University of Arkansas Medical Sciences
College of Health Related Professions
Department of Respiratory Care
Assistant Professor & Director of Clinical Education
Little Rock, Arkansas

Marcus Stowe, RRT
Ivy Tech State College
Indianapolis, Indiana

Laverne Yousey, MSTE, RRT
University of Akron
Allied Health
Akron, Ohio

## Text Objectives

The objectives of this text are to:

1. Prepare persons for the National Board for Respiratory Care (NBRC) Written Registry Examination for Advanced Respiratory Therapists (RRTs).
2. Assist respiratory therapy students in technician- and therapist-level programs with preparing for course examinations.
3. Prepare practitioners for legal credentialing (state) examinations.
4. Provide an organized approach for preparation for the Written Registry Examination.
5. Provide a self-assessment mechanism for credentialed respiratory therapy practitioners.
6. Assist respiratory therapy educators in developing evaluation instruments for course examinations.
7. Assist respiratory therapy educators with conducting review sessions for the Registry Examination for Advanced Respiratory Therapists.

## Organization of Book Content

This book consists of six chapters:

Introduction
Chapter 1: Test Preparation
Chapter 2: Pretest
Chapter 3: Clinical Data
Chapter 4: Equipment
Chapter 5: Therapeutic Procedures
Chapter 6: Posttest

## How To Use Each Chapter

### Introduction

The introduction provides the following information: (1) states this text's objectives, (2) explains how to use this review book, (3) describes the makeup and content areas contained in the NBRC Registry Examination for Advanced Respiratory Therapists (RRTs), (4) provides information about how to prepare for the Written Registry Examination, and (5) describes the three levels of questions contained on the Written Registry Examination.

Refer to the matrix of the examination to become familiar with the concepts that are presented on the credentialing examination. You must focus on the specific material described in each matrix item. Doing so makes your study time more efficient. Do not neglect this critical step in the credentialing examination review process. To assist you in this task, the questions in this book have been categorized into their content areas via the Written Registry Examination Matrix Scoring Form located in Chapters 2 through 6. You should use these forms as a prescription of study. Collate your results and focus your attention on the areas that require remediation.

### Chapter 1 • Test Preparation

Embarking on a credentialing examination review process requires a positive attitude. The content of Chapter 1 focuses your attention on the task at hand. As formidable an undertaking as the review process seems, a number of practical and relatively easy plans of action are presented to help alleviate your anxiety and stress. Suggestions for organizing a realistic timetable for using the examination review material presented in this text are provided. You are encouraged to implement the strategies provided for your use.

### Chapter 2 • Pretest (100 Items, Analyses, and References)

The pretest should be performed without the benefit of advance preparation. You should simply take it to establish a baseline for the measurement of your progress through this study guide. Make sure you allow yourself two hours of uninterrupted time to complete the pretest. That length of time is provided by the NBRC for this credentialing examination. Place yourself in a quiet, well-lighted, and well-ventilated area. Be seated on a chair with a back support at a desk or table.

The pretest offers you the opportunity to identify content areas that might require remediation. The pretest parallels the NBRC Written Registry Examination. The items on the pretest match the testing categories found on the Written Registry Examination. The following table indicates the content areas and the item distribution comprising the pretest.

Pretest Content Areas and Item Distribution

| Content Areas | Number of Items |
| --- | --- |
| I. Clinical Data | 17 |
| II. Equipment | 20 |
| III. Therapeutic Procedures | 63 |
| Total | 100 |

After completing the pretest, use the answer sheet provided in the book to determine your score. Use the Written Registry Examination Matrix Scoring Form located after the analysis to score each content category and to determine content areas that require remediation. Review and study the analyses of the questions that you have answered incorrectly and the analyses of the questions you might have gotten correct by answering with an *educated* guess. In other words, also review the analyses of any questions of which you are unsure.

After studying each question and analysis, refer to the Written Registry Examination Matrix located within Chapters 2 through 6. The matrix outlines all of the tasks that fall within the purview of the Written Registry Examination. You must become familiar with the range of knowledge and cognitive areas for which you are responsible on this credentialing examination. The manner in which to achieve this familiarity is to study the Written Registry Examination matrix, as well.

When you have reviewed the appropriate matrix categories, read and study the material indicated by the references. The references are provided to offer you a more detailed account of the concept associated with each question and analysis. By reading the matrix designation before proceeding to the references, you will be more focused on the information that is pertinent to the matrix category and less likely to go off on tangents as you read material in the references. After you have thoroughly reviewed the questions, analyses, matrix designations, and references, proceed to the next chapter.

## Chapter 3 • Clinical Data (212 Items, Analyses, and References)

Chapter 3 enables you to evaluate your knowledge in the three categories within this content area:

A. Review patient records and recommend diagnostic procedures.
B. Collect and evaluate additional clinical information.
C. Perform procedures, interpret results, and recommend modifications to the care plan.

Among the three categories encountered in the content area of clinical data, there are 79 matrix designations. Seventeen matrix items will be included on the Written Registry Examination.

Because there is no way to determine which 17 items relating to clinical data will appear on the examination, the candidate needs to experience questions from each matrix item. This chapter provides the candidate with practice questions that encompass all of the possible types that might be encountered on the actual examination.

In addition to thoroughly studying the questions, analyses, and references of the questions that were either incorrectly answered or answered correctly by guessing, you are encouraged to note the matrix designation of those questions and refer to the Written Registry Examination matrix for a clear description of the concept being tested. Remember to use the Written Registry Examination Matrix Scoring Form associated with the chapter to help identify areas of strength and weakness regarding clinical data.

Again, as with all of the other chapters, use the answer sheet provided at the beginning of each assessment. A minimum passing score for this assessment would be 159 correct out of 212 items, or 75%.

## Chapter 4 • Equipment (130 Items, Analyses, and References)

This chapter offers you the opportunity to evaluate your understanding of the two categories within this content area:

A. Select and obtain equipment; assure equipment cleanliness.
B. Assemble, check for proper function, correct equipment malfunctions, and perform quality control.

The two categories within this content area are represented by 115 matrix designations. Only 20 items from this section appear on the Written Registry Examination.

This chapter offers you an opportunity to sample the entire gamut of matrix items, because the assessment presented here contains 130 questions.

Again, you are urged to completely review the materials that require remediation and cross-reference the items to the Written Registry Matrix. Use the answer sheet located in front of the test and then employ the Written Registry Examination Matrix Scoring Form found after the analyses. A score of 75% would result from correctly answering 98 out of 130 items presented.

**Chapter 5 • Therapeutic Procedures (208 Items, Analyses, and References)**

This chapter enables you to evaluate your comprehension of the five categories within this content area:

A. Evaluate, monitor, and record the patient's response.
B. Maintain the airway, remove secretions, and assure ventilation and oxygenation.
C. Modify the therapy.
D. Perform emergency procedures.
E. Assist the physician in special procedures; conduct pulmonary rehabilitation/home care.

Therapeutic procedures contains five categories and has 77 matrix designations, 63 of which appear on the Written Registry Examination.

Chapter 5 provides you with 208 sample questions from this content area. Therefore, to achieve a passing score on this assessment, you must minimally answer 156 (75%) questions correctly. As before, careful attention to the remediation process and cross-referencing the questions to the Written Registry Examination Matrix should prepare you well for therapeutic procedures.

**Chapter 6 • Posttest (100 Items, Analyses, and References)**

The posttest is intended to provide you with feedback related to the remediation performed in response to the results obtained on the pretest. The posttest parallels the Written Registry Examination in terms of the content areas and the item distribution. The following table demonstrates the organization of the posttest:

Posttest Content Areas Item Distribution

| Content Areas | Number of Items |
|---|---|
| I. Clinical Data | 17 |
| II. Equipment | 20 |
| III. Therapeutic Procedures | 63 |
| Total | 100 |

Chapter 6 contains a posttest tailored after the Written Registry Examination. This evaluation tool represents the culmination of a substantial effort on the part of the candidate and of an exhaustive review of the Written Registry Examination Matrix.

The posttest should indicate the degree of progress you have made throughout the time that this review book was studied. The posttest should be approached seriously and with the confidence that should have developed over the past few weeks. As with the pretest, the posttest should be graded immediately, and for the final time, remediation (questions, analyses, and matrix) and cross-referencing must follow.

# Written Registry Examination Structure

The examination matrix is a detailed content outline describing the content categories appearing on the Written Registry Examination. The candidate needs to become familiar with the examination matrix. Keep in mind that the items appearing on the credentialing examination are developed from this outline.

The Written Registry Examination Matrix provides you with the information that is evaluated on this credentialing examination. The matrix of this test helps evaluate whether you possess the cognitive skills necessary to function as an Advanced Registered Respiratory Therapist (RRT).

# Written Registry Examination Matrix

The Written Registry Examination Matrix is composed of three major content areas:

I. Clinical Data
II. Equipment
III. Therapeutic Procedures

Each of these content areas is divided into a number of subcategories. The subcategories are subdivided into more specific content elements.

You should familiarize yourself with the following examination matrix as much as possible because the Written Registry Examination is based on it. You are encouraged to refer to this matrix throughout your preparation for the NBRC Written Registry Examination. As you work through each chapter in this book, you will notice each examination item has a specific matrix designation. Match that matrix designation with the content area identified on the matrix itself.

# NBRC Written Registry Examination for Advanced Respiratory Therapists (RRTs) Content Outline

This content outline is reprinted with permission of the copyright holder, the National Board For Respiratory Care, Inc., 8310 Nieman Rd, Lenexa, KS 66214. All rights reserved. Effective December 1999.

**I. Select, Review, Obtain, and Interpret Data**

SETTING: In any patient care setting, the advanced respiratory care therapist reviews existing clinical data, collects or recommends obtaining additional pertinent data. The therapist evaluates all data to determine the appropriateness of the prescribed respiratory care plan, and participates in the development of the respiratory care plan.

| | RECALL | APPLICATION | ANALYSIS |
|---|---|---|---|
| | 3 | 3 | 11 |
| **A. Review patient records and recommend diagnostic procedures.** | 1* | 1 | 3 |
| 1. Review existing data in patient's record: | | | |
| a. patient history [e.g., present illness, admission notes, respiratory care orders, progress notes] | X** | | |
| b. physical examination [e.g., vital signs, physical findings] | X | | |
| c. lab data [e.g., CBC, chemistries/electrolytes, coagulation studies, Gram stain, culture and sensitivities, urinalysis] | X | X | |
| d. pulmonary function and blood gas results | X | X | |
| e. radiological studies [e.g., X-rays of chest/upper airway, CT, MRI] | X | X | |
| f. monitoring data | | | |
| (1) fluid balance (intake and output) | | | |
| (2) pulmonary mechanics [e.g., maximum inspiratory pressure (MIP), vital capacity] | X | X | |
| (3) respiratory monitoring [e.g., rate, tidal volume, minute volume, I:E, inspiratory and expiratory pressures; flow, volume and pressure waveforms] | X | X | |
| (4) lung compliance, airway resistance, work of breathing | X | X | |
| (5) noninvasive monitoring [e.g., capnography, pulse oximetry, transcutaneous $O_2/CO_2$] | X | X | |
| g. results of cardiovascular monitoring | | | |
| (1) ECG, blood pressure, heart rate | X | X | |
| (2) hemodynamic monitoring [e.g., central venous pressure, cardiac output, pulmonary capillary wedge pressure, pulmonary artery pressures, mixed venous $O_2$, $C(a\text{-}\bar{v})O_2$, shunt studies ($\dot{Q}s/\dot{Q}t$)] | X | X | |
| h. maternal and perinatal/neonatal history and data [e.g., Apgar scores, gestational age, L/S ration, pre/post-ductal oxygenation studies] | X | | |
| i. other diagnostic studies [e.g., EEG, intracranial pressure monitoring, metabolic studies ($\dot{V}O_2$, $\dot{V}CO_2$, nutritional assessment), ventilation/perfusion scan, pulmonary angiography, sleep studies, other ultrasonography] | | | |
| 2. Recommend the following procedures to obtain additional data: | | | |
| a. CBC, electrolytes, other blood chemistries | | | |
| b. X-ray of chest and upper airway, CT scan, bronchoscopy, ventilation/perfusion lung scan, barium swallow | X | X | |
| c. Gram stain, culture and sensitivities | X | X | |
| d. Spirometry before and/or after bronchodilator, maximum voluntary ventilation, diffusing capacity, functional residual capacity, flow-volume loops, body plethysmography, nitrogen washout distribution test, total lung capacity, $CO_2$ response curve, closing volume, airway resistance, bronchoprovocation, maximum inspiratory pressure (MIP), maximum expiratory pressure (MEP) | X | X | |
| e. blood gas analysis, insertion of arterial, umbilical and/or central venous, pulmonary artery monitoring lines | X | X | |
| f. lung compliance, airway resistance, lung mechanics, work of breathing | X | X | |

*The number in each column is the number of items in that content area and cognitive level contained in each examination. For example, in category I.A., one item will be asked at the recall level, one item at the application level, and three items at the analysis level. The items could be asked relative to any tasks listed (1–2) under category I.A.

**Note: An "X" denotes the examination does NOT contain items for the given task at the cognitive level indicated in the respective column (Recall, Application, Analysis).

| | RECALL | APPLICATION | ANALYSIS |
|---|---|---|---|
| g. ECG, echocardiography, pulse oximetry, transcutaneous $O_2/CO_2$ monitoring | X | X | |
| h. $V_D/V_T$, $\dot{Q}s/\dot{Q}t$, cardiac output, cardiopulmonary stress testing | | | |
| **B. Collect and evaluate clinical information.** | **1** | **1** | **5** |
| 1. Assess patient's overall cardiopulmonary status by *inspection* to determine: | | | |
| a. general appearance, muscle wasting, venous distention, peripheral edema, diaphoresis, digital clubbing, cyanosis, capillary refill | X | X | |
| b. chest configuration, evidence of diaphragmatic movement, breathing pattern, accesory muscle activity, asymmetrical chest movement, intercostal and/or sternal retractions, nasal flaring, character of cough, amount and character of sputum | X | X | |
| c. transillumination of chest, Apgar score, gestational age | X | X | |
| 2. Assess patient's overall cardiopulmonary status by *palpation* to determine: | | | |
| a. heart rate, rhythm, force | X | X | |
| b. asymmetrical chest movements, tactile fremitus, crepitus, tenderness, secretions in the airway, tracheal deviation, endotracheal tube placement | X | X | |
| 3. Assess patient's overall cardiopulmonary status by *percussion* to determine diaphragmatic excursion and areas of altered resonance | X | X | |
| 4. Assess patient's overall cardiopulmonary status by *auscultation* to determine presence of: | | | |
| a. breath sounds [e.g., normal, bilateral, increased, decreased, absent, unequal, rhonchi or crackles (râles), wheezing, stridor, friction rub] | X | X | |
| b. heart sounds, dysrhythmias, murmurs, bruits | X | X | |
| c. blood pressure | X | X | |
| 5. Assess patient's learning needs [e.g., age and language appropriateness, education level, prior disease and medication knowledge] | X | X | |
| 6. Interview patient to determine: | | | |
| a. level of consciousness, orientation to time, place and person, emotional state, ability to cooperate | X | X | |
| b. presence of dyspnea and/or orthopnea, work of breathing, sputum | | | |

| | RECALL | APPLICATION | ANALYSIS |
|---|---|---|---|
| production, exercise tolerance and activities of daily living | X | X | |
| c. physical environment, social support systems, nutritional status | X | X | |
| 7. Review chest X-ray to determine: | | | |
| a. presence of, or changes in, pheumothorax or subcutaneous emphysema, other extra-pulmonary air, consolidation and/or atelectasis, pulmonary infiltrates | X | X | |
| b. presence and postion of foreign bodies | X | X | |
| c. position of endotracheal or tracheostomy tube, evidence of endotracheal or tracheostomy tube cuff hyperinflation | X | X | |
| d. position of chest tube(s), nasogastric and/or feeding tube, pulmonary artery catheter (Swan-Ganz), pacemaker, CVP, and other catheters | X | | |
| e. position of, or changes in, hemidiaphragms, hyperinflation, pleural fluid, pulmonary edema, mediastinal shift, patency and size of major airways | X | X | |
| 8. Review lateral neck X-ray to determine: | | | |
| a. presence of epiglottitis and subglottic edema | X | X | |
| b. presence or position of foreign bodies | X | X | |
| c. airway narrowing | X | X | |
| 9. Perform bedside procedures to determine: | | | |
| a. ECG, pulse oximetry, transcutaneous $O_2/CO_2$ monitoring, capnography, mass spectrometry | X | X | |
| b. tidal volume, minute volume, I:E | X | X | |
| c. blood gas analysis, $P(A-a)O_2$, alveolar ventilation, $V_D/V_T$, $\dot{Q}s/\dot{Q}t$, mixed venous sampling | X | X | |
| d. peak flow, maximum inspiratory pressure, maximum expiratory pressure, forced vital capacity, timed forced expiratory volumes [e.g., $FEV_1$], lung compliance, lung mechanics | X | X | |
| e. cardiac output, pulmonary capillary wedge pressure, central venous pressure, pulmonary artery pressures, fluid balance (intake and output) | | | |
| f. pulmonary vascular resistance and systemic vascular resistance | | | |
| g. apnea monitoring, sleep studies, respiratory impedance plethysmography | X | X | |
| h. tracheal tube cuff pressure, volume | X | X | |

| | RECALL | APPLICATION | ANALYSIS |
|---|---|---|---|
| 10. Interpret results of bedside procedures to determine: | | | |
|   a. ECG, pulse oximetry, transcutaneous $O_2/CO_2$ monitoring, capnography, mass spectrometry | X | X | |
|   b. tidal volume, minute volume, I:E | X | X | |
|   c. blood gas analysis, P(A-a)$O_2$, alveolar ventilation, $V_D/V_T$, Qs/Qt, mixed venous sampling | X | X | |
|   d. peak flow, maximum inspiratory pressure, maximum expiratory pressure, forced vital capacity, timed forced expiratory volumes [e.g., $FEV_1$], lung compliance, lung mechanics | X | X | |
|   e. cardiac output, pulmonary capillary wedge pressure, central venous pressure, pulmonary artery pressures, fluid balance (intake and output) | | | |
|   f. pulmonary vascular resistance and systematic vascular resistance | | | |
|   g. apnea monitoring, sleep studies, respiratory impedance plethysmography | X | X | |
|   h. tracheal tube cuff pressure, volume | X | X | |
| **C. Perform procedures and interpret results, determine appropriateness of and participate in developing and recommending modifications to respiratory care plan.** | 1 | 1 | 3 |
| 1. Perform and/or measure the following: | | | |
|   a. spirometry before and/or after bronchodilator, maximum voluntary ventilation, diffusing capacity, functional residual capacity, flow-volume loops, body plethysmography, nitrogen washout distribution test, total lung capacity, $CO_2$ response curve, closing volume, airway resistance | X | X | |
|   b. ECG, pulse oximetry, transcutaneous $O_2/CO_2$ monitoring | X | X | |
|   c. $V_D/V_T$, Qs/Qt, mixed venous sampling, C(a-v̄)$O_2$, cardiac output, pulmonary capillary wedge pressure, central venous pressure, pulmonary artery pressures, cardiopulmonary stress testing | | | |
|   d. fluid balance (intake and output) | | | |

| | RECALL | APPLICATION | ANALYSIS |
|---|---|---|---|
|   e. arterial sampling and blood gas analysis, co-oximetry, P(A-a)$O_2$ | X | X | |
|   f. sleep studies, metabolic studies [e.g., indirect calorimetry] | | | |
|   g. ventilator flow, volume, and pressure waveforms, lung compliance | X | X | |
| 2. Interpret results of the following: | | | |
|   a. spirometry before aad/or after bronchodilator, maximum voluntary ventilation, diffusing capacity, functional residual capacity, flow-volume loops, body plethysmography, nitrogen washout distribution test, total lung capacity, $CO_2$ response curve, closing volume, airway resistance, bronchoprovocation | X | X | |
|   b. ECG, pulse oximetry, transcutaneous $O_2/CO_2$ monitoring | X | X | |
|   c. $V_D/V_T$, Qs/Qt, mixed venous sampling, C(a-v̄)$O_2$, cardiac output, pulmonary capillary wedge pressure, central venous pressure, pulmonary artery pressures, cardiopulmonary stress testing | | | |
|   d. fluid balance (intake and output) | | | |
|   e. arterial sampling and blood gas analysis, co-oximetry, P(A-a)$O_2$ | X | X | |
|   f. peripheral venipuncture or insertion of intravenous line | | | |
|   g. sleep studies, metabolic studies [e.g., indirect calorimetry] | | | |
|   h. insertion of arterial and umbilical monitoring lines | | | |
|   i. ventilator flow, volume, and pressure waveforms, lung compliance | X | X | |
| 3. Determine the appropriateness of the prescribed respiratory care plan and recommend modifications where indicated: | | | |
|   a. perform respiratory care quality assurance | X | X | |
|   b. develop quality improvement program | X | X | |
|   c. review interdisciplinary patient and family care plan | X | X | |
| 4. Participate in development of respiratory care plan [e.g., case management, develop and apply protocols, disease management education] | X | X | |

Content Outline (Cont.)
*This content outline is reprinted with permission of the copyright holder, the National Board For Respiratory Care, Inc., 8310 Nieman Rd, Lenexa, KS 66214. All rights reserved. Effective July 1999*

| | RECALL | APPLICATION | ANALYSIS |
|---|---|---|---|
| **II. Select, Assemble and Check Equipment for Proper Function, Operation, and Cleanliness**<br><br>**SETTING:** In any patient care setting, the advanced respiratory therapist selects, assembles, and assures cleanliness of all equipment used in providing respiratory care. The therapist checks all equipment and corrects malfunctions. | 3 | 4 | 13 |
| **A. Select and obtain equipment and assure equipment cleanliness.** | 1 | 2 | 5 |
| 1. Select and obtain equipment appropriate to the respiratory care plan: | | | |
| a. oxygen administration devices | | | |
| (1) nasal cannula, mask, reservior mask (partial rebreathing, nonrebreathing), face tents, transtracheal oxygen catheter, oxygen conserving cannulas | X | X | |
| (2) air-entrainment devices, tracheostomy collar and T-piece, oxygen hoods and tents | X | X | |
| (3) CPAP devices | X | X | |
| b. humidifiers [e.g., bubble, passover, cascade, wick, heat moisture exchanger] | X | X | |
| c. aerosol generators [e.g., pneumatic nebulizer, ultrasonic nebulizer] | X | X | |
| d. resuscitation devices [e.g, manual resuscitator (bag-valve), pneumatic (demand-valve), mouth-to-valve mask resuscitator] | X | X | |
| e. ventilators | | | |
| (1) pneumatic, electric, microprocessor, fluidic | X | X | |
| (2) high frequency | | | |
| (3) noninvasive positive pressure | X | X | |
| f. artificial airways | | | |
| (1) oro- and nasopharyngeal airways | X | X | |
| (2) oral, nasal and double-lumen endotracheal tubes | X | X | |
| (3) tracheostomy tubes and buttons | X | X | |

| | RECALL | APPLICATION | ANALYSIS |
|---|---|---|---|
| (4) intubation equipment [e.g., laryngoscope and blades, exhaled $CO_2$ detection devices] | X | X | |
| (5) other airways [e.g., laryngeal mask airway (LMA), Esophageal Tracheal Combitube® (ETC)] | | | |
| g. suctioning devices [e.g., suction catheters, specimen collectors, oropharyngeal suction devices] | X | X | |
| h. gas delivery, metering and clinical analyzing devices | | | |
| (1) regulators, redcing valves, connectors and flowmeters, air/oxygen blenders, pulse-dose systems | X | X | |
| (2) oxygen concentrators, air compressors, liquid oxygen systems | X | X | |
| (3) gas cylinders, bulk systems and manifolds | X | X | |
| (4) capnograph, blood gas analyzer and sampling devices, co-oximeter, transcutaneous $O_2$/$CO_2$ monitor, pulse oximeter | X | X | |
| (5) CO, He, $O_2$ and specialty gas analyzers | X | X | |
| i. patient breathing circuits | | | |
| (1) IPPB, continuous mechanical ventilation | X | X | |
| (2) CPAP, PEEP valve assembly | X | X | |
| (3) H-valve assembly | | | X |
| j. environmental devices | | | |
| (1) incubators, radiant warmers | | | |
| (2) aerosol (mist) tents | X | X | |
| (3) scavenging systems | | X | X |
| k. positive expiratory pressure device (PEP) | | | |
| l. Flutter® mucous clearance device | | | X |
| m. other therapeutic gases [e.g., $O_2$/$CO_2$, He/$O_2$] | | | |
| n. manometers and gauges | | | |
| (1) manometers—water, mercury and aneroid, inspiratory/expiratory pressure meters, cuff pressure manometers | X | X | |
| (2) pressure transducers | X | X | |
| o. respirometers [e.g., flow-sensing devices (pneumotachometer), volume displacement] | X | X | |

| | RECALL | APPLICATION | ANALYSIS |
|---|---|---|---|
| p. electrocardiography devices [e.g., ECG oscilloscope monitors, ECG machines (12-lead), Holter monitors] | X | X | |
| q. hemodynamic monitoring devices | | | |
|    (1) central venous catheters, pulmonary artery catheters [e.g., Swan-Ganz], cardiac output, continuous $S\overline{v}O_2$ monitors | | | |
|    (2) arterial catheters | | | |
| r. vacuum systems [e.g., pumps, regulators, collection bottles, pleural drainage devices] | X | X | |
| s. metered dose inhalers (MDI), MDI spacers | X | X | |
| t. Small Particle Aerosol Generators (SPAG) | X | X | |
| u. bronchoscopes | X | X | |
| 2. Assure selected equipment cleanliness [e.g., select or determine appropriate agent and technique for disinfection and/or sterilization, perform procedures for disinfection and/or sterilization, monitor effectiveness of sterilization procedures] | X | X | |
| **B. Assemble and check equipment function, identify and correct equipment malfunctions, and perform quality control.** | **2** | **2** | **8** |
| 1. Assemble, check for proper function, and identify malfunctions of equipment: | | | |
|   a. oxygen administration devices | | | |
|    (1) nasal cannula, mask, reservoir mask (partial rebreathing, nonrebreathing), face tents, transtracheal oxygen catheter, oxygen conserving cannulas | X | X | |
|    (2) air-entrainment devices, tracheostomy collar and T-piece, oxygen hoods and tents | X | X | |
|    (3) CPAP devices | X | X | |
|   b. humidifiers [e.g., bubble, passover, cascade, wick, heat moisture exchanger] | X | X | |
|   c. aerosol generators [e.g., pneumatic nebulizer, ultrasonic nebulizer] | X | X | |
|   d. resuscitation devices [e.g., manual resuscitator (bag-valve), pneumatic (demand-valve), mouth-to-valve mask resuscitator] | X | X | |
|   e. ventilators | | | |
|    (1) pneumatic, electric, microprocessor, fluidic | X | X | |
|    (2) high frequency | | | |
|    (3) noninvasive positive pressure | X | X | |

| | RECALL | APPLICATION | ANALYSIS |
|---|---|---|---|
| f. artificial airways | | | |
|   (1) oro- and nasopharyngeal airways | X | X | |
|   (2) oral, nasal and double-lumen endotracheal tubes | X | X | |
|   (3) tracheostomy tubes and buttons | X | X | |
|   (4) intubation equipment [e.g., laryngoscope and blades, exhaled $CO_2$ detection devices] | X | X | |
| g. suctioning devices [e.g., suction catheters, speciment collectors, oropharyngeal suction devices] | X | X | |
| h. gas delivery, metering and clinical analyzing devices | | | |
|   (1) regulators, reducing valves, connectors and flowmeters, air/oxygen blenders, pulse-dose systems | X | X | |
|   (2) oxygen concentrators, air compressors, liquid oxygen systems | X | X | |
|   (3) gas cylinders, bulk, systems and manifolds | X | X | |
|   (4) capnograph, blood gas analyzer and sampling devices, co-oximeter, transcutaneous $O_2/CO_2$ monitor, pulse oximeter | X | X | |
|   (5) CO, He, $O_2$ and specialty gas analyzers | X | X | |
| i. patient breathing circuits | | | |
|   (1) IPPB, continuous mechanical ventilation | X | X | |
|   (2) CPAP, PEEP valve assembly | X | X | |
|   (3) H-valve assembly | | X | X |
| j. environmental devices | | | |
|   (1) incubators, radiant warmers | | | |
|   (2) aerosol (mist) tents | X | X | |
| k. positive expiratory pressure (PEP) device | | | |
| l. Flutter® mucous clearance device | | | X |
| m. other therapeutic gases [e.g., $O_2/CO_2$, $He/O_2$] | | | |
| n. manometers and gauges | | | |
|   (1) manometers—water, mercury and aneroid, inspiratory/expiratory pressure meters, cuff pressure manometers | X | X | |
|   (2) pressure transducers | | | |
| o. respirometers [e.g., flow-sensing devices (pneumotachometer), volume displacement] | X | X | |
| p. electrocardiography devices [e.g., ECG oscilloscope monitors, ECG machines (12-lead), Holter monitors] | X | X | |

| | RECALL | APPLICATION | ANALYSIS |
|---|:---:|:---:|:---:|
| q. hemodynamic monitoring devices | | | |
|   (1) central venous catheters, pulmonary artery catheters [e.g., Swan-Ganz], cardiac output, continuous $S\bar{v}O_2$ monitors | | | |
|   (2) arterial catheters | | | |
| r. vacuum systems [e.g., pumps, regulators, collection bottles, pleural drainage devices] | X | X | |
| s. bronchoscopes | | | X |
| 2. Take action to correct malfunctions of equipment: | | | |
|   a. oxygen administration devices | | | |
|     (1) nasal cannula, mask, reservoir mask (partial rebreathing, nonrebreathing), face tents, transtracheal oxygen catheter, oxygen conserving cannulas | X | X | |
|     (2) air-entrainment devices, tracheostomy collar and T-piece, oxygen hoods and tents | X | X | |
|     (3) CPAP devices | X | X | |
|   b. humidifiers [e.g., bubble, passover, cascade, wick, heat moisture exchanger] | X | X | |
|   c. aerosol generators [e.g., pneumatic nebulizer, ultrasonic nebulizer] | X | X | |
|   d. resuscitation devices [e.g., manual resuscitator (bag-valve), pneumatic (demand-valve), mouth-to-valve mask resuscitator] | X | X | |
|   e. ventilators | | | |
|     (1) pneumatic, electric, microprocessor, fluidic | X | X | |
|     (2) high frequency | | | |
|     (3) noninvasive positive pressure | X | X | |
|   f. artificial airways | | | |
|     (1) oro- and nasopharyngeal airways | X | X | |
|     (2) oral, nasal and double-lumen endotracheal tubes | X | X | |
|     (3) tracheostomy tubes and buttons | X | X | |
|     (4) intubation equipment [e.g., laryngoscope and blades, exhaled $CO_2$ detection devices] | X | X | |
|   g. suctioning devices [e.g., suction catheters, specimen collectors, oropharyngeal suction devices] | X | X | |
|   h. gas delivery, metering and clinical analyzing devices | | | |
|     (1) regulators, reducing valves, connectors and flowmeters, air/oxygen blenders, pulse-dose systems | X | X | |
|     (2) oxygen concentrators, air compressors, liquid oxygen systems | X | X | |

| | RECALL | APPLICATION | ANALYSIS |
|---|:---:|:---:|:---:|
|     (3) gas cylinders, bulk systems and manifolds | X | X | |
|     (4) capnograph, blood gas analyzer and sampling devices, co-oximeter, transcutaneous $O_2/CO_2$ monitor, pulse oximeter | X | X | |
|     (5) CO, He, $O_2$ and specialty gas analyzers | | | |
|   i. patient breathing circuits | | | |
|     (1) IPPB, continuous mechanical ventilation | X | X | |
|     (2) CPAP, PEEP valve assembly | X | X | |
|     (3) H-valve assembly | | | X |
|   j. environmental devices | | | |
|     (1) incubators, radiant warmers | | | X |
|     (2) aerosol (mist) tents | X | X | |
|   k. positive expiratory pressure (PEP) device | | | |
|   l. Flutter® mucous clearance device | | | X |
|   m. other therapeutic gases [e.g., $O_2/CO_2$, He/$O_2$] | | | |
|   n. manometers and gauges | | | |
|     (1) manometers—water, mercury and aneroid, inspiratory/expiratory pressure meters, cuff pressure manometers | X | X | |
|     (2) pressure transducers | | | |
|   o. respirometers [e.g., flow-sensing devices (pneumotachometer), volume displacement] | X | X | |
|   p. electrocardiography devices [e.g., ECG oscilloscope monitors, ECG machines (12-lead), Holter monitors] | | | |
|   q. hemodynamic monitoring devices | | | |
|     (1) central venous catheters, pulmonary artery catheters [e.g., Swan-Ganz], cardiac output, continuous $S\bar{v}O_2$ monitors | | | |
|     (2) arterial catheters | | | |
|   r. vacuum systems [e.g., pumps, regulators, collection bottles, pleural drainage devices] | X | X | |
|   s. Small Particle Aerosol Generators (SPAG) | | | X |
|   t. bronchoscopes | | | X |
| 3. Perform quality control procedures for: | | | |
|   a. blood gas analyzers and sampling devices, co-oximeters | X | X | |
|   b. pulmonary function equipment, ventilator volume/flow/pressure calibration | X | X | |
|   c. gas metering devices | X | X | |
|   d. noninvasive monitors [e.g., transcutaneous] | | | |

## III. Initiate, Conduct, and Modify Prescribed Therapeutic Procedures

**SETTING:** In any patient care setting, the RRT evaluates, monitors, and records the patient's response to care. The therapist maintains patient records and communicates with other healthcare team members. The therapist initiates, conducts, and modifies prescribed therapeutic procedures to achieve the desired objectives. The therapist provides care in emergency settings, assists the physician, and conducts pulmonary rehabilitation and homecare.

| | RECALL | APPLICATION | ANALYSIS |
|---|---|---|---|
| III. (total) | 6 | 8 | 49 |
| A. Evaluate, monitor, and record patient's response to respiratory care. | 2 | 3 | 13 |

A. **Evaluate, monitor, and record patient's response to respiratory care.**
  1. Evaluate and monitor patient's response to respiratory care:

| | RECALL | APPLICATION | ANALYSIS |
|---|---|---|---|
| a. recommend and review chest X-ray | X | X | |
| b. perform arterial puncture, capillary blood gas sampling, and venipuncture; obtain blood from arterial or pulmonary artery lines; perform transcutaneous $O_2/CO_2$, pulse oximetry, co-oximetry, and capnography monitoring | X | X | |
| c. observe changes in sputum production and consistency, note patient's subjective response to therapy and mechanical ventilation | X | X | |
| d. measure and record vital signs, monitor cardiac rhythm, evaluate fluid balance (intake and output) | X | X | |
| e. perform spirometry/determine vital capacity, measure lung compliance and airway resistance, interpret ventilator flow, volume, and pressure waveforms, measure peak flow | X | X | |
| f. determine and record central venous pressure, pulmonary artery pressures, pulmonary capillary wedge pressure and/or cardiac output | | | |

| | RECALL | APPLICATION | ANALYSIS |
|---|---|---|---|
| g. recommend measurement of electrolytes, hemoglobin, CBC and/or chemistries | | | |
| h. monitor mean airway pressure, adjust and check alarm systems, measure tidal volume, respiratory rate, airway pressures, I:E, and maximum inspiratory pressure (MIP) | X | X | |
| i. measure $FiO_2$ and/or liter flow | X | X | |
| j. monitor endotracheal or tracheostomy tube cuff pressure | X | X | |
| k. auscultate chest and interpret changes in breath sounds | X | X | |
| l. perform hemodynamic calculations (e.g., shunt studies ($\dot{Q}s/\dot{Q}t$), cardiac output, cardiac index, pulmonary vascular resistance and systemic vascular resistance, stroke volume] | | | |
| m. interpret hemodynamic calculations: | | | |
| (1) calculate and interpret $P(A-a)O_2$, $C(a-\bar{v})O_2$, $\dot{Q}s/\dot{Q}t$ | | | |
| (2) exhaled $CO_2$ monitoring, $V_D/V_T$ | | | |
| (3) cardiac output, cardiac index, pulmonary vascular resistance and systemic vascular resistance, stroke volume | | | |
| 2. Maintain records and communication: | | | |
| a. record therapy and results using conventional terminology as required in the healthcare setting and/or by regulatory agencies by noting and interpreting: | | | |
| (1) patient's response to therapy including the effects of therapy, adverse reactions, patient's subjective and attitudinal response to therapy | X | X | |
| (2) auscultatory findings, cough and sputum production and characteristics | X | X | |
| (3) vital signs [e.g., heart rate, respiratory rate, blood pressure, body temperature] | X | X | |
| (4) pulse oximetry, heart rhythm, capnography | X | X | |
| b. verify computations and note erroneous data | X | X | |

| | RECALL | APPLICATION | ANALYSIS |
|---|---|---|---|
| c. apply computer technology to patient management [e.g., ventilator waveform analysis, electronic charting, patient care algorithms] | | X | X |
| d. communicate results of therapy and alter therapy per protocol(s) | | X | X |
| **B. Conduct therapeutic procedures to maintain a patent airway, achieve adequate ventilation and oxygenation, and remove bronchopulmonary secretions.** | **1** | **1** | **10** |
| 1. Maintain a patent airway including the care of artificial airways: | | | |
| a. insert oro- and nasopharyngeal airway, select endotracheal or tracheostomy tube, perform endotracheal intubation, change tracheostomy tube, maintain proper cuff inflation, position of endotracheal or tracheostomy tube | X | X | |
| b. maintain adequate humidification | X | X | |
| c. extubate the patient | X | X | |
| d. properly position patient | X | X | |
| e. identify endotracheal tube placement by available means | X | X | |
| 2. Achieve adequate spontaneous and artificial ventilation: | | | |
| a. initiate and adjust IPPB therapy | X | X | |
| b. initiate and select appropriate settings for high frequency ventilation | | | |
| c. initiate and adjust ventilator modes [e.g., A/C, SIMV, pressure support ventilation (PSV), pressure control ventilation (PCV)] | X | X | |
| d. initiate and adjust independent (differential) lung ventilation | | | |
| 3. Remove bronchopulmonary secretions by instructing and encouraging bronchopulmonary hygiene techniques [e.g., coughing techniques, autogenic drainage, positive expiratory pressure device (PEP), intrapulmonary percussive ventilation (IPV), Flutter®, High Frequency Chest Wall Oscillation (HFCWO)] | X | X | |
| 4. Achieve adequate arterial and tissue oxygenation: | | | |
| a. initiate and adjust CPAP, PEEP, and noninvasive positive pressure | X | X | |
| b. initiate and adjust combinations of ventilatory techniques [e.g., SIMV, PEEP, PS, PCV] | X | X | |

| | RECALL | APPLICATION | ANALYSIS |
|---|---|---|---|
| c. position patient to minimize hypoxemia, administer oxygen (on or off ventilator), prevent procedure-associated hypoxemia [e.g., oxygenate before and after suctioning and equipment changes] | | X | X |
| **C. Make necessary modifications in therapeutic procedures based on patient response.** | **0** | **1** | **10** |
| 1. Modify IPPB: | | | |
| a. adjust sensitivity, flow, volume, pressure, $FiO_2$ | | X | X |
| b. adjust expiratory retard | | X | X |
| c. change patient—machine interface [e.g., mouthpiece, mask] | | X | X |
| 2. Modify patient breathing pattern during aerosol therapy | | X | X |
| 3. Modify oxygen therapy: | | | |
| a. change mode of administration, adjust flow, and $FiO_2$ | | X | X |
| b. set up an $O_2$ concentrator or liquid $O_2$ system | | X | X |
| 4. Modify specialty gas [e.g., $He/O_2$, $O_2/CO_2$] therapy [e.g., change mode of administration, adjust flow, adjust gas concentration] | | X | |
| 5. Modify bronchial hygiene therapy (e.g., alter position of patient, alter duration of treatment and techniques, coordinate sequence of therapies, alter equipment used and PEP therapy] | | X | X |
| 6. Modify artificial airway management: | | | |
| a. alter endotracheal or tracheostomy tube position, change endotracheal or tracheostomy tube | | X | X |
| b. initiate suctioning | | X | X |
| c. inflate and deflate the cuff | | X | X |
| 7. Modify suctioning: | | | |
| a. alter frequency and duration of suctioning | | X | X |
| b. change size and type of catheter | | X | X |
| c. alter negative pressure | | X | X |
| d. instill irrigating solutions | | X | X |
| 8. Modify mechanical ventilation: | | | |
| a. change patient breathing circuitry, change type of ventilator | | X | X |
| b. measure volume loss through chest tube(s) | | X | |
| c. change mechanical dead space | | X | X |

| | RECALL | APPLICATION | ANALYSIS |
|---|---|---|---|
| **D. Initiate, conduct, or modify respiratory care techniques in an emergency setting.** | 1 | 1 | 10 |
|   1. Treat cardiopulmonary collapse according to: | | | |
|     a. BCLS | X | X | |
|     b. ACLS | X | X | |
|     c. PALS | X | X | |
|     d. NRP | X | X | |
|   2. Treat tension pneumothorax | | | |
|   3. Participate in land/air patient transport | | | |
| **E. Assist physician, initiate, and conduct pulmonary rehabilitation.** | 2 | 2 | 6 |
|   1. Act as an assistant to the physician performing special procedures including: | | | |
|     a. bronchoscopy | X | X | |
|     b. thoracentesis | X | X | |
|     c. transtracheal aspiration | | | |
|     d. tracheostomy | X | X | |
|     e. cardiopulmonary stress testing | | | |
|     f. percutaneous needle biopsies of the lung | | | |
|     g. sleep studies | | | |
|     h. cardioversion | X | X | |
|     i. intubation | X | X | |
|     j. insertion of chest tubes | | | |
|     k. insertion of lines for invasive monitoring (e.g., central venous pressure, pulmonary artery catheters, Swan-Ganz, arterial lines] | | | |
|     l. conscious sedation | | | |
|   2. Initiate and conuct pulmonary rehabilitation and home care within the prescription: | | | |
|     a. monitor and maintain home respiratory care equipment, maintain apnea monitors | | | |
|     b. explain planned therapy and goals to patient in understandable terms to achieve optimal therapeutic outcome, counsel patient and family concerning smoking cessation, disease management | X | X | |
|     c. assure safety and infection control | X | X | |
|     d. modify respiratory care procedures for use in the home | X | X | |
|     e. implement and monitor graded exercise program | | | |
|     f. conduct patient education and disease management programs | X | X | |
| **TOTALS** | 12 | 15 | 73 |

# Level of Questions

On all of its credentialing examinations, the NBRC presents test items at three cognitive levels (recall, application, and analysis).

**RECALL:** Examination items written at this cognitive level test the ability to recall or recognize specific information. This information can be terminology, facts, principles, and so on. Information learned at the recall level involves remembering memorized material. The following is an example of a test item at the recall level:

The function of the body plethysmograph is based on _____ law.

A. Avogadro's
B. Boyle's
C. Charles'
D. Dalton's

**ANSWER: B**

**APPLICATION:** Examination questions posed at this cognitive level test the candidates's ability to relate concepts, principles, facts, or information to new or changing situations or mathematical problems. The two following items illustrate application-level questions:

1. The following data were obtained from a closed-circuit helium dilution study performed on a 64-year-old male:

Helium added: 650 ml
Percentage of initial helium: 9.5%
Percentage of final helium: 6.0%
Helium absorption factor: 100 ml
Collected gas temperature: 25°C

Calculate this person's functional residual capacity (FRC).

A. 4.1 L
B. 3.8 L
C. 3.0 L
D. 2.1 L

**ANSWER: A**

2. With which pulmonary disease is this functional residual capacity (FRC) value consistent?

A. asbestosis
B. adult respiratory distress syndrome (ARDS)
C. pulmonary emphysema
D. pneumonia

**ANSWER: C**

**ANALYSIS:** Test items presented at the analysis level evaluate the candidate's ability to analyze and/or synthesize information in order to arrive at a solution. The following question represents an example of an analysis-level item:

A patient is receiving volume-cycled mechanical ventilation in the control mode. Arterial blood gas (ABG) data reveal the following:

$PO_2$ 93 torr
$PCO_2$ 25 torr
pH 7.56
$HCO_3^-$ 22 mEq/liter
B.E. −1 mEq/liter

Which ventilator adjustment should be made at this time?

A. Institute 5 cm $H_2O$ PEEP.
B. Increase the $FIO_2$.
C. Increase the tidal volume.
D. Decrease the ventilatory rate.

**ANSWER: D**

# Written Registry Examination Item Format

The Written Registry Examination is composed of two types of questions: multiple choice and multiple true–false, or K-type. At various points throughout the examination, you will encounter questions that refer to diagrams, waveforms, or tracings. Again, these questions follow the multiple-choice and multiple true–false formats.

The instructions for the Written Registry Advanced Practitioner Examination read as follows:

**DIRECTIONS:** Each of the following questions or incomplete statements is followed by four suggested answers or completions. Select one that is best in each case and then blacken the corresponding space on the answer sheet.

### Multiple-Choice Questions

**EXAMPLE:** On an electrocardiogram (ECG), the T wave represents:

A. atrial depolarization.
B. ventricular depolarization.
C. ventricular repolarization.
D. atrial repolarization.

The one best response is C.

Multiple-choice test items require the candidate to choose *the one best response* from four plausible selections. The three selections that are not correct answers are called *distractors*. The style of the multiple-choice test item is constructed in such a manner as to present all four choices as plausible responses. The candidate must determine which selection represents the one best response.

The phrase "one best response" refers to the choice that, among those presented, most accurately completes the stem of the question. The best response might not actually be the precise answer; however, among the four selections available, it represents the best choice.

### Multiple True–False (K-Type) Questions

**EXAMPLE:** Which pathologic conditions are associated with a decreased tactile fremitus?

I. atelectasis
II. pneumothorax
III. thickened pleura
IV. pleural effusion

A. I, III only
B. II, IV only
C. II, III, IV only
D. I, III, IV only

The correct response is C.

With this type of question, the candidate must select the statements that accurately, or correctly, refer to or describe the stem. The statements range in number from three to five and are designated as Roman numerals. All of the true statements relating to the stem must be selected.

The process of elimination is easier to employ with this type of question than with a regular multiple-choice question. For example, referring to the sample question, suppose you were certain that III and IV were true concerning the stem and that I was false, but you were uncertain about II. You could automatically eliminate A and D knowing that I was false. Choice B could be eliminated because it does not contain III, which you know is true. Because no selection is provided listing II and III only, C represents the logical choice.

As you read through the responses that are available, you should indicate the true responses with some kind of mark (such as X or T). You will save time by not having to reread certain selections.

### Situational Sets

Questions 1, 2, and 3 refer to the following data:

A patient is receiving mechanical ventilation via a Siemens Servo 900C. The ventilator settings include the following:

ventilatory rate: 12 breaths/min.
minute ventilation ($\dot{V}_E$): 8 L/min.
inspiratory time percent ($T_{I\%}$): 20%

1. Calculate the tidal volume delivered by the ventilator.

   A. 333 ml
   B. 666 ml
   C. 830 ml
   D. 1,500 ml

2. Calculate this patient's inspiratory time.

   A. 0.75 sec.
   B. 1.25 sec.
   C. 1.33 sec.
   D. 2.00 sec.

3. Calculate this patient's inspiratory:expiratory (I:E) ratio.

   A. 2:1
   B. 1:1
   C. 1:2
   D. 1:3

   **ANSWERS:** 1 = B
                   2 = B
                   3 = D

You must read the scenario and review the data carefully when presented with situational sets. Responses to previous questions must be kept in mind as responses to ensuing questions within the same situational set are considered. For example, in the situational set given, the calculation of the inspiratory time in Question 2 was needed to determine the I:E ratio in Question 3.

# General Written Registry Examination Information

1. Every word in the stem of each question is essential and meaningful. No extraneous information is found in the stem. Each bit of information is noteworthy. Do not "read more into" the question than that which is presented. Accept each question for what it states.
2. All data reported on the examination are assumed to have been obtained under standard pressure conditions (i.e., 760 mm Hg or torr) *unless otherwise specified* in the stem of the question or a scenario referring to a sequence of questions.
3. Pressures are generally reported in terms of the unit *torr.* One torr equals 1 mm Hg.

4. Whenever you perform calculations, do not insert the numerical values only into the equation used. Insert the appropriate unit along with the numerical value. Following this policy enables you to cancel some of the units in the course of the calculation. Generally, you should end up with some number accompanied by a unit. If that unit is consistent with the unit that is required in the answer, you are more likely to have the correct answer. Additionally, incorporating units into the equation improves the likelihood of arriving at the correct answer.

You are allowed two hours to complete the 115 questions on the NBRC Written Registry Examination. The score that you receive is based on the percentage of correct responses for 100 questions.

The candidate who is taking the Written Registry Examination will encounter 15 pretest items on the examination. These pretest items have been included by the NBRC because of instant examination scoring and computer-based testing. Pretesting enables the NBRC to continuously introduce new test items, and it facilitates the candidates receiving instant scores.

Using a process termed *embedded pretesting*, the NBRC collects data on new questions that might appear as scored items on future exams. Pretesting by the NBRC assures that candidates' scores are based on firm measurement methodologies.

Pretesting involves inserting a number of new (previously unused) questions throughout the exam. These questions do not contribute to the candidate's score on the Written Registry Examination. At the same time, they do not influence the candidate's pass-fail status. The previously unused questions are interspersed throughout the examination, causing candidates to answer them carefully and thoughtfully.

Statistical analysis is applied to these new questions, and those items that meet certain statistical standards will likely appear on future credentialing examinations as bona fide questions.

To maintain secure examinations that parallel current standards of clinical practice, new questions must continuously be developed. Pretesting ensures this outcome, because it is an accepted psychometric methodology. Therefore, as you work through the examination, do not labor too long over questions that appear difficult. Use your time efficiently. If a question seems too difficult, move on to the next question. Then, when you reach the end of the examination, return to the question(s) with which you had difficulty. You do not want to waste time pondering a question that you might not be able to answer.

The NBRC allows you to write in the examination booklet. If you need to perform calculations, write formulas, or jot down any mnemonics, feel free to do so on the booklet. There are also blank pages located at the end of the booklet that can be used for this purpose.

Your responses are made on a separate answer sheet that is graded. You need at least two No. 2 pencils (soft lead) to complete the examination. Bring three No. 2 pencils for safe measure. You are instructed to completely darken the response that you select.

**EXAMPLE:** Which of the following University of South Alabama graduates have gone on to play major-league baseball?

I. Juan Pierre (Rockies)
II. Luis Gonzalez (Diamondbacks)
III. Jon Leiber (Cubs)
IV. Sammy Sosa (Cubs)

A. I, II only
B. II, III, IV only
C. I, II, III only
D. III, IV only

ANSWER FORMAT

[A] [B] [■] [D]

When you complete the examination, review only those questions that you definitely were not able to answer. Do not change any answers unless you are absolutely certain that your initial response is wrong. If you are uncertain about an answer that you have made, do not change the answer, because (assuming that you prepared well for this examination) you have likely made the correct choice. Your first inclination is ordinarily correct based on the fact that you prepared for this test.

Make sure that you do not leave any items unanswered. If you do, those unanswered questions will be recorded as incorrect responses.

# Written Registry Examination Preparation

### Study Hints

When you use this book to prepare for the Written Registry Examination, establish a timetable for complete review of the material. The timetable you establish should be realistic, taking your work and social schedules into consideration. Additionally, your timetable should include the time that you require to read and study the questions and analyses as well as the time that you need to read and study appropriate references.

> **NOTE:** It is not necessary to have all the references listed here. Two or three of the standard texts should be sufficient.

A suggested schedule for the completion of this study guide is shown next. Start at least five weeks before the Written Registry Examination.

| Time | Chapter |
|------|---------|
| Week 1 | 2. Pretest (100 items, analyses, and references) |
| Week 2 | 3. Clinical Data (212 items, analyses, and references) |
| Week 3 | 4. Equipment (130 items, analyses, and references) |
| Week 4 | 5. Therapeutic Procedures (208 items, analyses, and references) |
| Week 5 | 6. Posttest (100 items, analyses, and references) |
| Week 6 | NBRC Written Registry Examination |

Keep in mind that this examination represents a critical stage in your professional career. Successful completion of this examination is essential to your professional growth. You owe it to yourself to impose strict measures of self-discipline and to adhere to your established timetable. Good luck with your preparation, and good luck on the NBRC Written Registry Examination.

# CHAPTER 1 ————————— TEST PREPARATION

by William F. Galvin, MSED, RRT, CPFT

Successfully completing the credentialing examination is probably the most important professional goal of any aspiring Registered Respiratory Therapist (RRT). Although many graduates believe that the completion of a formal educational program guarantees the ultimate attainment of the Certified Respiratory Therapist (CRT) and/or the Registered Respiratory Therapist (RRT) credential, National Board for Respiratory Care (NBRC) statistics prove otherwise. What accounts for success is complex and difficult to determine. Success is likely to occur, however, when the candidate has graduated from an educational training program characterized by:

- A well-developed, well-designed curriculum of science and mathematics courses, a blend of effective communication and critical-thinking skills, and a sound, comprehensive respiratory care curriculum (as depicted in the current NBRC matrix). The foregoing essential items represent *academic preparation*.

Academic preparation is only one of four components deemed necessary for the successful completion of the credentialing examinations. Another important component for success involves serious physical considerations, such as the following:

- Fitness, endurance, appropriate and satisfactory sleep, and adherence to healthy nutritional standards. This component of the process is *physical preparation*.

NBRC examination candidates should not take the importance of such considerations lightly. A third essential ingredient is somewhat more of an excuse than poor performance and is thus out of one's control. This concept relates to attitudinal preparation issues and concerns such as the following:

- The need to develop self-assurance, strong feelings of likely success on the examination, and essentially overcoming the feelings of anxiety and "butterflies." In other words, this prepara-

tion involves overcoming the feeling that one will perform poorly under pressure.

These feelings or attitudes can be a means of mobilization into action. One can use this nervous energy productively in order to plan a strategy that entails periods of focused study, content review, and preparation. The last and probably most critical ingredient is the primary focus of this chapter. That focus includes the following:

- Using all of those little tricks, such as "creative guessing" or "playing the odds," time management, knowing whether to change your first answer, and knowing what to do when you absolutely do not know an answer

We call this last point *test-taking strategies and techniques*, or simply *being testwise*. This component might separate a failing grade from a passing grade. This chapter assists you in maximizing your efforts and demonstrates how to take advantage of every opportunity in order to successfully complete the examination process. A balance or blend of all four components constitutes the guidelines for success. We now discuss each of these guidelines.

## Academic Preparation

Being academically prepared to sit for the NBRC Written Registry Examination entails having learned and retained the information comprising the scope of practice for the RRT. Exposure to a well-developed and comprehensive curriculum is essential. Thus, the biggest problem faced by most unsuccessful candidates is the learning-forgetting process. The forgetting process is very powerful, and research indicates that the forgetting curve is inverse (whereby the units of material recalled decrease with the passage of time). Some researchers have shown that the average person forgets as much as 50% of material initially learned after only 20 minutes. Other research studies have demonstrated that more than 75% of material is forgotten after 31 days. In short, the greatest amount of forgetting occurs directly after finishing the learning task. After that initial loss, forgetting diminishes. When studies determined what was responsible for the forgetting process, it was theorized that time was not the culprit but rather what happens in the course of time that determines the degree of forgetting. The researchers have come to call this phenomenon the *interference theory*. Interference theory refers to the constant bombardment of our senses with incredibly numerous new thoughts and information. We are essentially overloaded and unable to remember or recall this voluminous supply of material. To overcome this problem (i.e., decelerate forgetting and accelerate learning), we need to employ certain tactics: (1) observation, (2) repetition/recitation, and (3) association.

*Observation* refers to the need to see, hear, or somehow consciously encounter material to be learned. How often have you forgotten someone's name? This problem might result from not hearing the person's name in the first place. You might have been in awe of the surroundings or of the circumstances during the introduction and might not have focused your attention on the person's name. No recollection occurs because you directed your attention elsewhere, and the person's name never became imprinted. In other cases, you might have been too embarrassed to ask the person to repeat his name. The point is that the person's name was never etched in your mind.

Another example involves not remembering where you parked your car. You might have been in a hurry to get to the stadium for a big game, or you might have been late for a movie. In either case, you neglected to consciously observe where you had parked. There was an interference in the learning process.

You can use *repetition/recitation* to overcome the forgetting process by employing spaced repetition or repeated recitation. For example, if you were asked to solve the multiplication problem $2 \times 4$, you would likely say the answer is "8." If you were asked to solve $4 \times 3$, your answer would probably be 12. If confronted with the problem $17 \times 14$, however, you would no doubt be momentarily silent. In all likelihood, you learned the multiplication tables in elementary school and were exposed to tables up to, but not beyond, 12. You learned the product of two numbers by means of rote memorization, spaced repetition, or repeated recitation. You were drilled over and over again until the material was imprinted on your mind. Knowing the number of days in a month refers to the same process. You might have learned the mnemonic, "Thirty days hath September, April, June, and November . . . ." You

probably still sing that little jingle in your mind when you are trying to determine the number of days in a particular month. If you have the need to learn something or to retain a piece of information, you must first observe or hear it. Then, you need to repeat or recite it for extended periods. The literature strongly supports the notion that frequent and short study intervals strengthen the learning process and help overcome the forgetting process.

The last tactic, *association*, entails coupling the material to be learned with something that has meaning or that is related to the information in question. For example, if you were asked to outline the country Ireland, the likelihood is that you would not be able to do so. If you were asked to draw Italy, however, you would probably be able to sketch a fairly good representation of that country. Why would you be more able to outline Italy than Ireland? The answer lies in the fact that people associate the shape of Italy with a boot, and that association provides the basis for remembering the shape of that country. Associations can be powerful tools to enhance your ability to remember information. You should develop associations in your practice of respiratory care and in the context of preparing for the credentialing examination.

In summary, as you prepare for the NBRC Written Registry Examination, you should observe, repeat/recite, and associate information to strengthen your learning process. If you are attempting to learn the concept of *oxygen transport*, you would be well served by reading the text dealing with this concept. After listing the essential components of oxygen transport, you should recite these components repeatedly. Finally, associate this concept with an everyday example of something that is simple and easy to comprehend. Respiratory care educators frequently use the train-cargo analogy to make the oxygen transport concept more relevant to their students. The educators generally represent the oxygen as the cargo, carried by the hemoglobin (which is the boxcar). You strengthen your learning whenever you can visualize, observe, repeat/recite, and associate concepts with simple and practical examples.

Another important component of academic preparation is the development of a study schedule. You should employ the support of your family, friends, and colleagues in determining the best time to study. Soliciting their support can assist you in your effort to adhere to your schedule. The purpose for engaging their support is to provide you with a source of encouragement. Do not forget to engender your own support as well. Consider all of the positive aspects that are derived from the hard work and effort that you will put forth to achieve the goal of becoming an RRT (i.e., personal satisfaction, prestige, higher salary, career mobility, job security, more opportunities, etc.). Many forces should drive your motivation. Once you have all of this support and develop your timetable for studying, adhere to it. Avoid succumbing to the temptation of procrastination. The sacrifices that you make now will pay dividends in the future.

After establishing a test-preparation timetable, select an area conducive to studying. Also, identify a time of day when you are at your peak performance. Being at your peak mental level allows you to maximize your study effort. You should also match your learning style with your study methodology. Some people are visual learners; others are auditory; and still others are tactile. Choose a study method that is compatible with your learning style. Visual learners should carefully select texts and written material that are best suited to their needs. Reading the material in this review book and the references listed offers the visual learner the opportunity to prepare for the Written Registry Examination by identifying areas of strength and weakness. One can then overcome deficiencies by further reading and review.

Auditory learners can tape questions, analyses, and matrix designations. Then they can listen to audiocassettes at home, while traveling in the car, or while lying in bed. Tactile learners should take advantage of time at work. This type of learner can best prepare for the equipment portion of the examination by obtaining as much hands-on experience as possible. For example, one can study equipment in the process of disassembly and reassembly and practice troubleshooting on ventilators and other equipment.

Regardless of your learning style, do not overlook the opportunities in the workplace. This environment is a fertile area for learning. Identify mentors at your institution and request their advice and counsel. Discuss commonly encountered cases and treatment modalities with them. Avoid wasting time on the unusual cases or bizarre situations because they are unlikely to appear on the Written Registry Examination. When you work with your patients, consider aspects such as physical assessment, adverse reactions to therapy, rationale for the therapy, and so on. Make a conscious effort to learn something new and to review something every day at work. Spend that extra time reading charts, reviewing laboratory studies, and/or working up the patient's case. Reviewing and learning opportunities abound at the workplace. Take advantage of the situation.

# Physical Preparation

As we previously stated, physical preparation is probably one of the more overlooked components in preparing for an examination. How often have you noticed an increased number of students in the library during the week of final examinations? As you recall this scene, consider the physical appearance of these students (or that of yourself, if you were among them). You are probably recollecting unshaven faces, faces with dark circles under the eyes, a general unkempt and disheveled appearance—people who probably have not slept much or at all recently and who likely have not had a decent meal in days. They resemble refugees fleeing a war zone. (Whatever happened to the image of the care free college student enjoying the tranquility and leisure of the college campus?) Attention must be given to physical needs. This period (preparing for the credentialing examination) is a time of increased stress —a time of tremendous mental demand. If you were preparing to participate in an important athletic event, you would not neglect your physical needs. You would get sufficient sleep, eat the proper foods, and become fine-tuned like a precise, high-performance engine. The high-performance needs of your body must not be overlooked even though you are not preparing for an athletic event. You must create a balance between your mental and physical demands. Study for appropriate time intervals, take breaks, engage in physical activity (walking, jogging, etc.), get adequate sleep, and eat proper foods. You want to avoid feeling fatigued, irritable, and physically sick just before the examination. If you experience some of these adverse effects, you might jeopardize your performance on the credentialing examination. You can avoid these consequences by developing a well-planned master study schedule, eating properly and nutritiously, giving serious thought to your physical needs, and declining to work a double shift the day before the examination. Do not underestimate the value of physical preparation. Nurture your body as well as your mind to decrease the likelihood of physical illness and to improve your chances of better performance on the Written Registry Examination.

# Testwiseness

How often have you heard someone say, "I simply cannot take exams." You must shed this notion. Taking tests is a fact of life. Thus far, test taking is the only means to become credentialed. Possessing good test-taking skills is not genetic; rather it is a learned behavior that all people, including you, can master.

Where does the NBRC obtain the material appearing on the credentialing examination? Before this question is answered, let's make an analogy with an examination pertaining to another subject matter—history. Assume you were about to sit for an examination dealing with U.S. history. You would certainly expect to receive direction from the professor regarding the scope of the subject matter for the examination. Will the examination pertain to the American Revolution, the Civil War, the Great Depression, and so on? You would expect to be informed of the limitations or the boundaries of this examination.

Now, to answer the question initially posed, the NBRC formulates the questions appearing on the Written Registry Examination from the Written Registry Examination Matrix. This matrix is the product of a nationwide Job Analysis Survey conducted by the NBRC to determine the tasks performed by the advanced RRT. The Written Registry Examination Matrix appears throughout the various chapters of this text to inculcate the matrix designations in the test candidates.

This book offers you an organized approach to preparing for the Written Registry Examination by exhaustively reviewing the foundation on which this credentialing examination is based. You have in your hands the result of a painstaking effort to outline in detail every matrix designation included on the Written Registry Examination Matrix. You must familiarize yourself with the material comprising this examination.

Once you become familiar with the matrix items, you will likely find it unnecessary to say, "I simply cannot take exams." Success requires preparation, and preparation requires effort. By expending a great effort toward preparing for this examination, you can increase the likelihood of success. You must make the sacrifices to prepare for success.

The NBRC has recently revised the matrices of its credentialing examinations. Significant changes in the matrix of the Written Registry Examination have been made. The percentages of items from the three major categories on the examination are as follows:

- Clinical data: 17%
- Equipment: 20%
- Therapeutic procedures: 63%

The revised NBRC Written Registry Examination Matrix specifies that 12% of the test questions are at the recall level. Fifteen percent (15%) are application level, and 73% are analysis level. Therefore, you must know

more than plain facts. You must be able to apply your knowledge to clinical situations and analyze clinical problems.

For example, test items are unlikely to ask you to identify normal values for pulmonary function studies or hemodynamic monitoring. You should anticipate applying your knowledge of normal values to first analyze data and then to arrive at a diagnosis or recommend a therapeutic intervention. Essentially, you must be able to take the information and knowledge that you have and apply it to a higher level of understanding and demonstrate critical thinking skills to successfully complete the Written Registry Examination.

We urge you to heed these significant changes in the credentialing examination matrix because they appear to coincide with the evolution of clinical practice guidelines and therapist-driven protocols. The changes also dovetail with the demand for more critical thinking and independent judgment on the part of the advanced RRT.

The majority of the test items also now emphasize analysis as well as therapeutic procedures. Because of this emphasis, you would be best served by first assessing your knowledge and skills in these sections and then developing a study plan that maximizes your time and personal needs. This text, which contains questions, analyses, references, and matrix designations, can aid in the assessment process.

# Attitudinal Preparation

This section pertains to emotional or attitudinal preparation which is generally given too much attention by many test takers. They often use the emotional aspect surrounding the examination process as an excuse. We refer to sayings such as, "I just cannot take exams" or "I have test anxiety." Although test anxiety is an actual occurrence, it is more likely a rare phenomenon than a common reality. The real problem includes fear of failure, lack of preparation, and ultimately not believing in yourself. We all have a tendency to be hard on ourselves and to dwell on our weaknesses and deficiencies rather than on our strengths and accomplishments.

Academic preparation is the ultimate key. Once you employ the tactics presented thus far—academic preparation, physical preparation, and sound test-taking strategies—the final ingredient (attitude) generally takes care of itself. The formula for success is to believe in yourself. It simply comes down to the self-fulfilling prophecy. We all have a tendency to move in the direction of our dominant thought. Whether our dominant thought is positive or negative, the results are likely to follow in that direction. We are products of our inner thoughts and inner beliefs. If you believe you can accomplish something, more often than not, you will. Sports literature is replete with such examples. Years ago, a baseball player was pitching in a critical game in the World Series. He had runners on base and was pitching against a player notorious for being a good high-and-outside fastball hitter. The pitcher's manager called time out, left the dugout, approached the mound, and said to the pitcher, "Whatever you do, don't pitch it high and outside!" With that he walked off the mound and returned to the dugout. The pitcher with the ball in his hand repeatedly said to himself, "High and outside, high and outside: I know I'm not supposed to pitch it high and outside." Well, guess what happened? The next pitch was high and outside, and the batter hit the ball out of the park.

People have a tendency to move in the direction of their dominant thought. You cannot motivate someone with the reverse of an idea. In this case, the pitcher's dominant thought was "high and outside," and he moved in the direction of his dominant thought. We generally perform in accord with our own inner and long-developed beliefs. If we believe we can do something, we ordinarily can. Being emotionally and attitudinally prepared means you have invested months of time and energy, sticking to a conscientious and well-developed strategy. When you prepare, you improve the likelihood of acquiring the prerequisite academic knowledge.

The purpose of this chapter is to provide you with the essential ingredients for successful examination performance. The intent is to stimulate and motivate you to incorporate these tools into your study strategy. What you need to do at this point is establish a master timetable and study plan that you can employ over the next several weeks. Incorporate the principles provided here as you establish your personal game plan. When you have determined your study schedule, you should be prepared to include all of the components of this text to assess your strengths and weaknesses and to focus on the areas that require remediation. Congratulations. You are on the road to attaining the RRT credential.

**PURPOSE:** The pretest contained here is your first step toward preparing for the Written Registry Examination. The content of the pretest parallels that which you will encounter on the Written Registry Examination offered by the National Board for Respiratory Care (NBRC). You will encounter 100 test items that match the Written Registry Examination Matrix. The content areas included on the pretest are as follows:

- Clinical data (17 items)
- Equipment (20 items)
- Therapeutic procedures (63 items)

Remember to allow yourself 2 (uninterrupted) hours for the pretest and use the answer sheet located on the next page. Score the pretest soon after you complete it. Begin reviewing the pretest analyses and references and the NBRC matrix designations as soon as you have a reasonable block of time available.

# Pretest Answer Sheet

**DIRECTIONS:**     Darken the space under the selected answer.

|      | A | B | C | D |      |      | A | B | C | D |
|------|---|---|---|---|------|------|---|---|---|---|
| 1.   | ❏ | ❏ | ❏ | ❏ |      | 25.  | ❏ | ❏ | ❏ | ❏ |
| 2.   | ❏ | ❏ | ❏ | ❏ |      | 26.  | ❏ | ❏ | ❏ | ❏ |
| 3.   | ❏ | ❏ | ❏ | ❏ |      | 27.  | ❏ | ❏ | ❏ | ❏ |
| 4.   | ❏ | ❏ | ❏ | ❏ |      | 28.  | ❏ | ❏ | ❏ | ❏ |
| 5.   | ❏ | ❏ | ❏ | ❏ |      | 29.  | ❏ | ❏ | ❏ | ❏ |
| 6.   | ❏ | ❏ | ❏ | ❏ |      | 30.  | ❏ | ❏ | ❏ | ❏ |
| 7.   | ❏ | ❏ | ❏ | ❏ |      | 31.  | ❏ | ❏ | ❏ | ❏ |
| 8.   | ❏ | ❏ | ❏ | ❏ |      | 32.  | ❏ | ❏ | ❏ | ❏ |
| 9.   | ❏ | ❏ | ❏ | ❏ |      | 33.  | ❏ | ❏ | ❏ | ❏ |
| 10.  | ❏ | ❏ | ❏ | ❏ |      | 34.  | ❏ | ❏ | ❏ | ❏ |
| 11.  | ❏ | ❏ | ❏ | ❏ |      | 35.  | ❏ | ❏ | ❏ | ❏ |
| 12.  | ❏ | ❏ | ❏ | ❏ |      | 36.  | ❏ | ❏ | ❏ | ❏ |
| 13.  | ❏ | ❏ | ❏ | ❏ |      | 37.  | ❏ | ❏ | ❏ | ❏ |
| 14.  | ❏ | ❏ | ❏ | ❏ |      | 38.  | ❏ | ❏ | ❏ | ❏ |
| 15.  | ❏ | ❏ | ❏ | ❏ |      | 39.  | ❏ | ❏ | ❏ | ❏ |
| 16.  | ❏ | ❏ | ❏ | ❏ |      | 40.  | ❏ | ❏ | ❏ | ❏ |
| 17.  | ❏ | ❏ | ❏ | ❏ |      | 41.  | ❏ | ❏ | ❏ | ❏ |
| 18.  | ❏ | ❏ | ❏ | ❏ |      | 42.  | ❏ | ❏ | ❏ | ❏ |
| 19.  | ❏ | ❏ | ❏ | ❏ |      | 43.  | ❏ | ❏ | ❏ | ❏ |
| 20.  | ❏ | ❏ | ❏ | ❏ |      | 44.  | ❏ | ❏ | ❏ | ❏ |
| 21.  | ❏ | ❏ | ❏ | ❏ |      | 45.  | ❏ | ❏ | ❏ | ❏ |
| 22.  | ❏ | ❏ | ❏ | ❏ |      | 46.  | ❏ | ❏ | ❏ | ❏ |
| 23.  | ❏ | ❏ | ❏ | ❏ |      | 47.  | ❏ | ❏ | ❏ | ❏ |
| 24.  | ❏ | ❏ | ❏ | ❏ |      | 48.  | ❏ | ❏ | ❏ | ❏ |

| | | | | | | | | | |
|---|---|---|---|---|---|---|---|---|---|
| 49. | ❏ | ❏ | ❏ | ❏ | 75. | ❏ | ❏ | ❏ | ❏ |
| 50. | ❏ | ❏ | ❏ | ❏ | 76. | ❏ | ❏ | ❏ | ❏ |
| 51. | ❏ | ❏ | ❏ | ❏ | 77. | ❏ | ❏ | ❏ | ❏ |
| 52. | ❏ | ❏ | ❏ | ❏ | 78. | ❏ | ❏ | ❏ | ❏ |
| 53. | ❏ | ❏ | ❏ | ❏ | 79. | ❏ | ❏ | ❏ | ❏ |
| 54. | ❏ | ❏ | ❏ | ❏ | 80. | ❏ | ❏ | ❏ | ❏ |
| 55. | ❏ | ❏ | ❏ | ❏ | 81. | ❏ | ❏ | ❏ | ❏ |
| 56. | ❏ | ❏ | ❏ | ❏ | 82. | ❏ | ❏ | ❏ | ❏ |
| 57. | ❏ | ❏ | ❏ | ❏ | 83. | ❏ | ❏ | ❏ | ❏ |
| 58. | ❏ | ❏ | ❏ | ❏ | 84. | ❏ | ❏ | ❏ | ❏ |
| 59. | ❏ | ❏ | ❏ | ❏ | 85. | ❏ | ❏ | ❏ | ❏ |
| 60. | ❏ | ❏ | ❏ | ❏ | 86. | ❏ | ❏ | ❏ | ❏ |
| 61. | ❏ | ❏ | ❏ | ❏ | 87. | ❏ | ❏ | ❏ | ❏ |
| 62. | ❏ | ❏ | ❏ | ❏ | 88. | ❏ | ❏ | ❏ | ❏ |
| 63. | ❏ | ❏ | ❏ | ❏ | 89. | ❏ | ❏ | ❏ | ❏ |
| 64. | ❏ | ❏ | ❏ | ❏ | 90. | ❏ | ❏ | ❏ | ❏ |
| 65. | ❏ | ❏ | ❏ | ❏ | 91. | ❏ | ❏ | ❏ | ❏ |
| 66. | ❏ | ❏ | ❏ | ❏ | 92. | ❏ | ❏ | ❏ | ❏ |
| 67. | ❏ | ❏ | ❏ | ❏ | 93. | ❏ | ❏ | ❏ | ❏ |
| 68. | ❏ | ❏ | ❏ | ❏ | 94. | ❏ | ❏ | ❏ | ❏ |
| 69. | ❏ | ❏ | ❏ | ❏ | 95. | ❏ | ❏ | ❏ | ❏ |
| 70. | ❏ | ❏ | ❏ | ❏ | 96. | ❏ | ❏ | ❏ | ❏ |
| 71. | ❏ | ❏ | ❏ | ❏ | 97. | ❏ | ❏ | ❏ | ❏ |
| 72. | ❏ | ❏ | ❏ | ❏ | 98. | ❏ | ❏ | ❏ | ❏ |
| 73. | ❏ | ❏ | ❏ | ❏ | 99. | ❏ | ❏ | ❏ | ❏ |
| 74. | ❏ | ❏ | ❏ | ❏ | 100. | ❏ | ❏ | ❏ | ❏ |

# Pretest Assessment

**DIRECTIONS:**  Each of the following questions or incomplete statements is followed by four suggested answers or completions. Select the one that is best in each case and then blacken the corresponding space on the answer sheet found in the front of this chapter. Good luck.

1. While performing ventilator rounds in the intensive care unit (ICU), the RRT perceives via percussion an area of hyperresonance on the chest wall of a multiple trauma victim who is receiving mechanical ventilation. What is the likely cause of this physical finding?

   A. pleural effusion
   B. consolidation
   C. pneumothorax
   D. hemothorax

2. Calculate the percent shunt in a patient who has a pulmonary artery catheter in place. The blood gas data shown were obtained after the patient breathed 100% oxygen for 30 minutes:

   | Arterial | Venous |
   |----------|--------|
   | $PO_2$ 555 torr | $PO_2$ 38 torr |
   | $PCO_2$ 35 torr | $PCO_2$ 43 torr |
   | pH 7.37 | pH 7.30 |
   | $HCO_3^-$ 20 mEq/liter | $HCO_3^-$ 20 mEq/liter |
   | $SO_2$ 100% | $SO_2$ 65% |
   | Hb 19 g% | Hb 19 g% |

   Assume a normal respiratory quotient, a normal body temperature, and normal atmospheric pressure.

   A. 2.5%
   B. 3.3%
   C. 9.6%
   D. 12.3%

3. Chest assessment indicates that retained secretions have caused atelectasis of the right middle lobe in a 45-year-old, non-smoking patient. The patient has received postural drainage therapy and has used the directed cough technique. Both therapeutic measures have been ineffective. What should the RRT recommend to help remove the secretions and to facilitate the reversal of the atelectasis?

   A. encouraging the patient to cough more vigorously
   B. initiating incentive spirometry
   C. increasing the patient's $FIO_2$
   D. hydrating the patient and using positive expiratory pressure (PEP) therapy

4. An oxygen flow meter set at 10 L/min. is being used to deliver an 80% helium–20% oxygen gas mixture to a patient experiencing laryngeal edema. What is the actual flow rate being delivered by the oxygen flow meter?

   A. 6 L/min.
   B. 10 L/min.
   C. 18 L/min.
   D. 24 L/min.

5. A patient's serum electrolyte report indicates a potassium concentration of 3.8 mEq/liter. Which statement reflects this value?

   A. The patient is receiving diuretic therapy.
   B. The patient has a hypokalemic metabolic alkalosis.
   C. The patient requires potassium supplementation.
   D. The potassium concentration is normal.

6. After which of the following procedures should the RRT recommend a portable anteroposterior chest radiograph?

   I. bronchoscopy
   II. pulmonary artery catheter insertion
   III. removal of the inner cannula and addition of the decannulation cannula of a fenestrated tracheostomy tube
   IV. nasogastric feeding tube insertion

   A. I, II only
   B. III, IV only
   C. I, II, IV only
   D. I, II, III, IV

7. The RRT receives a call from a home care patient who states that her oxygen concentrator has stopped

operating. The patient is instructed to switch to the backup H cylinder. The pressure gauge of the H cylinder indicates 2,000 psig. The flow rate at which it will operate will be 2.5 L/min. How long will this cylinder last?

A. 41.9 hours
B. 34.6 hours
C. 32.1 hours
D. 26.5 hours

8. The RRT enters the room of a tracheotomized patient. The patient has a foam-cuffed or Kamen–Wilkenson tracheostomy tube in place. The RRT notices that the pilot balloon port is open. What action should she take at this time?

A. Inflate 1 cc of air into the pilot balloon port and cap it.
B. Aspirate the air from the cuff, inflate 3 cc of air through the pilot balloon port, then cap it.
C. No action is necessary.
D. Perform the minimum occluding volume procedure, then cap the pilot balloon port.

9. Which cardiac dysrhythmia(s) is(are) treatable via synchronized cardioversion?

I. sinus bradycardia
II. supraventricular tachycardia
III. ventricular fibrillation
IV. ventricular tachycardia

A. III only
B. II, III, IV only
C. II, IV only
D. I only

10. Pursed-lip breathing might provide expiratory resistance during mild exercise. Which type of patient is most likely to benefit from this maneuver?

A. patients with air trapping associated with chronic obstructive pulmonary disease (COPD)
B. patients with alveolar infiltrates associated with acute infection
C. patients with alveolar or interstitial fibrosis
D. patients with thoracic wall deformities

11. A 45-year-old patient with status asthmaticus is receiving continuous mechanical ventilation. The patient's acid-base status is indicated as follows:

$PaCO_2$ 65 torr
pH 7.19

What should the RRT do at this time?

A. Add 50 to 100 cc of mechanical dead space.
B. Institute 10 cm $H_2O$ of positive end-expiratory pressure (PEEP).
C. Recommend that $HCO_3^-$ be given intravenously (I.V.).
D. Increase either the tidal volume or the ventilatory rate.

12. The RRT is about to perform an arterial puncture procedure on a COPD patient whose oxygen delivery device was changed from a nasal cannula to an air-entrainment mask. The RRT obtains a negative modified Allen test from the patient's right arm. What action should the RRT take at this time?

A. Obtain the arterial blood sample from the right radial artery.
B. Obtain the arterial blood sample from the patient's right brachial artery.
C. Perform the modified Allen test on the patient's left hand.
D. Obtain the arterial blood sample from the patient's left radial artery.

13. Which of the following drugs can be given via the endotracheal tube during a code?

I. atropine
II. isoproterenol
III. epinephrine
IV. sodium bicarbonate

A. I only
B. I, III only
C. II, IV only
D. I, II, III, IV

14. Which statement(s) refer(s) to the function of a constant-flow ventilator?

I. Inspiratory time will increase if the patient's lung compliance decreases.
II. As the patient's airway resistance increases, the delivered flow rate will gradually decrease.
III. Increasing back pressure in the system reduces the machine's flow rate.
IV. Neither a change in the patient's lung compliance nor a change in airway resistance will result in a change in the flow rate.

A. II, III only
B. IV only
C. I only
D. I, III only

15. An ultrasonic nebulizer is being used intermittently for sputum induction on a cystic fibrosis patient. The RRT notices that *not* much mist is coming from the ultrasonic nebulizer. What should the RRT do to increase the mist production of the ultrasonic nebulizer?

    I.   Increase the blower fan speed.
    II.  Heat the water in the couplant.
    III. Adjust the frequency of the power unit.
    IV.  Add water to the couplant compartment.

    A. I, III only
    B. I, IV only
    C. II, III only
    D. III, IV only

16. A COPD patient has undergone a laparotomy and is receiving full mechanical ventilatory support. His arterial blood gases (ABGs) on an $F_1O_2$ of 0.30 at this time indicate

    $PO_2$ 70 torr
    $PCO_2$ 55 torr
    pH 7.33
    $HCO_3^-$ 28 mEq/liter
    B.E. 4 mEq/liter

    The decision is to place this patient on a Briggs adaptor at 35% $O_2$ for a weaning trial. At the time weaning began, his spontaneous ventilatory rate was 16 breaths/min. After 5 minutes, the ventilatory rate increased to 25 breaths/min., at which time paradoxical breathing was observed. After 20 minutes into the weaning trial, ABG data revealed the following:

    $PO_2$ 68 torr
    $PCO_2$ 65 torr
    pH 7.25
    $HCO_3^-$ 28 mEq/liter
    B.E. 4 mEq/liter

    Paradoxical breathing continued. He became tachycardic, diaphoretic, and agitated. What should the RRT do at this time?

    A. Recommend pressure-control inverse-ratio ventilation.
    B. Initiate airway-release pressure ventilation.

    C. Reconnect the patient to the ventilator before weaning.
    D. Increase the $F_1O_2$ of the Briggs adaptor to 0.40.

17. Which mode of mechanical ventilation is depicted on the pressure-time tracing shown in Figure 2-1?

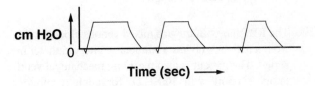

Figure 2-1: Pressure-time tracing.

    A. controlled mechanical ventilation
    B. assisted mechanical ventilation
    C. intermittent mandatory ventilation (IMV)
    D. pressure-support ventilation (PSV)

18. A patient is receiving controlled mechanical ventilation with the following settings:

    mode: control
    $F_1O_2$: 1.0
    peak inspiratory pressure (PIP): 55 cm $H_2O$
    PEEP: 15 cm $H_2O$

    The patient's ventilation and oxygenation statuses are not improving with this mode of ventilation. Therefore, the RRT is about to institute pressure control ventilation (PCV). Which of the following settings should he initially establish with this new mode of ventilation?

    A. $F_1O_2$: 1.0; PIP: 55 cm $H_2O$; PEEP 15 cm $H_2O$
    B. $F_1O_2$: 0.60; PIP: 15 cm $H_2O$; PEEP 10 cm $H_2O$
    C. $F_1O_2$: 1.0; PIP: 27 cm $H_2O$; PEEP 7 cm $H_2O$
    D. $F_1O_2$: 0.40; PIP: 30 cm $H_2O$; PEEP 0 cm $H_2O$

19. In the process of assisting a physician with inserting a pulmonary artery catheter, the RRT observes the electrocardiogram on the cardiac monitor (Figure 2-2)).

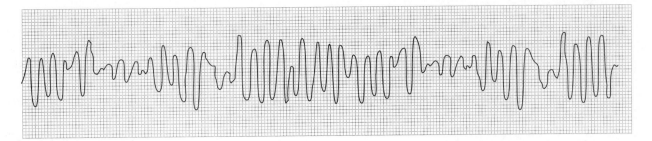

Figure 2-2: ECG tracing.

What should the RRT recommend at this time?

A. immediately withdrawing the pulmonary artery catheter
B. deflating the balloon immediately
C. continuing with the procedure
D. starting cardiac compressions

20. The RRT has withdrawn a mixed venous blood sample from a patient who has a pulmonary artery catheter inserted. The patient is also receiving mechanical ventilatory support with 100% $O_2$ for adult respiratory distress syndrome (ARDS) caused by gram-negative sepsis.

Analysis of the blood sample reveals the following:

$P\bar{V}O_2$ 55 torr
$P\bar{V}CO_2$ 46 torr
pH 7.30
$S\bar{V}O_2$ 80%
blood lactate 3.6 mmoles/liter

What is the likely cause of these data?

A. These are normal mixed venous blood values.
B. The patient recently had a left ventricular myocardial infarction.
C. The patient is experiencing peripheral microcirculation shunting.
D. The patient might have just received a dose of corticosteroids.

21. The RRT has just intubated an adult female patient with an 8-mm, internal-diameter endotracheal (ET) tube. What size catheter would be most appropriate to use when performing tracheobronchial suctioning on this patient?

A. 8 Fr
B. 10 Fr
C. 12 Fr
D. 14 Fr

22. While checking the ventilator of an ARDS patient, the RRT hears the high pressure alarm sounding during each inspiration. The RRT auscultates the right hemithorax and hears no breath sounds. Percussion on the right side reveals hyperresonance. The RRT notices the patient's trachea is shifted toward the left. What action should the RRT take at this time?

A. Decompress the right hemithorax with a 19-gauge needle.
B. Begin manually resuscitating the patient with 100% oxygen.

C. Reduce the tidal volume and increase the high pressure limit.
D. Assess the patient for right endobronchial intubation.

23. While assisting a physician performing a thoracentesis, the RRT is asked to provide the physician with a needle for anesthetizing the periosteum of the rib. What size needle would be appropriate for the RRT to obtain?

A. 0.28 gauge
B. 0.25 gauge
C. 0.22 gauge
D. 0.19 gauge

24. The capnograph shown in Figure 2-3 was obtained from a patient receiving controlled mechanical ventilation. What is the likely cause of the change in this recording from Tracing A to Tracing B?

A. PEEP was instituted.
B. The ventilatory rate was decreased.

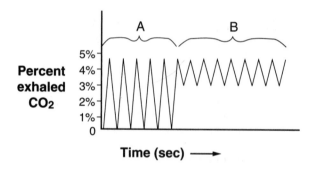

Figure 2-3: Capnograph tracing.

C. The exhalation valve has malfunctioned.
D. Mechanical dead space was added to the ventilator circuitry.

25. The RRT is using capnography in conjunction with endotracheal intubation. As he advances the ET tube, he notices that the capnograph is indicating 0.03%. What is the significance of this value as it relates to the intubation procedure?

A. The ET tube might have been inserted into the esophagus.
B. The ET tube was likely inserted into the right mainstem bronchus.

C. The ET tube has been properly placed through the glottic opening.

D. This reading indicates that the patient has a severe respiratory acidosis.

26. The RRT is calibrating a 7-liter volume wedge spirometer with a 3-liter calibration syringe. After displacing the volume from the syringe into the spirometer in the span of 5 seconds, she notices that the volume recorded is 2.70 liters. Which of the following situations might have accounted for this reading?

I. The syringe might *not* have been completely filled before the calibration maneuver.
II. The wedge spirometer might have a leak.
III. The RRT injected the volume from the syringe too slowly.
IV. The patient hose between the syringe and the wedge spirometer was not attached.

A. I, II only
B. II, III, IV only
C. I, IV only
D. I, II, IV only

27. The RRT is working in the coronary care unit (CCU) and suspects that a microprocessor ventilator malfunction is occurring with a patient who is receiving controlled mechanical ventilation. What procedures should she *sequentially* perform?

I. Disconnect the patient from the ventilator and provide ventilation via a manual resuscitator.
II. Clinically assess the patient for level of consciousness, breathing activity, changes in system pressure, and unusual patient and/or machine sounds.
III. Check all tubing connections, humidifier seal, IMV/PEEP valves, and so on.
IV. Replace the ventilator.

A. I, II, III, IV
B. II, I, III, IV
C. III, II, I, IV
D. I, IV, II, III

28. While performing ventilator rounds in the surgical ICU, the RRT observes the pressure-time waveform shown in Figure 2-4.

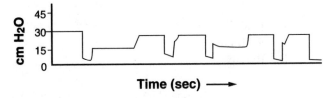

**Figure 2-4:** Pressure-time tracing.

Based on this observation, what can the RRT determine?

A. that auto-PEEP is present
B. that the tidal volume is set too low
C. that the high pressure alarm is set too high
D. that the patient is having a difficult time cycling on the ventilator

29. An elderly female patient in the hospital has a metered-dose inhaler (MDI) ordered for two puffs of albuterol QID. The patient has been using an MDI at home for the past several months as prescribed by her physician. Upon admission to the hospital, the RRT notes that the patient has a great deal of difficulty timing the activation of the MDI just prior to taking a breath. Which of the following alterations in technique should the RRT try at this time?

A. Replace the MDI with a small-volume nebulizer powered by a room air compressor.
B. Demonstrate the procedure and have the patient practice using the MDI with a spacer.
C. Replace the MDI with intermittent positive pressure breathing (IPPB) therapy to allow inspiratory nebulization only.
D. Have the patient place the MDI mouthpiece in her mouth before activating the MDI.

30. The RRT is setting up an oxygen-delivery system for a home care patient. The system includes a 40-liter liquid oxygen reservoir that weighs approximately 100 pounds. How many liters of gaseous oxygen will be available from this unit?

A. 860 L
B. 2,250 L
C. 25,300 L
D. 34,400 L

31. The RRT enters the ICU to check the ventilator of a patient who has a pulmonary artery catheter in place. A pulmonary artery pressure waveform is displayed on the monitor. Upon taking a second look at the monitor, the RRT suddenly notices that the waveform has changed to reflect a pulmonary capillary wedge pressure pattern. What action should be taken at this time?

A. The catheter should be withdrawn until the pulmonary artery pressure waveform reappears.
B. A venous blood sample should be obtained and the venous oxygen content should be determined.
C. The catheter's balloon should be inflated.
D. The catheter should be further advanced until the tracing changes.

32. Based on the quality-control data (Figure 2-5) obtained from a Severinghaus electrode in a blood-gas analyzer, determine the nature of the problem associated with the electrode.

**A.**

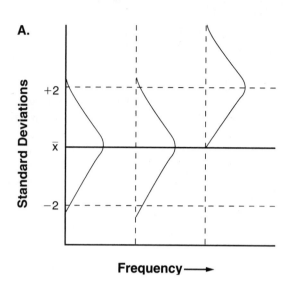

**B.**

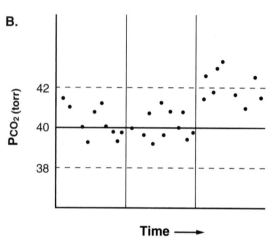

**Figure 2-5:** Quality control data obtained from a Severinghaus electrode.

   A. The electrode has experienced a random error.
   B. The electrode has developed an accuracy problem.
   C. The Severinghaus electrode has developed a precision problem.
   D. The electrode has experienced a trending problem.

33. Calculate the $C(a-\bar{v})O_2$ based on the data given as follows:

$\dot{V}O_2$ 250 ml/min.
C.O. 5 liters/min.

   A. 2.5 vol%
   B. 5.0 vol%
   C. 5.5 vol%
   D. 7.0 vol%

34. Chest radiographs of which of the following clinical disorders are likely to display air bronchograms?

   I. interstitial edema
   II. interstitial hemorrhage
   III. atelectasis
   IV. pneumonia

   A. I, II, III, IV
   B. I, II, IV only
   C. I, IV only
   D. I, II, III only

35. What should the RRT recommend when a patient has a large-volume pleural effusion or has continuously accumulating intrapleural fluid?

   A. pleural needle aspiration
   B. chest tube insertion
   C. transtracheal needle aspiration
   D. pleural biopsy

36. Which of the following clinical interventions are appropriate for the treatment of carbon monoxide poisoning?

   I. The administration of oxygen under normobaric conditions.
   II. The administration of oxygen under hyperbaric conditions.
   III. The administration of carbogen (5% $CO_2$ and 95% $O_2$) to increase the minute ventilation.
   IV. Endotracheal intubation of an apneic victim along with hyperventilation via a manual resuscitator and oxygen administration.

   A. II, IV only
   B. I, III, IV only
   C. I, II, IV only
   D. I, II, III only

37. A patient receiving assisted mechanical ventilation is observed using his accessory muscles of ventilation and demonstrating labored breathing. Which ventilator-related condition(s) can cause this problem?

   I. a high inspiratory flow rate
   II. an increased sensitivity setting
   III. the presence of auto-PEEP
   IV. an I:E ratio of 1:2

   A. I, IV only
   B. I only
   C. II, III only
   D. III only

38. A neonate in the neonatal intensive care unit (NICU) is receiving humidified oxygen via a large, enclosed oxyhood operating at a source gas flow of 3 L/min. ABG

analysis reveals a $PCO_2$ of 56 torr. What should the RRT do at this time?

A. Institute nasal continuous positive airway pressure (CPAP).
B. Lower the temperature of the humidified oxygen delivered to the oxyhood.
C. Increase the oxygen flowrate to 6 L/min.
D. Place the patient and the oxyhood at 3 L/min. in an incubator.

39. An ARDS patient who has an ideal body weight (IBW) of 155 pounds is receiving mechanical ventilation via a volume ventilator. The physician asks the RRT to establish inverse-ratio ventilation at an I:E ratio of 2:1, with an inspiratory time of 2 seconds. What peak inspiratory flow rate ($V_I$) setting should the RRT establish to achieve the requested I:E ratio?

A. 10 to 16 L/min.
B. 14 to 21 L/min.
C. 21 to 32 L/min.
D. 28 to 42 L/min.

40. Which device is the most appropriate to use to assess the oxygenation status of a carbon monoxide poisoning victim?

A. pulse oximeter
B. oxygen analyzer
C. ABG analyzer
D. co-oximeter

41. Before being administered an aerosolized $\beta_2$ agonist, a patient exhibited loud, high-pitched wheezing heard during inspiration and expiration. Which of the following auscultatory findings would be considered an improvement resulting from breathing this aerosolized medication?

A. early inspiratory crackles
B. less loud and lower-pitched wheezing heard only during exhalation
C. lower-pitched inspiratory wheezes and late inspiratory crackles
D. polyphonic expiratory wheezing and loud, high-pitched inspiratory wheezing

42. A patient receiving mechanical ventilation through a 9.0 mm I.D. oral ET tube displays the following data:

inspired tidal volume: 800 ml
expired tidal volume: 400 ml
PIP: 25 cm $H_2O$
ET tube cuff pressure: 5 cm $H_2O$

Which of the following actions needs to be taken at this time?

I. The minimal leak technique is being used, therefore *no* action is necessary.
II. The cuff should be reinflated to a pressure of 50 cm $H_2O$.
III. If a cuff leak is present, the endotracheal tube must be replaced.
IV. The tidal volume setting must be increased.

A. I only
B. II only
C. III only
D. III, IV only

43. PEP therapy can be recommended for which of the following conditions?

I. sputum retention that is *not* responsive to coughing
II. air trapping without sputum retention
III. history of a pulmonary problem that has been successfully treated with postural drainage

A. I only
B. II only
C. III only
D. I, III only

44. Through which of the following methods can ventricular fibrillation be recognized?

I. palpation of an abnormal, racing, thready pulse
II. observation of consistently wide QRS complexes on the ECG monitor
III. palpation of a rapid pulse
IV. observation of distorted and irregular complexes on the ECG tracing

A. I, II, III, IV
B. I only
C. IV only
D. II, III only

45. The following data were obtained from a 75-kg patient receiving mechanical ventilation:

mode: SIMV
$FIO_2$: 0.40
tidal volume: 800 ml
SIMV rate: 8 breaths/min.
inspiratory flow: 60 L/min.
PIP: 50 cm $H_2O$
plateau pressure: 40 cm $H_2O$
PEEP/CPAP: 0 cm $H_2O$
spontaneous rate: 15 breaths/min.
spontaneous inspiratory flow: 1.0 L/sec.

ABG data reveal the following:

$PO_2$ 73 torr
$PCO_2$ 35 torr
pH 7.43

HCO$_3^-$ 24 mEq/liter
B.E. 0 mEq/liter

The RRT notices that the patient is using accessory neck muscles with each spontaneous inspiration and that there are intercostal and substernal retractions at the same time. What should the RRT recommend?

A. initiating PEEP/CPAP
B. initiating pressure support
C. increasing the tidal volume to 900 ml
D. increasing the SIMV rate to 10 breaths/min.

46. Which factor(s) influence(s) the volume delivered to a patient via a pressure-limited, time-cycled mechanical ventilator?

I. the inspiratory time
II. the inspiratory flow rate
III. the pressure limit
IV. the patient's time constant

A. I, II, III, IV
B. II, III only
C. I, IV only
D. I, II, IV only

47. An overweight, 80-kg, 60-year-old female enters the emergency department complaining of a rapid heart beat. She is pale, diaphoretic, and tachypneic. She also complains of a crushing chest pain. Her ECG and vital signs are shown as follows:

ECG: ventricular tachycardia
heart rate: 120 beats/min.
blood pressure: 95/65 torr
palpable pulse: 100 beats/min.
ventilatory rate: 30 breaths/min.

Oxygen is started by nasal cannula at 4 L/min., and an I.V. access is established. What is the definitive clinical therapy for this patient?

A. lidocaine 75–100 mg I.V. push, followed by 2 mg/min. lidocaine I.V. drip
B. defibrillation with 200 watt-seconds (w-sec), followed by 300 w-sec, followed by 360 w-sec if the preceding shocks do *not* work
C. cardioversion with 200 w-sec, followed by 200 to 300 w-sec, followed by 360 w-sec if the preceding shocks are unsuccessful
D. adenosine 6 mg rapid I.V. push, followed by 12 mg I.V. push if there is *no* initial response

48. Calculate the percent shunt in a patient who, after breathing an F$_I$O$_2$ of 1.0 for 20 minutes, has the following arterial and mixed venous blood-gas data. The patient has a normal respiratory quotient and a normal body temperature and a hemoglobin concentration of 17 g%. Assume normal ambient conditions.

| ARTERIAL | MIXED VENOUS |
| --- | --- |
| PaO$_2$ 500 torr | P$\bar{v}$O$_2$ 70 torr |
| PaCO$_2$ 60 torr | P$\bar{v}$CO$_2$ 65 torr |
| pH 7.34 | pH 7.32 |
| SaO$_2$ 100% | S$\bar{v}$O$_2$ 85% |

A. 13.68%
B. 10.71%
C. 8.89%
D. 8.33%

49. An adult patient's resting cardiac index is calculated to be 3.5 L/min/m$^2$. This value can be interpreted as follows:

A. normal
B. below normal
C. above normal
D. incompatible with life

50. A 5-day-old, term infant requires a capillary blood gas. The infant's heel is arterialized, prepped, and punctured. The following room air data are obtained:

PaO$_2$ 68 torr
PaCO$_2$ 33 torr
pH 7.39
HCO$_3^-$ 20 mEq/liter
B.E. 4 mEq/liter

Interpretation of these results would indicate the following:

A. the infant has an uncompensated respiratory alkalosis with hypoxemia.
B. the capillary blood gases are normal.
C. the infant should immediately receive 30% oxygen via an oxyhood.
D. a laboratory error has occurred and the values are inconsistent with capillary blood gases.

51. For which of the following conditions would BiPAP® be most appropriate to recommend?

I. ARDS
II. refractory hypoxemia
III. nocturnal hypoventilation
IV. sleep apnea

A. I, II only
B. III, IV only
C. I, II, IV only
D. II, III, IV only

52. A physician writes an order for the RRT to perform pulse oximetry on a patient receiving supplemental oxygen. Which of the following conditions or situations might produce erroneous data?

A. The patient is hypercapneic.
B. The patient is hypotensive.
C. The patient is alkalotic.
D. The patient is polycythemic.

53. A patient rescued from a burning building has been brought to the emergency department. His ventilatory rate is 28 breaths/min. His breath sounds are clear, but he is complaining of shortness of breath. He does *not* have singed nasal hair, *nor* does he have carbonaceous sputum. Which of the following methods of monitoring oxygenation are necessary in this patient to adequately assess oxygenation?

   A. $PtcO_2$ monitoring
   B. pulse oximetry
   C. arterial blood gas results
   D. co-oximetry

54. While a physician is performing a bronchoscopic biopsy on an intubated patient, bleeding at the biopsy site occurs. The physician asks the RRT to obtain medication to help arrest the bleeding. Which of the following medications should be chosen?

   A. atropine
   B. lidocaine
   C. acetylcysteine
   D. epinephrine

55. Which suction catheter(s) would be best suited for evacuating thick, tenacious secretions from the tracheobronchial tree?

   I. Argyle Aero-Flo tip suction catheter
   II. whistle-tip suction catheter
   III. open-end, angular-tip suction catheter
   IV. open-end, perpendicular-tip suction catheter

   A. I, II only
   B. III only
   C. II, IV only
   D. III, IV only

56. A patient who has gram-negative pneumonia of the right lung has just been admitted to the ICU to receive mechanical ventilation. From all diagnostic and clinical data, the left lung has *no* pathology. What should the RRT recommend at this time?

   A. Intubate the patient with a high-volume, low-pressure cuffed tube.
   B. Intubate the patient with a low-volume, high-pressure cuffed tube and provide mechanical ventilation.
   C. Intubate the patient with a double-lumen tube to achieve independent lung ventilation.
   D. Tracheotomize the patient and insert a tracheostomy tube.

57. A patient is receiving volume-limited mechanical ventilation in the control mode. The peak airway pressure is 60 cm $H_2O$. The physician requests that the RRT initiate pressure-control ventilation to reduce the mean airway pressure. The initial pressure-control setting should be:

   A. 10 cm $H_2O$.
   B. 20 cm $H_2O$.
   C. 40 cm $H_2O$.
   D. 55 cm $H_2O$.

58. A 65-year-old asthmatic with chronic bronchitis and a 20-pack-per-year smoking history enters the emergency department. Upon auscultation, the RRT perceives bilaterally diminished breath sounds and wheezes at end-exhalation over both lung bases. Various clinical and physiological data are presented as follows:

ventilatory rate: 35 breaths/min.
heart rate: 120 beats/min.
blood pressure: 185/95 torr

The patient is using his accessory muscles of ventilation and is orthopneic.

ABG on 2 L/min. of oxygen via a nasal cannula reveal the following:

$PO_2$ 33 torr
$PCO_2$ 112 torr
pH 7.12
$HCO_3^-$ 35 mEq/liter
B.E. 10 mEq/liter

What should the RRT do at this time?

   A. Administer a bronchodilator to relieve the patient's bronchospasm.
   B. Intubate and mechanically ventilate the patient.
   C. Intubate the patient and institute CPAP.
   D. Administer oxygen by way of a Venturi mask at 30%.

59. Which of the following statements accurately refers to the administration of sodium bicarbonate ($NaHCO_3$) during cardiopulmonary resuscitation (CPR)?

   A. $NaHCO_3$ should be administered to completely correct the base deficit.
   B. The potential benefits of $NaHCO_3$ administration outweigh its deleterious effects.
   C. The administration of $NaHCO_3$ enhances the effect of defibrillation.
   D. $NaHCO_3$ administration should be considered only after defibrillation, compressions, and ventilation have been employed.

60. A patient has a pulmonary artery catheter in place. The following hemodynamic pressures have been recorded:

proximal port: 10 mm Hg

distal port: 22 mm Hg/14 mm Hg

distal port, balloon inflated: 9 mm Hg

Which of these pressure measurements is equal to the central venous pressure?

A. 22 mm Hg

B. 14 mm Hg

C. 10 mm Hg

D. 9 mm Hg

61. The RRT is performing a pre- and postbronchodilator study on a patient (Table 2-1). The patient has been given two puffs of Atrovent. Fifteen minutes later, the postbronchodilator forced vital capacity maneuver was performed. The pre- and postbronchodilator data are shown in Table 2–1 below.

Which of the following conditions contributed to the cause of this data?

A. The amount of Atrovent administered was insufficient.

B. The postbronchodilator study was performed too soon after the medication was given.

C. A different bronchodilator should have been used.

D. The patient is unresponsive to bronchodilators.

62. Which of the following measurements must the RRT perform while assisting at a bronchoscopy?

   I. heart rate

  II. ventilatory rate

 III. oxygen saturation

 IV. end-tidal $PCO_2$

A. I, II, III, IV

B. I, II, III only

C. II, III only

D. IV only

63. A patient is being mechanically ventilated with a ventilator classified as a pressure controller. How will the patient's tidal volume be affected if the patient's lung compliance decreases?

A. The tidal volume will be unaffected.

B. The tidal volume will increase.

C. The tidal volume will decrease.

D. The tidal volume will fluctuate with each breath.

64. Which of the following factors affect the end-tidal $CO_2$ measurements obtained by capnography?

   I. fraction of inspired oxygen

  II. alveolar ventilation

 III. ventilation–perfusion ratio

 IV. cardiac output

A. III, IV only

B. II, IV only

C. II, III, IV only

D. I, II only

65. Prior to receiving mechanical ventilation, a patient had a $V_D/V_T$ ratio of 0.45. The $V_D/V_T$ ratio rose to 0.55 after positive pressure mechanical ventilation was instituted. What might have accounted for the increase in this ratio?

A. The positive pressure mechanical ventilation caused the elevation.

B. The patient might have developed pneumonia.

C. The patient might be hypervolemic.

D. The patient's cardiac output increased.

66. An RRT receives an order to administer, via an ultrasonic nebulizer, 0.30 ml of metaproterenol in 4 ml of normal saline to a chronic bronchitic who has a reversible component to his pulmonary pathology. What should the RRT do in this situation?

A. Administer the treatment as ordered.

B. Inform the prescribing physician that the medication dosage is too high.

C. Suggest to the physician that an intermittent small-volume nebulizer be used.

D. Suggest to the physician that less diluent needs to be used.

67. Fetal lung maturity is denoted by a lecithin–sphingomyelin ratio of at least ___ along with the presence of ___ in the amniotic fluid.

A. 1:3; phosphatidylcholine

B. 1:2; phosphatidylinositol

**Table 2-1**

| PARAMETERS | PREDICTED | Prebronchodilator | | Postbronchodilator | |
|---|---|---|---|---|---|
| | | ACTUAL | % PRED | ACTUAL | % PRED |
| FVC | 5.28 L | 4.11 L | 78% | 4.13 L | 78% |
| FEV1 | 3.24 L | 2.43 L | 75% | 2.49 L | 77% |
| FEV$_3$ | 4.85 L | 3.88 L | 80% | 4.92 L | 81% |
| PEFR | 9.59 L/sec. | 7.29 L/sec. | 76% | 7.30 L/sec. | 76% |
| FEF$_{25-75\%}$ | 4.40 L/sec. | 3.04 L/sec. | 69% | 3.10 L/sec. | 70% |
| FEF$_{75-85\%}$ | 1.09 L/sec. | 0.76 L/sec. | 70% | 0.81 L/sec. | 74% |

C. 1:1; phosphatidylcholine

D. 2:1; phosphatidyglycerol

68. The data shown in Table 2-2 were obtained by the RRT monitoring a patient who was receiving volume-cycled positive-pressure ventilation:

**Table 2-2**

| TIME | PIP | $P_{plateau}$ |
|------|-----|-----------|
| 0700 | 30 cm $H_2O$ | 20 cm $H_2O$ |
| 0800 | 32 cm $H_2O$ | 20 cm $H_2O$ |
| 0900 | 34 cm $H_2O$ | 20 cm $H_2O$ |
| 1000 | 38 cm $H_2O$ | 20 cm $H_2O$ |
| 1100 | 40 cm $H_2O$ | 20 cm $H_2O$ |

How should the RRT evaluate these data?

A. The patient is experiencing retained secretions.

B. The patient's lungs are becoming more difficult to inflate.

C. The patient is developing intrapulmonary shunting.

D. The patient should be given conscious sedation.

69. A patient is about to receive pressure-control inverse-ratio ventilation (PC-IRV). What combination of medications should the RRT recommend for this patient?

A. *d*-tubocurarine and pentobarbital

B. diazapam and pancuronium bromide

C. morphine and fentanyl

D. midazolam and succinylcholine

70. The RRT notices that a chest tube draining a hemothorax via a three-bottle pleural drainage system is occluded. What action can she take to relieve this obstruction?

A. Clamp the chest tube between the occlusion and the chest wall until sufficient negative pressure develops to evacuate the obstruction.

B. Gently milk the chest tube from the chest wall toward the drainage-collection bottle.

C. Increase the suction pressure.

D. Increase the water level in the suction-control bottle.

71. While working with a patient suspected of having pneumonia, the RRT obtains a sputum sample that contains pus cells and is foul smelling. How should the RRT describe this sputum sample in the patient's chart?

A. as viscous and tenacious

B. as purulent and fetid

C. as mucoid

D. as yellow-green and blood-tinged

72. Which of the following pathophysiologic conditions can cause a widened $P(A\text{-}a)O_2$?

I. alveolarcapillary membrane diffusion defect

II. intrapulmonary shunting

III. ventilation–perfusion abnormalities

IV. hyperventilation

A. I, II, III only

B. I, II only

C. II, III, IV only

D. III, IV only

73. A near-drowning victim is receiving pressure-support ventilation at a level of 30 cm $H_2O$. A tidal volume of 10 ml/kg is being delivered. After being mechanically ventilated in this mode for 48 hours, the patient suddenly exhibits refractory hypoxemia, decreased lung compliance, and tachypnea. Chest radiography at this time reveals pulmonary infiltrates in all lung fields. Which mode of mechanical ventilation would be appropriate at this time?

A. BiPAP® ventilation in the timed mode

B. pressure-support ventilation at 5 cm $H_2O$

C. PC-IRV

D. SIMV at a rate of 6 breaths/min.

74. A patient being treated for an acute asthma attack is having her blood pressure taken by the RRT. The RRT measures a drop of 10 mm Hg in the patient's systolic pressure during inspiration. How should the RRT record this finding in the patient's chart?

A. as pulsus paradoxus

B. as pulsus alternans

C. as pulsus interruptus

D. as Korotkoff sounds

75. The patient's ability to perform incentive spirometry effectively would require which of the following subjective responses?

A. orientation to place

B. orientation to time

C. awareness of environment

D. patient cooperation

76. A postoperative patient is receiving 50% oxygen at 15 L/min. via an all-purpose nebulizer. The oxygen saturation has fallen to 90%, and the patient's minute ventilation is 14.9 L/min. Which of the following recommendation(s) would be appropriate to increase the total flow to the patient to deliver 50% oxygen?

I. Bleed-in 5 L/min. oxygen to the all-purpose nebulizer.

II. Institute dual all-purpose nebulizers at 50% operating at 15 L/min.

III. Switch to a gas-injection nebulizer with an oxygen flow rate set at 22 L/min. and an air flow meter set at 37 L/min.

A. I, II, III
B. III only
C. II only
D. II, III only

77. How will hemodynamic measurements be affected if the pulmonary artery catheter transducer is placed below the phlebostatic axis after the transducer has been zeroed?

A. As long as the transducer was zeroed, the data will be reliable.
B. The pressure measurements will fluctuate.
C. The data obtained will read erroneously higher.
D. *No* data will be available.

78. An asthmatic patient having an acute attack is admitted to the hospital. He receives a chest X-ray that shows considerable air trapping. Another chest film is taken about 35 minutes following a nebulized albuterol treatment. If the treatment was effective, which of the following changes would be expected if the second X-ray is compared to the admitting X-ray?

A. The lungs would be more hypertranslucent in the post-therapy chest film.
B. The heart shadow would appear smaller than in the pretherapy chest film.
C. The hemidiaphragms would appear flatter than they did in the pretherapy chest film.
D. The intercostal spaces would be narrower in the post-therapy chest film.

79. Which medication(s) has(have) been effective in the treatment of obstructive sleep apnea?

I. naloxone
II. protriptyline
III. pyridostigmine
IV. aminophylline

A. I, II only
B. I, III only
C. III, IV only
D. II only

80. A 27-year-old male enters the emergency department with labored breathing, a ventilatory rate of 30 breaths/min., a pulse of 100 beats/min., and chest pain. Assessment of the patient reveals that he has shaking chills, decreased movement of the right chest, and increased fremitus in the right base, which was also dull to percussion. Auscultation indicates coarse crackles and wheezes in the right base. He has a strong, productive cough bringing up thick, brown sputum. His body temperature is 103.5°F, and his white blood cell (WBC) count is 25,000/mm³.

ABGs show the following:

$PO_2$ 70 mm Hg
$PCO_2$ 30 mm Hg
pH 7.34

What should the RRT recommend for this patient at this time?

A. ET intubation and mechanical ventilation
B. continuous aerosol mask at 30% $O_2$ and chest physiotherapy
C. continuous positive airway pressure at an $FIO_2$ of 0.60
D. nasal cannula at 2 L/min.

81. While the RRT is performing chest physiotherapy on an elderly patient with pneumonia for involvement of the posterior basal segments, the patient says, "I'm having a hard time breathing." What should the RRT do at this time?

A. Apply percussion with less force.
B. Place the patient in a different position.
C. Deliver 2 liters/min. of oxygen via a nasal cannula and continue the treatment.
D. Instill 3 cc of normal saline and perform nasotracheal suctioning.

82. The volume-pressure loop shown in Figure 2-6 was obtained from a patient who was receiving controlled mechanical ventilation.

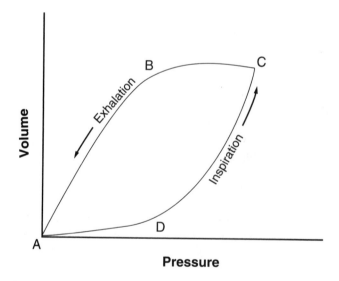

**Figure 2-6:** Volume-pressure curve.

Which of the following points (shown in Figure 2-7 A–D) on the curve represent inflection points?

A. A and C
B. A and D
C. B and D
D. B and C

83. The hatched area under which pressure-time tracing (Figure 2-7 A–D) represents the mean airway pressure?

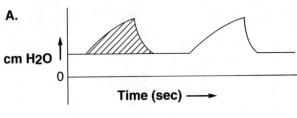

**A.**

cm H2O

0

Time (sec) ⟶

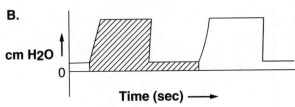

**B.**

cm H2O

0

Time (sec) ⟶

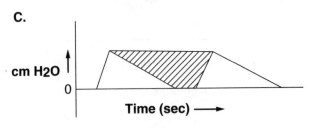

**C.**

cm H2O

0

Time (sec) ⟶

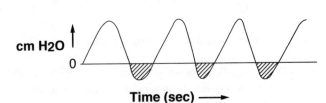

**D.**

cm H2O

0

Time (sec) ⟶

**Figure 2-7:** Pressure-time waveform.

A. 2-7 A
B. 2-7 B
C. 2-7 C
D. 2-7 D

84. Based on the pressure waveform shown in Figure 2-8, which ventilator setting adjustment has been instituted?

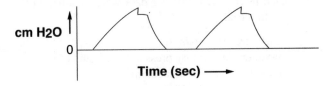

cm H2O

0

Time (sec) ⟶

**Figure 2-8:** Pressure waveform.

A. expiratory retard
B. increased PIP
C. inspiratory hold
D. increased high-pressure limit

85. Which radiologic view would be most helpful in confirming the presence of a pleural effusion?

A. anteroposterior supine
B. posteroanterior upright
C. lateral decubitus
D. posteroanterior supine

86. At what lung volume is it generally recommended that a patient actuate a metered-dose inhaler (MDI)?

A. at functional residual capacity (FRC)
B. at residual volume (RV)
C. at total lung capacity (TLC)
D. at resting, end inspiration

87. A 51-year-old woman receiving continuous mechanical ventilation following a cardiac arrest has a Swan–Ganz catheter in place. Her hemodynamic data are as follows:

pulmonary capillary wedge pressure: 7 mm Hg
mean pulmonary artery pressure: 35 mm Hg
heart rate: 115 beats/min.
blood pressure: 95/45 mm Hg
cardiac output: 4.1 L/min.
body surface area (BSA): 2.3 m$^2$

Which hemodynamic measurements would be below normal based on the preceding data?

I. cardiac index
II. stroke volume
III. mixed venous oxygen
IV. central venous pressure

A. I, II, III only
B. II, III, IV only
C. I, III only
D. I, II only

88. A 2-year-old girl enters the emergency department drooling and presenting with respiratory distress and stridor. The physician believes the child has epiglottitis. Tonsillitis and foreign body obstruction cannot be ruled out, however. Which of the following diagnostic procedures should the RRT recommend?

A. fiberoptic bronchoscopy
B. direct laryngoscopy
C. impedance plethysmography
D. lateral neck radiograph

89. An ARDS patient is receiving mechanical ventilation with the following settings:

mode: pressure-control ventilation
pressure-control level: 20 cm $H_2O$
ventilatory rate: 12 breaths/min.
I:E ratio: 1:1
$FIO_2$: 0.50
PEEP: 15 cm $H_2O$

The patient's exhaled tidal volume is 6 ml/kg.
ABG data reveal the following:

$PO_2$ 62 torr
$PCO_2$ 55 torr
pH 7.28

The physician wants a $PaCO_2$ of 40 to 45 torr. What
ventilator setting change would the RRT recommend?

A. increasing the ventilatory rate to 20 breaths/min.
B. increasing the PEEP to 20 cm $H_2O$
C. increasing the pressure-control level to 25 cm $H_2O$
D. increasing the I:E ratio to 2:1

90. A patient who has left ventricular failure would likely
benefit from which of the following medications?

I. cardiac glycosides
II. diuretics
III. angiotensin-converting enzyme inhibitors
IV. antidysrhythmics

A. I, II, III, IV
B. II, III, IV only
C. II, III only
D. I, II, IV only

91. Through which port or channel is a mixed venous blood
sample obtained via a pulmonary artery catheter?

A. balloon-inflation channel
B. proximal channel
C. distal channel
D. thermistor channel

92. What action should be taken if the PCWP waveform
becomes nonphasic while a wedge-pressure tracing is
being obtained?

A. Continue obtaining the PCWP measurement.
B. Remove the catheter from the patient immediately.
C. Inflate more air into the balloon.
D. Deflate the balloon.

93. The RRT is asked to recommend a nondepolarizing,
neuromuscular blocking agent for a patient who is
about to be mechanically ventilated in the control
mode. Which of the following medications would she
suggest?

I. pancuronium bromide
II. succinylcholine chloride
III. gallamine triethiodide
IV. *d*-tubocurarine

A. I, II, III, IV
B. II, III only
C. I, IV only
D. I, III, IV only

94. What is the significance of the small curved line (arrow) at the origin of the volume-pressure loop shown
in Figure 2-9?

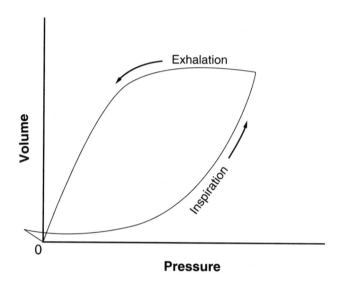

**Figure 2-9:** Volume-pressure curve.

A. a patient-triggered mechanical ventilation breath
B. PEEP
C. auto-PEEP
D. volume compressed in the ventilator tubing

95. During cardiopulmonary resuscitation, the RRT observes the cardiac monitor displaying the following
electrocardiogram (Figure 2-10).

What action should she recommend?

A. I.V. administration of bicarbonate
B. intracardiac epinephrine
C. cardioversion
D. defibrillation

96. A patient receiving mechanical ventilatory support is
being weaned via Briggs adaptor trials. The physician's order calls for the initial trials to be 15 minutes
each hour. The following data were obtained before
the first trial.

heart rate: 80 beats/min.
maximum inspiratory pressure: −25 cm $H_2O$
ventilatory rate: 18 breaths/min.
vital capacity: 10 ml/kg
$FIO_2$: 0.40
$SpO_2$: 94%

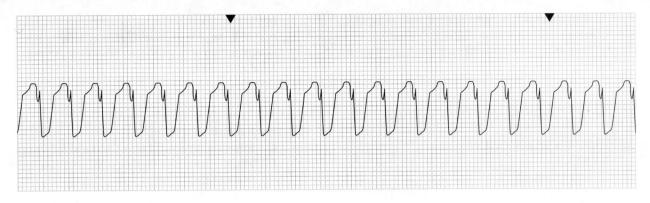

**Figure 2-10:** ECG tracing.

After breathing 10 minutes via the Briggs adaptor, the measurements shown as follows were obtained:

heart rate: 100 beats/min
maximum inspiratory pressure: −13 cm $H_2O$
ventilatory rate: 28 breaths/min
vital capacity: 7 ml/kg
$FIO_2$: 0.40
$SpO_2$: 86%

What should the RRT do at this time?

A. Continue with the weaning procedure and monitor the patient.
B. Reconnect the patient to the mechanical ventilator.
C. Nebulize a bronchodilator inline with the Briggs adaptor.
D. Add 50 cc more of reservoir tubing to the distal end of the Briggs adaptor.

97. The RRT has plotted the quality-control data reported by the $PCO_2$ electrode throughout the shift on the Levey–Jennings chart (Figure 2-11).

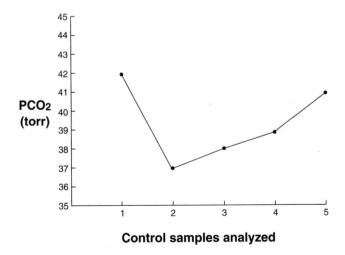

**Figure 2-11:** $PCO_2$ electrode quality-control data.

Based on the graph generated, what should the RRT do?

A. Do *nothing* because the data points all lie within the normal standard deviation limit.
B. A random error has oczcurred and it should be ignored.
C. Clean the electrode because protein has likely accumulated.
D. Check the electrode membrane for the presence of air bubbles.

98. A patient who is receiving controlled, volume-cycled ventilation is suspected of having a bronchopleural fistula. The RRT is asked to recommend a different form of ventilation. His recommendation should be to institute:

A. SIMV
B. assist-control ventilation
C. high-frequency jet ventilation
D. pressure-support ventilation

**Questions 99 and 100 refer to the same patient.**

99. A 55-year-old patient is being hemodynamically monitored in the CCU. She displays the following measurements:

pulmonary artery systolic pressure: 48 torr
pulmonary artery diastolic pressure: 38 torr
pulmonary capillary wedge pressure: 30 torr
systemic arterial systolic pressure: 100 torr
systemic arterial diastolic pressure: 70 torr
central venous pressure: 13 torr

The RRT auscultates the patient's chest and perceives bilateral, late-inspiratory crackles especially prominent in the dependent regions of the lungs. Evaluate these hemodynamic results.

A. The patient is developing ARDS.
B. The patient is experiencing left ventricular failure.

C. The patient is exhibiting signs of right ventricular failure.

D. The patient is developing systemic hypertension.

100. The RRT has been asked to evaluate a patient for extubation. The patient was evaluated as follows:

PaO$_2$ 80 torr on an FIO$_2$ 0.30
SaO$_2$ 94%
positive gag reflex

positive cuff-leak test
patient is capable of raising his head off the bed
patient is alert and coughs deeply while suctioned
MEP 75 cm H$_2$O

Based on these findings, what should the RRT do?

A. Reinitiate mechanical ventilation.
B. Extubate the patient.
C. Maintain the patient on a T-piece at 40% oxygen.
D. Monitor the patient for the next few hours, and re-evaluate him.

# Pretest Matrix Categories

1. IB3
2. IIIA1m(1)
3. IIIC5
4. IIB2h(1)
5. IIIA1g
6. IIIA1a
7. IIIE2a
8. IIB2f(3)
9. IIID1b
10. IIIA1h
11. IIIA1h
12. IIIA1b
13. IIID1b
14. IIB1e(1)
15. IIB2c
16. IIIB2c
17. IA1f(3)
18. IIIB2c
19. IIB2q
20. IC2c
21. IIA1g
22. IIID2
23. IIIE1b
24. IA1f(5)
25. IIIB1e

26. IIB3b
27. IIB2e(1)
28. IA1f(3)
29. IIIC2
30. IIIE2a
31. IIIA1f
32. IIB3a
33. IIIA1m(1)
34. IB7a
35. IIIE1j
36. IIA1a
37. IIIA1h
38. IIIC3a
39. IIIB2c
40. IIA1h(4)
41. IIIA1k
42. IIIB1a
43. IIIB3
44. IIIA1d
45. IIIB4b
46. IIB2e(1)
47. IIID1b
48. IIIA1m(1)
49. IIIA1m(3)
50. IC2e

51. IIIB4a
52. IIB2h(4)
53. IIIA1b
54. IIIE1a
55. IIIC7b
56. IIA1f(2)
57. IIIB2c
58. IIIB1a
59. IIID1b
60. IIIA1f
61. IC2a
62. IIIE1a
63. IIIB2c
64. IIB1h(4)
65. IIIA1m(2)
66. IIA1c
67. IA1h
68. IIIA1e
69. IIIB2c
70. IIB2r
71. IA1f(4)
72. IIIA1m(1)
73. IIIB2c
74. IB2a
75. IB6a

76. IIIC3a
77. IIB2n(2)
78. IIIA1a
79. IIIE1g
80. IIIC5
81. IIIC5
82. IIIA1e
83. IA1f(3)
84. IC2i
85. IB7e
86. IIIE2b
87. IIIA1m
88. IB8a
89. IIIB2c
90. IIID1b
91. IIIE1k
92. IIB1q(1)
93. IIIE1l
94. IIIA1e
95. IIID1b
96. IIIA1h
97. IIIB2h(4)
98. IIIC8a
99. IA1g(2)
100. IIIB1c

# Chapter 2 Pretest Written Registry Examination Matrix Scoring Form

| CONTENT AREA | PRETEST ITEM NUMBER | PRETEST CONTENT AREA SCORE | |
|---|---|---|---|
| **I. CLINICAL DATA** | | | |
| A. Review patient records; recommend diagnostic procedures. | 17,24,28,67,71,83,99 | $\frac{}{7} \times 100 = \_\_\_\_\%$ | |
| B. Collect and evaluate additional clinical information. | 1,34,74,75,85,88 | $\frac{}{6} \times 100 = \_\_\_\_\%$ | $\frac{}{17} \times 100 = \_\_\_\_\%$ |
| C. Perform procedures, interpret results, and assist in care plan. | 20,50,61,84 | $\frac{}{4} \times 100 = \_\_\_\_\%$ | |
| **II. EQUIPMENT** | | | |
| A. Select, obtain, and assure cleanliness. | 21,36,40,56,66 | $\frac{}{5} \times 100 = \_\_\_\_\%$ | $\frac{}{20} \times 100 = \_\_\_\_\%$ |
| B. Assemble, check for proper function, identify and/or correct malfunctions, and perform quality control. | 4,8,14,15,19,26,27,32,46, 52,64,70,77,92,97 | $\frac{}{15} \times 100 = \_\_\_\_\%$ | |
| **III. THERAPEUTIC PROCEDURES** | | | |
| A. Evaluate, monitor, and record patient's response. | 2,5,6,10,11,12,31,33,37, 41,44,48,49,53,60,65,68, 72,78,82,87,94,96 | $\frac{}{23} \times 100 = \_\_\_\_\%$ | |
| B. Maintain airway, remove secretions, and assure ventilation and tissue oxygenation. | 16,18,25,39,42,43,45,51, 57,58,63,69,73,89,100 | $\frac{}{15} \times 100 = \_\_\_\_\%$ | |
| C. Modify therapy/make recommendations based on patient's response. | 3,13,29,38,55,76,80, 81,98 | $\frac{}{9} \times 100 = \_\_\_\_\%$ | $\frac{}{63} \times 100 = \_\_\_\_\%$ |
| D. Perform emergency procedures. | 9,22,47,59,90,95 | $\frac{}{6} \times 100 = \_\_\_\_\%$ | |
| E. Assist physician and conduct pulmonary rehabilitation/home care. | 7,23,30,35,54,62,79,86, 91,93 | $\frac{}{10} \times 100 = \_\_\_\_\%$ | |

# NBRC Written Registry Examination for Advanced Respiratory Therapists (RRTs) Content Outline

*This content outline is reprinted with permission of the copyright holder, the National Board For Respiratory Care, Inc., 8310 Nieman Rd, Lenexa, KS 66214. All rights reserved. Effective December 1999.*

## I. Select, Review, Obtain, and Interpret Data

**SETTING:** In any patient care setting, the advanced respiratory care therapist reviews existing clinical data and collects or recommends obtaining additional pertinent clinical data. The therapist evaluates all data to determine the appropriateness of the prescribed respiratory care plan, and participates in the development of the respiratory care plan.

| | RECALL | APPLICATION | ANALYSIS |
|---|---|---|---|
| I. Select, Review, Obtain, and Interpret Data | 3 | 3 | 11 |
| A. Review patient records and recommend diagnostic procedures. | 1* | 1 | 3 |
| 1. Review existing data in patient's record: | | | |
| a. patient history [e.g., present illness, admission notes, respiratory care orders, progress notes] | X** | | |
| b. physical examination [e.g., vital signs, physical findings] | X | | |
| c. lab data [e.g., CBC, chemistries/electrolytes, coagulation studies, Gram stain, culture and sensitivities, urinalysis] | X | X | |
| d. pulmonary function and blood gas results | X | X | |
| e. radiological studies [e.g., X-rays of chest/upper airway, CT, MRI] | X | X | |
| f. monitoring data | | | |
|   (1) fluid balance (intake and output) | | | |
|   (2) pulmonary mechanics [e.g., maximum inspiratory pressure (MIP), vital capacity] | X | X | |
|   (3) respiratory monitoring [e.g., rate, tidal volume, minute volume, I:E, inspiratory and expiratory pressures; flow, volume and pressure waveforms] | X | X | |
|   (4) lung compliance, airway resistance, work of breathing | X | X | |

| | RECALL | APPLICATION | ANALYSIS |
|---|---|---|---|
|   (5) noninvasive monitoring [e.g., capnography, pulse oximetry, transcutaneous $O_2/CO_2$] | | X | X |
| g. results of cardivascular monitoring | | | |
|   (1) ECG, blood pressure, heart rate | | X | X |
|   (2) hemodynamic monitoring [e.g., central venous pressure, cardiac output, pulmonary capillary wedge pressure, pulmonary artery pressures, mixed venous $O_2$, $C(a-\bar{v})O_2$, shunt studies $(\dot{Q}s/\dot{Q}t)$] | | X | X |
| h. maternal and perinatal/neonatal history and data [e.g., Apgar scores, gestational age, L/S ration, pre/post-ductal oxygenation studies] | | X | |
| i. other diagnostic studies [e.g., EEG, intracranial pressure monitoring, metabolic studies ($\dot{V}O_2$, $\dot{V}CO_2$, nutritional assessment), ventilation/perfusion scan, pulmonary angiography, sleep studies, other ultrasonography] | | | |
| 2. Recommend the following procedures to obtain additional data: | | | |
| a. CBC, electrolytes, other blood chemistries | | | |
| b. X-ray of chest and upper airway, CT scan, bronchoscopy, ventilation/perfusion lung scan, barium swallow | | X | X |
| c. Gram stain, culture and sensitivities | | X | X |
| d. Spirometry before and/or after bronchodilator, maximum voluntary ventilation, diffusing capacity, functional residual capacity, flow-volume loops, body plethysmography, nitrogen washout distribution test, total lung capacity, $CO_2$ response curve, closing volume, airway resistance, bronchoprovocation, maximum inspiratory pressure (MIP), maximum expiratory pressure (MEP) | | X | X |
| e. blood gas analysis, insertion of arterial, umbilical and/or central venous, pulmonary artery monitoring lines | | X | X |
| f. lung compliance, airway resistance, lung mechanics, work of breathing | | X | X |

*The number in each column is the number of items in that content area and cognitive level contained in each examination. For example, in category I.A., one item will be asked at the recall level, one item at the application level, and three items at the analysis level. The items could be asked relative to any tasks listed (1–2) under category I.A.

**Note: An "X" denotes the examination does NOT contain items for the given task at the cognitive level indicated in the respective column (Recall, Application, Analysis).

| | RECALL | APPLICATION | ANALYSIS |
|---|---|---|---|
| g. ECG, echocardiography, pulse oximetry, transcutaneous $O_2/CO_2$ monitoring | X | X | |
| h. $V_D/V_T$, Qs/Qt, cardiac output, cardiopulmonary stress testing | | | |
| **B. Collect and evaluate clinical information.** | **1** | **1** | **5** |
| 1. Assess patient's overall cardiopulmonary status by *inspection* to determine: | | | |
| a. general appearance, muscle wasting, venous distention, peripheral edema, diaphoresis, digital clubbing, cyanosis, capillary refill | X | X | |
| b. chest configuration, evidence of diaphragmatic movement, breathing pattern, accesory muscle activity, asymmetrical chest movement, intercostal and/or sternal retractions, nasal flaring, character of cough, amount and character of sputum | X | X | |
| c. transillumination of chest, Apgar score, gestational age | X | X | |
| 2. Assess patient's overall cardiopulmonary status by *palpation* to determine: | | | |
| a. heart rate, rhythm, force | X | X | |
| b. asymmetrical chest movements, tactile fremitus, crepitus, tenderness, secretions in the airway, tracheal deviation, endotracheal tube placement | X | X | |
| 3. Assess patient's overall cardiopulmonary status by *percussion* to determine diaphragmatic excursion and areas of altered resonance | X | X | |
| 4. Assess patient's overall cardiopulmonary status by *auscultation* to determine presence of: | | | |
| a. breath sounds [e.g., normal, bilateral, increased, decreased, absent, unequal, rhonchi or crackles (râles), wheezing, stridor, friction rub] | X | X | |
| b. heart sounds, dysrhythmias, murmurs, bruits | X | X | |
| c. blood pressure | X | X | |
| 5. Assess patient's learning needs [e.g., age and language appropriateness, education level, prior disease and medication knowledge] | X | X | |
| 6. Interview patient to determine: | | | |
| a. level of consciousness, orientation to time, place and person, emotional state, ability to cooperate | X | X | |
| b. presence of dyspnea and/or orthopnea, work of breathing, sputum | | | |

| | RECALL | APPLICATION | ANALYSIS |
|---|---|---|---|
| production, exercise tolerance and activities of daily living | X | X | |
| c. physical environment, social support systems, nutritional status | X | X | |
| 7. Review chest X-ray to determine: | | | |
| a. presence of, or changes in, pneumothorax or subcutaneous emphysema, other extra-pulmonary air, consolidation and/or atelectasis, pulmonary infiltrates | X | X | |
| b. presence and postion of foreign bodies | X | X | |
| c. position of endotracheal or tracheostomy tube, evidence of endotracheal or tracheostomy tube cuff hyperinflation | X | X | |
| d. position of chest tube(s), nasogastric and/or feeding tube, pulmonary artery catheter (Swan-Ganz), pacemaker, CVP, and other catheters | X | | |
| e. position of, or changes in, hemidiaphragms, hyperinflation, pleural fluid, pulmonary edema, mediastinal shift, patency and size of major airways | X | X | |
| 8. Review lateral neck X-ray to determine: | | | |
| a. presence of epiglottitis and subglottic edema | X | X | |
| b. presence or position of foreign bodies | X | X | |
| c. airway narrowing | X | X | |
| 9. Perform bedside procedures to determine: | | | |
| a. ECG, pulse oximetry, transcutaneous $O_2/CO_2$ monitoring, capnography, mass spectrometry | X | X | |
| b. tidal volume, minute volume, I:E | X | X | |
| c. blood gas analysis, P(A-a)$O_2$, alveolar ventilation, $V_D/V_T$, Qs/Qt, mixed venous sampling | X | X | |
| d. peak flow, maximum inspiratory pressure, maximum expiratory pressure, forced vital capacity, timed forced expiratory volumes [e.g., $FEV_1$], lung compliance, lung mechanics | X | X | |
| e. cardiac output, pulmonary capillary wedge pressure, central venous pressure, pulmonary artery pressures, fluid balance (intake and output) | | | |
| f. pulmonary vascular resistance and systemic vascular resistance | | | |
| g. apnea monitoring, sleep studies, respiratory impedance plethysmography | X | X | |
| h. tracheal tube cuff pressure, volume | X | X | |

| | RECALL | APPLICATION | ANALYSIS |
|---|:---:|:---:|:---:|
| 10. Interpret results of bedside procedures to determine: | | | |
|   a. ECG, pulse oximetry, transcutaneous $O_2/CO_2$ monitoring, capnography, mass spectrometry | X | X | |
|   b. tidal volume, minute volume, I:E | X | X | |
|   c. blood gas analysis, P(A-a)$O_2$, alveolar ventilation, $V_D/V_T$, Qs/Qt, mixed venous sampling | X | X | |
|   d. peak flow, maximum inspiratory pressure, maximum expiratory pressure, forced vital capacity, timed forced expiratory volumes [e.g., $FEV_1$], lung compliance, lung mechanics | X | X | |
|   e. cardiac output, pulmonary capillary wedge pressure, central venous pressure, pulmonary artery pressures, fluid balance (intake and output) | | | |
|   f. pulmonary vascular resistance and systematic vascular resistance | | | |
|   g. apnea monitoring, sleep studies, respiratory impedance plethysmography | X | X | |
|   h. tracheal tube cuff pressure, volume | X | X | |
| **C. Perform procedures and interpret results, determine appropriateness of and participate in developing and recommending modifications to respiratory care plan.** | **1** | **1** | **3** |
|   1. Perform and/or measure the following: | | | |
|     a. spirometry before and/or after bronchodilator, maximum voluntary ventilation, diffusing capacity, functional residual capacity, flow-volume loops, body plethysmography, nitrogen washout distribution test, total lung capacity, $CO_2$ response curve, closing volume, airway resistance | X | X | |
|     b. ECG, pulse oximetry, transcutaneous $O_2/CO_2$ monitoring | X | X | |
|     c. $V_D/V_T$, Qs/Qt, mixed venous sampling, C(a-$\bar{v}$)$O_2$, cardiac output, pulmonary capillary wedge pressure, central venous pressure, pulmonary artery pressures, cardiopulmonary stress testing | | | |
|     d. fluid balance (intake and output) | | | |

| | RECALL | APPLICATION | ANALYSIS |
|---|:---:|:---:|:---:|
|     e. arterial sampling and blood gas analysis, co-oximetry, P(A-a)$O_2$ | X | X | |
|     f. sleep studies, metabolic studies [e.g., indirect calorimetry] | | | |
|     g. ventilator flow, volume, and pressure waveforms, lung compliance | X | X | |
|   2. Interpret results of the following: | | | |
|     a. spirometry before aad/or after bronchodilator, maximum voluntary ventilation, diffusing capacity, functional residual capacity, flow-volume loops, body plethysmography, nitrogen washout distribution test, total lung capacity, $CO_2$ response curve, closing volume, airway resistance, bronchoprovocation | X | X | |
|     b. ECG, pulse oximetry, transcutaneous $O_2/CO_2$ monitoring | X | X | |
|     c. $V_D/V_T$, Qs/Qt, mixed venous sampling, C(a-$\bar{v}$)$O_2$, cardiac output, pulmonary capillary wedge pressure, central venous pressure, pulmonary artery pressures, cardiopulmonary stress testing | | | |
|     d. fluid balance (intake and output) | | | |
|     e. arterial sampling and blood gas analysis, co-oximetry, P(A-a)$O_2$ | X | X | |
|     f. peripheral venipuncture or insertion of intravenous line | | | |
|     g. sleep studies, metabolic studies [e.g., indirect calorimetry] | | | |
|     h. insertion of arterial and umbilical monitoring lines | | | |
|     i. ventilator flow, volume, and pressure waveforms, lung compliance | X | X | |
|   3. Determine the appropriateness of the prescribed respiratory care plan and recommend modifications where indicated: | | | |
|     a. perform respiratory care quality assurance | X | X | |
|     b. develop quality improvement program | X | X | |
|     c. review interdisciplinary patient and family care plan | X | X | |
|   4. Participate in development of respiratory care plan [e.g., case management, develop and apply protocols, disease management education] | X | X | |

| | RECALL | APPLICATION | ANALYSIS |
|---|---|---|---|
| **II. Select, Assemble, and Check Equipment for Proper Function, Operation, and Cleanliness** | | | |
| **SETTING:** In any patient care setting, the advanced respiratory therapist selects, assembles, and assures cleanliness of all equipment used in providing respiratory care. The therapist checks all equipment and corrects malfunctions. | 3 | 4 | 13 |
| **A. Select and obtain equipment and assure equipment cleanliness.** | 1 | 2 | 5 |
| 1. Select and obtain equipment appropriate to the respiratory care plan: | | | |
| a. oxygen administration devices | | | |
| (1) nasal cannula, mask, reservior mask (partial rebreathing, nonrebreathing), face tents, transtracheal oxygen catheter, oxygen conserving cannulas | X | X | |
| (2) air-entrainment devices, tracheostomy collar and T-piece, oxygen hoods and tents | X | X | |
| (3) CPAP devices | X | X | |
| b. humidifiers [e.g., bubble, passover, cascade, wick, heat moisture exchanger] | X | X | |
| c. aerosol generators [e.g., pneumatic nebulizer, ultrasonic nebulizer] | X | X | |
| d. resuscitation devices [e.g, manual resuscitator (bag-valve), pneumatic (demand-valve), mouth-to-valve mask resuscitator] | X | X | |
| e. ventilators | | | |
| (1) pneumatic, electric, microprocessor, fluidic | X | X | |
| (2) high frequency | | | |
| (3) noninvasive positive pressure | X | X | |
| f. artificial airways | | | |
| (1) oro- and nasopharyngeal airways | X | X | |
| (2) oral, nasal and double-lumen endotracheal tubes | X | X | |
| (3) tracheostomy tubes and buttons | X | X | |

| | RECALL | APPLICATION | ANALYSIS |
|---|---|---|---|
| (4) intubation equipment [e.g., laryngoscope and blades, exhaled $CO_2$ detection devices] | X | X | |
| (5) other airways [e.g., laryngeal mask airway (LMA), Esophageal Tracheal Combitube® (ETC)] | | | |
| g. suctioning devices [e.g., suction catheters, specimen collectors, oropharyngeal suction devices] | X | X | |
| h. gas delivery, metering and clinical analyzing devices | | | |
| (1) regulators, redcing valves, connectors and flowmeters, air/oxygen blenders, pulse-dose systems | X | X | |
| (2) oxygen concentrators, air compressors, liquid oxygen systems | X | X | |
| (3) gas cylinders, bulk systems and manifolds | X | X | |
| (4) capnograph, blood gas analyzer and sampling devices, co-oximeter, transcutaneous $O_2$/$CO_2$ monitor, pulse oximeter | X | X | |
| (5) CO, He, $O_2$ and specialty gas analyzers | X | X | |
| i. patient breathing circuits | | | |
| (1) IPPB, continuous mechanical ventilation | X | X | |
| (2) CPAP, PEEP valve assembly | X | X | |
| (3) H-valve assembly | | | X |
| j. environmental devices | | | |
| (1) incubators, radiant warmers | | | |
| (2) aerosol (mist) tents | X | X | |
| (3) scavenging systems | | X | X |
| k. positive expiratory pressure device (PEP) | | | |
| l. Flutter® mucous clearance device | | | X |
| m. other therapeutic gases [e.g., $O_2$/$CO_2$, He/$O_2$] | | | |
| n. manometers and gauges | | | |
| (1) manometers—water, mercury and aneroid, inspiratory/expiratory pressure meters, cuff pressure manometers | X | X | |
| (2) pressure transducers | X | X | |
| o. respirometers [e.g., flow-sensing devices (pneumotachometer), volume displacement] | X | X | |

| | RECALL | APPLICATION | ANALYSIS |
|---|---|---|---|
| p. electrocardiography devices [e.g., ECG oscilloscope monitors, ECG machines (12-lead), Holter monitors] | X | X | |
| q. hemodynamic monitoring devices | | | |
|   (1) central venous catheters, pulmonary artery catheters [e.g., Swan-Ganz], cardiac output, continuous S$\overline{v}$O$_2$ monitors | | | |
|   (2) arterial catheters | | | |
| r. vacuum systems [e.g., pumps, regulators, collection bottles, pleural drainage devices] | X | X | |
| s. metered dose inhalers (MDI), MDI spacers | X | X | |
| t. Small Particle Aerosol Generators (SPAG) | X | X | |
| u. bronchoscopes | X | X | |
| 2. Assure selected equipment cleanliness [e.g., select or determine appropriate agent and technique for disinfection and/or sterilization, perform procedures for disinfection and/or sterilization, monitor effectiveness of sterilization procedures] | X | X | |
| **B. Assemble and check equipment function, identify and correct equipment malfunctions, and perform quality control.** | **2** | **2** | **8** |
| 1. Assemble, check for proper function, and identify malfunctions of equipment: | | | |
| a. oxygen administration devices | | | |
|   (1) nasal cannula, mask, reservoir mask (partial rebreathing, nonrebreathing), face tents, transtracheal oxygen catheter, oxygen conserving cannulas | X | X | |
|   (2) air-entrainment devices, tracheostomy collar and T-piece, oxygen hoods and tents | X | X | |
|   (3) CPAP devices | X | X | |
| b. humidifiers [e.g., bubble, passover, cascade, wick, heat moisture exchanger] | X | X | |
| c. aerosol generators [e.g., pneumatic nebulizer, ultrasonic nebulizer] | X | X | |
| d. resuscitation devices [e.g., manual resuscitator (bag-valve), pneumatic (demand-valve), mouth-to-valve mask resuscitator] | X | X | |
| e. ventilators | | | |
|   (1) pneumatic, electric, microprocessor, fluidic | X | X | |
|   (2) high frequency | | | |
|   (3) noninvasive positive pressure | X | X | |

| | RECALL | APPLICATION | ANALYSIS |
|---|---|---|---|
| f. artificial airways | | | |
|   (1) oro- and nasopharyngeal airways | X | X | |
|   (2) oral, nasal and double-lumen endotracheal tubes | X | X | |
|   (3) tracheostomy tubes and buttons | X | X | |
|   (4) intubation equipment [e.g., laryngoscope and blades, exhaled CO$_2$ detection devices] | X | X | |
| g. suctioning devices [e.g., suction catheters, speciment collectors, oropharyngeal suction devices] | X | X | |
| h. gas delivery, metering and clinical analyzing devices | | | |
|   (1) regulators, reducing valves, connectors and flowmeters, air/oxygen blenders, pulse-dose systems | X | X | |
|   (2) oxygen concentrators, air compressors, liquid oxygen systems | X | X | |
|   (3) gas cylinders, bulk, systems and manifolds | X | X | |
|   (4) capnograph, blood gas analyzer and sampling devices, co-oximeter, transcutaneous O$_2$/CO$_2$ monitor, pulse oximeter | X | X | |
|   (5) CO, He, O$_2$ and specialty gas analyzers | X | X | |
| i. patient breathing circuits | | | |
|   (1) IPPB, continuous mechanical ventilation | X | X | |
|   (2) CPAP, PEEP valve assembly | X | X | |
|   (3) H-valve assembly | | X | X |
| j. environmental devices | | | |
|   (1) incubators, radiant warmers | | | |
|   (2) aerosol (mist) tents | X | X | |
| k. positive expiratory pressure (PEP) device | | | |
| l. Flutter® mucous clearance device | | | X |
| m. other therapeutic gases [e.g., O$_2$/CO$_2$, He/O$_2$] | | | |
| n. manometers and gauges | | | |
|   (1) manometers—water, mercury and aneroid, inspiratory/expiratory pressure meters, cuff pressure manometers | X | X | |
|   (2) pressure transducers | | | |
| o. respirometers [e.g., flow-sensing devices (pneumotachometer), volume displacement] | X | X | |
| p. electrocardiography devices [e.g., ECG oscilloscope monitors, ECG machines (12-lead), Holter monitors] | X | X | |

| | RECALL | APPLICATION | ANALYSIS |
|---|---|---|---|
| q. hemodynamic monitoring devices | | | |
| (1) central venous catheters, pulmonary artery catheters [e.g., Swan-Ganz], cardiac output, continuous $s\bar{v}O_2$ monitors | | | |
| (2) arterial catheters | | | |
| r. vacuum systems [e.g., pumps, regulators, collection bottles, pleural drainage devices] | X | X | |
| s. bronchoscopes | | | X |
| 2. Take action to correct malfunctions of equipment: | | | |
| a. oxygen administration devices | | | |
| (1) nasal cannula, mask, reservoir mask (partial rebreathing, nonrebreathing), face tents, transtracheal oxygen catheter, oxygen conserving cannulas | X | X | |
| (2) air-entrainment devices, tracheostomy collar and T-piece, oxygen hoods and tents | X | X | |
| (3) CPAP devices | X | X | |
| b. humidifiers [e.g., bubble, passover, cascade, wick, heat moisture exchanger] | X | X | |
| c. aerosol generators [e.g., pneumatic nebulizer, ultrasonic nebulizer] | X | X | |
| d. resuscitation devices [e.g., manual resuscitator (bag-valve), pneumatic (demand-valve), mouth-to-valve mask resuscitator] | X | X | |
| e. ventilators | | | |
| (1) pneumatic, electric, microprocessor, fluidic | X | X | |
| (2) high frequency | | | |
| (3) noninvasive positive pressure | X | X | |
| f. artificial airways | | | |
| (1) oro- and nasopharyngeal airways | X | X | |
| (2) oral, nasal and double-lumen endotracheal tubes | X | X | |
| (3) tracheostomy tubes and buttons | X | X | |
| (4) intubation equipment [e.g., laryngoscope and blades, exhaled $CO_2$ detection devices] | X | X | |
| g. suctioning devices [e.g., suction catheters, specimen collectors, oropharyngeal suction devices] | X | X | |
| h. gas delivery, metering and clinical analyzing devices | | | |
| (1) regulators, reducing valves, connectors and flowmeters, air/oxygen blenders, pulse-dose systems | X | X | |
| (2) oxygen concentrators, air compressors, liquid oxygen systems | X | X | |

| | RECALL | APPLICATION | ANALYSIS |
|---|---|---|---|
| (3) gas cylinders, bulk systems and manifolds | X | X | |
| (4) capnograph, blood gas analyzer and sampling devices, co-oximeter, transcutaneous $O_2/CO_2$ monitor, pulse oximeter | X | X | |
| (5) CO, He, $O_2$ and specialty gas analyzers | | | |
| i. patient breathing circuits | | | |
| (1) IPPB, continuous mechanical ventilation | X | X | |
| (2) CPAP, PEEP valve assembly | X | X | |
| (3) H-valve assembly | | | X |
| j. environmental devices | | | |
| (1) incubators, radiant warmers | | | X |
| (2) aerosol (mist) tents | X | X | |
| k. positive expiratory pressure (PEP) device | | | |
| l. Flutter® mucous clearance device | | | X |
| m. other therapeutic gases [e.g., $O_2/CO_2$, $He/O_2$] | | | |
| n. manometers and gauges | | | |
| (1) manometers—water, mercury and aneroid, inspiratory/expiratory pressure meters, cuff pressure manometers | X | X | |
| (2) pressure transducers | | | |
| o. respirometers [e.g., flow-sensing devices (pneumotachometer), volume displacement] | X | X | |
| p. electrocardiography devices [e.g., ECG oscilloscope monitors, ECG machines (12-lead), Holter monitors] | | | |
| q. hemodynamic monitoring devices | | | |
| (1) central venous catheters, pulmonary artery catheters [e.g., Swan-Ganz], cardiac output, continuous $S\bar{v}O_2$ monitors | | | |
| (2) arterial catheters | | | |
| r. vacuum systems [e.g., pumps, regulators, collection bottles, pleural drainage devices] | X | X | |
| s. Small Particle Aerosol Generators (SPAG) | | | X |
| t. bronchoscopes | | | X |
| 3. Perform quality control procedures for: | | | |
| a. blood gas analyzers and sampling devices, co-oximeters | X | X | |
| b. pulmonary function equipment, ventilator volume/flow/pressure calibration | X | X | |
| c. gas metering devices | X | X | |
| d. noninvasive monitors [e.g., transcutaneous] | | | |

Columns: RECALL | APPLICATION | ANALYSIS

## III. Initiate, Conduct, and Modify Prescribed Therapeutic Procedures

**SETTING:** In any patient care setting, the RRT evaluates, monitors, and records the patient's response to care. The therapist maintains patient records and communicates with other healthcare team members. The therapist initiates, conducts, and modifies prescribed therapeutic procedures to achieve the desired objectives. The therapist provides care in emergency settings, assists the physician, and conducts pulmonary rehabilitation and homecare.

| Item | RECALL | APPLICATION | ANALYSIS |
|---|---|---|---|
| III. (total) | 6 | 8 | 49 |
| A. Evaluate, monitor, and record patient's response to respiratory care. | 2 | 3 | 13 |
| 1. Evaluate and monitor patient's response to respiratory care: | | | |
| a. recommend and review chest X-ray | X | X | |
| b. perform arterial puncture, capillary blood gas sampling, and venipuncture; obtaion blood from arterial or pulmonary artery lines; perform transcutaneous $O_2/CO_2$, pulse oximetry, co-oximetry, and capnography monitoring | X | X | |
| c. observe changes in sputum production and consistency, note patient's subjective response to therapy and mechanical ventilation | X | X | |
| d. measure and record vital signs, monitor cardiac rhythm, evaluate fluid balance (intake and output) | X | X | |
| e. perform spirometry/determine vital capacity, measure lung compliance and airway resistance, interpret ventilator flow, volume, and pressure waveforms, measure peak flow | X | X | |
| f. determine and record central venous pressure, pulmonary artery pressures, pulmonary capillary wedge pressure and/or cardiac output | | | |

| Item | RECALL | APPLICATION | ANALYSIS |
|---|---|---|---|
| g. recommend measurement of electrolytes, hemoglobin, CBC and/or chemistries | | | |
| h. monitor mean airway pressure, adjust and check alarm systems, measure tidal volume, respiratory rate, airway pressures, I:E, and maximum inspiratory pressure (MIP) | X | X | |
| i. measure $F_IO_2$ and/or liter flow | X | X | |
| j. monitor endotracheal or tracheostomy tube cuff pressure | X | X | |
| k. auscultate chest and interpret changes in breath sounds | X | X | |
| l. perform hemodynamic calculations [e.g., shunt studies ($\dot{Q}s/\dot{Q}t$), cardiac output, cardiac index, pulmonary vascular resistance and systemic vascular resistance, stroke volume] | | | |
| m. interpret hemodynamic calculations: | | | |
| (1) calculate and interpret $P(A-a)O_2$, $C(a-\bar{v})O_2$, $\dot{Q}s/\dot{Q}t$ | | | |
| (2) exhaled $CO_2$ monitoring, $V_D/V_T$ | | | |
| (3) cardiac output, cardiac index, pulmonary vascular resistance and systemic vascular resistance, stroke volume | | | |
| 2. Maintain records and communication: | | | |
| a. record therapy and results using conventional terminology as required in the healthcare setting and/or by regulatory agencies by noting and interpreting: | | | |
| (1) patient's response to therapy including the effects of therapy, adverse reactions, patient's subjective and attitudinal response to therapy | X | X | |
| (2) auscultatory findings, cough and sputum production and characteristics | X | X | |
| (3) vital signs [e.g., heart rate, respiratory rate, blood pressure, body temperature] | X | X | |
| (4) pulse oximetry, heart rhythm, capnography | X | X | |
| b. verify computations and note erroneous data | X | X | |

| Content | RECALL | APPLICATION | ANALYSIS |
|---|---|---|---|
| c. apply computer technology to patient management [e.g., ventilator waveform analysis, electronic charting, patient care algorithms] |  | X | X |
| d. communicate results of therapy and alter therapy per protocol(s) |  | X | X |
| **B. Conduct therapeutic procedures to maintain a patent airway, achieve adequate ventilation and oxygenation, and remove bronchopulmonary secretions.** | 1 | 1 | 10 |
| 1. Maintain a patent airway including the care of artificial airways: |  |  |  |
| a. insert oro- and nasopharyngeal airway, select endotracheal or tracheostomy tube, perform endotracheal intubation, change tracheostomy tube, maintain proper cuff inflation, position of endotracheal or tracheostomy tube |  | X | X |
| b. maintain adequate humidification |  | X | X |
| c. extubate the patient |  | X | X |
| d. properly position patient |  | X | X |
| e. identify endotracheal tube placement by available means |  | X | X |
| 2. Achieve adequate spontaneous and artificial ventilation: |  |  |  |
| a. initiate and adjust IPPB therapy |  | X | X |
| b. initiate and select appropriate settings for high frequency ventilation |  |  |  |
| c. initiate and adjust ventilator modes (e.g., A/C, SIMV, pressure support ventilation (PSV), pressure control ventilation (PCV)) |  | X | X |
| d. initiate and adjust independent (differential) lung ventilation |  |  |  |
| 3. Remove bronchopulmonary secretions by instructing and encouraging bronchopulmonary hygiene techniques (e.g., coughing techniques, autogenic drainage, positive expiratory pressure device (PEP), intrapulmonary percussive ventilation (IPV), Flutter®, High Frequency Chest Wall Oscillation (HFCWO)) |  | X | X |
| 4. Achieve adequate arterial and tissue oxygenation: |  |  |  |
| a. initiate and adjust CPAP, PEEP, and noninvasive positive pressure |  | X | X |
| b. initiate and adjust combinations of ventilatory techniques [e.g., SIMV, PEEP, PS, PCV] |  | X | X |

| Content | RECALL | APPLICATION | ANALYSIS |
|---|---|---|---|
| c. position patient to minimize hypoxemia, administer oxygen (on or off ventilator), prevent procedure-associated hypoxemia [e.g., oxygenate before and after suctioning and equipment changes] |  | X | X |
| **C. Make necessary modifications in therapeutic procedures based on patient response.** | 0 | 1 | 10 |
| 1. Modify IPPB: |  |  |  |
| a. adjust sensitivity, flow, volume, pressure, $F_IO_2$ |  | X | X |
| b. adjust expiratory retard |  | X | X |
| c. change patient—machine interface [e.g., mouthpiece, mask] |  | X | X |
| 2. Modify patient breathing pattern during aerosol therapy |  | X | X |
| 3. Modify oxygen therapy: |  |  |  |
| a. change mode of administration, adjust flow, and $F_IO_2$ |  | X | X |
| b. set up an $O_2$ concentrator or liquid $O_2$ system |  | X | X |
| 4. Modify specialty gas [e.g., $He/O_2$, $O_2/CO_2$] therapy [e.g., change mode of administration, adjust flow, adjust gas concentration] |  | X |  |
| 5. Modify bronchial hygiene therapy [e.g., alter position of patient, alter duration of treatment and techniques, coordinate sequence of therapies, alter equipment used and PEP therapy] |  | X | X |
| 6. Modify artificial airway management: |  |  |  |
| a. alter endotracheal or tracheostomy tube position, change endotracheal or tracheostomy tube |  | X | X |
| b. initiate suctioning |  | X | X |
| c. inflate and deflate the cuff |  | X | X |
| 7. Modify suctioning: |  |  |  |
| a. alter frequency and duration of suctioning |  | X | X |
| b. change size and type of catheter |  | X | X |
| c. alter negative pressure |  | X | X |
| d. instill irrigating solutions |  | X | X |
| 8. Modify mechanical ventilation: |  |  |  |
| a. change patient breathing circuitry, change type of ventilator |  | X | X |
| b. measure volume loss through chest tube(s) |  | X |  |
| c. change mechanical dead space |  | X | X |

| | RECALL | APPLICATION | ANALYSIS |
|---|---|---|---|
| **D. Initiate, conduct, or modify respiratory care techniques in an emergency setting.** | **1** | **1** | **10** |
| 1. Treat cardiopulmonary collapse according to: | | | |
|    a. BCLS | X | X | |
|    b. ACLS | X | X | |
|    c. PALS | X | X | |
|    d. NRP | X | X | |
| 2. Treat tension pneumothorax | | | |
| 3. Participate in land/air patient transport | | | |
| **E. Assist physician, initiate, and conduct pulmonary rehabilitation.** | **2** | **2** | **6** |
| 1. Act as an assistant to the physician performing special procedures including: | | | |
|    a. bronchoscopy | X | X | |
|    b. thoracentesis | X | X | |
|    c. transtracheal aspiration | | | |
|    d. tracheostomy | X | X | |
|    e. cardiopulmonary stress testing | | | |
|    f. percutaneous needle biopsies of the lung | | | |
|    g. sleep studies | | | |
|    h. cardioversion | X | X | |
|    i. intubation | X | X | |
|    j. insertion of chest tubes | | | |
|    k. insertion of lines for invasive monitoring [e.g., central venous pressure, pulmonary artery catheters, Swan-Ganz, arterial lines] | | | |
|    l. conscious sedation | | | |
| 2. Initiate and conuct pulmonary rehabilitation and home care within the prescription: | | | |
|    a. monitor and maintain home respiratory care equipment, maintain apnea monitors | | | |
|    b. explain planned therapy and goals to patient in understandable terms to achieve optimal therapeutic outcome, counsel patient and family concerning smoking cessation, disease management | X | X | |
|    c. assure safety and infection control | X | X | |
|    d. modify respiratory care procedures for use in the home | X | X | |
|    e. implement and monitor graded exercise program | | | |
|    f. conduct patient education and disease management programs | X | X | |
| **TOTALS** | **12** | **15** | **73** |

# Pretest Answers and Analyses

**NOTE:** The references listed after each analysis are numbered and keyed to the reference list located at the end of this section. The first number indicates the text. The second number indicates the page where you can find information about the questions. For example, (1:114, 187) means that on pages 114 and 187 of reference 1, information about the question will be found. Frequently, it will be necessary to read beyond the page number indicated to obtain complete information. Therefore, reference to the question will be found either on the page indicated or on subsequent pages.

**IB3**

1. C. Percussion over the chest wall produces four general percussion notes: (1) resonant (normal lungs), (2) hyperresonant (pneumothorax and emphysema), (3) dull (pleural effusion, consolidation, hemothorax, and atelectasis), and (4) flat (extensive atelectasis).

   Percussion is one component of the physical assessment of the chest. The others are inspection, palpation, and auscultation.

   (1:310)(9:79–80).

**IIIAIm(I)**

2. B. A simple calculation to use is the classic shunt equation. This equation also enables easier understanding and comprehension of the shunt concept.

   Mathematically, it is shown as

   $$\frac{\dot{Q}_S}{\dot{Q}_T} = \frac{C\dot{c}O_2 - CaO_2}{C\dot{c}O_2 - C\bar{v}O_2}$$

$\dot{Q}_s$ = shunted cardiac output (C.O.) (L/min.)

$\dot{Q}_T$ = total C.O. (L/min.)

$C\dot{c}O_2$ = end-pulmonary capillary oxygen content (vol%)

$CaO_2$ = total arterial oxygen content (vol%)

$C\bar{v}O_2$ = total venous oxygen content (vol%)

Figure 2-12 illustrates the relationship among the factors present in the classic shunt equation.

From the diagram, one should see that $\dot{Q}_T$ (total C.O.) is the sum of $\dot{Q}_S$ (shunted output) and $\dot{Q}_C$ (capillary output). Hence,

$$\dot{Q}_T = \dot{Q}_S + \dot{Q}_C$$

STEP 1: Calculate the $PAO_2$ (alveolar oxygen tension) that represents the end-pulmonary capillary oxygen tension ($P\dot{c}O_2$) in mm Hg or torr. The alveolar air equation is needed for this calculation. A normal respiratory quotient is assumed, therefore R equals 0.8. A normal body temperature (37°C)

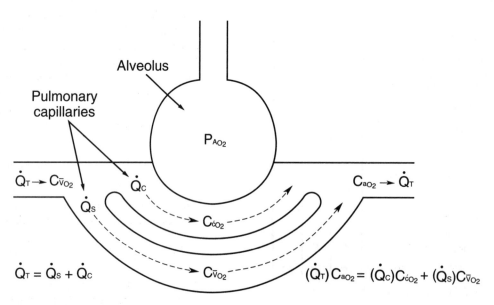

**Figure 2-12:** Total ($Q_T$), capillary ($Q_C$), and shunted ($Q_S$) cardiac output.

$$PAO_2 = FIO_2(P_B - P_{H_2O}) - PACO_2\left(FIO_2 + \frac{1 - FIO_2}{R}\right)$$

is also assumed, consequently, the $P_{H_2O}$ equals 47 torr. The assumed normal barometric pressure is 760 torr.

$$PAO_2 = 1.0(760 \text{ torr} - 47 \text{ torr}) - 35 \text{ torr*}\left(1.0 + \frac{1 - 1.0}{0.8}\right)^{**}$$

$$= 713 \text{ torr} - 35 \text{ torr}$$

$$= 678 \text{ torr}$$

*The $Pa\overline{C}O_2$ can substitute for the $PACO_2$.

**When the $FIO_2$ is 1.0, the factor $\left(FIO_2 + \dfrac{1 - FIO_2}{R}\right)$ will always equal 1.

Assuming complete equilibration across the alveolar-capillary membrane, the end-pulmonary capillary oxygen tension will be 678 torr.

STEP 2: Calculate the $Cc'O_2$.

$$Cc'O_2 = \text{combined } O_2 + \text{dissolved } O_2$$

$$= (19 \text{ g\%} \times 1.34 \text{ ml } O_2/\text{g Hb} \times 1.0)$$
$$+ (678 \text{ torr} \times 0.003 \text{ vol\%/torr})$$

$$= 25.46 \text{ vol\%} + 2.03 \text{ vol\%}$$

$$= 27.49 \text{ vol\%}$$

STEP 3: Calculate the $CaO_2$.

$$CaO_2 = \text{combined } O_2 + \text{dissolved } O_2$$

$$= (19 \text{ g\%} \times 1.34 \text{ ml } O_2/\text{g Hb} \times 1.0)$$
$$+ (555 \text{ torr} \times 0.003 \text{ vol\%/torr})$$

$$= 25.46 \text{ vol\%} + 1.67 \text{ vol\%}$$

$$= 27.13 \text{ vol\%}$$

STEP 4: Calculate the $C\overline{v}O_2$.

$$C\overline{v}O_2 = \text{combined } O_2 + \text{dissolved } O_2$$

$$= (19 \text{ g\%} \times 1.34 \text{ ml } O_2/\text{g Hb} \times 0.65)$$
$$+ (38 \text{ torr} \times 0.003 \text{ vol\%/torr})$$

$$= 16.55 \text{ vol\%} + 0.11 \text{ vol\%}$$

$$= 16.66 \text{ vol\%}$$

STEP 5: Calculate the $\dot{Q}_S/\dot{Q}_T$.

$$\frac{\dot{Q}_S}{\dot{Q}_T} = \frac{Cc'O_2 - CaO_2}{Cc'O_2 - C\overline{v}O_2}$$

$$\frac{\dot{Q}_S}{\dot{Q}_T} = \frac{27.49 \text{ vol\%} - 27.13 \text{ vol\%}}{27.49 \text{ vol\%} - 16.66 \text{ vol\%}}$$

$$= \frac{0.36 \text{ vol\%}}{10.83 \text{ vol\%}}$$

$$= 0.33 \text{ or}$$
$$0.33 \times 100 = 3.3\%$$

(1:929–930), (10:272), (17:46–51).

**IIIC5**

3. D. This patient did not respond favorably to postural drainage and directed cough for the removal of tracheobronchial secretions. Therefore, right middle lobe atelectasis remains. Having the patient cough more vigorously would not be appropriate because the directed cough technique employs a rather forceful cough. Perhaps the forced expiratory technique (FET) or huffing would be useful (they are also called active cycle of breathing and autogenic drainage).

Incentive spirometry is not intended to remove tracheobronchial secretions. It is useful, however, for reversing or preventing atelectasis.

In this case, using aerosol or high humidity therapy with PEP might be more effective.

(1:794, 803, 805, 807).

**IIB2h(I)**

4. C. When an 80% helium–20% oxygen gas mixture is being administered by an oxygen flow meter, the liter flow rate needs to be calculated because the helium–oxygen mixture is less dense than oxygen by itself. Therefore, the flow meter will indicate a reading lower than the actual flow rate. To determine the flow rate of an 80% helium–20% oxygen mixture being delivered by an oxygen flow meter, the following calculation must be performed

$$\left(\begin{array}{c}\text{conversion}\\\text{factor}\end{array}\right)\left(\begin{array}{c}\text{oxygen flow}\\\text{meter setting}\end{array}\right) = \text{80-20 He-O}_2 \text{ flow rate}$$

Because the conversion factor of this gas mixture is 1.8, the calculation becomes the following:

$$(1.8)(10 \text{ L/min.}) = 18 \text{ L/min.}$$

Therefore, setting the oxygen flow meter at 10 L/min. will deliver approximately 18 L/min. of an 80–20 heliox gas mixture.

On the other hand, if the RRT were asked to determine the appropriate flow rate setting for an oxygen flow meter being used to administer an 80-20 helium–oxygen gas mixture, the formula must be rearranged as follows:

$$\frac{\left(\begin{array}{c}\text{prescribed 80-20}\\\text{He-O}_2\text{ flow rate}\end{array}\right)}{\text{conversion factor}} = \text{flow rate setting on O}_2\text{ flow meter}$$

For example, if the order stated that 18 L/min. of an 80–20 helium–oxygen gas mixture were to be the source of the gas flow rate, the flow rate setting on an oxygen flow meter would be determined in the following manner:

$$\frac{18\text{ L/min.}}{1.8} = 10\text{ L/min.}$$

The conversion factors for other heliox gas mixtures are 1.6 and 1.4 for 70% helium–30% oxygen and 60% helium–40% oxygen, respectively.

(1:768–769), (13:59–60).

## IIAIg

5. D. Serum or extracellular potassium ($K^+$) normally is within the range of 3.5 to 5.0 mEq/liter. The vast majority of the body's potassium (142 mEq/liter) resides in the intracellular compartment. When the extracellular $K^+$ level begins to diminish, $K^+$ from the intracellular environment makes up the deficit. In other words, $K^+$ ions migrate from the cells and enter the plasma.

This $K^+$ redistribution process causes the serum $K^+$ level to be regarded with caution, however, because a normal extracellular $K^+$ concentration can mask a depleting intracellular $K^+$ level. Whenever the extracellular $K^+$ concentration is low, the clinician should suspect a depletion of the intracellular $K^+$ level.

Another aspect that clouds the interpretation of the $K^+$ concentration is that $K^+$ enters the intracellular space during acidemia and leaves the intracellular environment during alkalemia. Again, in some conditions, a low-serum $K^+$ concentration might only mean that $K^+$ has diffused into the cells and has not been lost from the body.

Maintaining normal intracellular and extracellular levels of $K^+$ are important because $K^+$ and $H^+$ are involved with $Na^+$ reabsorption in the kidneys. Ordinarily, there is a balance between the exchange of $K^+$ and $H^+$ for reabsorbed $Na^+$. If $K^+$ levels are low, more $H^+$ will be secreted from the renal tubules as $Na^+$ contin-

ues to be reabsorbed. Low levels of $K^+$ can eventually lead to an excessive loss of $H^+$, thereby producing the acid-base imbalance termed *hypokalemic metabolic alkalosis*.

A variety of diuretics is associated with an excessive loss of $K^+$. These diuretics require that the patient receive $K^+$ supplementation to prevent an iatrogenically induced hypokalemic metabolic alkalosis.

(1:253, 254, 334), (4:230, 254, 274).

## IIIA1a

6. C. The RRT should recommend a portable anteroposterior (AP) chest radiograph following the completion of the procedures listed below.

1) nasotracheal or orotracheal intubation
   - Verification of the location of the distal tip of the endotracheal tube in relation to the carina is essential for adequate ventilation of the patient.
2) pulmonary artery catheter (PAC) insertion
   - Verification of the location of the distal tip of the PAC in relation to the pulmonary circulation is essential for the procurement of reliable and valid hemodynamic data.
3) bronchoscopy
   - Radiographic evaluation of the procedure is necessary to assist with determining the effects of the procedure on the patient.
4) nasogastric feeding tube insertion
   - Radiographic assessment is essential to verify the tube's location in the stomach and small intestine.
5) chest tube insertion
   - Verification of the position and function of chest tubes is required for the evacuation of fluid and/or air from the intrapleural space.
6) central venous pressure (CVP) line insertion
   - Evaluation of the position of the tip of the CVP catheter is necessary for the same reasons for the PAC.
7) thoracentesis
   - The effect of the procedure on the patient's lung function and status must be evaluated with a portable AP chest x-ray.

Performing a portable AP chest x-ray on a patient who has had the inner cannula of a fenestrated tracheostomy tube removed and the decannulation cannula of the tube inserted is not critical to the procedure or its outcome. Assessment of the effects of these actions can be performed by observation of the patient's response and by measuring ventilatory data.

(1:594), (9:165–168).

7. A. The oxygen flow duration (minutes) formula is shown as follows:

$$O_2 \text{ flow duration} = \frac{\left(\substack{\text{pressure} \\ \text{gauge reading}}\right)\left(\substack{\text{conversion} \\ \text{factor}}\right)}{(\text{liter flow})}$$

The conversion factor for an H cylinder is 3.14 L/psig.

STEP 1: Calculate the duration in minutes:

$$\text{flow duration} = \frac{(2,000 \text{ p̶s̶i̶g̶})(3.14 \text{ L̶/p̶s̶i̶g̶})}{(2.5 \text{ l̶i̶t̶e̶r̶s̶}/\text{minute})}$$

$$= \frac{6,280}{2.5 \text{ min.}^{-1}}$$

$$= 2,512 \text{ min.}$$

STEP 2: Convert minutes to hours:

$$\text{hours} = \frac{2,512 \text{ m̶i̶n̶}}{60 \text{ m̶i̶n̶}/\text{hour}}$$

$$= 41.87 \text{ hours}$$

(1:721–722), (13:45–46).

8. C. The Kamen–Wilkenson (Bivona cuff) or foam cuff self-inflates with atmospheric air causing foam expansion. Before the tube is inserted, air must be aspirated from the cuff by a syringe (collapses foam), and the pilot balloon port is then capped. Once the tube is in position, the pilot balloon port is opened and the cuff is inflated (foam expands) with air at atmospheric pressure. The polyurethane foam cuff expands (self-inflates) until it contacts the tracheal wall. Minimum or low pressure exists inside the cuff.

Personnel working with a patient who has a Kamen–Wilkenson tube inserted must know the mechanics of operation of the cuff inflation for this tube.

Injecting air into the cuff by personnel unfamiliar with this type of tube will elevate intracuff pressure, which would likely have adverse consequences for the patient.

(5:240), (13:175–176).

9. C. Supraventricular tachycardia and ventricular tachycardia are two tachyarhythmias that are treatable with synchronized cardioversion. When performing synchronized cardioversion, the applied depolarization is timed to coincide with the R wave of the dysrhythmia.

The ECG strip shown in Figure 2-13 below illustrates supraventricular tachycardia (SVT).

The ECG tracing shown in Figure 2-14 (page 56) indicates where (R wave) the synchronized cardioversion should be applied to an SVT pattern to convert it to a normal sinus rhythm.

Defibrillation is the asynchronous (untimed) application of depolarization to a disorganized dysrhythmia (e.g., ventricular fibrillation).

(1:657).

10. A. Pursed-lip breathing provides expiratory resistance in spontaneously breathing patients. This maneuver might raise the intraluminal pressures in the airway and prevent or reduce air trapping. By this mechanism, pursed-lip breathing increases the expiratory time and promotes more complete lung emptying. Pursed-lip breathing is especially useful in COPD patients.

(9:69), (16:167, 537).

11. D. A person who has an acute asthmatic episode but does not respond favorably to the usual regimen of medications on the standard therapeutic modalities is said to have status asthmaticus.

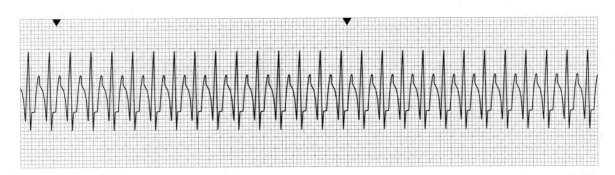

**Figure 2-13:** Supraventricular tachycardia (SVT).

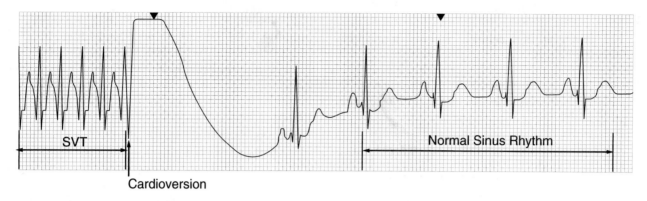

**Figure 2-14:** Cardioversion of SVT cardioverted to a normal sinus rhythm.

Arterial blood gas analysis varies according to the stage of the asthmatic episode. During the initial attack, the patient characteristically exhibits hypocapnia, hypoxemia, and alkalemia (acute respiratory alkalosis). At some time further along in the episode, the patient's hypoxemia persists or worsens, whereas the arterial $CO_2$ and pH tend to normalize. In the late stage (essentially status asthmaticus), the hypoxemia worsens and hypercapnia and acidemia are displayed.

It is generally near the onset of the late stage when the decision is made to intubate and mechanically ventilate the patient. This stage actually represents acute ventilatory failure.

The current approach to treating the situation posed here is to reduce the arterial $PCO_2$ (i.e., to normalize the $PCO_2$), and in so doing correct the pH. At this stage of the patient's condition, the $HCO_3^-$ is not appreciably increased because the kidneys have not had time to retain more $HCO_3^-$ (compensate). Recall that mechanical ventilation was recently instituted. What is conventionally expected here is for ventilator adjustments to be made to lower the arterial $PCO_2$.

The arterial $PCO_2$ can generally be lowered by increasing the patient's alveolar ventilation ($\dot{V}_A$), which is a function of the tidal volume and the ventilatory rate. Two schools of thought conflict here, however. One advocates using low-tidal volumes (8 to 10 ml/kg) because of the hyperinflation associated with this condition. The other is a proponent of large tidal volumes (15 to 20 ml/kg) and inspiratory flow rates half of normal for that person.

Ordinarily, the decision of which setting to increase is based on the current ventilation rate and tidal volume. Adjusting the setting that will least influence the mean intrathoracic pressure should be performed first.

To further complicate matters, Daioli found that these patients can be successfully treated while allowing hypoventilation. Arterial $PCO_2$ values have been allowed to rise in the 90 mm Hg range. The rationale for this approach is that the risk of barotrauma associated with attempts to lower the arterial $PCO_2$ is minimized or avoided altogether.

(10:236–237), (15:717–719), (16:1124).

**IIIA1b**

12. C. The purpose of the modified Allen test is to evaluate the status of a patient's collateral circulation to the hand. A positive modified Allen test indicates the patient has adequate collateral circulation through the arteries (radial and ulnar) serving the hand. A negative result, however, documents inadequate blood flow through the radial and ulnar arteries of the hand being tested.

Therefore, if a negative modified Allen test is obtained from one hand, the RRT should perform the same test on the other hand to determine its suitability for an arterial puncture.

Because performing an arterial puncture on the brachial artery has more complications associated with it compared to the radial site, obtaining the blood sample from the brachial artery before evaluating the other hand is inadvisable.

(3:302–304), (9:121).

**IIID1b**

13. B. Epinephrine, lidocaine, and atropine have all been approved for endotracheal (ET) administration. Bioavailability of these drugs by ET tube administration is similar to the I.V. route. Sodium bicarbonate is not used for ET instillation during codes because the volume of the drug needed to effectively buffer the blood would be rather significant. During cardiopulmonary resuscitation, sodium bicarbonate is most efficiently administered I.V.

Isoproterenol hydrochloride is a drug that is administered I.V. to ellicit a positive inotropic (increased myocardial contractility) and positive chronotropic (increased heart rate) effect. It is also a vasodilator. Isoproterenol is not administered endotracheally.

("Guidelines 2000 for Cardiopulmonary Resuscitation and Emergency Cardiovascular Care," *American Heart Assoc.,* pages I–121, I-123, and I-130).

### IIB1e(1)

14. B. A constant-flow ventilator maintains a relatively constant flow rate throughout the inspiratory phase.

The pressure differential between that generated by the ventilator and the pressure in the lungs is extraordinarily high at end inspiration. Therefore, the pressure change throughout inspiration across the ventilator–patient system is practically neglible. Consequently, no variation occurs in the gas flow pattern, and the flow rate remains essentially constant despite a decreased pulmonary compliance or an increased airway resistance.

The pressure and flow waveforms associated with a constant-flow (generator) ventilator under normal lung-compliance and airway-resistance conditions are depicted in Figure 2-15.

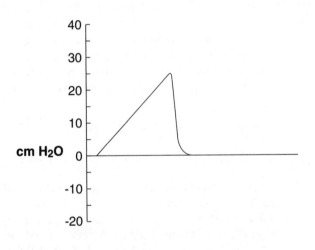

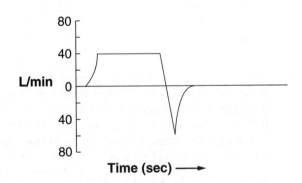

**Figure 2-15:** Pressure and flow waveforms developed by a constant-flow ventilator (generator) under normal lung-compliance and airway-resistance conditions.

The waveforms (pressure and flow) illustrated in Figure 2-16 represent the result of ventilating lungs that are more stiff (decreased lung compliance). The pressure curve reflects a higher inflation pressure, which is demonstrated by the steeper and greater amplitude of the pressure tracing. The flow tracing remains constant under these conditions despite the increased magnitude of pressure.

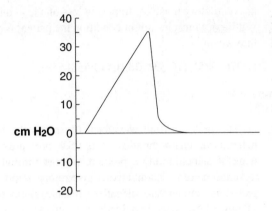

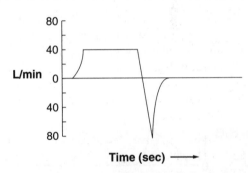

**Figure 2-16:** Pressure and flow waveforms obtained from a constant-flow ventilator (generator) under conditions of decreased pulmonary compliance. Note that the amplitude and steepness of the pressure curve are increased, reflecting the response to ventilating stiffer lungs. The flow curve remains constant despite the pressure changes.

(5:351–354), (10:54–56).

### IIB2c

15. B. An ultrasonic nebulizer's mist output will increase when (1) the blower fan speed is increased, (2) the water level in the coupling compartment is at an adequate level, and (3) the amplitude of the unit is increased.

(5:154), (13:121, 296, 669).

### IIIB2c

16. C. The ABG data as well as the other signs (paradoxical breathing, tachycardia, diaphoresis, and agitation) indicate that the patient is not capable of sustaining spontaneous ventilations at this time. The appropriate action is to reconnect the patient to the mechanical ventilator as he was before the weaning trial began.

The patient should be informed of the actions taking place and should be allowed to rest. After appropriate time has elapsed and the patient has become stable once again, switching the patient from full ventilatory support to SIMV or to SIMV with pressure-support ventilation (PSV) might be useful. Partial ventilatory support might allow the patient to gradually strengthen his ventilatory muscles. Imposing less of a load on the ventilatory muscles might condition the patient for future weaning.

(1:976–985), (10:331–332), (15:558–559).

### IA1f(3)

17. D. The pressure-time waveform illustrates the PSV mode. The characteristics of a PSV pressure-time waveform include (1) a pressure plateau throughout inspiration, (2) a spontaneous inspiratory effort depicted as a downward (negative pressure) deflection, (3) irregularly spaced tidal volumes, and (4) differing-sized tidal volumes.

The pressure-time waveforms for controlled mechanical ventilation, assisted mechanical ventilation, and intermittent mandatory ventilation (IMV) are illustrated in Figure 2-17.

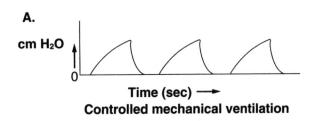

**A.**

cm $H_2O$

Time (sec) ⟶
**Controlled mechanical ventilation**

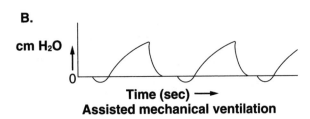

**B.**

cm $H_2O$

Time (sec) ⟶
**Assisted mechanical ventilation**

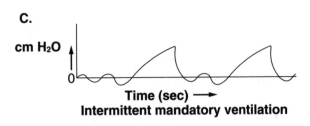

**C.**

cm $H_2O$

Time (sec) ⟶
**Intermittent mandatory ventilation**

**Figure 2-17:** Pressure-time waveforms: (a) controlled mechanical ventilation, (b) assisted mechanical ventilation, (c) intermittent mandatory ventilation

(1:864, 877, 979), (10:85, 199, 214, 331), (15:960).

### IIIB2c

18. C. PCV is time-cycled. The tidal volume that the patient receives is determined by the lung compliance, airway resistance, PIP, inspiratory time, and auto-PEEP if applicable.

When a patient is switched to PCV, the initial settings usually include an $FiO_2$ of 1.0, a PIP approximately one-half of the PIP on the previous mode, and a PEEP about one-half that on the previous mode if that PEEP level was greater than 8 cm $H_2O$. If the PEEP was less than 8 cm $H_2O$ on the previous mode, no PEEP is necessary during PCV. Initially, the I:E ratio is set at 1:2 or less. If necessary, the inspiratory time is eventually set to exceed expiratory time. In such cases, the mode of ventilation is termed PCV with an inverse I:E ratio (i.e., PCIRV).

(1:837, 875, 876), (10:198–199, 214–215).

### IIB2q

19. A. Ventricular fibrillation requires immediate catheter withdrawal and defibrillation. During pulmonary artery catheter insertion, premature ventricular contractions (PVCs) or ventricular tachycardia are not uncommon. Whenever a life-threatening dysrhythmia (e.g., ventricular fibrillation) develops during the procedure, however, generally the catheter must be withdrawn.

(1:331, 652, 653), (16:814–815, 853).

### IC2c

20. C. Sepsis is known to cause peripheral vascular shunting. This condition results in tissue oxygen deprivation and the buildup of lactic acid (lactate ions) caused by anaerobic metabolism. Additionally, because the arterial blood is not allowed to deliver an adequate supply of oxygen (caused by the altered peripheral microcirculation), mixed venous blood exhibits an inordinately higher $P\bar{v}O_2$ and $S\bar{v}O_2$. The normal $P\bar{v}O_2$ and $S\bar{v}O_2$ values are 40 torr and 70%–75%, respectively.

Other indices, such as $SaO_2$, cardiac output (C.O.), and blood lactate levels, need to be evaluated because mixed venous blood analysis alone renders insufficient data. The normal blood lactate level ranges between 0.5 mmole/liter and 2.5 mmoles/liter. The normal C.O. output ranges between 4 to 8 L/min., and the normal $SaO_2$ ranges between 95% to 97.5%.

(1:207, 225, 232, 345, 511), (15:534), (16:176, 255, 326).

### IIA1g

21. C. French sizes actually represent the outer circumference of a suction catheter (or artificial airway),

whereas the internal diameter is measured in millimeters (mm). The relationship of circumference to diameter is given by the formula:

$$C = \pi d$$

where

C = circumference
$\pi$ = 3.14
d = diameter (outer)

The following expression can be conveniently used to obtain the French size. The value 3 in the expression is an approximation of pi, i.e., 3.14.

French gauge = 3 × outer diameter (mm)

The customary clinical guideline is that the outer diameter (O.D.) of a suction catheter should not exceed one-half the inner diameter (I.D.) of the ET tube. The ET tube in this problem is 8.0 mm I.D. Therefore,

STEP 1: Use the formula that converts French size to the metric system.

$$\frac{\text{French gauge}}{3.0} = \text{external diameter (mm)}$$

STEP 2: Insert the known values and determine the external diameter in millimeters.

$$\frac{12 \text{ Fr}}{3.0} = \text{external diameter (mm)}$$

4.0 mm = external diameter

For optimum secretion removal, it is desirable to use the largest suction catheter possible without violating the rule stated previously. The appropriate French gauge would be determined by solving the equation previously given (Fr gauge = 3 × outer diameter). Therefore,

$$\text{Fr gauge} = 3 \times 4.00 \text{ mm (O.D.)}$$
$$= 12 \text{ Fr}$$

The most appropriate suction catheter to use for suctioning an 8.0 mm I.D. ET tube is a 12 Fr size.

The RRT must keep in mind, however, that this guideline does not apply to all clinical situations. For example, if a patient has thick, tenacious secretions, a suction catheter with an external diameter larger than one-half the ET tube's I.D. might be needed to effectively remove tracheobronchial secretions. Similarly, in the case of neonates, larger suction catheters need to be used or else secretions would be difficult to evacuate.

(13:182), (16:604).

## IIID2

22. A. A tension pneumothorax is a medical emergency and must be treated immediately. Keep in mind a pneumothorax developing during positive pressure ventilation always becomes a tension pneumothorax. The signs of a tension pneumothorax are (1) diminished or absent breath sounds on the affected side, (2) a hyperresonant percussion note on the affected side, (3) mediastinal shift toward the contralateral (unaffected) lung, (4) decreased cardiac output, (5) hypotension with tachycardia, and (5) hypoxemia.

The immediate insertion of chest tubes is required to relieve a tension pneumothorax. If chest tubes cannot be inserted immediately, then rapid decompression of the lung is accomplished via the insertion of a 19-gauge needle into the second or third anterior intercostal space at the nipple line.

(1:485), (9:179, 260, 264), (15:974, 1090).

## IIIE1b

23. C. During thoracentesis, the puncture site must be completely anesthetized. The areas of the puncture site that must be anesthetized are (1) the skin, (2) the periosteum of the rib, and (3) the pleura. The procedure must be completely painless. Specific needle sizes are generally used for applying local anesthesia to the different areas of the puncture site.

A 0.25-gauge (small-bore) needle is usually used to anesthetize the skin. The large-bore, 0.22-gauge needle is ordinarily used for the rib periosteum. The actual size of the needle used for aspirating the pleural effusion should be 0.22 gauge or larger depending on the volume and nature of the effusion.

(1:145, 480, 482), (15:636).

## IA1f (5)

24. D. Any time the capnograph demonstrates a tracing above the baseline (0.0% $CO_2$), the patient is experiencing rebreathing of his own exhaled gas. If the exhalation valve in the ventilator tubing malfunctions, the patient might be at risk of rebreathing his own expirate. The capnograph would probably not reflect this condition, however, because the continuous cycling on of the ventilator would flush the ventilator tubing of any exhaled gas. Furthermore, with the ventilator in the control mode, the patient is not breathing; therefore, he would not be depositing any expirate in the ventilator circuitry for the capnometer to sense. In this

case, the capnograph would register essentially 0.0% exhaled carbon dioxide.

On the other hand, the addition of mechanical dead space to the patient's circuit (control mode only) produces the capnometry tracing shown in Figure 2-18, as the patient rebreathes a portion of his exhaled $CO_2$.

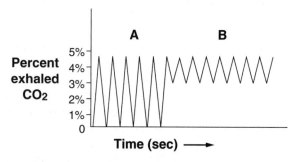

**Figure 2-18:** Capnometry tracing (a) normal capnogram, and (b) patient rebreathing carbon dioxide.

The portion of the tracing on the left represents a normal capnogram. The percent of exhaled carbon dioxide approximately ranges from 0.0% to more than 5.0%. The tracing on the right indicates that the percent of exhaled carbon dioxide is not returning to 0.0% (baseline). Carbon dioxide is being retained by the patient.

(1:363–367), (9:290–291), (10:101–103).

**IIIB1b**

25. A. When capnography is used in conjunction with endotracheal intubation, the capnograph will indicate a rapid rise in the percentage of the exhaled carbon dioxide. The readout will generally change abruptly from about 0.03% to 5.6%, indicating that the room air carbon dioxide percentage (0.03%) in the ET tube has been replaced by carbon dioxide-laden gas from the patient's lungs. In other words, the ET tube has been inserted through the patient's glottis, and the capnograph is measuring the percentage of the patient's exhaled carbon dioxide.

If the ET tube is advanced and the capnograph continues to reflect room air carbon dioxide values, it is likely that the tube has been inserted into the esophagus.

Whenever capnography is used during the ET intubation procedure, proper ET tube location and position must be confirmed either via fiber-optic laryngoscopy or by portable chest X-ray.

(1:363–367), (10:101–103).

**IIB3b**

26. A. According to the recommendations made by the American College of Chest Physicians (ACCP) and the American Thoracic Society (ATS), a 7-liter volume

spirometer is accurate if the measured volume is ±3.0% of the calibrated volume (i.e., 2.91 to 3.09 liters).

| + 3.0% of Calibrated Volume | − 3.0% of Calibrated Volume |
|:---:|:---:|
| 3.00 L | 3.00 L |
| + 0.09 L | − 0.09 L |
| 3.09 L | 2.91 L |

Therefore, the measured volume in this example is unacceptable because it represents a 10% error.

$$\frac{2.70 \text{ L}}{3.00 \text{ L}} \times 100 = 10.0\%$$

A number of factors can cause the measured volume to deviate from the calibrated volume by more than ±3.0%. These factors include (1) a leak in the spirometer, (2) incomplete filling or emptying of the calibration syringe, (3) excessively high flow rates during volume injection, and (4) loose connections between the calibration syringe and the spirometer.

The flow-rate range for a 7-liter volume spirometer is 0 to 12 L/sec. The flow rate (0.6 L/sec.) used by the therapist in this case was adequate.

$$\frac{\text{volume}}{\text{time}} = \text{flow rate}$$

$$\frac{3.0 \text{ L}}{5.0 \text{ sec.}} = 0.6 \text{ L/sec.}$$

Most spirometer manufacturers suggest at least three syringe injection times: (1) 0.5 to 1.0 sec., (2) 1.0 to 1.5 sec., and (3) 5.0 to 5.5 sec.

Omitting the patient hose during the calibration procedure does not affect the volume injected. It merely prevents evaluating the hose for leaks that might not be visibly noted.

(6:297–301), (11:378–382).

**IIB2e(1)**

27. B. When an RRT suspects that a ventilator is malfunctioning, the first appropriate response is to evaluate the patient's level of consciousness, color, breathing activity, inspiratory effort, and so on. Any unusual patient and/or machine sounds should be noted. The system pressure manometer also should be observed. An increasing PIP is indicative of an obstruction. A decreasing PIP indicates a volume leak or a disconnection. If you believe that the equipment is malfunctioning, the ventilator should be disconnected from the patient, and ventilation via a manual resuscitator should be provided. A manual resuscitator must be kept in proximity of the ventilator at all times. A thorough check of all tubing connections should then be performed along

with equipment function. If the malfunction cannot be corrected, the ventilator must be replaced. During this process, the patient should be reassured and comforted.

(10:306–307).

## IA1f(3)

28. A. The appearance of a pressure plateau (arrows) on the pressure-time waveform shown in Figure 2-19 indicates the presence of auto-PEEP.

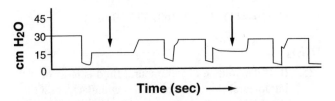

**Figure 2-19:** Pressure-time tracing showing the presence (arrows) of auto-PEEP.

The pressure plateau occurred when the exhalation valve was closed immediately before the delivery of the next ventilator breath. The presence of a gas under pressure within the lungs during exhalation produces the pressure plateau.

(1:951–953), (10:87).

## IIIC2

29. B. The next step in working with this patient would be to determine whether the use of a spacer would allow the patient to better coordinate her breathing with the activation of the MDI. When a patient uses a spacer, the MDI is activated and then the spacer mouthpiece is placed in the mouth and a deep breath is taken. Most spacers have one-way valves to prevent the patient from exhaling into the medication chamber prior to inspiration. A small-volume nebulizer would be needed for this patient only if the patient is unable to properly use the MDI with a spacer.

(1:689–690), (13:147–148).

## IIIE2a

30. D. The formula for calculating the volume of gaseous oxygen from a liquid system is as follows:

$$\begin{pmatrix} \text{volume of} \\ \text{gaseous} \\ \text{oxygen} \\ \text{(L)} \end{pmatrix} = \begin{pmatrix} \text{liquid weight-gas} \\ \text{volume oxygen} \\ \text{conversion factor} \\ \text{(L/lb)} \end{pmatrix} \begin{pmatrix} \text{liquid oxygen} \\ \text{reservoir} \\ \text{weight} \\ \text{(lb)} \end{pmatrix}$$

Because a 40-liter liquid oxygen system weighs about 100 pounds, and because the liquid weight–gas volume oxygen conversion factor is 344 L/lb, the calculation becomes

$$\begin{pmatrix} \text{volume of} \\ \text{gaseous oxygen} \\ \text{(L)} \end{pmatrix} = (344 \text{ L/lb})(100 \text{ lb})$$

$$= 34,400 \text{ L}$$

Because one cubic foot of liquid oxygen yields 860 cubic feet of gaseous oxygen, more oxygen is clinically available from the liquid state than from the gaseous state.

The liquid oxygen continuously vaporizes in a liquid oxygen system. Therefore, oxygen in the gas phase is present above the liquid oxygen. The weight of the entire liquid system must be considered when one attempts to calculate the duration of flow from a liquid oxygen system. Because the liquid oxygen continuously vaporizes, the pressure gauge on the liquid oxygen system will always indicate 20 to 25 psig until the liquid phase is depleted. From that point, only the gas phase will exist, and the pressure gauge will reflect lower readings as the gaseous oxygen is used.

(1:1115), (4:27–29), (13:48–49).

## IIIA1f

31. A. A pulmonary artery catheter with the balloon inflated is advanced to the pulmonary artery until it achieves the wedge position. Once hemodynamic data are obtained, the balloon is deflated and a normal pulmonary artery pressure tracing is observed.

The problem with which the RRT is confronted in this instance is not highly unusual. The pulmonary artery catheter has inadvertently migrated into the wedge position. The catheter needs to be pulled back until the wedge-pressure waveform disappears and the pulmonary artery pressure tracing reappears.

Allowing the tip of the pulmonary artery catheter to remain in the wedge position for a prolonged time increases the potential of a pulmonary infarction.

(1:943–946), (9:346–347), (10:127–128), (15:529–533).

## IIB3a

32. B. In general, quality-control data help identify random errors and systematic errors. A random error is an isolated occurrence or result beyond the control limits. A single, random error can be disregarded but might be a harbinger of the onset of a problem. Quite often, a single, random error is ignored. The occurrence of frequent random errors is called dispersion.

Systematic errors are recurring deviations beyond the mean. They can occur either within or outside the control limits. A sudden change in the measurements resulting in a clustering of data in a specific region on a

Levy-Jennings chart is called shifting. Trending is a systematic error characterized by a gradual change in measurements.

These aforementioned errors are also described as problems with the accuracy of the measuring device or the precision of the instrument. How close the measured results come to the actual or true value refers to accuracy.

Precision reflects the dispersion of numerous measurements. For example, an instrument measuring $\pm 8$ standard deviations (S.D.s) from the mean is less precise than one consistently measuring $\pm 5$ S.D.s.

The data from the carbon dioxide (Severinghaus) electrode given in the problem reflects an accuracy problem as a shift in the mean (as reflected by the changes in the frequency of distribution) occurred.

(3:323–325), (4:48–49).

## IIIA1m(1)

33. B. Use the Fick equation to calculate the arterial mixed venous oxygen content difference [$C(a-\bar{v})O_2$] when given the oxygen consumption ($\dot{V}O_2$) and the cardiac output ($\dot{Q}_T$).

The Fick equation is as follows:

$$\dot{Q}_T = \frac{\dot{V}O_2}{C(a - \bar{v})O_2}$$

To solve for the $C(a-\bar{v})O_2$,

$$C(a - \bar{v})O_2 = \frac{\dot{V}O_2}{\dot{Q}_T} = \frac{250 \text{ ml/min}}{5 \text{ liters/min}}$$

$$= \frac{50 \text{ ml } O_2}{100 \text{ ml-bld}} = 0.5 \text{ ml } O_2/100 \text{ ml bld}$$

$$= 5.0 \text{ vol\%}$$

(1:225–226, 930), (9:323–324).

## IB7a

34. A. Normally, air within the bronchi is not seen on a chest radiograph. The reason is because the bronchi are ordinarily air filled and are surrounded by air-filled aveoli. Therefore, no contrast exists between these two lung areas.

Air bronchograms on a chest radiograph result from the contrast between air-filled bronchi and adjacent fluid-filled lungs. When this situation develops, the contrast between these two conditions becomes greater, making the hyperlucent bronchi appear on the chest X-ray.

Pathologic conditions that are associated with the appearance of air bronchograms on a chest roentgeno-

gram include interstitial edema, hemorrhage, pneumonia, and atelectasis. The presence of air bronchograms indicates that the pathology is in the lungs, not in the intrapleural space. As the fluid level in the alveoli increases and enters the airways, air bronchograms will be absent because no contrast exists between the fluid in the bronchi and the fluid in the surrounding alveoli. Similarly, when an obstructed bronchus is the cause of atelectasis, air bronchograms will be absent. With the collapse of lung tissue distal to the obstruction, no contrast between the two areas will exist.

(1:410–411), (9:162–163), (15:604).

## IIIE1j

35. B. If the volume of intrapleural fluid is large or if the intrapleural fluid continues to accumulate, chest tubes should be placed for drainage. The chest tubes are generally inserted at the level of the sixth or seventh intercostal space along either the midaxillary or posterior axillary lines. The selected area must be liberally anesthetized with a local anesthetic. The procedure for chest-tube insertion is also called *tube thoracostomy*.

(1:482, 487), (9:265–266), (15:1092–1093).

## IIA1h

36. C. Carbon monoxide (CO) is a tasteless, odorless gas. It can be breathed unknowingly and can cause dangerous consequences. Carbon monoxide in the blood shifts the oxyhemoglobin dissociation curve to the left, thereby interfering with the release of oxygen at the tissue level. It also interferes with oxygen transport because hemoglobin has an affinity for CO that is 210 times greater than for oxygen ($O_2$).

Treatment of CO poisoning centers around oxygen administration and hyperventilation. Therefore, it would be appropriate to administer either hyperbaric or nomobaric $O_2$ to a CO-poisoning victim depending on the carboxyhemoglobin (COHb) level in the blood. Carboxyhemoglobin blood levels can be measured via co-oximetry with blood samples obtained from either arterial or venous blood. Similarly, if a CO-inhalation victim was apneic, it would be appropriate to intubate, oxygenate, and hyperventilate the patient to help remove the CO from the blood as rapidly as possible.

In either case, oxygen administration greatly reduces the half-life of CO in the blood. For example, the half-life ($t\frac{1}{2}$) of CO is approximately 1.0 hour when the victim breaths 100% $O_2$ at 1 atmosphere, compared with a $t\frac{1}{2}$ of 5.3 hours while breathing room air (21% $O_2$) at 1 atmosphere. Under hyperbaric conditions (3 atmospheres), the $t\frac{1}{2}$ is reduced to 23 minutes. Because oxygenation of the patient is critical, 100% $O_2$ should be administered immediately until the patient's COHb% is determined. Hyperbaric intervention is generally indicated when the COHb% is 40% or greater.

Table 2-3 outlines the relationship among the $F_ICO$, the COHb%, and the patient's response.

(1:764-765), (15:320, 940, 1107–1109).

## IIIA1h

37.   D. Auto-PEEP generally develops when there is insufficient time devoted to exhalation. Too short an expiratory time prevents adequate emptying of the lungs. Consequently, the ensuing breath begins before the previous exhalation is completed.

Auto-PEEP can develop in patients who have normal lung characteristics (airway resistance and compliance) when a prolonged inspiratory time is used, when high-minute ventilation is employed, or when a small-caliber ET tube has been inserted.

Patients who have chronic airflow obstruction frequently experience auto-PEEP when inordinately high-tidal volumes (greater than 12 ml/kg of ideal body weight) are used or when high ventilatory rates are present.

The following measures can be taken to reduce auto-PEEP: (1) increasing the inspiratory flow rate, (2) increasing the expiratory time, (3) decreasing the inspiratory time, (4) employing a reduced ventilatory rate, and (5) using a lower tidal volume. Additionally, the use of low-compliance ventilatory circuits and large-caliber ET tubes are effective in reducing auto-PEEP.

(1:917, 951–953), (10:153–154, 155–156), (15:901–907).

## IIIC3a

38.   C. Based on the information presented, it is reasonable to assume that the infant is experiencing hypercapnia and that hypoxemia is a likely subsequent development. The hypercapnia can be attributed to the low oxygen flow rate (3 L/min.) to the oxyhood. Oxyhoods should be operated at flow rates between 6 to 8 L/min.

The purpose of these flow rates is to purge the enclosure of the neonate's exhaled carbon dioxide.

In this situation, the oxyhood is being operated at an oxygen flow rate of 3 L/min. This flow rate is too low, thereby resulting in the neonate rebreathing his exhaled carbon dioxide. The appropriate action at this time would be to increase the oxygen flow rate to the oxyhood and evaluate the patient's response to this adjustment by performing an arterial puncture in about 15 minutes.

(5:80–82), (13:79–81).

## IIIB2c

39.   C. Because no tidal volume was given in this situation, the guideline for estimating an initial tidal volume must be used. The guideline states that based on the patient's IBW, a 10 to 15 cc tidal volume range can be given per kilogram. The patient here was stated to have an IBW of 155 pounds. Therefore, his IBW in kilograms is determined as follows:

$$IBW\ (kg) = \frac{155\ \text{lbs}}{2.2\ \text{lbs/kg}}$$
$$= 70\ kg$$

It is estimated that this patient can receive a tidal volume ($V_T$) of 700 to 1,050 cc.

$$(70\ \text{kg})(10\ \text{cc/kg}) = 700\ cc\ or\ 0.7\ L$$

or

$$(70\ \text{kg})(15\ \text{cc/kg}) = 1,050\ cc\ or\ 1.05\ L$$

The following formula can be applied to determine the peak inspiratory flow rate ($\dot{V}_I$):

$$\dot{V}_I = \frac{V_T}{T_I}$$
$$= \frac{0.70\ L}{2\ sec.}$$
$$= 0.35\ L/sec.$$

**Table 2-3** Effects of Carbon Monoxide Poisoning

| $F_ICO$ | COHb% | Response in healthy adult |
|---|---|---|
| 0.0 | 0.3 to 0.7 | No effect |
| 0.003 | 1 to 5 | Selective increase in blood flow to vital organs to compensate for reduced $O_2$-carrying capacity |
| 0.007 | 5 to 10 | Visual light threshold increased, dyspnea on vigorous exercise, dilation of cutaneous blood vessels |
| 0.012 | 10 to 20 | Abnormal vision evoked response, dyspnea on mild exertion, throbbing headache |
| 0.022 | 20 to 30 | Marked headache, irritability, easy fatiguability, poor judgment, diminished vision and fine manual dexterity, nausea/vomiting |
| 0.035–0.052 | 30 to 40 | Severe headache, nausea/vomiting, confusion, syncope on exertion |
| 0.082–0.122 | 50 to 60 | Intermittent convulsions, ventilatory failure, coma, death if prolonged exposure |
| 0.199 | 70 to 80 | Coma, rapidly fatal |

or

$$= 0.35 \text{ L/sec.} \times 60 \text{ sec./min.} = 21 \text{ L/min.}$$

If the larger range of $V_T$ is used, the $\dot{V}_I$ needed would be as follows:

$$\dot{V}_I = \frac{1.05 \text{ L}}{2 \text{ sec.}}$$

$$= 0.525 \text{ L/sec.}$$

or

$$= 0.525 \text{ L/sec} \times 60 \text{ sec/min.}$$

$$= 31.5 \text{ L/min.}$$

(1:896–897), (10:207–208).

## IA1h(4)

40. D. Co-oximeters measure four different types of hemoglobin: (1) oxyhemoglobin, (2) reduced hemoglobin, (3) methemoglobin, and (4) carboxyhemoglobin. These four types of hemoglobin are measured spectrophotometrically by using monochromatic light at four different wavelengths.

The co-oximeter is the only device that measures carboxyhemoglobin (COHb) levels. Therefore, its use in evaluating the oxygenation status of a suspected CO-poisoning victim is invaluable.

A pulse oximeter will render erroneously high $SaO_2$ readings in the presence of COHb because this device cannot distinguish $HbO_2$ from COHb. A pulse oximeter measures only two wavelengths of light (red and infrared for deoxyhemoglobin and oxyhemoglobin, respectively).

Transcutaneous oxygen monitoring and arterial blood gas analysis provide measurement of the partial pressure of dissolved oxygen. In CO poisoning, the dissolved oxygen tension generally remains normal. That is why CO-poisoning victims frequently do not hyperventilate. Their peripheral chemoreceptors (aortic and carotid bodies) do not send hyperventilatory signals to their medulla because the arterial $PO_2$ is generally normal.

(1:358–359), (15:493).

## IIIA1k

41. B. Wheezes result from rapid vibrations of airway walls. Air moving at high velocity through partially obstructed airways causes the airways to begin vibrat-

ing. Wheezing can be heard during inspiration or exhalation or both.

Wheezes are described as continuous, musical sounds. Depending on the degree of vibrations, wheezing can be loud and high-pitched or less loud and lower-pitched. Wheezing can also be characterized as monophonic or polyphonic.

Monophonic wheezing occurs when one partially obstructed airway produces a single note. Polyphonic wheezing develops when multiple partially obstructed airways concurrently vibrate and produce many musical sounds.

If the patient in this question exhibited less loud and lower-pitched wheezes during exhalation after the $\beta_2$ agonist (bronchodilator) treatment, the treatment would be deemed successful. Because the intensity of wheezing is related to the gas flow past the airway obstruction or narrowing, the RRT must not entirely rely on changes in the intensity of wheezing to evaluate a patient's response to a bronchodilator. Very often, the sound of the wheezing might intensify because of increased air flow.

(1:313–314), (9:84–85).

## IIIB1a

42. C. A large air leak is occurring somewhere in the system. The problem appears to be a leak in the cuff of the ET tube. The cuff should be reinflated to achieve a seal with a cuff pressure of less than 25 cm $H_2O$ if possible. If the cuff continues to leak, the ET tube must be replaced. If the minimal leak (minimum occluding volume) technique was being used, the cuff pressure would be much higher than 5 cm $H_2O$.

(1:609–610), (5:264–266).

## IIIB3

43. D. According to the American Association for Respiratory Care (AARC) Clinical Practice Guidelines, indications for PEP therapy include sputum retention not responsive to coughing and a history of a pulmonary problem that has been successfully treated with postural drainage.

("American Association for Respiratory Care Clinical Practice Guidelines: Use of Positive Airway Pressure Adjuncts to Bronchial Hygiene," *Respiratory Care, 38*(5), 516–519).

## IIIA1d

44. C. The ECG tracing shown in Figure 2-20 demonstrates *ventricular fibrillation displaying complete distortion*

and irregularity of the complexes. No palpable pulse is present during ventricular fibrillation. During ventricular tachycardia, however, the ECG displays a rapid rate and wide QRS complexes.

(1:652–653), (15:1119–1120).

**IIIB4b**

45. B. This patient has an increased work of breathing that might have been caused by an inadequate inspiratory gas flow during spontaneous breathing. Pressure-support ventilation (PSV) can reduce the work of breathing associated with SIMV demand valves, ventilator circuits, and artificial airways. During PSV, the patient establishes his own tidal volume, ventilatory rate, inspiratory time, and peak inspiratory flow rate. The only setting that is controlled by the RRT is the level of pressure support.

(1:864), (10:85, 199), (15:960–961).

**IIB2e(1)**

46. A. The designation *time-cycled* describes the variable that is responsible for terminating inspiration. The following four factors are ordinarily responsible for ending inspiration: (1) flow, (2) pressure, (3) volume, or (4) time.

The *pressure-limited* classification refers to the variable that cannot be exceeded during the mechanical inspiratory phase. This variable is not the cycling factor, however. The following four factors can be limited during mechanical inspiration: (1) flow, (2) pressure, (3) volume, or (4) time.

Therefore, a mechanical ventilator classified as a pressure-limited, time-cycled device will sustain a preset pressure (pressure-limited) during the inspiratory phase and will terminate inspiration at a preset inspiratory time (time-cycled).

The following four factors determine the volume delivered by a pressure-limited, time-cycled ventilator:

(1) the inspiratory flow rate, (2) the preset pressure limit, (3) the inspiratory time, and (4) the patient's ventilation time constant.

The ventilation time constant is calculated by multiplying the patient's airway resistance by the lung compliance:

$$\text{time constant} = (\text{airway resistance})(\text{lung compliance})$$
$$= (cmH_2O/L/sec)(L/cmH_2O)$$
$$= \text{second}$$

(1:843–845), (10:79–82, 84).

**IIID1b**

47. C. The patient presents with ventricular tachycardia and hemodynamic compromise (decreased blood pressure, tachypnea, chest pain, and diaphoresis). She also exhibits potential electromechanical disassociation indicated by differences between the monitored heart rate and the palpable pulse rate. The electrical heart rate or monitored rate is 120 beats/min., whereas the palpable heart rate is 100 beats/min. In this situation, rapid electrical shock is necessary. The treatment of choice is cardioversion. The energy levels and sequences must conform with current advanced cardiac life support (ACLS) standards (i.e., cardioversion with 200 joules, or w-sec, followed by 200 to 300 w-sec and then followed by 360 w-sec if the preceding shocks were unsuccessful). Had the patient been pulseless, the initial treatment would be defibrillation.

(1:653–657), (15:1120–1121), (16:859, 866–867), ("Guidelines 2000 for Cardiopulmonary Resuscitation and Emergency Cardiovascular Care," page I-92).

**IIIA1m(1)**

48. C.

STEP 1: Calculate the $P_{A}O_2$ by using the alveolar air equation:

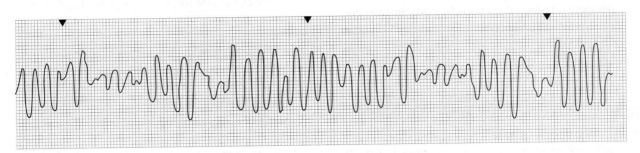

**Figure 2-20:** Ventricular fibrillation. Note the complete distortion and irregularity of complexes.

$$P_{AO_2} = F_{IO_2}(P_B - P_{H_2O}) - PaCO_2\left(F_{IO_2} + \frac{1 - F_{IO_2}}{R}\right)$$

$$= 1.0(760 \text{ torr} - 47 \text{ torr}) - 60 \text{ torr}\left(1 + \frac{1 - 1.0}{0.8}\right)$$

$$= 713 \text{ torr} - 60 \text{ torr}$$

$$= 653 \text{ torr}$$

STEP 2: Calculate the end pulmonary capillary oxygen content (CcO2).

$$C\acute{c}O_2 = [(S\acute{c}O_2)(1.34 \text{ ml } O_2/\text{g Hb})([Hb])$$

$$+ P_{AO_2}(0.003 \text{ vol\%/torr})]$$

$$= (1.0)(1.34 \text{ ml } O_2/\text{g Hb})(17 \text{ g}/100 \text{ ml})$$

$$+ 653 \text{ torr } (0.003 \text{ vol\%/torr})$$

$$= 22.78 \text{ vol\%} + 1.96 \text{ vol\%}$$

$$= 24.74 \text{ vol\%}$$

STEP 3: Calculate the total arterial oxygen content (CaO2).

$$CaO_2 = (SaO_2)(1.34 \text{ ml } O_2/\text{g Hb})([Hb])$$

$$+ P_{AO_2}(0.003 \text{ vol\%/torr})$$

$$= (1.0)(1.34 \text{ ml } O_2/\text{g Hb})(17 \text{ g}/100 \text{ ml})$$

$$+ 500 \text{ torr } (0.003 \text{ vol\%/torr})$$

$$= 22.78 \text{ vol\%} + 1.50 \text{ vol\%}$$

$$= 24.28 \text{ vol\%}$$

STEP 4: Calculate the total mixed venous oxygen content (C$\bar{v}$O2).

$$C\bar{v}O_2 = (S\bar{v}O_2)(1.34 \text{ ml } O_2/\text{g Hb})([Hb])$$

$$+ P\bar{v}O_2 (0.003 \text{ vol\%/torr})$$

$$= (85\%)(1.34 \text{ ml } O_2/\text{g Hb})(17 \text{ g}/100 \text{ ml})$$

$$+ 70 \text{ torr } (0.003 \text{ vol\%/torr})$$

$$= 19.36 \text{ vol\%} + 0.21 \text{ vol\%}$$

$$= 19.57 \text{ vol\%}$$

STEP 5: Calculate the shunt by using the following shunt equation:

$$\frac{\dot{Q}_S}{\dot{Q}_T} = \frac{C\acute{c}O_2 - CaO_2}{C\acute{c}O_2 - C\bar{v}O_2}$$

$$= \frac{24.74 \text{ vol\%} - 24.28 \text{ vol\%}}{24.74 \text{ vol\%} - 19.57 \text{ vol \%}} = \frac{0.46 \text{ vol\%}}{5.17 \text{ vol\%}}$$

$$= 0.0889, \text{ or } 8.89\%$$

(1:930), (9:295), (10:272), (17:46–51).

49. A. The cardiac index (C.I.) is calculated as follows:

$$C.I. = \frac{C.O. \text{ (L/min)}}{BSA \text{ (m}^2)}$$

Because the C.I. is based on the patient's body surface area (BSA), it can be used to compare patients of different sizes. The C.O. is not a standardized measurement and varies significantly among patients of different sizes. Therefore, standardizing the C.I. of normal persons enables for meaningful comparisons among different size persons. The normal range of the C.I. is 2.5 to 4.2 liters/min/m$^2$.

(1:949), (9:309), (10:119, 136).

**IC2e**

50. B. Table 2-4 provides normal capillary blood gas value ranges for an infant 72 hours after birth.

**Table 2-4** Normal Capillary Blood Values 72 Hours After Birth

| MEASUREMENT | NORMAL RANGE |
| --- | --- |
| $PaO_2$ | 62 to 92 mm Hg |
| $PaCO_2$ | 32 to 41 mm Hg |
| pH | 7.34 to 7.42 |
| $HCO_3^-$ | 19 to 23 mEq/liter |

Because all of the values obtained from the capillary blood gas sample are within normal limits, the data are acceptable for a room air blood gas. In infants who are more than 48 hours old, capillary blood samples from an appropriately "arterialized" heel roughly correlate with arterial samples in terms of pH, $PCO_2$, and $HCO_3^-$. The capillary $PO_2$ is affected by numerous factors and is not considered to be a reliable indicator of arterial $PO_2$ values.

Figure 2-21 illustrates the proper technique and locations for obtaining capillary samples.

(4:19), (18:106–107).

**IIIB4a**

51. B. BiPAP ventilation is a form of noninvasive ventilation (i.e., applied mask). It actually is sometimes described as noninvasive PSV. It is not intended for patients requiring full ventilatory support.

BiPAP is useful in the treatment of sleep apnea and nocturnal hypoventilation. BiPAP has also been used in the CCU in the management of respiratory failure in an attempt to avoid ET intubation and conventional

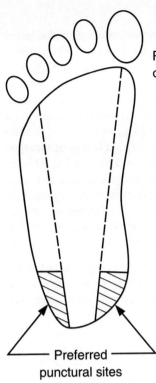

Proper technique for obtaining a capillary sample:

- Wrap heel in a wet, warm cloth (45°C).
- Wait 7 minutes.
- Lance the heel in the preferred area. (Do not dig or slice!)
- Collect only free-flowing blood.
- Do *not* collect blood smeared over the heel.

Preferred punctural sites

**Figure 2-21:** Proper technique and locations for obtaining capillary samples. Note the preferred puncture sites (hatched areas).

mechanical ventilation. Again, BiPAP should not be used with patients who require high levels of ventilatory support and/or high levels of PEEP or CPAP.

(1:563–564, 866, 910), (10:89–90, 201, 217).

**IIB2h(4)**

52. B. Pulse oximetry is a noninvasive method of measuring the arterial oxygen saturation (SaO$_2$). Pulse oximetry incorporates the use of red and infrared wavelengths of light. A light-emitting diode (LED) is housed in the probe of the pulse oximeter. The LED transmits red and infrared light. As the probe is applied to a finger, red and infrared light pass through the patient's skin. As these wavelengths of light pass through the skin, they are absorbed by muscle, skin, and adipose tissue. These tissues are viewed by the probe as a constant factor. This factor is referred to as the *absorption component*. Portions of this transmitted red and infrared light are also absorbed by the hemoglobin in circulation. Specifically, the saturated (oxygenated) hemoglobin absorbs the infrared and red light, whereas the desaturated (deoxygenated) hemoglobin absorbs red light.

The measurement of the SaO$_2$ depends on a pulsatile arterial blood flow. The constant absorption of red and infrared wavelengths is disregarded. The constant ab-

sorption component includes the skin, muscle, adipose tissue, and venous blood, which is normally non-pulsatile.

There are a number of conditions for which pulse oximetry renders erroneous data. These conditions include (1) hypotension, (2) cardiac arrest, (3) hypothermia, and (4) cardiopulmonary bypass. In the case of hypotension, the patient's pulse will tend to be weak or imperceptible. Because the accuracy of pulse oximetry requires a pulsatile arterial blood flow, hypotension will likely render erroneous data.

(1:359, 362, 928–929), (6:144–146, 183–184, 276–279), (10:96–99).

**IIIA1b**

53. D. Co-oximetry is indicated for this patient. Although his symptoms do not indicate a respiratory burn because there are no signs of singed nasal hair, carbonaceous sputum, or stridorous breath sounds, it is highly likely that he has inhaled carbon monoxide—a by-product of the incomplete burning of carbon-based substances.

The PtcO$_2$ monitoring only reflects the partial pressure of oxygen within the capillaries underneath the heated polarographic electrode that is applied to the skin. The PaO$_2$ and PtcO$_2$ highly correlate in the neonate because the increase in the PO$_2$ caused by heating is balanced by the decrease in PO$_2$ caused by (a) the consumption of oxygen by the skin and (b) the diffusion of oxygen across the skin. The PtcO$_2$/PaO$_2$ ratio decreases with age and with cardiac output. The PtcO$_2$ monitoring does not track the oxygen content because it does not reflect hemoglobin saturation.

Pulse oximetry utilizes a noninvasive spectrophotometer to determine the relationship of oxyhemoglobin to reduced hemoglobin. Numerous factors affect the accuracy of the pulse oximeter, including the following:

- carboxyhemoglobin
- methemoglobin
- fetal hemoglobin
- motion
- vascular dyes
- ambient light
- dark skin pigmentation
- nail polish

Arterial blood gases report hemoglobin saturation; however, this value is calculated based on the PaO$_2$, pH, and PaCO$_2$. Methemoglobin and carboxyhemoglobin are not reflected in the calculated arterial oxygen saturation (SaO$_2$) obtained via an arterial blood gas.

The most accurate method of tracking the levels of carboxyhemoglobin and oxyhemoglobin is with a co-oximeter. The principle of operation is related to the

Beer–Lambert law, which states that the amount of light absorbed by a substance is directly related to the concentration of the substance. The co-oximeter uses various wavelengths of light to measure the concentrations of oxyhemoglobin, reduced hemoglobin, carboxyhemoglobin, and methemoglobin.

(1:349, 354–356, 358), (6:134), (9:227), (10:102, 104), (15:492), (16:274–275, 1092)., (Hess, D., and Kacmarek, R. M., "Monitoring Oxygenation," *Respiratory Care, 38,* 646–671).

### IIIE1a

54. D. Epinephrine in the strength of about 1:20,000 should be instilled directly at the bleeding site. Epinephrine, which has both alpha and beta effects, is a potent vasoconstrictor. Generally, 10 cc or less is sufficient to stop the bleeding. In some cases, the bleeding is greater and will require additional boluses of epinephrine. If significant bleeding is anticipated, epinephrine is instilled before the biopsy is performed.

(8:326), (15:643).

### IIIC7b

55. D. Both types of open-end suction catheters (angular cut or perpendicular cut) are best suited for the removal of thick, tenacious secretions from the tracheobronchial tree. Caution must be exercised with both of these catheters, however, because the entire negative pressure will be applied through the single opening at the catheter's tip. The angular cut offers a larger surface area exposed to the suction pressure compared with the perpendicular cut. In either case, if the open end impinges against the airway wall, suction must be terminated immediately to prevent respiratory mucosal damage.

Other types of suction catheters are designed to minimize the risk of respiratory mucosal damage by having one or more additional openings (holes) near the tip of the catheter. For example, the whistle-tip suction catheter has an angular-cut tip and an opening on the side wall of the catheter near the tip. This alignment of openings is an attempt to reduce the risk of catheter impingement against the mucosal surface. Either hole can adhere to the airway wall, however.

The Argyle Aero-Flo tip suction catheter contains a raised (integral) ring at the tip and four side holes. The raised tip decreases the chances of the catheter adhering to the airway wall. Suction catheters with multiple holes are less likely to be as effective as open-end tip catheters for the removal of thick, tenacious secretions.

(1:616–617), (5:279–281), (7:511–512).

### IIA1f(2)

56. C. A double-lumen ET tube (endobronchial tube) is designed to provide independent ventilation of either the right or left lung. In the situation posed here, a double-lumen ET tube will enable right endobronchial intubation. The portion of the double-lumen ET tube that is inserted into the right mainstem bronchus has a cuff that requires inflation to create a seal for ventilation of the right lung. The second lumen of this type tube resides in the trachea and is also cuffed. This lumen provides for ventilation of the normal left lung. Caution must be exercised to prevent the improper insertion of the double-lumen ET tube further into the right mainstem bronchus to avoid occluding the right upper lobe segmental bronchus.

The double-lumen ET tube is also used for enabling the nonintubated lung to collapse to facilitate surgery or for the intubated lung to enhance the removal of secretions.

(15:828–829).

### IIIB2c

57. C. The initial pressure-control level should be approximately $\frac{1}{2}$ to $\frac{2}{3}$ that used during conventional volume ventilation. This pressure setting should generate a tidal volume in the range of about 400 to 600 ml.

(1:837, 875, 909–910), (10:198–199).

### IIIB1a

58. B. This patient is experiencing acute ventilatory failure, as revealed by the arterial blood gas and acid-base data. The patient is likely a chronic $CO_2$ retainer, evidenced by the high bicarbonate level (normally 22 to 24 mEq/liter) and the fact that he has a 20-pack-year smoking history. This bicarbonate level is probably not much higher than this patient's usual value because it takes hours to days for the bicarbonate level to compensate for increased arterial $PCO_2$ levels.

This patient's acid-base status can be categorized as acute ventilatory failure with hypoxemia superimposed on chronic ventilatory failure. Therefore, this patient requires ET intubation and mechanical ventilation.

Whenever a patient presents with respiratory distress, serial arterial blood gas measurements (perhaps every 30 to 45 minutes) should be taken to determine whether a trend toward ventilatory failure is occurring. Frequent monitoring of the patient's ventilatory rate, pulse, blood pressure, and tidal volume must also take place. Acute ventilatory failure can occur rather rapidly, however.

(1:445–446), (10:232–235).

59.  D.  During cardiopulmonary resuscitation, alveolar ventilation is the cornerstone of the acid-base balance. Carbon dioxide can be effectively removed via artificial ventilation, thereby correcting for a respiratory acidosis.

Regarding the administration of $NaHCO_3$ during a cardiac arrest, sufficient data are available demonstrating that $NaHCO_3$ does not enhance the outcome of defibrillation. In fact, it causes the oxyhemoglobin curve to shift leftward (increased oxyhemoglobin affinity). Paradoxically, $NaHCO_3$ administration can result in an acidosis caused by the production of $CO_2$ from the following reaction:

$$HCO_3^- + H^+ \rightarrow H_2CO_3 \rightarrow H_2O + CO_2$$

Sodium bicarbonate administration in a cardiac arrest situation is suggested only after defibrillation, cardiac compressions, intubation, ventilation, and more than one trial of epinephrine have been unsuccessfully employed. When $NaHCO_3$ is used, 1 mEq/kg should be administered as the initial dose. Ensuing administrations should be given every 10 minutes and at one-half the initial dose. Because an iatrogenically induced alkalosis is a threat, any calculated base deficit must not be completely corrected.

("Guidelines 2000 for Cardiopulmonary Resuscitation and Emergency Cardiovascular Care," page I-133).

60.  C.  A quadruple-lumen pulmonary artery catheter is used for measuring pressures within the right atrium, pulmonary artery, and the pulmonary capillary bed. In addition, RRTs can connect the catheter to a computer that is used to measure cardiac outputs based on the thermodilution method.

Most pulmonary artery catheters in use today have a quadruple lumen. The shortest line extending from the catheter body is usually red and has a two-way stopcock attached to it. This line is used to inflate the balloon at the distal tip of the catheter in order to obtain pulmonary capillary wedge-pressure readings. Because no flow is occurring distal to the balloon when the balloon is inflated, the pressure reading from the lumen opening at the distal tip of the catheter (PA) corresponds to the pressure within the left atrium and left ventricle (when the mitral valve opens).

The next longest line is blue and is labeled either *proximal* or *RA* (right atrium). This lumen opens at a point approximately 30 centimeters from the distal tip, within the right atrium. Connecting this port to a pressure transducer will enable continuous monitoring of right-atrial pressures. Pressures from the proximal port also reflect the central venous pressure (CVP), which provides information regarding the fluid status of the patient, and right ventricular, end-diastolic pressure.

The next line is usually yellow and is labeled either *distal* or *PA* (pulmonary artery). This lumen opens at the distal tip and is used for measuring pulmonary artery systolic and diastolic pressures as well as pulmonary capillary wedge pressures when the balloon on the catheter tip is inflated. This port is used for the withdrawal of mixed venous blood, which is necessary for the calculation of shunt fractions and cardiac outputs via the Fick method.

The fourth lumen contains a wire from a small thermistor bead located approximately 4 centimeters from the catheter tip and connected to a thermodilution cardiac output computer. Additional models of catheters have venous infusion ports, A-V sequential pacing electrodes, and optical sensors for monitoring mixed venous saturation.

The diagram shown in Figure 2-22 summarizes the components of a quadruple-lumen pulmonary artery catheter.

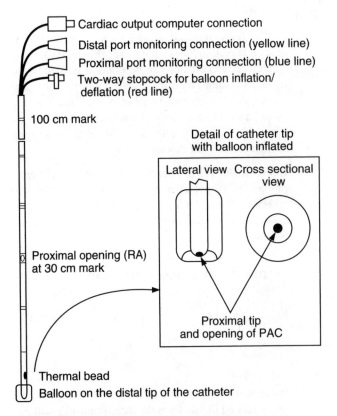

**Figure 2-22:**  Components of a quadruple-lumen pulmonary artery catheter.

(1:943–948), (10:122–124), (15:529–530).

61. B. Atrovent (ipratropium bromide) is ordinarily administered by way of a metered dose inhaler (MDI). Each puff of the MDI dispenses 0.02 mg of Atrovent. Two puffs is the usual recommendation; however, 4 to 6 puffs can be given if indicated.

It takes Atrovent at least 30 minutes to take effect. In some situations, up to 90 minutes is required for maximum bronchodilatation to occur. The RRT did not wait long enough after giving the bronchodilator. Therefore, no judgment can be made regarding the efficacy of this drug or concerning the patient's responsiveness to it. The test needs to be repeated.

(1:455, 577–579, 689), (15:181–183).

62. B. The responsibility for monitoring the patient's cardiopulmonary status sometimes lies with the RRT assisting with the bronchoscopy procedure. Measurements that need to be monitored include the ventilatory rate, the heart rate, and the patient's oxygen saturation. At the same time, the RRT must monitor the ECG.

(1:623–625), (15:628–635).

63. C. The following four variables can be control variables: (1) pressure, (2) volume, (3) flow, and (4) time. Therefore, a ventilator can be either a pressure controller, a volume controller, a flow controller, or a time controller. The control variable is unaffected by the compliance and resistance characteristics of the lungs. The other variables will vary with changes in lung compliance and airway resistance.

If a ventilator is a pressure controller and the patient's pulmonary compliance decreases, the patient's tidal volume will also decrease and the pressure will remain constant. This relationship is based on the following formula:

$$C_L = \frac{V}{P} \quad \textbf{(Remember, P is constant.)}$$

Rearranging the formula to solve for the constant P,

$$P = \frac{V}{C_L}, \text{ or } k = \frac{V}{C_L}$$

Because the volume and the lung compliance are directly related in this formula, the volume (V) will decrease when $C_L$ decreases. Conversely, when $C_L$ increases, V will increase proportionately to maintain the constant P.

(1:836–840), (5:368–371), (10:75–76), (13:368–372).

64. C. Capnography is a noninvasive method providing the continuous measurement of the end-tidal carbon dioxide tension ($P_{ET}CO_2$) via infrared or mass spectrometry. The utility of measuring the $P_{ET}CO_2$ is that under normal and stable cardiovascular conditions, it reflects the alveolar $CO_2$ tension and in turn the arterial $CO_2$ tension. The usual difference between the $PaCO_2$ and the $P_{ET}CO_2$ is less than 3 torr. This gradient widens as a result of the influence of a variety of factors.

For example, a low cardiac output causes less metabolically produced $CO_2$ to be delivered to the pulmonary circulation for gas exchange, thereby causing the $PaCO_2$ to become much greater than the $P_{ET}CO_2$. Likewise, ventilation–perfusion ($\dot{V}_A/\dot{Q}_C$) mismatches produce an increased disparity between these two measurements.

Similarly, alveolar ventilation out of phase with the level of $CO_2$ production ($\dot{V}CO_2$) widens the $PaCO_2$-$P_{ET}CO_2$ gradient. Some infants experience an increased $PaCO_2$ as a result of the added dead space of the $CO_2$ sensor. Tachypneic infants might breathe too rapidly for an accurate measure to be made. Aside from being independent of tissue perfusion and displaying waveforms reflecting cardiopulmonary conditions, capnography is associated with a variety of technical difficulties.

(1:364–366, 984), (10:99–102), (15:460–463).

65. A. The dead space–tidal volume ratio is ordinarily around 0.30. This value is based on an anatomic dead space volume of 150 cc and a tidal volume of 500 cc (i.e., 150 cc/500 cc = 0.30). Patients who receive positive pressure mechanical ventilation experience an increased $V_D/V_T$ ratio because of the increased ventilation to the nongravity-dependent (less-perfused) regions of the lung. Because of this phenomenon, the $V_D/V_T$ ratio for positive pressure mechanically ventilated patients usually ranges from 0.40 to 0.60.

(1:212–213), (17:25–29).

66. C. An ultrasonic nebulizer is not routinely used for medication delivery because the vibrational energy of the high-frequency waves is a threat to the disruption of the chemical structure of the medication. It would be more appropriate in this situation to use an intermittent small-volume nebulizer.

Because of the high aerosol output (up to about 6 ml/min.), ultrasonic nebulizers are primarily used for sputum induction. These devices should be used for continuous aerosol delivery because fluid retention will likely be a problem.

(1:698), (13:121–122, 143), (15:804).

## IA1h

67. D. Pulmonary surfactant begins to appear in the lungs at about 22 to 24 weeks' gestation. Most of this surface active material is in storage, however, with little present in the alveolar lining layer. Pulmonary surfactant is synthesized and secreted by the alveolar type II cells, which comprise about 5% of the alveolar surface.

Lecithin and sphingomyelin are phospholipids that appear in the amniotic fluid in differing amounts and at different times during gestation. Sphingomyelin is the first of these two phospholipids to appear. Its concentration in the amniotic fluid remains relatively constant from about 18 to 34 weeks' gestation. On the contrary, lecithin shows up around 32 to 34 weeks' gestation. When the *lecithin/sphingomyelin* (L/S) ratio is at least 2:1, lung maturity is implied.

The L/S ratio is quite reliable in the absence of surfactant-deficiency disease. In pregnancies complicated by diabetes, for example, the L/S ratio is less reliable. A third phospholipid (i.e., phosphatidylglycerol [PG]) appears in the amniotic fluid at 35 to 36 weeks' gestation. The presence of PG in the amniotic fluid has increased the predictability of the L/S ratio determination.

(1:1001), (15:29), (18:6–7).

## IIIA1e

68. A. When a mechanical ventilator delivers a tidal volume to a patient, the peak inspiratory pressure (PIP) developed in the process consists of two pressures: (1) the pressure generated to overcome airway resistance and (2) the pressure developed to inflate the lungs. The pressure generated to overcome airway resistance ($P_{Raw}$) is the difference between the PIP and the plateau pressure ($P_{plateau}$). That is,

$$P_{Raw} = PIP - P_{plateau}$$

The pressure developed to inflate the lungs, or the $P_{plateau}$, is obtained by an inflation hold (inspiratory pause).

During mechanical ventilation of a patient, the changes in PIP, $P_{plateau}$, and $P_{Raw}$ provide information about the patient's lung status. The RRT can determine whether the patient's lung compliance changes, and whether the patient's airway resistance changes, or both.

Again, specifically, if the difference between the PIP and the $P_{plateau}$ widens, airway resistance has increased.

For example, if the $P_{plateau}$ remains constant as the PIP increases, the $P_{Raw}$ increases. Consequently, airway resistance increases.

If the pressure developed to inflate the lungs ($P_{plateau}$) increases, pulmonary compliance decreases (i.e., the lungs become more stiff).

(1:937), (10:256–257).

## IIIB2c

69. B. Pressure-control inverse-ratio ventilation (PC-IRV) is characterized by an inspiratory time longer than the expiratory time. In the process, inspiration begins before the previous exhalation ends. This inspiratory:expiratory (I:E) ratio is incompatible with spontaneous ventilation. Therefore, when PC-IRV is to be initiated, the patient must be sedated and paralyzed to accommodate this mode of ventilation.

An appropriate combination of medications to use is a benzodiazapine and a neuromuscular blocking agent. The benzodiazapine *diazapam* and the competitive neuromuscular blocking agent *pancuronium bromide* would effectively allow for PC-IRV.

(1:518–519, 827, 876), (10:156, 215–216, 278, 286–287).

## IIB2r

70. B. To check for chest-tube patency, the RRT should turn off the vacuum source. If the water level in the water-seal bottle fluctuates during the patient's ventilatory cycle, the chest tube is patent (Figure 2-23).

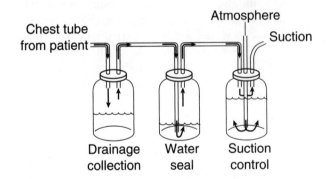

**Figure 2-23:** Three-bottle water-seal system.

However, if the water level in the water-seal bottle remains stationary, the chest tube is obstructed. The obstruction can usually be cleared by gently milking the chest tube from the point of its insertion at the chest wall toward the suction drainage bottle. Excessive subatmospheric pressures can be generated in the process, therefore this procedure must be performed carefully.

(1:482, 487), (15:1093–1094).

## IA1f(4)

71. B. When charting results of sputum induction, the RRT should note the following variables: (1) the volume of the sample, (2) the time the sample was obtained, (3) the consistency and viscosity of the sample, (4) whether or not the sputum is purulent, and (5) the absence or presence of blood in the sample.

The description of sputum relates to certain pulmonary diseases. For example, purulent green or yellow sputum is often found in pneumonia, cystic fibrosis, bronchitis, bronchiectasis, and lung abscess patients. Mucoid sputum is clear and characteristic of asthma. Fetid sputum is rank or foul in odor. Rancid also describes sputum that has an offensive odor.

(9:28, 112).

## IIIA1m(1)

72. A. The normal (room air) alveolar–arterial oxygen tension gradient [i.e., P(A-a)O$_2$] ranges from 8 mm Hg to 14 mm Hg. In the presence of 100% O$_2$, the P(A-a)O$_2$ ranges from 25 mm Hg to 65 mm Hg.

Three general pathophysiologic conditions are often responsible for the widening or increasing of the P(A-a)O$_2$: (1) alveolarcapillary membrane-diffusion defect, (2) ventilation–perfusion abnormalities, and (3) intrapulmonary shunting.

A number of pulmonary pathologies can adversely influence the alveolar-capillary membrane. For example, the pneumoconiosis silicosis caused by the inhalation of free silica, a fibrogenic dust, can result in a thickening of the alveolar-capillary membrane that will widen the P(A-a)O$_2$. Ventilation–perfusion defects are characterized by alveoli that are partially obstructed and receive compromised ventilation. These alveoli continue to receive pulmonary capillary blood flow, however. This type of ventilation–perfusion defect is termed *perfusion in excess of ventilation—or shunt effect* or *venous admixture*. This situation will also widen the room air P(A-a)O$_2$.

Finally, intrapulmonary shunting (specifically, capillary shunting) increases the P(A-a)O$_2$ because oxygen cannot enter unventilated alveoli and diffuse across the alveolar-capillary membrane to enter the pulmonary capillary blood.

The P(A-a)O$_2$ provides a means for estimating a patient's shunt fraction. For example, when a patient breathes an F$_1$O$_2$ of 1.00, a 1.0% shunt is estimated for every 10 mm Hg to 15 mm Hg P(A-a)O$_2$. Therefore, if a patient had an alveolar PO$_2$ of 465 mm Hg and an arterial PO$_2$ of 325 mm Hg, the estimated percent shunt would range from 9.3% to 14.0%. Note the following calculations:

STEP 1: Calculate the P(A-a)O$_2$.

$$P(A\text{-}a)O_2 = PAO_2 - PaO_2$$
$$= 465 \text{ mm Hg} - 325 \text{ mm Hg}$$
$$= 140 \text{ mm Hg}$$

STEP 2: Estimate the percent shunt.

$$\frac{140 \text{ mm Hg}}{15 \text{ mm Hg}} \sim 9.3\%$$

or

$$\frac{140 \text{ mm Hg}}{10 \text{ mm Hg}} = 14.0\%$$

Additionally, having the patient breathe an F$_1$O$_2$ of 1.00 often enables the clinician to determine the cause of the widened room air alveolar arterial oxygen tension gradient. Under most circumstances, the P(A-a)O$_2$ will decrease with the administration of 100% O$_2$ if the hypoxemia is caused by either ventilation–perfusion defects or by a diffusion impairment. In the face of intrapulmonary shunting, the P(A-a)O$_2$ will increase with the administration of 100% O$_2$.

(1:217, 234–235, 821, 929), (15:100–103, 945–946).

## IIIB2c

73. C. This patient has developed adult respiratory distress syndrome (ARDS). Near drowning is one of the etiologic factors associated with ARDS. In this condition, there often is a 12- to 48-hour latent period during which the patient appears to be making an uneventful recovery from the event that caused his hospitalization. Suddenly, as a result of pulmonary vascular permeability, the patient develops refractory hypoxemia. The presence of pulmonary infiltrates causes the inactivation of pulmonary surfactant, resulting in decreased lung compliance. The increased elastic recoil of the lung reduces the functional residual capacity (FRC) and produces an increased ventilatory rate. Chest radiography reveals diffuse pulmonary infiltrates (i.e., lung "whiteout").

PC-IRV would be an appropriate choice of mechanical ventilation because it would tend to increase the mean airway pressure ($\overline{P}_{aw}$). Improved oxygenation in ARDS has been linked to increased $\overline{P}_{aw}$. The increased $\overline{P}_{aw}$ helps increase the FRC, improve the distribution of ventilation, and decrease intrapulmonary shunting.

The Siemens Servo 900C has the capability of providing both PSV and PC-IRV.

(1:508–509, 516–518), (15:335, 956, 959, 961).

## IB2a

74. A. Patients with asthma sometimes display a sign called *paradoxical pulse* or *pulsus paradoxicus*. This sign is identified when the patient's systolic blood pressure during exhalation is greater than during inspiration (by 10 torr or more).

Normally, the strength of a spontaneously breathing person's pulse decreases during inspiration. When the strength of the pulse diminishes substantially during spontaneous breathing, pulsus paradoxicus might be present.

(1:290, 304, 308), (9:258–260), (15:265, 675).

## IB6a

75. D. Evaluation of a patient's sensorium or mental status involves four components: (1) level of consciousness, (2) orientation to time and place, (3) emotional state, and (4) cooperation. Each of these aspects of a patient's mental status has a number of components.

The different levels of consciousness include alertness, confusion, lethargy, and comatose. A patient is oriented to time and place if he accurately responds to questions referring to the date and his location. The patient's emotional state can be evaluated by asking the patient to explain and describe how he feels. At the same time, the RRT must closely observe and record the patient's physical response to questioning.

The patient's ability to perform therapeutic maneuvers or diagnostic procedures can be assessed by determining and observing the patient's ability to follow instructions.

(1:301–302), (9:54–55, 270–271), (15:423).

## IIIC3a

76. D. The total delivered flow rate from the all-purpose nebulizer set at 50% oxygen operating at 15 L/min. is 40.5 L/min. This total delivered flow rate is based on an air–oxygen ratio of 1.7:1 for 50% oxygen. The patient would be receiving 25.5 L/min. of air and 15 L/min. of oxygen, hence a total flow rate of 40.5 L/min.

The total delivered flow rate provided by the two all-purpose nebulizers, both set at 50% and operating at 15 L/min., would be twice the original setup. Hence, 40.5 L/min. plus 40.5 L/min. would render a total delivered flow rate of 81 L/min. This arrangement would more than meet the patient's estimated inspiratory flow rate of $4 \times \dot{V}_E$, or $4 \times 14.9$ L/min.

The gas-injected nebulizer (GIN) would provide 22 L/min. of oxygen and 37 L/min. of air for a total delivered flow rate of 59 L/min. This setup would closely meet the patient's estimated inspiratory flow requirements of almost 60 L/min.

(5:146–148), (15:879, 882–883).

## IIB2n(2)

77. C. When the pulmonary artery catheter (PAC) transducer is zeroed, it must be set at the patient's phlebostatic axis. The phlebostatic axis is the mid-chest along the anterior axillary line (level of the right atrium). Once the PAC transducer is zeroed in this position, it must not be moved. For example, if it is moved below the phlebostatic axis after zeroing, the hemodynamic measurements will be erroneously high. The converse is likewise true.

(14:165–170, 296).

## IIIA1a

78. D. During an asthma attack, air trapping is a significant problem, causing alterations in the ventilation–perfusion ratio and adversely affecting the patient's arterial blood gas results. Because of the increased airway resistance ($R_{aw}$), expiratory times are prolonged. Because the airways are more narrowed from the mucosal edema, increased secretions, and bronchoconstriction associated with the asthmatic attack, however, air trapping occurs and exhalation is incomplete.

Research has shown that an expiratory time of 4 tau ($\tau$) ventilation time constant is necessary to assure adequate emptying of the lungs. Because $\tau$ is calculated by multiplying the patient's $R_{aw}$ by his compliance ($C_{LT}$), factors that will increase the $R_{aw}$ or $C_{LT}$ will compromise the lungs' capability to return to their normal FRC. Air trapping will result in an increased FRC, flattened hemidiaphragms, and increased intercostal spaces. The chest X-ray might be normal, however.

Additional signs and symptoms of an acute asthma attack include wheezing, use of accessory muscles, pulsus paradoxus, sinus tachycardia, and premature ventricular complexes.

When hyperaeration (air trapping) is present, the intercostal spaces widen. Therefore, if the bronchodilator was effective, the bronchoconstriction would be relieved and the air trapping would be reduced. By reducing the air trapping, the intercostal spaces will tend to retract (i.e., normalize).

(10:37–38, 358), (15:215–217), (17:320–324).

## IIIE1g

79. D. Protriptyline, a tricyclic antidepressant, has shown to decrease the rate of occurrence of apneic episodes

associated with obstructive sleep apnea. Naloxone (narcotic antagonist) reverses the activity of morphine and is used for the reversal of respiratory depression in newborns. Pyridostigmine (Mestinon) is an anticholinesterase medication used to treat myasthenia gravis. Aminophylline (methylxanthine) is a bronchodilator via phosphodiesterase inhibition. Aminophylline, which is primarily theophylline, has generalized central nervous system effects.

(8:149, 353, 357), (15:752).

## IIIC5

80. B. This patient exhibits the signs and symptoms of bacterial pneumonia. In addition to identifying the microorganism so that the appropriate antibiotic can be prescribed, treatment should be directed toward bronchial hygiene and oxygenation.

The best response here was to administer continuous aerosol therapy to facilitate secretion removal along with CPT. An $FIO_2$ of 0.30 appears to be a reasonable starting point based on arterial blood gas (ABG) data.

CPAP, in conjunction with bronchopulmonary hygiene techniques, is another therapeutic approach, as is the inclusion of incentive spirometry. In the case described, however, CPAP does not seem to be indicated because oxygenation is not that bad. I.V. fluids are also indicated in pneumonia.

(15:345–348).

## IIIC5

81. B. The patient here is presumed to be in the Trendelenburg position (head down at a 45-degree angle) on his stomach for the drainage of the posterior basal segments. Because the patient is complaining of difficulty breathing (dyspnea), the RRT should stop the therapy and place the patient in a position enabling him to "catch" his breath. Once the patient feels ready to resume the treatment, the RRT should modify the position. Perhaps the patient might tolerate a less acute angle, or maybe the patient should be placed flat on his stomach.

(1:799), (*Respiratory Care* 36:1418–1426, 1991).

## IIIA1e

82. C. All volume-pressure loops have at least two inflection points. Generally, one occurs during inspiration and the other occurs during exhalation. An inflection point usually is present as a distinct alteration in the slope of each line. In this problem, the inflection points are easily discerned as point D during inspiration and point B during exhalation as shown in Figure 2-24.

If an inflection point is difficult to identify, drawing lines along relatively straight segments of the inspiratory and expiratory limbs provides for its identifica-

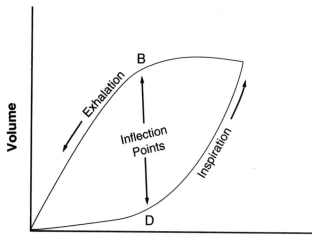

**Figure 2-24:** Volume-pressure loop demonstrating two inflection points B and D.

tion. The inflection point in such cases approximately resides where the drawn lines intersect. Figure 2-25 illustrates how to locate less obvious inflection points.

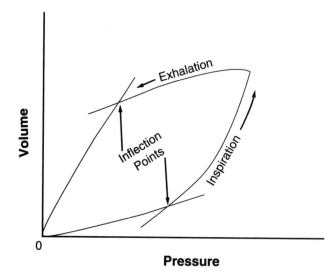

**Figure 2-25:** Volume-pressure loop illustrating the method for identifying inflection point location.

Inflection points are believed to represent alveolar recruitment during inspiration and alveolar derecruitment during exhalation.

(9:289).

## IA1f(3)

83. B. The mean airway pressure ($\overline{P}_{aw}$) is the pressure throughout the airways from the beginning of one inspiration to the start of the ensuing inspiration. Ordinarily, increases in the $\overline{P}_{aw}$ improve oxygenation.

Sizable increases in the $\bar{P}_{aw}$, however, are associated with the occurrence of barotrauma.

A number of factors influence the $\bar{P}_{aw}$: (1) the peak inspiratory pressure (PIP), (2) the inspiratory time ($T_I$), (3) the ventilatory rate (f), and (4) positive end-expiratory pressure (PEEP).

The formula used to calculate the $\bar{P}_{aw}$ is as follows:

$$\bar{P}_{aw} = K(PIP - PEEP)(T_I \div TCT) + PEEP$$

where

$\bar{P}_{aw}$ = mean airway pressure (cm $H_2O$)

*K = waveform constant

PIP = peak inspiratory pressure (cm $H_2O$)

PEEP = positive end-expiratory pressure (cm $H_2O$)

$T_I$ = inspiratory time (sec.)

TCT = total cycle time (sec.)

(10:144–147) (17:136–137).

*K equals 0.5 for triangular pressure waveform, whereas K equals 1.0 for a rectangular pressure waveform.

## IC2i

84. C. The pressure waveform illustrated here demonstrates the initiation of an inspiratory hold maneuver during IPPV (Figure 2-26).

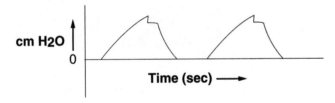

**Figure 2-26:** Pressure waveform.

This technique simulates a breath-holding maneuver, and is intended to "hold" the air in the lungs at end inspiration. This maneuver improves the distribution of the inspired gas throughout the lungs.

When an inspiratory hold is instituted, the pressure manometer on the ventilator indicates the plateau or static pressure. This pressure represents the pressure developed to maintain the lungs inflated with the tidal volume just delivered. Other terms synonymous with inspiratory hold are *inflation hold, inspiratory pause,* and *end-inspiratory pause.*

(1:845, 879), (10:85, 146, 213), (15:968, 975).

## IB7E

85. C. A variety of fluid types can collect in the intrapleural space. These fluids include exudates, transudates, blood, chyle, and pus.

The appearance of a pleural effusion on a chest X-ray will depend on the amount of fluid present in the intrapleural space. The appearance can range from blunting of the costophrenic angle and the meniscus sign for small-volume pleural effusions to "whiteout" on the affected side and obscuring of the hemidiaphragm for large fluid volumes in the intrapleural space.

In the absence of loculation and adhesions causing intrapleural fluid trapping, placing the patient on the involved side will cause the fluid to shift to the most gravity-dependent area of the thorax. This radiologic view is termed the *lateral decubitus* view. Note the lateral decubitus view shown in the radiograph (Figure 2-27) on page 76.

The lateral decubitus radiograph presented there is a large volume pleural effusion; therefore, the "whiteout" is on the gravity-dependent side. By having the patient lie on the affected side, the pleural effusion has shifted, as evidenced again by the "whiteout" on the gravity-dependent side. The fact that the effusion has shifted because the patient assumed this position indicates that loculations and adhesions are lacking. The hemidiaphragm on the affected side is also obliterated.

(1:406, 477–481).

## IIIE2b

86. A. Metered dose inhalers (MDIs) are subject to incorrect use. Controversy exists concerning a number of aspects related to the technique for using an MDI.

One of the issues concerns the lung volume at which an MDI should be actuated. Some clinicians favor MDI activation at high lung volumes. Others propose its actuation at low lung volumes. The generally accepted volume deemed appropriate for MDI actuation is at FRC.

(1:689), (5:147), (15:810–811).

## IIIA1m

87. A. Based on the cardiovascular data presented, the stroke volume, CI, and mixed-venous oxygen would be decreased in this situation.

By rearranging the formula generally used for calculating the C.O., one can calculate the stroke volume (SV). For example,

$$SV = \frac{C.O.}{HR}$$

After converting the C.O. to ml/min. (4.1 L/min. × 1,000 ml/liter = 4,100 ml/min.), the SV is

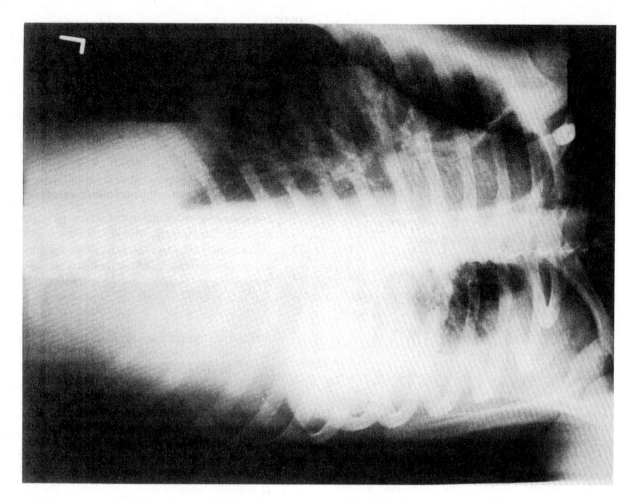

**Figure 2-27:** Lateral decubitis radiographic view of pleural effusion, demonstrating "whiteout" on the gravity-dependent side. The hemidiaphragm on the affected side is obliterated.

$$SV = \frac{4,100 \text{ ml/min}}{115 \text{ beats/min}}$$

$$= 36 \text{ ml/beat}$$

Normal SV ranges between 50 and 80. The cardiac index CI is determined as shown:

$$CI = \frac{C.O.}{\text{body surface area (BSA)}}$$

$$= \frac{4.1 \text{ L/min.}}{2.3 \text{ m}^2}$$

$$= 1.78 \text{ L/min./m}^2$$

A normal CI ranges between 2.8 and 4.5 L/min./m$^2$.

Based on the following Fick equation, mixed venous oxygen ($C\bar{v}O_2$) decreases when the C.O. ($\dot{Q}_T$) decreases if the oxygen consumption ($\dot{V}O_2$) and the arterial oxygen level ($CaO_2$) remain constant:

$$\dot{Q}_T = \frac{\dot{V}O_2}{CaO_2 - C\bar{v}O_2}$$

Rearranging to solve for the mixed venous oxygen content,

$$C\bar{v}O_2 = CaO_2 - \frac{\dot{V}O_2}{\dot{Q}_T}$$

By applying two sets of values to this rearranged Fick equation, one can numerically evidence what has been stated here qualitatively. For example, using normal values for the factors involved,

$\dot{V}O_2$: 250 ml/min.

$\dot{Q}_T$: 5 L/min. or 5,000 ml/min.

$CaO_2$: 20 vol% (20 ml $O_2$/100 ml plasma)

Then, solving for the $C\bar{v}O_2$,

$$C\bar{v}O_2 = \left(\frac{20\ ml}{100\ ml}\right) - \left(\frac{250\ ml/min.}{5,000\ ml/min.}\right)$$

$$= 0.20 - 0.05$$

$$= 0.15\ or\ 15\ vol\%\ or\ 15\ ml\ O_2/100\ ml\ plasma$$

What would be the effect on the $C\bar{v}O_2$ if the $\dot{Q}_T$ was halved (2.5 L/min. or 2,500 ml/min.) while the $\dot{V}O_2$ and $CaO_2$ remained constant?

$$C\bar{v}O_2 = \left(\frac{20\ ml}{100\ ml}\right) - \left(\frac{250\ ml/min.}{2,500\ ml/min.}\right)$$

$$= 0.20 - 0.10$$

$$= 0.10\ or\ 10\ vol\%\ or\ 10\ ml\ O_2/100\ ml\ plasma$$

As the $\dot{V}O_2$ and $CaO_2$ remained constant and as the $\dot{Q}_T$ was halved, the $C\bar{v}O_2$ decreased. Notice also that the $CaO_2 - C\bar{v}O_2$ doubled when the $\dot{Q}_T$ was halved.

(1:225–226, 930), (14:326), (17:58, 87, 135).

### IB8a

88. D. Epiglottitis and croup are two frequent causes of airway obstruction in infants and small children. Epiglottitis is caused by a bacterial infection of the supraglottic area, whereas croup is caused by a viral infection of the subglottic region. Because the caliber of an infant's or a small child's airway is relatively narrow compared with that of an adult, acute epiglottitis is potentially a life-threatening airway obstruction.

Characterized by abrupt onset, stridor, and dysphagia, acute epiglottitis demands a rapid diagnosis and the immediate establishment of an artificial airway. A lateral neck X-ray illustrating a broad, flat epiglottis which appears as the size of an adult's thumb confirms the diagnosis. Until an airway is established, pharyngeal examination, positioning the patient supine, or other diagnostic procedures are contraindicated because they can result in total airway occlusion.

(1:1038–1040), (18:196–201).

### IIIB2c

89. C. An increase in the pressure-control level to 25 cm $H_2O$ should increase the tidal volume and decrease the $PaCO_2$ without overinflation at this patient's lung compliance. An arterial $PO_2$ of 62 torr at an $FIO_2$ of 0.50 does not indicate the need to increase the PEEP.

(1:827, 875–876), (10:198–199, 214–215), (15:995).

### IIID1b

90. A. Left ventricular failure is often pharmacologically treated with cardiac glycosides, diuretics, antihypertensives (e.g., angiotensin converting enzyme [ACE] inhibitors), and antidysrhythmics. Cardiac glycosides (e.g., digoxin) have a positive inotropic effect. Positive inotropism refers to the drug's ability to strengthen the myocardial contractility. Diuretics such as furosemide (Lasix) help maintain body-fluid balance by causing the excretion of urine. Numerous antihypertensive medications are available to normalize the blood pressure. These drugs include (1) diuretics, (2) central-acting anti-adrenergics, (3) peripherally acting anti-adrenergics, (4) beta-adrenergic blockers, (5) alpha- and beta-adrenergic blockers, (6) direct-acting vasodilators, and (7) ACE inhibitors.

Antidysrhythmics are sometimes used to reduce myocardial irritability. Cardiac stimulants and anticoagulants are sometimes included in the pharmacologic management of left-ventricular failure.

(14:296–297, 412–417, 429–430).

### IIIE1k

91. C. Whenever a mixed-venous blood sample is obtained from a pulmonary artery catheter, the syringe is attached to the distal channel or distal injection port.

Because the pulmonary artery catheter tip generally rests near the vicinity where gas exchange is occurring, caution must be taken against aspirating the sample too rapidly. Rapid sample aspiration increases the potential for diluting venous blood with arterialized pulmonary capillary blood, yielding a blood sample that has erroneously high oxygenation levels. When patients are receiving positive pressure ventilation with a high $FIO_2$, this situation is especially true. The recommended rate of withdrawal is less than 3 cc/min.

(14:277), (15:534).

### IIB1q(1)

92. D. Whenever the pulmonary capillary wedge-pressure (PCWP) waveform becomes nonphasic, the balloon needs to be deflated immediately. The appearance of a nonphasic PCWP waveform can indicate that the balloon is overinflated or eccentrically inflated (with the balloon extending over the catheter's tip).

The potential hazard associated with balloon tip overinflation or eccentric inflation is the rupture of the pulmonary artery. Although this complication is rare, it has a high mortality rate.

The following situations and conditions have a higher risk for pulmonary artery rupture: (1) anticoagulation therapy, (2) pulmonary hypertension, (3) cardiopulmonary bypass, and (4) advanced age (generally older than 60 years).

(14:310), (15:537).

## IIIE1l

93. D. Pancuronium bromide (Pavulon), gallamine triethiodide (Flaxedil), and tubocurarine chloride (*d*-tubocurarine) are classified as nondepolarizing neuromuscular blocking agents or competitive blockers. These medications paralyze muscles by competing for acetylcholine at the receptor sites on the postsynaptic membrane at the neuromuscular junction.

Succinylcholine chloride (Anectine) is a depolarizing neuromuscular blocking agent. Depolarization of the muscle membrane occurs, thus preventing muscle stimulation. The postsynaptic membrane is maintained in a refractory state.

(2:592–593), (8:299), (15:230).

## IIIA1e

94. A. The small loop near the origin of the volume-pressure loop represents a patient-assisted, or triggered, positive pressure breath. The more sensitive the ventilator, the less the small curved line projects to the left (because once inspiration is triggered, the curve travels rightward and into the positive pressure range to the right of the *y*-axis). The area to the left of the *y*-axis represents negative or subatmospheric pressure.

If the small curve representing patient effort required to trigger the ventilator is large and deflected far to the left, the patient is being required to generate excessive subatmospheric pressure to trigger the ventilator.

(10:49).

## IIID1b

95. D. The dysrhythmia showing on the cardiac monitor is ventricular tachycardia. The rapid rate (greater than 200 beats/min.) associated with this dysrhythmia results in a decreased C.O. It represents a life-threatening situation and must be treated immediately. Treatment can include lidocaine, procainamide, or bretylium, which are antidysrhythmic medications. If the antidysrhythmic drug given fails to convert the ventricular tachycardia to a normal sinus rhythm, immediate defibrillation is warranted.

Ventricular tachycardia is generally preceded by premature ventricular contractions (PVCs). Actually, a run of three or more consecutive PVCs constitutes ventricular tachycardia. PVCs often indicate that the myocardium is in a heightened state of excitability.

(1:652).

## IIIA1h

96. B. During T-piece ventilator weaning trials, patients frequently become fatigued and require additional time on the mechanical ventilator. T-piece trials entail removing the patient from mechanical ventilation for progressively longer times. Each time the patient demonstrates signs of fatigue, mechanical ventilation is reinstituted. Eventually, the patient assumes more and more responsibility for his own work of breathing and becomes weaned from mechanical ventilation.

(1:976–977), (10:331–332).

## IIB2h(4)

97. B. The $PCO_2$ electrode has a normal range of $\pm 2$ standard deviations from the mean. The mean is 40 torr, and each standard deviation is equivalent to 1 torr. Therefore, when a quality-control solution is injected into the $PCO_2$ electrode, the acceptable range is 38 to 42 torr. Any value less than 38 torr or greater than 42 torr with the control solution represents a situation that is out of control.

In this instance, however, analysis of the second quality-control check resulted in a datum point below 2 standard deviations from the mean. The analyzed control sample produced a $PCO_2$ value of 37 torr, which is 3 standard deviations from the mean. Because the other four quality-control checks were in control, the second analysis represents a random error and probably can be disregarded.

Protein contamination of the electrode and electrode aging cause trending, whereas air bubbles beneath the electrode membrane can produce shifting.

(1:351–352), (5:310–312), (6:311–314).

## IIIC8a

98. C. A bronchopleural fistula is a form of barotrauma characterized by the development of a communication between the intrapleural space and the lung parenchyma. When this condition develops while a patient is receiving conventional mechanical ventilation, significant portions of the delivered volume can be lost, thereby further compromising lung inflation. Therefore, the patient will likely experience deteriorating $\dot{V}_A/\dot{Q}_C$ ratios and suffer progressive atelectasis.

High-frequency jet ventilation (HFJV) is associated with low peak inspiratory pressure (PIP) and small tidal volumes ($V_T$). Consequently, in the face of a bronchopleural fistula, the airway pressures that develop tend to be low. It is likely that the airway pressures developed with HFJV will be less than the critical opening pressure of the bronchopleural fistula. As a result, more ventilation will enter the lungs and less will escape through the fistula. As long as the PIP remains less than the critical opening pressure of the bronchopleural fistula, air will flow to the lungs and none will be lost through the fistula.

(1:1023 Box 43–8), (10:368–369).

## IA1g(2)

99. B. Normal mean pulmonary capillary wedge pressure (PCWP) is between 6 and 12 torr, and normal central venous pressure (CVP) is between 1 and 7 torr. In this patient, both the mean PCWP (30 torr) and CVP (13 torr) are high, which is consistent with the development of left-ventricular failure. Pulmonary artery pressures (PAP) are likewise high, indicating pulmonary vascular engorgement. The mean PAP is:

$$PAP = \frac{48 \text{ torr} + (2)20 \text{ torr}}{3}$$
$$= 29.3 \text{ torr}$$

Normal mean PAP is between 10 and 22 torr.

Furthermore, auscultation of the lungs reveals bilateral, late inspiratory crackles, which lends further evidence to the existence of fluid in the lungs and the presence of pulmonary edema caused by the left ventricular failure.

(1:948), (9:348, 349–352).

## IIIB1c

100. B. Numerous criteria are used to evaluate a patient's readiness for extubation. The primary criterion for extubation is the resolution of the cause for the patient being intubated and ventilated in the first place.

The patient in this question complies with the following measures used to assess a patient's readiness for extubation:

1) $PaO_2$ 80 torr on an $F_IO_2$ of 0.30 and $SaO_2$ of 94% (CRITERION: $PaO_2 > 60$ torr or an $SaO_2 > 90\%$ on an $F_IO_2$ of $\leq 0.50$ with no PEEP)
2) positive gag reflex (patient has an airway protection mechanism; minimal risk for aspiration exists)
3) positive cuff-leak test (patient has minimal risk of an upper-airway obstruction)
4) patient is capable of raising his head off the bed (patient has an airway protection mechanism; minimal risk for aspiration exists)
5) patient is alert and coughing deeply while suctioned (patient has the ability to adequately clear pulmonary secretions)

(1:612–613).

# References

1. Scanlan, C., Spearman, C., and Sheldon, R., *Egan's Fundamentals of Respiratory Care*, 7th ed., Mosby, Inc., St. Louis, MO, 1999.

2. Kacmarek, R., Mack, C., and Dimas, S., *The Essentials of Respiratory Care*, 3rd ed., Mosby-Year Book, Inc., St. Louis, MO, 1990.

3. Shapiro B., Peruzzi, W., and Kozlowska-Templin, R., *Clinical Applications of Blood Gases*, 5th ed., Mosby-Year Book, Inc., St. Louis, MO, 1994.

4. Malley, W., *Clinical Blood Gases: Application and Noninvasive Alternatives*, W.B. Saunders Co., Philadelphia, PA, 1990.

5. White, G., *Equipment Theory for Respiratory Care*, 3rd ed., Delmar Publishers, Inc., Albany, NY, 1999.

6. Ruppel, G., *Manual of Pulmonary Function Testing*, 7th ed., Mosby-Year Book, Inc., St. Louis, MO, 1998.

7. Barnes, T., *Core Textbook of Respiratory Care Practice*, 2nd ed., Mosby-Year Book, Inc., St. Louis, MO, 1994.

8. Rau, J., *Respiratory Care Pharmacology*, 5th ed., Mosby-Year Book, Inc., St. Louis, MO, 1998.

9. Wilkins, R., Sheldon, R., and Krider, S., *Clinical Assessment in Respiratory Care*, 4th ed., Mosby, St. Louis, MO, 2000.

10. Pilbeam, S., *Mechanical Ventilation: Physiological and Clinical Applications*, 3rd ed., Mosby-Year Book, Inc., St. Louis, MO, 1998.

11. Madama, V., *Pulmonary Function Testing and Cardiopulmonary Stress Testing*, 2nd ed., Delmar Publishers, Inc., Albany, NY, 1998.

12. Koff, P., Eitzman, D., and New, J., *Neonatal and Pediatric Respiratory Care*, 2nd ed., Mosby-Year Book, Inc., St. Louis, MO, 1993.

13. Branson, R., Hess, D., and Chatburn, R., *Respiratory Care Equipment*, J.B. Lippincott, Co., Philadelphia, PA, 1995.

14. Darovic, G., *Hemodynamic Monitoring: Invasive and Noninvasive Clinical Application*, 2nd ed., W.B. Saunders Company, Philadelphia, PA, 1995.

15. Pierson, D, and Kacmarek, R., *Foundations of Respiratory Care*, Churchill Livingston, Inc., New York, NY, 1992.

16. Burton, et al., *Respiratory Care: A Guide to Clinical Practice*, 4th ed., Lippincott-Raven Publishers, Philadelphia, PA, 1997.

17. Wojciechowski, W., *Respiratory Care Sciences: An Integrated Approach*, 3rd ed., Delmar Publishers, Inc., Albany, NY, 2000.

18. Aloan, C., *Respiratory Care of the Newborn and Child*, 2nd ed., Lippincott-Raven Publishers, Philadelphia, PA, 1997.

19. Dantzker, D., MacIntyre, N., and Bakow, E., *Comprehensive Respiratory Care*, W.B. Saunders Company, Philadelphia, PA, 1998.

20. Farzan, S., and Farzan, D., *A Concise Handbook of Respiratory Diseases*, 4th ed., Appleton & Lange, Stamford, CT, 1997.

**PURPOSE:** This chapter consists of 212 items intended to assess your understanding and comprehension of subject matter contained in the clinical data portion of the Written Registry Examination. In this chapter, you are required to answer questions regarding the following activities:

A. Reviewing patient records and recommending diagnostic procedures
B. Collecting and evaluating clinical information
C. Performing procedures and interpreting results, determining the appropriateness of and participating in developing and recommending modifications to the respiratory care plan.

> **NOTE:** Please refer to the examination matrix key located at the end of this chapter. This examination matrix key will enable you to identify the specific areas in the Clinical Data section of the Written Registry Examination Matrix that require remediation, based on your performance on the test items in this chapter.

Use the answer sheet located at the front of this chapter to record your answers as you work through questions relating to clinical data.

Remember to study the analyses that follow the questions in this chapter. The purpose of each analysis is to present you with the rationale for the correct answer (and in many instances, reasons are given for why the distractors are incorrect). The references at the end of each analysis provide you with resources to seek more information regarding each question and its associated Written Registry Examination Matrix item.

You are *not* expected, or even recommended, to attempt to complete this chapter in one sitting because of the large number of questions located here. Rather, you are encouraged to work at your own pace and answer however many questions you feel comfortable completing. As a suggestion, you might consider completing this chapter in four sessions (i.e., 53 questions and analyses at a time).

The following timetable might assist you:

SESSION 1: 1 to 53 questions, analyses, and matrix items
SESSION 2: 54 to 106 questions, analyses, and matrix items
SESSION 3: 107 to 159 questions, analyses, and matrix items
SESSION 4: 160 to 212 questions, analyses, and matrix items

# Clinical Data Answer Sheet

**DIRECTIONS:** Darken the space under the selected answer.

| | A | B | C | D | | | A | B | C | D |
|---|---|---|---|---|---|---|---|---|---|---|
| 1. | ❏ | ❏ | ❏ | ❏ | | 25. | ❏ | ❏ | ❏ | ❏ |
| 2. | ❏ | ❏ | ❏ | ❏ | | 26. | ❏ | ❏ | ❏ | ❏ |
| 3. | ❏ | ❏ | ❏ | ❏ | | 27. | ❏ | ❏ | ❏ | ❏ |
| 4. | ❏ | ❏ | ❏ | ❏ | | 28. | ❏ | ❏ | ❏ | ❏ |
| 5. | ❏ | ❏ | ❏ | ❏ | | 29. | ❏ | ❏ | ❏ | ❏ |
| 6. | ❏ | ❏ | ❏ | ❏ | | 30. | ❏ | ❏ | ❏ | ❏ |
| 7. | ❏ | ❏ | ❏ | ❏ | | 31. | ❏ | ❏ | ❏ | ❏ |
| 8. | ❏ | ❏ | ❏ | ❏ | | 32. | ❏ | ❏ | ❏ | ❏ |
| 9. | ❏ | ❏ | ❏ | ❏ | | 33. | ❏ | ❏ | ❏ | ❏ |
| 10. | ❏ | ❏ | ❏ | ❏ | | 34. | ❏ | ❏ | ❏ | ❏ |
| 11. | ❏ | ❏ | ❏ | ❏ | | 35. | ❏ | ❏ | ❏ | ❏ |
| 12. | ❏ | ❏ | ❏ | ❏ | | 36. | ❏ | ❏ | ❏ | ❏ |
| 13. | ❏ | ❏ | ❏ | ❏ | | 37. | ❏ | ❏ | ❏ | ❏ |
| 14. | ❏ | ❏ | ❏ | ❏ | | 38. | ❏ | ❏ | ❏ | ❏ |
| 15. | ❏ | ❏ | ❏ | ❏ | | 39. | ❏ | ❏ | ❏ | ❏ |
| 16. | ❏ | ❏ | ❏ | ❏ | | 40. | ❏ | ❏ | ❏ | ❏ |
| 17. | ❏ | ❏ | ❏ | ❏ | | 41. | ❏ | ❏ | ❏ | ❏ |
| 18. | ❏ | ❏ | ❏ | ❏ | | 42. | ❏ | ❏ | ❏ | ❏ |
| 19. | ❏ | ❏ | ❏ | ❏ | | 43. | ❏ | ❏ | ❏ | ❏ |
| 20. | ❏ | ❏ | ❏ | ❏ | | 44. | ❏ | ❏ | ❏ | ❏ |
| 21. | ❏ | ❏ | ❏ | ❏ | | 45. | ❏ | ❏ | ❏ | ❏ |
| 22. | ❏ | ❏ | ❏ | ❏ | | 46. | ❏ | ❏ | ❏ | ❏ |
| 23. | ❏ | ❏ | ❏ | ❏ | | 47. | ❏ | ❏ | ❏ | ❏ |
| 24. | ❏ | ❏ | ❏ | ❏ | | 48. | ❏ | ❏ | ❏ | ❏ |

|      | A | B | C | D |      |      | A | B | C | D |
|------|---|---|---|---|------|------|---|---|---|---|
| 49.  | ❑ | ❑ | ❑ | ❑ | 78.  | ❑ | ❑ | ❑ | ❑ |
| 50.  | ❑ | ❑ | ❑ | ❑ | 79.  | ❑ | ❑ | ❑ | ❑ |
| 51.  | ❑ | ❑ | ❑ | ❑ | 80.  | ❑ | ❑ | ❑ | ❑ |
| 52.  | ❑ | ❑ | ❑ | ❑ | 81.  | ❑ | ❑ | ❑ | ❑ |
| 53.  | ❑ | ❑ | ❑ | ❑ | 82.  | ❑ | ❑ | ❑ | ❑ |
| 54.  | ❑ | ❑ | ❑ | ❑ | 83.  | ❑ | ❑ | ❑ | ❑ |
| 55.  | ❑ | ❑ | ❑ | ❑ | 84.  | ❑ | ❑ | ❑ | ❑ |
| 56.  | ❑ | ❑ | ❑ | ❑ | 85.  | ❑ | ❑ | ❑ | ❑ |
| 57.  | ❑ | ❑ | ❑ | ❑ | 86.  | ❑ | ❑ | ❑ | ❑ |
| 58.  | ❑ | ❑ | ❑ | ❑ | 87.  | ❑ | ❑ | ❑ | ❑ |
| 59.  | ❑ | ❑ | ❑ | ❑ | 88.  | ❑ | ❑ | ❑ | ❑ |
| 60.  | ❑ | ❑ | ❑ | ❑ | 89.  | ❑ | ❑ | ❑ | ❑ |
| 61.  | ❑ | ❑ | ❑ | ❑ | 90.  | ❑ | ❑ | ❑ | ❑ |
| 62.  | ❑ | ❑ | ❑ | ❑ | 91.  | ❑ | ❑ | ❑ | ❑ |
| 63.  | ❑ | ❑ | ❑ | ❑ | 92.  | ❑ | ❑ | ❑ | ❑ |
| 64.  | ❑ | ❑ | ❑ | ❑ | 93.  | ❑ | ❑ | ❑ | ❑ |
| 65.  | ❑ | ❑ | ❑ | ❑ | 94.  | ❑ | ❑ | ❑ | ❑ |
| 66.  | ❑ | ❑ | ❑ | ❑ | 95.  | ❑ | ❑ | ❑ | ❑ |
| 67.  | ❑ | ❑ | ❑ | ❑ | 96.  | ❑ | ❑ | ❑ | ❑ |
| 68.  | ❑ | ❑ | ❑ | ❑ | 97.  | ❑ | ❑ | ❑ | ❑ |
| 69.  | ❑ | ❑ | ❑ | ❑ | 98.  | ❑ | ❑ | ❑ | ❑ |
| 70.  | ❑ | ❑ | ❑ | ❑ | 99.  | ❑ | ❑ | ❑ | ❑ |
| 71.  | ❑ | ❑ | ❑ | ❑ | 100. | ❑ | ❑ | ❑ | ❑ |
| 72.  | ❑ | ❑ | ❑ | ❑ | 101. | ❑ | ❑ | ❑ | ❑ |
| 73.  | ❑ | ❑ | ❑ | ❑ | 102. | ❑ | ❑ | ❑ | ❑ |
| 74.  | ❑ | ❑ | ❑ | ❑ | 103. | ❑ | ❑ | ❑ | ❑ |
| 75.  | ❑ | ❑ | ❑ | ❑ | 104. | ❑ | ❑ | ❑ | ❑ |
| 76.  | ❑ | ❑ | ❑ | ❑ | 105. | ❑ | ❑ | ❑ | ❑ |
| 77.  | ❑ | ❑ | ❑ | ❑ | 106. | ❑ | ❑ | ❑ | ❑ |

|      | A | B | C | D |      | A | B | C | D |
|------|---|---|---|---|------|---|---|---|---|
| 107. | ❏ | ❏ | ❏ | ❏ | 136. | ❏ | ❏ | ❏ | ❏ |
| 108. | ❏ | ❏ | ❏ | ❏ | 137. | ❏ | ❏ | ❏ | ❏ |
| 109. | ❏ | ❏ | ❏ | ❏ | 138. | ❏ | ❏ | ❏ | ❏ |
| 110. | ❏ | ❏ | ❏ | ❏ | 139. | ❏ | ❏ | ❏ | ❏ |
| 111. | ❏ | ❏ | ❏ | ❏ | 140. | ❏ | ❏ | ❏ | ❏ |
| 112. | ❏ | ❏ | ❏ | ❏ | 141. | ❏ | ❏ | ❏ | ❏ |
| 113. | ❏ | ❏ | ❏ | ❏ | 142. | ❏ | ❏ | ❏ | ❏ |
| 114. | ❏ | ❏ | ❏ | ❏ | 143. | ❏ | ❏ | ❏ | ❏ |
| 115. | ❏ | ❏ | ❏ | ❏ | 144. | ❏ | ❏ | ❏ | ❏ |
| 116. | ❏ | ❏ | ❏ | ❏ | 145. | ❏ | ❏ | ❏ | ❏ |
| 117. | ❏ | ❏ | ❏ | ❏ | 146. | ❏ | ❏ | ❏ | ❏ |
| 118. | ❏ | ❏ | ❏ | ❏ | 147. | ❏ | ❏ | ❏ | ❏ |
| 119. | ❏ | ❏ | ❏ | ❏ | 148. | ❏ | ❏ | ❏ | ❏ |
| 120. | ❏ | ❏ | ❏ | ❏ | 149. | ❏ | ❏ | ❏ | ❏ |
| 121. | ❏ | ❏ | ❏ | ❏ | 150. | ❏ | ❏ | ❏ | ❏ |
| 122. | ❏ | ❏ | ❏ | ❏ | 151. | ❏ | ❏ | ❏ | ❏ |
| 123. | ❏ | ❏ | ❏ | ❏ | 152. | ❏ | ❏ | ❏ | ❏ |
| 124. | ❏ | ❏ | ❏ | ❏ | 153. | ❏ | ❏ | ❏ | ❏ |
| 125. | ❏ | ❏ | ❏ | ❏ | 154. | ❏ | ❏ | ❏ | ❏ |
| 126. | ❏ | ❏ | ❏ | ❏ | 155. | ❏ | ❏ | ❏ | ❏ |
| 127. | ❏ | ❏ | ❏ | ❏ | 156. | ❏ | ❏ | ❏ | ❏ |
| 128. | ❏ | ❏ | ❏ | ❏ | 157. | ❏ | ❏ | ❏ | ❏ |
| 129. | ❏ | ❏ | ❏ | ❏ | 158. | ❏ | ❏ | ❏ | ❏ |
| 130. | ❏ | ❏ | ❏ | ❏ | 159. | ❏ | ❏ | ❏ | ❏ |
| 131. | ❏ | ❏ | ❏ | ❏ | 160. | ❏ | ❏ | ❏ | ❏ |
| 132. | ❏ | ❏ | ❏ | ❏ | 161. | ❏ | ❏ | ❏ | ❏ |
| 133. | ❏ | ❏ | ❏ | ❏ | 162. | ❏ | ❏ | ❏ | ❏ |
| 134. | ❏ | ❏ | ❏ | ❏ | 163. | ❏ | ❏ | ❏ | ❏ |
| 135. | ❏ | ❏ | ❏ | ❏ | 164. | ❏ | ❏ | ❏ | ❏ |

|      | A | B | C | D |      | A | B | C | D |
|------|---|---|---|---|------|---|---|---|---|
| 165. | ❏ | ❏ | ❏ | ❏ | 189. | ❏ | ❏ | ❏ | ❏ |
| 166. | ❏ | ❏ | ❏ | ❏ | 190. | ❏ | ❏ | ❏ | ❏ |
| 167. | ❏ | ❏ | ❏ | ❏ | 191. | ❏ | ❏ | ❏ | ❏ |
| 168. | ❏ | ❏ | ❏ | ❏ | 192. | ❏ | ❏ | ❏ | ❏ |
| 169. | ❏ | ❏ | ❏ | ❏ | 193. | ❏ | ❏ | ❏ | ❏ |
| 170. | ❏ | ❏ | ❏ | ❏ | 194. | ❏ | ❏ | ❏ | ❏ |
| 171. | ❏ | ❏ | ❏ | ❏ | 195. | ❏ | ❏ | ❏ | ❏ |
| 172. | ❏ | ❏ | ❏ | ❏ | 196. | ❏ | ❏ | ❏ | ❏ |
| 173. | ❏ | ❏ | ❏ | ❏ | 197. | ❏ | ❏ | ❏ | ❏ |
| 174. | ❏ | ❏ | ❏ | ❏ | 198. | ❏ | ❏ | ❏ | ❏ |
| 175. | ❏ | ❏ | ❏ | ❏ | 199. | ❏ | ❏ | ❏ | ❏ |
| 176. | ❏ | ❏ | ❏ | ❏ | 200. | ❏ | ❏ | ❏ | ❏ |
| 177. | ❏ | ❏ | ❏ | ❏ | 201. | ❏ | ❏ | ❏ | ❏ |
| 178. | ❏ | ❏ | ❏ | ❏ | 202. | ❏ | ❏ | ❏ | ❏ |
| 179. | ❏ | ❏ | ❏ | ❏ | 203. | ❏ | ❏ | ❏ | ❏ |
| 180. | ❏ | ❏ | ❏ | ❏ | 204. | ❏ | ❏ | ❏ | ❏ |
| 181. | ❏ | ❏ | ❏ | ❏ | 205. | ❏ | ❏ | ❏ | ❏ |
| 182. | ❏ | ❏ | ❏ | ❏ | 206. | ❏ | ❏ | ❏ | ❏ |
| 183. | ❏ | ❏ | ❏ | ❏ | 207. | ❏ | ❏ | ❏ | ❏ |
| 184. | ❏ | ❏ | ❏ | ❏ | 208. | ❏ | ❏ | ❏ | ❏ |
| 185. | ❏ | ❏ | ❏ | ❏ | 209. | ❏ | ❏ | ❏ | ❏ |
| 186. | ❏ | ❏ | ❏ | ❏ | 210. | ❏ | ❏ | ❏ | ❏ |
| 187. | ❏ | ❏ | ❏ | ❏ | 211. | ❏ | ❏ | ❏ | ❏ |
| 188. | ❏ | ❏ | ❏ | ❏ | 212. | ❏ | ❏ | ❏ | ❏ |

# Clinical Data Assessment

**DIRECTIONS:** Each of the following questions or incomplete statements is followed by four suggested answers or completions. Select the one that is best in each case and then blacken the corresponding space on the answer sheet found in the front of this chapter. Good luck.

1. Which of the ventilator-pressure tracings in Figure 3-1 (A–D) represents continuous positive pressure ventilation (CPPV) in the control mode with positive end-expiratory pressure (PEEP)?

**A.**

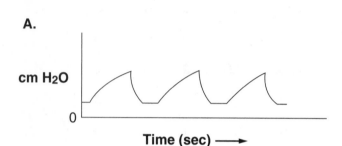

**B.**

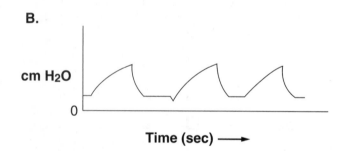

**C.**

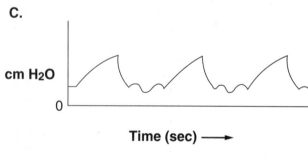

**D.**

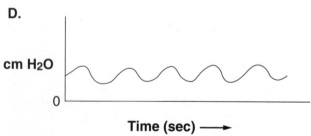

**Figure 3-1 (A–D)**

2. Which of the following types of equipment would enable the measurement of the transpulmonary pressure, which can be used to calculate pulmonary compliance?

    I. fiber-optic bronchoscope
    II. intraesophageal balloon
    III. transcutaneous $PO_2$ electrode
    IV. co-oximeter

    A. I, II only
    B. II only
    C. II, III, IV only
    D. I, IV only

3. A 15-month-old baby is brought to the emergency department dyspneic, coughing, and displaying wheezes audible to the unaided ear. Chest X-rays reveal a slight rightward mediastinal and cardiac shift and overaeration of the left lower lobe. A left-lateral decubitus view indicates that the left lower lobe remains more inflated than the left upper lobe. What problem is this child likely experiencing?

    A. left lower lobe pneumonia
    B. acute bronchial asthma
    C. subglottic stenosis
    D. foreign-body aspiration

4. A 42-year old Black female in ventilatory failure entered the emergency department at approximately 5:00 P.M. She was ultimately admitted to the respiratory intensive care unit and was placed on a mechanical ventilator. Her ABG values in the emergency room were:

    $PO_2$ 55 mm Hg
    $PCO_2$ 60 mm Hg
    pH 7.22
    $HCO_3^-$ 29 mEq/liter
    B.E. 5 mEq/liter

    The patient's husband informed the medical personnel that his wife complained of general fatigue and muscle weakness, especially in her legs. The husband also described his wife as experiencing diplopia, ptosis, dysphonia, and dysphagia. He expressed that these signs and symptoms were rarely present in the early morning hours or after his wife took a nap. They seemed to appear more regularly late in the day. Medical personnel also were informed that the patient had not had any bacterial or viral infections for a few years. What is the probably diagnosis of this patient?

A. Guillain–Barré syndrome
B. postinfectious polyneuritis
C. myasthenia gravis
D. amyotrophic lateral sclerosis

5. A patient receiving mechanical ventilation has just had a transtracheal aspiration procedure performed. A chest radiograph was obtained 10 minutes after the procedure. The chest film revealed multiple linear lucencies within the cervical musculature and the adipose tissue around the neck. Which condition is likely occurring?

A. pneumothorax
B. air embolism
C. subcutaneous emphysema
D. bilateral upper lobe atelectasis

6. The spirometric data in Table 3-1 were obtained during a pre- and postbronchodilator study. What interpretation can be made based on these data?

**Table 3-1**

| Spirometric Measurement | Prebronchodilator | Postbronchodilator |
|---|---|---|
| FVC | 3.24 L | 3.29 L |
| $FEV_1$ | 2.25 L | 2.34 L |
| $FEV_1$/FVC | 69% | 71% |
| $FEF_{25\%-75\%}$ | 1.65 L/sec. | 1.72 L/sec. |

A. Insufficient data are available for an interpretation to be made.
B. The patient has reversible obstructive airway disease.
C. The patient shows an insignificant response to bronchodilator administration.
D. The patient has a restrictive lung abnormality.

7. Calculate the static compliance by using the data from the tracings presented. The three tracings are (A) pressure time, (B) flow time, and (C) volume time (Figure 3-2, A–C).

A. 15 cc/cm $H_2O$
B. 17 cc/cm $H_2O$

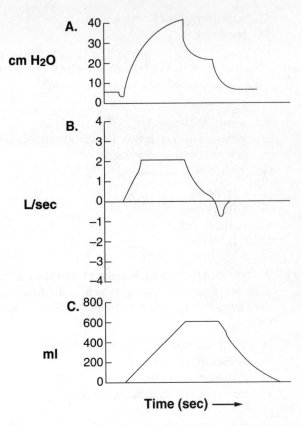

**Figure 3-2:** Pressure-time tracing, (B) flow-time tracing, and (C) volume-time tracing.

C. 30 cc/cm $H_2O$
D. 40 cc/cm $H_2O$

8. Which of the following observations would likely be made by an RRT inspecting the chest wall of a pulmonary emphysema patient?

A. equal anteroposterior and transverse chest-wall diameters
B. paradoxical chest-wall movement
C. respiratory alternans
D. anterior protrusion of the sternum

9. Which of the following diseases is consistent with the radiographic and physical findings listed as follows?

• mild to moderate airway obstruction
• signs of anxiety
• normal pharynx
• lateral neck X-ray: steeple sign
• normal epiglottis
• anteroposterior chest X-ray: subglottic narrowing
• barking cough and stridor

A. acute epiglottitis
B. asthma

C. acute laryngotracheobronchitis
D. bronchiolitis

10. Which of the following electrophysiologic characteristics are associated with sinus bradycardia?

   I. regular rhythm
   II. normal QRS complex
   III. increased interval between ventricular depolarization and atrial depolarization
   IV. regular pulse rate interval

   A. I, II, IV only
   B. I, III, IV only
   C. II, III, IV only
   D. I, II, III, IV

11. A 15-year-old asthmatic is being evaluated to determine his ability to exercise. Which of the following maneuvers or diagnostic procedures would render useful data?

   A. maximum voluntary ventilation (MVV)
   B. methacholine challenge
   C. maximum inspiratory pressure (MIP)
   D. carbon monoxide diffusing capacity

12. The RRT is reviewing a chest radiograph displaying the following findings:

   • cardiac enlargement
   • interstitial and alveolar infiltrates
   • Kerley B lines
   • peribronchial cuffing

   These roentgenographic findings are diagnostic of the following:

   A. pneumomediastinum.
   B. right middle-lobe pneumonia.
   C. pulmonary edema.
   D. pulmonary emphysema.

13. Which percussion note is characteristic of air trapping in the lungs?

   A. normal
   B. flat
   C. dull
   D. hyperresonant

14. Which flow-volume loop in Figure 3-3 represents a restrictive disorder?

   A. A
   B. B
   C. C
   D. D

15. A coronary care unit (CCU) patient has the following hemodynamic values:

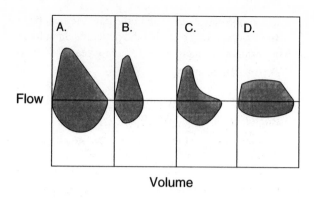

Flow

Volume

**Figure 3-3:** Flow-volume loops.

pulmonary artery systolic pressure: 15 mm Hg
pulmonary artery diastolic pressure: 11 mm Hg
pulmonary capillary wedge pressure (PCWP): 5 mm Hg
central venous pressure (CVP): 3 mm Hg
heart rate: 175 beats/min.
cardiac index (C.I.): 2.1 L/min./m²

The physician has asked the RRT to interpret this data. What interpretation would be most appropriate?

   A. pulmonary hypertension
   B. left ventricular infarction
   C. hypovolemia
   D. adult respiratory distress syndrome

16. After endotracheal intubation, proper tube placement should be assessed by which procedures?

   I. auscultation of the chest
   II. observation for equal bilateral chest expansion
   III. observation for adequate cough mechanism
   IV. portable chest X-ray

   A. I, II, IV only
   B. I, IV only
   C. II, III only
   D. IV only

17. An intensive care unit postoperative thoracotomy patient displays the following arterial blood gas and acid-base data while breathing 40% oxygen via an aerosol mask:

PO₂ 60 mm Hg
PCO₂ 30 mm Hg
pH 7.40
HCO₃⁻ 18 mEq/liter
B.E. −6 mEq/liter

Which of the following bedside procedures would enable the RRT to determine the cause of this patient's hypoxemia?

A. shunt study
B. capnography
C. pulse oximetry
D. metabolic study

18. A patient was found in his closed garage with the engine of his automobile running. He was taken immediately to the emergency department. His carboxyhemoglobin (COHb) percentage was found to be 35%. Which of the following mechanisms would need to be used to provide this patient's tissues with 5 vol% oxygen?

A. 100% $O_2$ under normobaric conditions via a non-rebreathing mask
B. ET intubation with 100% $O_2$ administered through a volume ventilator under ambient conditions
C. Tracheotomy with 100% $O_2$ administered by means of a volume ventilator at 2 atmosphere absolute (ATA) of pressure in a hyperbaric chamber
D. 80% $O_2$ under 3 ATA of pressure

19. Which of the following physiologic components influence the $D_{L_{CO}}$ value derived from either the steady state or the single-breath, lung-diffusion capacity study?

I. blood bicarbonate level
II. pulmonary capillary blood volume
III. rate of reaction between carbon monoxide and hemoglobin
IV. diffusion capacity of the alveolar-capillary membrane

A. I, II, III, IV
B. II, III only
C. I, IV only
D. II, III, IV only

20. Which precordial lead(s) display(s) positive electrocardiographic tracing(s)?

I. $V_6$
II. $V_4$
III. $V_5$
IV. $V_1$

A. III, IV only
B. II only
C. I, II, III only
D. III only

21. Calculate the dead space volume/tidal volume ratio for a patient having an end-tidal carbon dioxide tension of 44 torr and mean exhaled carbon dioxide tension of 33 torr.

A. 0.11
B. 0.13

C. 0.21
D. 0.25

22. The RRT, performing ICU ventilator rounds, observes that the right thorax of a mechanically ventilated patient is more expanded than the left. The patient's apical pulse is shifted to the left, and there are significantly decreased breath sounds on the right side. What action is appropriate at this time?

A. Perform an ABG.
B. Call for a STAT chest radiograph.
C. Perform a thoracentesis.
D. Increase the tidal volume.

23. Which statement(s) is(are) correct concerning the arterial pressure tracing shown in Figure 3-4?

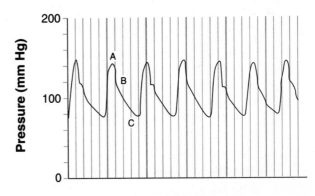

Figure 3-4: Arterial pressure tracing.

I. Point A on the tracing represents systolic pressure.
II. Point B coincides with the sudden closure of the aortic valve.
III. Point C depicts diastolic pressure.

A. II, III only
B. I, III only
C. II only
D. I, II, III

24. A patient's $S\bar{v}O_2$ is being continuously monitored via fiberoptic reflectance oximetry incorporated in a 5-lumen pulmonary artery catheter. The $S\bar{v}O_2$ value currently displayed is 87%. Which of the following conditions might account for this value? (Assume a normal $\dot{V}O_2$ and $CaO_2$.)

I. increased blood lactate levels
II. wedged pulmonary artery catheter
III. C.O. greater than normal
IV. cyanide poisoning

A. II, III only
B. II, III, IV only

C. I, III, IV only

D. I, II, IV only

25. Which of the following diseases are associated with muscle wasting?

   I. chronic bronchitis

   II. pulmonary emphysema

   III. cystic fibrosis

   IV. asthma

A. II, III only

B. III, IV only

C. I, II only

D. II, III, IV only

26. While assessing a patient's breathing by inspection, the RRT sees the patient's abdomen moving inward on inspiration and outward on exhalation. What is the significance of this observation?

A. This abdominal movement is characteristic of normal tidal breathing.

B. The patient may be experiencing diaphragmatic fatigue.

C. This ventilatory pattern is described as Pendelluft breathing.

D. The patient's abdominal muscles might be paralyzed.

27. On an electrocardiogram, the T wave represents:

A. atrial depolarization.

B. ventricular depolarization.

C. ventricular repolarization.

D. atrial repolarization.

28. Which of the following clinical conditions would cause a mediastinal shift toward the involved lung?

   I. pleural effusion

   II. pulmonary consolidation

   III. atelectasis

   IV. pulmonary fibrosis

   V. pneumothorax

A. II, III, IV only

B. I, II, V only

C. I, III, IV, V only

D. III, IV only

29. An RRT is reviewing the records of a patient who is receiving oxygen therapy. The patient has *no* history of dysoxia or ARDS. The RRT is asked to identify the best indicator of the presence or absence of hypoxia. The most appropriate response is the:

A. arterial $PO_2$.

B. total arterial oxygen content.

C. mixed venous $PO_2$.

D. static compliance.

30. Which of the following situations can produce erroneous results for the $FEF_{25\%-75\%}$ obtained from a forced vital capacity (FVC) maneuver?

A. maximum forced expiratory effort to residual volume

B. termination of the forced exhalation between the FRC and the residual volume

C. complete exhalation to residual with a submaximal effort

D. incomplete inspiratory effort less than total lung capacity (TLC) before maximal exhalation to residual volume

31. The RRT is asked to evaluate the results of a diagnostic sleep study. Which of the following guidelines would the RRT use to determine the existence of sleep apnea?

A. three or more apneic episodes per hour, each lasting at least 6 seconds

B. five or more apneic episodes per hour, each lasting at least 10 seconds

C. five or more apneic episodes per hour, each lasting at least 15 seconds

D. eight or more apneic episodes per hour, each lasting at least 8 seconds

32. Which route is most appropriate for obtaining a mixed venous blood sample?

A. venipuncture from any vein conveniently available

B. withdrawal from a venous line

C. withdrawal from a pulmonary artery catheter

D. venipuncture of the femoral vein

33. Determine a person's body surface area if her C.I. is 3.4 L/min./m² and her C.O. is 6.7 L/min.

A. 0.50 m²

B. 1.97 m²

C. 3.30 m²

D. 10.10 m²

34. Calculate the amount of reduced hemoglobin in a patient who has the following clinical data while breathing room air:

$PaO_2$ 30 torr

$PaCO_2$ 90 torr

pH 7.25

[Hb] 20 g%

$SaO_2$ 51%

$S\bar{v}O_2$ 45%

A. 5.0 g%
B. 8.5 g%
C. 10.4 g%
D. 12.0 g%

35. A 2-year-old child has just had a sweat test performed, and the sweat chloride concentration was determined to be 28 mEq/liter. What possible diagnosis can be made?

A. normal value
B. bronchiectasis
C. cystic fibrosis
D. bronchiolitis

36. A patient who has venous distention of the internal jugular vein 3 cm above the sternal angle while lying supine with his head elevated 45° is likely to have:

A. right ventricular failure.
B. normal venous pressure.
C. decreased venous return.
D. right ventricular hypertrophy.

37. While performing percussion of the diaphragm on an adult patient, the RRT determines that the right hemidiaphragm comes to rest at the T-9 level posteriorly at end-tidal exhalation while the left hemidiaphragm stops at T-10 posteriorly. This finding is consistent with:

A. left hemidiaphragmatic paralysis.
B. right hemidiaphragmatic paralysis.
C. bilateral diaphragmatic paralysis.
D. normal diaphragmatic positioning.

38. Which flow waveform (Figure 3-5, A–D) produced under high airway-pressure conditions represents that associated with a volume-cycled, constant-flow generator that generates moderate internal pressures?

39. The first heart sound ($S_1$) and second heart sound ($S_2$) are created by which of the following cardiac events?

A. distension of the heart walls
B. vibrations of the ventricular walls
C. tensing of the papillary muscles
D. closure of the heart valves

**A.**

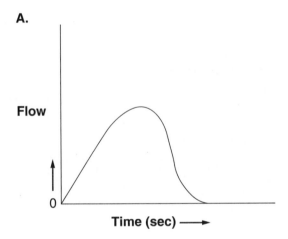

**B.**

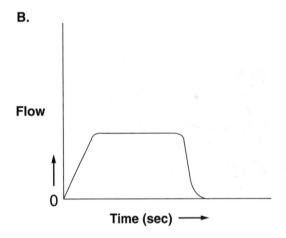

**C.**

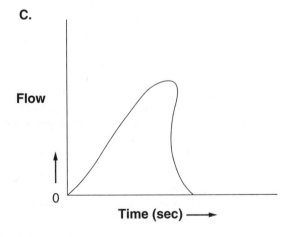

**D.**

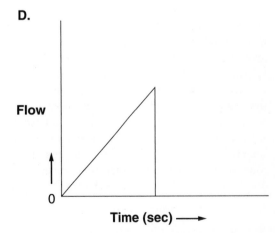

**Figure 3-5 (A–D)**

40. What does II represent on the %N₂ volume tracing illustrated in Figure 3-6?

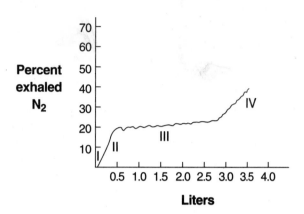

**Figure 3-6:** Percent exhaled nitrogen-volume tracing (single-breath nitrogen-elimination test).

A. expired gas from the oral and nasal cavities and the trachea
B. expired gas from the lung apices
C. mixed expired bronchial and alveolar gas
D. gas expired from the lower zones of the lungs

41. Calculate the inspiratory:expiratory ratio for a time-cycled, pressure-limited ventilator with the following settings:

- ventilatory rate: 60 breaths/min.
- inspiratory flow: 10 L/min.
- inspiratory time: 0.5 sec.
- F$_I$O$_2$: 0.60

A. 1:1
B. 1:2
C. 1:3
D. 1:3.5

42. A 24-year-old female enters the emergency room displaying tachypnea. The RRT notes the following findings during chest physical assessment. Inspection reveals limited chest movement of the left thorax, and palpation indicates decreased left chest excursion. The trachea is found to be shifted to the right, and vocal fremitus is diminished over the left lower lobe. Dull percussion notes are perceived over the left lower lobe. Auscultation of this area reveals diminished breath sounds. A pleural friction rub is occasionally noted over the left lower lobe when the patient breathes deeply. What is this patient experiencing?

A. a left-sided pneumothorax
B. right lower lobe atelectasis
C. a left-sided pleural effusion
D. left lower lobe atelectasis

43. Which of the following statements accurately refers to airway obstruction?

   I. A small airway obstruction is generally less symptomatic than a large airway obstruction.
   II. A partial airway obstruction can lead to hyperinflation distal to the point of obstruction.
   III. Flaring of the alae nasi and the use of accessory muscles of ventilation can indicate airway obstruction.
   IV. Airway obstruction does not affect the patient's acid-base status.

A. I, II, III, IV
B. I, IV only
C. I, II, III only
D. II, IV only

44. Which of the following sets of blood gas data reflect normal, mixed venous blood values?

A. PO$_2$ 40 torr; PCO$_2$ 47 torr; pH 7.37; SO$_2$ 75%
B. PO$_2$ 50 torr; PCO$_2$ 50 torr; pH 7.31; SO$_2$ 65%
C. PO$_2$ 55 torr; PCO$_2$ 40 torr; pH 7.35; SO$_2$ 60%
D. PO$_2$ 55 torr; PCO$_2$ 35 torr; pH 7.38; SO$_2$ 50%

45. Which of the ventilator-pressure tracings in Figure 3-7 (A–D) on page 93 represents synchronized intermittent mandatory ventilation (SIMV)?

46. Bronchial breath sounds heard during auscultation of the lung periphery are caused by:

   I. a pleural effusion.
   II. fibrosis.
   III. atelectasis.
   IV. consolidation.

A. I, III only
B. II, IV only
C. III, IV only
D. I, II only

47. A transcutaneous oxygen electrode placed on an infant's upper right arm is consistently indicating a PtcO$_2$ value 20 torr higher than the arterial PO$_2$ obtained from an umbilical artery catheter. What is a possible explanation for this occurrence?

A. The sensor temperature is set too low.
B. The sensor has been placed on edematous tissue.
C. Air bubbles have gotten between the skin and the sensor.
D. Right-to-left shunting through a patent ductus arteriosus is occurring.

48. Which of the following clinical conditions displays the thumb sign on neck roentgenography?

A. subglottic stenosis
B. laryngotracheobronchitis

**A.**

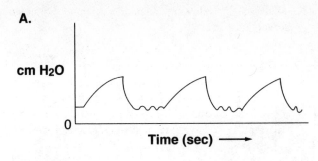

cm H₂O

0

Time (sec) ⟶

**B.**

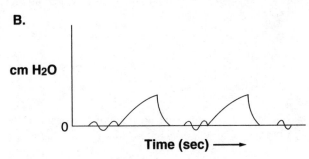

cm H₂O

0

Time (sec) ⟶

**C.**

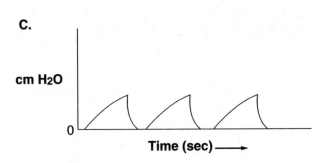

cm H₂O

0

Time (sec) ⟶

**D.**

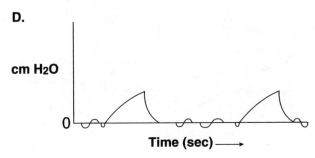

cm H₂O

0

Time (sec) ⟶

**Figure 3-7 (A–D)**

    C. epiglottitis
    D. laryngomalacia

49. A patient enters the emergency room displaying the following room air arterial blood gas data:

$PO_2$ 40 torr
$PCO_2$ 65 torr
pH 7.18

Which clinical condition matches this data?

    A. early stage of an asthmatic episode
    B. acute ventilatory failure
    C. diabetic ketoacidosis
    D. chronic ventilatory failure

50. A patient receiving volume-controlled, mechanical ventilation has experienced a $\dot{V}_A/\dot{Q}_C$ ratio increase as a consequence. What might be a reason for this phenomenon?

    A. re-established circulation
    B. impeded venous return
    C. increased ventilatory rate
    D. absorption atelectasis caused by an increased $FIO_2$

51. The RRT is asked to review the records of an ICU patient who has a possible empyema. To confirm the diagnosis, a specimen must be collected and sent to the lab. Which type of specimen is most likely to be evaluated?

    A. blood
    B. pleural fluid
    C. sputum
    D. urine

52. Which ECG (Figure 3-8, A–D on page 94) reflects a dysrhythmia indicating a need for immediate defibrillation?

53. The waveform depicted was generated as a pulmonary artery catheter and was floated into position (Figure 3-9 on page 95). What does Section B of the tracing represent?

    A. pulmonary capillary wedge pressure
    B. pulmonary artery pressure
    C. right atrial pressure
    D. right ventricular pressure

54. Which resuscitative measure is indicated at delivery for a vigorous neonate with light, thin meconium in the amniotic fluid?

    A. intubation and controlled mechanical ventilation
    B. aggressive pharyngeal suctioning
    C. bag-mask ventilation with oxygen
    D. no resuscitative measure

55. An RRT notes a high-pitched sound heard during the expiration of a patient in the pediatric emergency room. This sound is most likely:

    A. wheezing.
    B. grunting.
    C. snoring.
    D. stridor.

56. Generally, which intracuff pressure range will prevent arterial blood flow from entering the tracheal wall in an intubated patient?

    A. 10 to 15 torr
    B. 15 to 20 torr
    C. 20 to 25 torr
    D. 30 to 35 torr

**A.**

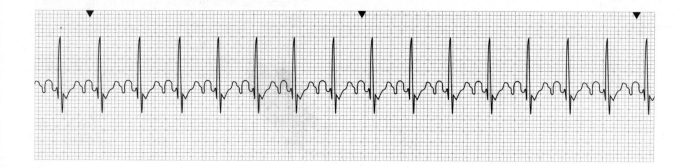

**B.**

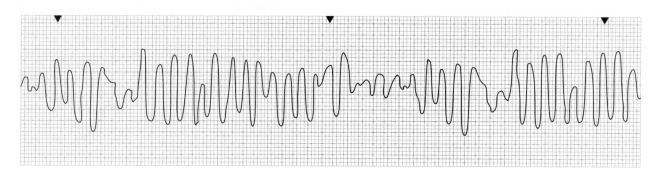

**C.**

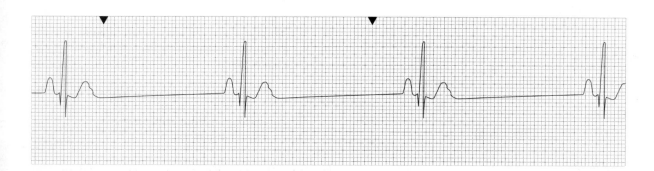

**D.**

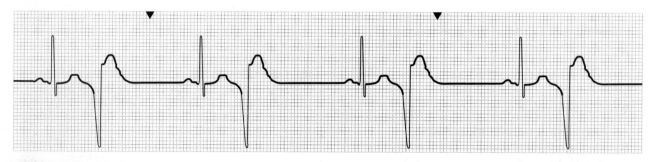

**Figure 3-8 (A–D)**

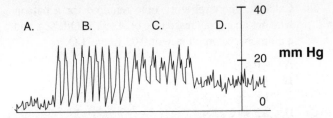

A.    B.    C.    D.

40

20    **mm Hg**

0

**Figure 3-9:** Pulmonary artery catheter waveforms.

57. The RRT is about to mechanically ventilate a postoperative thoracotomy patient. The minute ventilation is set at 10 L/min. and the ventilatory rate is 12 breaths/min. The SIMV rate is also established at 12 breaths/min. Calculate the inspiratory time % that will achieve an inspiratory time of 1.65 sec.

    A. 67%
    B. 60%
    C. 33%
    D. 25%

58. Which of the following signs and symptoms are associated with sleep apnea?

    I.   nocturnal enuresis
    II.  abnormal motor activity during sleep
    III. hypersomnalence
    IV.  hypertension

    A. I, II, III, IV
    B. I, III only
    C. II, IV only
    D. I, II, III only

59. Which of the following breathing patterns are associated with diaphragmatic dysfunction or fatigue?

    I.   respiratory alternans
    II.  paradoxical chest-wall movement
    III. Pendelluft breathing
    IV.  abdominal paradox

    A. I, II, III only
    B. I, III, IV only
    C. I, IV only
    D. II, III only

60. A diagnosed myasthenia gravis patient is exhibiting the signs and symptoms of her disease. The physician asks the RRT to recommend a medication that can distinguish between a myasthenic crisis and a cholinergic crisis. Which of the following drugs would the RRT recommend?

    A. edrophonium chloride
    B. neostygmine methylsulfate
    C. pyridostigmine
    D. Mestinon

61. Which of the following signs would likely be seen in a state of early septic shock?

    I.   fever
    II.  markedly increased C.O.
    III. low systemic vascular resistance
    IV.  tachypnea

    A. I, II, III, IV
    B. I, IV only
    C. II, III, IV only
    D. I, III only

62. A 38-year-old Caucasian female enters the emergency room displaying the following signs and symptoms: (1) chills and fever, (2) cough, (3) increased white blood cell count, and (4) pleuritic pain. The patient complains of coughing up copious amounts of purulent, foul-smelling, foul-tasting, blood-tinged sputum. Sputum cultures indicate anaerobes and mixed flora. The patient also claims that she has not experienced any weight loss, anorexia, or dyspnea. Amphoric breath sounds can be heard upon auscultation of the right anterior upper chest. Which of the following clinical conditions is the probable diagnosis?

    A. pulmonary neoplasm
    B. bronchiectasis
    C. pleural effusion
    D. lung abscess

63. The Silverman score is useful for evaluating which of the following neonatal conditions?

    A. cyanosis
    B. respiratory distress
    C. congenital cardiac defects
    D. pulmonary surfactant deficiency

64. A 165-pound Guillain–Barré patient has been monitored by the RRT for the past 4 hours. The maximum inspiratory pressure (MIP) and forced vital capacity (FVC) values obtained over this course of time are listed in Table 3-2.

**Table 3-2**

| Time | Ventilatory Measurement | Value |
|------|------------------------|-------|
| 11:00 A.M. | MIP | −45 cm $H_2O$ |
|  | FVC | 4.5 L |
| 12:10 P.M. | MIP | −40 cm $H_2O$ |
|  | FVC | 4.0 L |
| 1:15 P.M. | MIP | −30 cm $H_2O$ |
|  | FVC | 3.0 L |
| 2:05 P.M. | MIP | −15 cm $H_2O$ |
|  | FVC | 0.75 L |

The 2:05 P.M. entries represent the latest data obtained. What therapeutic intervention should the RRT recommend?

A. intubation and mechanical ventilation
B. administration of 28% oxygen via a Venturi mask
C. administration of 50% oxygen via a Briggs adaptor
D. bag-mask ventilation with 100% oxygen

65. Which of the following pulmonary function tests would be the most useful in determining the degree of alveolar wall impairment in pulmonary emphysema patients?

A. single-breath nitrogen washout
B. carbon monoxide lung-diffusion study
C. routine spirometry
D. closed-system helium dilution

66. The following slow-speed capnograph tracing was obtained from a Guillain–Barré patient who is being mechanically ventilated in the control mode (Figure 3-10). What has occurred during Segment B of this tracing?

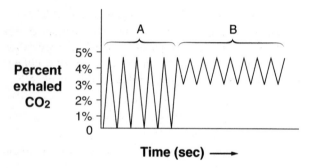

**Figure 3-10:** Slow-speed capnograph tracing.

A. The $F_IO_2$ was increased.
B. The ventilatory rate was increased.
C. Mechanical dead space was added.
D. The ventilatory rate was decreased.

67. Given the following hemodynamic data, calculate the C.O. for this patient, who is being invasively hemodynamically monitored.

pulmonary artery systolic pressure: 20 mm Hg
pulmonary artery diastolic pressure: 14 mm Hg
mean pulmonary artery pressure: 16 mm Hg
pulmonary artery wedge pressure: 11 mm Hg
oxygen consumption: 250 ml/min.
arterial–venous oxygen content difference: 5.0 vol%

A. 3.5 L/min.
B. 4.0 L/min.
C. 4.5 L/min.
D. 5.0 L/min.

68. Calculate the expiratory time required for a patient who has an airway resistance of 30 cm $H_2O$/L/sec. and a pulmonary compliance of 0.02 L/cm $H_2O$.

A. 0.6 sec.
B. 1.6 sec.
C. 1.8 sec.
D. 2.5 sec.

69. The RRT is auscultating the thorax of a patient who has an abundant amount of chest hair. The RRT perceives crackles. What should he do at this time?

A. Record the presence of crackles.
B. Moisten the chest hair so it becomes somewhat matted, and reauscultate.
C. Auscultate with the bell instead of with the diaphragm.
D. Shave a portion of the patient's chest to remove some of the hair, and reauscultate.

70. Which $V_D/V_T$ ratio range is acceptable when evaluating a mechanically ventilated patient for weaning?

A. $> 0.40$
B. $> 0.30$
C. $< 0.60$
D. $< 0.40$

71. An arterial blood gas (ABG) obtained from a normal preterm infant 1 hour following birth reveals:

$PO_2$ 65 torr
$PCO_2$ 45 torr
pH 7.34

Which intervention is appropriate based on these ABG findings?

A. *No* intervention is necessary.
B. Administer sodium bicarbonate.
C. Institute oxygen via an oxyhood.
D. Institute nasal CPAP.

72. Which of the following evaluation procedures are useful in determining whether a patient can be successfully weaned from mechanical ventilation?

I. vital capacity
II. sensorium
III. dead space–tidal volume ratio
IV. maximum inspiratory pressure

A. I, II, III, IV
B. I, III, IV only
C. II, III, IV only
D. I, III only

73. During auscultation, an RRT perceives a high-pitched sound as a patient in the pediatric emergency department inspires. Which type of sound has the RRT likely heard?

A. wheezing
B. grunting
C. snoring
D. stridor

74. What is the local response to a regional increase in alveolar dead space ventilation?

   A. Alveolar $CO_2$ tension increases.
   B. The alveolar partial pressure of $CO_2$ decreases.
   C. Blood $HCO_3^-$ concentration increases.
   D. The partial pressure of alveolar oxygen decreases.

75. Anatomically, where can cyanosis generally be perceived?

   I. ear lobes
   II. conjunctiva
   III. lips
   IV. digits

   A. I, II, III, IV
   B. III, IV only
   C. II, III, IV only
   D. I, II only

76. Which of the following statements are true about the following diagram (Figure 3-11)?

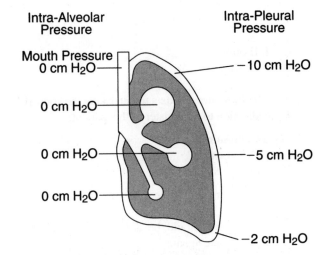

**Figure 3-11:** Lung pressures at FRC.

   I. The transpulmonary pressure gradient in the lung bases is greater than in the apicies.
   II. The transpulmonary pressure-gradient differences cause alveoli in the bases to contain a greater volume at FRC than the apical alveoli.
   III. When compared with the apices, any given inspiratory pressure change in the bases is accompanied by a greater volume change.
   IV. The elastance is greater in the apices than in the bases of the upright, normal lung.

A. I, III, IV only
B. II, IV only
C. III, IV only
D. I, III only

77. Which of the following conditions are likely to cause an abnormal elevation of the right hemidiaphragm?

   I. pulmonary emphysema
   II. right phrenic nerve damage
   III. fibrosis or scarring of the right lung
   IV. left-sided pneumothorax

   A. I, II only
   B. II, III only
   C. III, IV only
   D. I, II, III, IV

78. Which method of determining the FRC of a pulmonary emphysema patient will render the largest FRC value?

   A. closed-circuit helium dilution
   B. open-circuit nitrogen washout
   C. body plethysmography
   D. single-breath nitrogen washout

79. While performing tracheal palpation on an orally intubated patient receiving mechanical ventilation, the RRT notices that the patient is exhibiting rightward tracheal deviation. Which of the following clinical conditions might be responsible for this situation?

   A. consolidation of the left lower lobe
   B. atelectasis of the right upper lobe
   C. tension pneumothorax on the right side
   D. slippage of the ET tube into the right mainstem bronchus

80. Calculate the inspiratory flow rate delivered by a time-cycled, volume-limited, constant-flow generator when the preset volume is 800 cc and the inspiratory time is 1.2 sec.

   A. 30 L/min.
   B. 35 L/min.
   C. 40 L/min.
   D. 55 L/min.

81. Which of the pressure waveforms in Figure 3-12 (A–D) on page 98 contains an inspiratory hold?

82. Central venous pressure (CVP) measurements are being taken while a patient is receiving mechanical ventilation. How will these values be affected by positive pressure ventilation?

   A. If the patient is receiving control-mode ventilation, the CVP measurements will be normal.
   B. If the patient is receiving pressure-support ventilation, the CVP readings will be low.

**A.**

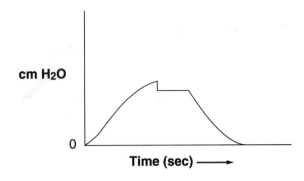

cm H₂O

Time (sec) →

**B.**

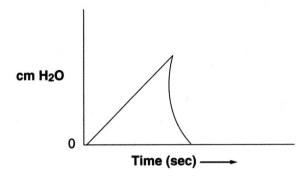

cm H₂O

Time (sec) →

**C.**

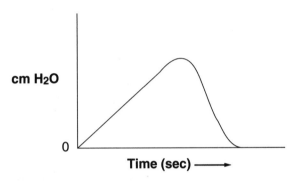

cm H₂O

Time (sec) →

**D.**

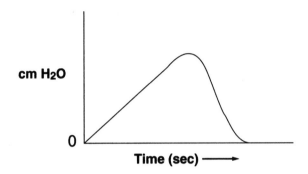

cm H₂O

Time (sec) →

**Figure 3-12 (A–D)**

C. CVP measurements during mechanical ventilation will be high only if PEEP is employed.

D. CVP readings will be high during positive pressure ventilation.

83. While reviewing a patient's chart, the RRT notices that a Gram's stain was performed on a sputum sample that was described as "rusty-colored." The Gram's stain results indicate that the sputum contained encapsulated, lancet-shaped, gram-positive diplococci. Which microorganism matches this description?

A. *Staphylococcus aureus*
B. *Streptococcus pneumoniae*
C. *Klebsiella pneumoniae*
D. *Haemophilus influenzae*

84. Which of the following physical examination techniques would be helpful in assessing and evaluating underlying lung structure and function as well as airway secretions?

I. percussion
II. palpation
III. tactile fremitus
IV. auscultation

A. I, II, IV only
B. II, III, IV only

C. I, II only
D. I, II, III, IV

85. Evaluate the following data to determine the appropriate medication to administer to this patient:

$\dot{V}O_2$ 250 ml/min.
$CaO_2$ 19.5 vol%
$C\bar{v}O_2$ 14.5 vol%

A. The patient should be given a positive inotropic agent.
B. The patient should be administered a positive chronotropic agent.
C. The patient should be administered a beta-one blocker.
D. *No* medication is indicated in this situation.

86. A young man with a history of human immunodeficiency virus infection presents in the emergency department with fever, chills, and weight loss. A sputum sample is obtained for culture and sensitivity, Gram staining, and acid-fast staining. The results are positive for an acid-fast bacillus *Mycobacterium avium-intracellulare*. This finding would lead the RRT to suspect:

A. gram-negative pneumonia.
B. atypical tuberculosis.

C. viral pneumonia.

D. fungal pneumonia.

87. At what lung level should a maximum inspiratory pressure maneuver be performed?

A. total lung capacity

B. end-tidal inspiration

C. FRC

D. residual volume

88. The evaluation in the emergency department of a 36-year-old, febrile, male patient with tachycardia reveals the following information:

ABG data and blood data are as follows:

$PO_2$ 69 mm Hg

$PCO_2$ 33 mm Hg

pH 7.47

$HCO_3^-$ 23 mEq/liter

B.E. −1 mEq/liter

[Hb] 14 g%

HCT 45%

WBC 20,000/$mm^3$

Which of the following laboratory tests would be most appropriate to further evaluate this patient?

A. cardiac enzymes

B. electrolytes

C. sputum culture and sensitivity

D. urinalysis

89. Which of the following statements most accurately describes the normal ventilation–perfusion relationship between the bases and apices?

A. The bases receive more ventilation than perfusion.

B. The lung apices receive more perfusion than ventilation.

C. The apices receive more perfusion than the bases.

D. The apices receive more ventilation than perfusion.

90. Dividing the oxygen consumption by the difference in the total oxygen content in the arterial blood from the total oxygen content in the mixed venous blood provides for the calculation of the:

A. tissue oxygen delivery.

B. tissue oxygen extraction.

C. cardiac output.

D. cardiac index.

91. Interpret the ECG pattern presented in Figure 3-13.

A. Mobitz II

B. Wenckebach

C. third-degree AV block

D. first-degree AV block

92. From a chest radiograph, how can a right lower lobe pneumonia be distinguished from a right middle-lobe pneumonia?

A. In a right middle-lobe pneumonia, the right hemidiaphragm is obscured.

B. When a right middle-lobe pneumonia is present, both the right heart border and right hemidiaphragm are obscured.

C. In the presence of a right middle-lobe pneumonia, the right heart border is obscured whereas the right hemidiaphragm is distinct.

D. In the presence of a right lower lobe pneumonia, both the right heart border and the right hemidiaphragm are obscured.

93. An adult patient is exhibiting an increased work of breathing. Where on the thorax can the RRT inspect for retractions?

I. along the sternum

II. between the ribs

III. below the lower margin of the ribs

IV. above the clavicles

A. II, III only

B. I, III, IV only

C. II, III, IV only

D. II, IV only

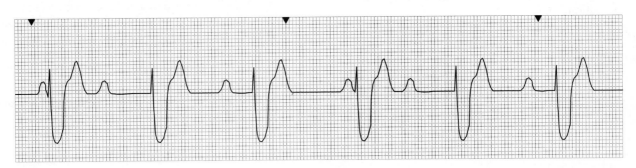

**Figure 3-13:** ECG tracing.

94. A 26-year-old diabetic primagravida has just given birth to a 1,200-g male infant of 33 weeks' gestation. Observation of the infant indicates that he is grunting on exhalation; has nasal flaring, sternal, and intercostal retractions; and is cyanotic. His ventilatory rate is 20 breaths/min. Auscultation of the chest reveals diminished breath sounds. The chest roentgenogram shows a symmetric reticulogranular pattern and a general loss of lung volume. What is the probable diagnosis of this neonate?

A. primary apnea
B. hyaline membrane disease
C. Wilson–Mikity syndrome
D. epiglottitis

95. Calculate the ventilation time constant given the following data. (Assume that a square-flow waveform is being used.)

peak inspiratory pressure: 40 cm $H_2O$
plateau pressure: 20 cm $H_2O$
tidal volume: 800 cc (measured at the ET tube)
PEEP: 5 cm $H_2O$
inspiratory flow rate: 50 L/min.
inspiratory time: 1 sec.

A. 1.27 seconds
B. 0.95 second
C. 0.79 second
D. 0.33 second

96. Which of the following respiratory conditions is consistent with the radiologic finding of tracheal dilatation?

A. croup
B. ET tube cuff hyperinflation
C. pneumothorax
D. tracheal stenosis

97. The neonatologist suspects that an infant has persistent pulmonary hypertension of the newborn. Which diagnostic procedure should the RRT recommend?

A. arterial and venous blood gases
B. transcutaneous oxygen and carbon dioxide monitoring
C. pre- and postductal transcutaneous oxygen monitoring
D. thermodilution C.O. study

98. Why does blood drawn from an umbilical artery catheter in neonates who have a patent ductus arteriosus sometimes reflect a low arterial oxygen saturation?

A. Because of anatomic differences among neonates.
B. Because air embolization is a frequent complication when drawing blood from the catheter.

C. Because of the location of the arterial catheter.
D. Because fibrin frequently accumulates at the tip of the arterial catheter.

99. A person is being evaluated for the source of recurrent pulmonary infections. He has a history of intravenous drug abuse. His current chest radiograph shows a diffuse interstitial pneumonic process. Definitive information to determine whether this is *Pneumocystis carinii* can be obtained by:

A. flexible fiberoptic bronchoscopic biopsy.
B. thoracentesis.
C. bronchography.
D. a lateral decubital view of the chest.

100. The RRT has been monitoring both the static and peak pressures of a patient receiving mechanical ventilation. The data pertaining to these two measurements are plotted on the following graph, where static pressure is represented by the solid line and the peak pressure is reflected by the dashed line (Figure 3-14).

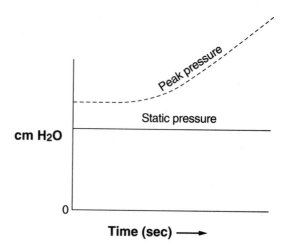

Figure 3-14: Static and peak pressures; peak pressure (dashed line) and static pressure (solid line).

Based on this graph, what is occurring with this patient?

A. The patient has developed excessive secretions.
B. The patient has developed a pulmonary embolism.
C. The ET tube has slipped into the right mainstem bronchus.
D. Massive atelectasis has occurred.

101. A 40-year-old female complains of dyspnea at rest and an impaired ability to carry out normal daily activities. Which of the following diagnostic procedures would provide the most useful information?

A. single-breath nitrogen elimination
B. flow-volume loop
C. maximum expiratory pressure
D. 7-minute nitrogen washout

102. To evaluate diaphragmatic movement, the RRT can estimate the range of excursion by:

A. holding the ulnar surface of his hand against the posterior thorax and noting where vibrations are felt while the patient repeats "ninety-nine."
B. holding both hands against the patient's posterior lower thorax and noting how far they spread laterally as the patient maximally inhales.
C. percussing small increments in a vertical, mid-scapular line downward on the posterior thorax and noting where resonant percussive notes cease during inhalation, and where resonant percussive notes resume on exhalation.
D. palpating along the lower region of the anterior thorax until the point where crepitance is noted.

103. Which of the following statements refer to CPAP being used to treat sleep apnea?

I. Use of the CPAP device for several nights reduces the number of apneic episodes during ensuing nights, even when the patient stops using the device.
II. The mask used covers both the nose and the mouth of the patient.
III. The appropriate CPAP level can often be determined during sleep studies.
IV. Despite the use of CPAP, the patient can still maintain a negative intrapharyngeal pressure during inspiration.

A. I, II, III only
B. II, IV only
C. I, III only
D. II, III, IV only

104. Which of the following conditions are associated with an elevated PCWP?

I. hypervolemia
II. right ventricular infarction
III. left ventricular infarction
IV. ARDS

A. I, III, IV only
B. II, III only
C. I, III only
D. III, IV only

105. Which of the following factors influence the compressible volume in a ventilator circuit for a volume-cycled ventilator?

I. the system compliance
II. the inspiratory:expiratory ratio
III. the $FiO_2$
IV. the pressure generated in the system

A. I, IV only
B. II, III, IV only
C. I, II, III only
D. I, II only

106. Purulent sputum is often associated with which disease conditions?

I. bronchiectasis
II. cystic fibrosis
III. pneumonia
IV. chronic bronchitis

A. I, II, IV only
B. I, IV only
C. II, III only
D. I, II, III, IV

107. Anatomic dead space is best described as:

A. physiologic dead space minus alveolar dead space.
B. alveoli receiving ventilation but no perfusion.
C. alveolar dead space minus physiologic dead space.
D. intrapulmonary shunting.

108. A 38-year-old Caucasian female was hospitalized and was convalescing comfortably from fractures of bones in both legs resulting from a skiing accident. The patient had no history of cardiopulmonary disease or smoking. Two days later, the patient suddenly became dyspneic, tachypneic, and cyanotic. Adventitious breath sounds—crackles and rhonchi—were heard upon auscultation of the chest. The patient exhibited a diminished sensorium and petechiae on her chest and neck. What is the probable diagnosis?

A. fat embolization
B. acute myocardial infarction
C. tension pneumothorax
D. aspiration pneumonitis

109. The ECG monitor displays the pattern shown in Figure 3-15 on page 102 while the balloon tip of a pulmonary artery catheter is in the right ventricle during the catheter's insertion. What should the RRT recommend at this time?

A. begin cardiac compressions
B. withdraw the pulmonary artery catheter immediately
C. continue advancing the pulmonary artery catheter
D. cardiovert the patient immediately

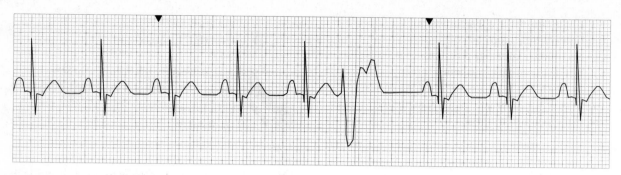

**Figure 3-15:** ECG tracing.

110. Calculate the $FEV_{1\%}$ based on the spirometry data given in Table 3-3.

**Table 3-3**

| Parameter | Actual | Predicted |
|-----------|--------|-----------|
| FVC | 7.60 L | 5.26 L |
| $FEV_1$ | 5.64 L | 4.26 L |
| $FEV_3$ | 7.29 L | 5.10 L |
| PEFR | 13.54 L/sec. | 9.00 L/sec. |

    A. 56%
    B. 74%
    C. 80%
    D. 86%

111. Which of the following conditions would contraindicate the use of transcutaneous $PO_2/PCO_2$ monitoring of a patient's respiratory status?

    A. methemoglobinemia
    B. decreased perfusion
    C. irregular ventilatory patterns
    D. anemia

112. During an interview, a patient informs the RRT of experiencing shortness of breath without exertion and that she feels confined to the house because of her dyspnea. To what grade of dyspnea is this complaint equivalent?

    A. Grade I
    B. Grade III
    C. Grade IV
    D. Grade V

113. Determine the dead space–tidal volume ratio for a patient who has a dissolved arterial carbon dioxide tension of 40 mm Hg and a mean exhaled carbon dioxide tension of 28 mm Hg.

    A. 1.3
    B. 0.7
    C. 0.5
    D. 0.3

114. A patient is suspected of having maldistribution of ventilation. Which of the following diagnostic procedures would be useful in providing data to help determine the degree of nonuniformity of ventilation?

    A. diffusing capacity
    B. volume of isoflow
    C. maximum voluntary ventilation
    D. single-breath nitrogen-elimination test

115. Which condition(s) is(are) likely to be associated with a decreased tactile fremitus?

    I. consolidation
    II. obesity
    III. muscularity
    IV. pneumothorax

    A. II, III, IV only
    B. I only
    C. II, III only
    D. IV only

116. According to the Fick equation, when the $\dot{V}O_2$ remains constant, the C.O. ___ as the $CaO_2\text{-}C\bar{v}O_2$ gradient ___.

    I. increases; increases
    II. decreases; decreases
    III. increases; decreases
    IV. decreases; increases

    A. III only
    B. II only
    C. II, III only
    D. III, IV only

117. The presence of meconium in the amniotic fluid is usually indicative of:

A.  necrotizing enterocolitis.
B.  an intrauterine asphyxial episode.
C.  persistent pulmonary hypertension of the newborn.
D.  an infant's predisposition toward the development of bronchopulmonary dysplasia.

118. The RRT is monitoring the cardiopulmonary status of a 33-year-old ARDS patient who is receiving continuous mechanical ventilation and has a pulmonary artery catheter inserted. The waveform shown in Figure 3-16 has been continuously displayed on the monitor. What should the RRT do at this time?

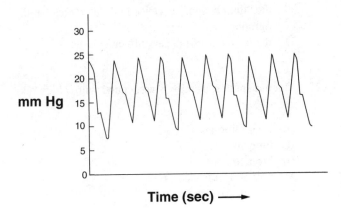

**Figure 3-16:**  Pulmonary artery catheter waveform.

A.  Do *nothing* because the waveform signifies pulmonary artery pressure.
B.  Withdraw the catheter a few centimeters because it has drifted into the wedge position.
C.  Deflate the balloon because the waveform is displaying PAWP.
D.  Advance the catheter because it appears to have been pulled into the right atrium.

119. A 9-year-old girl who suffers from allergic (extrinsic) asthma is about to be discharged from the hospital. The RRT is asked to recommend a prophylactic medication useful for the treatment of this condition. Which drug should he recommend?

A.  racemic epinephrine
B.  procainamide
C.  cromolyn sodium
D.  n-acetylcysteine

120. Which of the following diagnostic studies would be most beneficial in aiding in the definitive diagnosis of pulmonary embolism?

A.  chest X-ray
B.  ECG

C.  $\dot{V}/\dot{Q}$ scan
D.  prothrombin time

121. A 4-foot, 10 inch, 11-year-old girl is performing a bedside forced vital capacity (FVC) maneuver. Her predicted and actual values are shown in Table 3-4.

**Table 3-4**

| Parameter | Predicted | Actual |
|---|---|---|
| FVC | 2.10 L | 1.97 L |
| FEV$_1$ | 1.81 L | 1.76 L |
| PEFR | 3.41 L/sec. | 3.10 L/sec. |
| FEV$_1$/FVC | 83% | 89.3% |
| FEF$_{200-1200}$ | 3.03 L/sec. | 2.66 L/sec. |
| FEF$_{25\%-75\%}$ | 2.89 L/sec. | 1.85 L/sec. |
| FEV$_T$ | | 6.51 sec. |

What interpretation can be made from these data?

A.  The patient might *not* have comprehended the instructions.
B.  The patient has a small airway obstruction.
C.  The patient has an upper airway obstruction.
D.  A bronchodilator would *not* be useful in this situation.

122. While performing palpation of a patient's trachea, the RRT notices that the patient is exhibiting tracheal deviation to the left. Which of the following clinical conditions might be associated with this situation?

A.  pleural effusion in the left intrapleural space
B.  air trapping of the left upper lobe
C.  atelectasis of the left upper lobe
D.  tension pneumothorax on the left side

123. An automobile mechanic was found unconscious in the garage where he worked. When he entered the emergency department, an RRT placed a pulse oximeter probe on his finger and obtained an arterial saturation of 98%. What should the RRT do at this time?

A.  Obtain a blood sample from the patient and place it in a co-oximeter.
B.  Re-perform the pulse oximetry.
C.  Apply a transcutaneous oxygen electrode to the patient's chest.
D.  Measure the patient's end-tidal carbon dioxide tension.

124. Which of the waveforms shown in Figure 3-17 (A–D) on page 104 are characteristic of pressure-controlled ventilation?

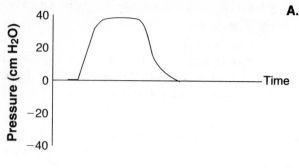

**A.**

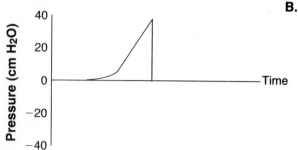

**B.**

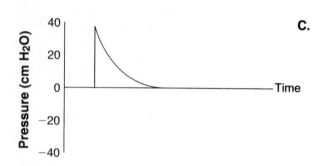

**C.**

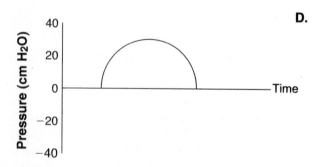

**D.**

**Figure 3-17 (A–D)**

A. nasal cannula at 3 L/min.
B. simple mask at 8 L/min.
C. air-entrainment mask at 28%
D. aerosol mask at 40%

125. A COPD patient enters the emergency department with an acute exacerbation. ABG analysis reveals the following data:

PO$_2$ 50 torr
PCO$_2$ 70 torr
pH 7.25
HCO$_3^-$ 30 mEq/liter
B.E. 6 mEq/liter

Which oxygen-delivery device would be appropriate for this patient at this time?

126. The RRT is asked to assist in the evaluation of a child suspected of having epiglottitis. Which of the following findings would assist in the differential diagnosis and provide a positive result for epiglottitis?

A. a "steeple sign," as viewed in an anteroposterior radiograph of the chest
B. presence of a "barky" cough
C. the "thumb sign," as viewed in a lateral neck radiograph
D. the presence of the parainfluenza virus

127. Mucoid sputum usually is associated with which disease(s)?

I. cystic fibrosis
II. lung abscess
III. bronchial asthma
IV. bronchogenic carcinoma
V. chronic bronchitis

A. III only
B. I only
C. III, IV only
D. III, V only

128. A 2-year-old Caucasian child with a history of frequent pulmonary infections, abnormal stool, cough productive of green sputum, and a general appearance of being malnourished is being evaluated. Among other studies, the RRT would be particularly interested in obtaining a:

I. serum potassium level.
II. sweat chloride level.
III. serum calcium level.

A. I, II only
B. II only
C. I, III only
D. I only

129. In the process of viewing a patient's chest radiographs, the RRT observes the presence of (1) large lung volumes, (2) flattened diaphragms, (3) increased retrosternal air space, (4) a small heart, and (5) increased intercostal spaces. What is this patient's likely diagnosis?

A. pneumothorax
B. pulmonary emphysema

C. bronchiectasis
D. chronic bronchitis

130. A positive sweat chloride test for diagnosing cystic fibrosis shows a chloride concentration of:

A. > 30 mEq/liter
B. > 40 mEq/liter
C. > 50 mEq/liter
D. > 60 mEq/liter

131. The pulmonary function data in Table 3-5 were obtained from a 41-year-old, 77-kg male who has a 3-year history of tachypnea.

**Table 3-5**

| Lung Volumes, Capacities/Flows | Actual | % Predicted |
|---|---|---|
| FVC | 3.61 L | 70 |
| RV | 1.01 L | 61 |
| FRC | 2.01 L | 61 |
| TLC | 4.50 L | 70 |
| FEV$_1$/FVC | 83% | |
| PEF | 9.66 L/sec. | 96 |

Which of the following conditions are consistent with these data?

I. pulmonary emphysema
II. chronic bronchitis
III. kyphoscoliosis
IV. asbestosis

A. I, III only
B. III, IV only
C. II, III, IV only
D. I, II only

132. What is the likely cause of capillary refill requiring 5 seconds?

A. hypoperfusion
B. hypertension
C. increased capillary osmotic pressure
D. systemic vasodilatation

133. Which clinical condition(s) is(are) associated with usage of the inspiratory accessory muscles of ventilation?

I. increased pulmonary compliance
II. increased airway resistance
III. decreased chest-wall compliance
IV. eucapnia

A. I, IV only
B. II, III only
C. III only
D. I, II only

134. A 33-year-old Black male from South Carolina enters his physician's office complaining of general malaise, dyspnea, and a nonproductive cough. Breath sounds are found to be normal. Chest X-rays reveal bilateral hilar adenopathy and diffuse alveolar infiltrates. Pulmonary function data are shown in Table 3-6.

What is the probable diagnosis of this patient?

A. sarcoidosis
B. pulmonary edema
C. asthma
D. hypersensitivity pneumonitis

135. Anatomically, where should a pulmonary artery catheter be placed to measure PCWP?

A. right atrium
B. right ventricle
C. pulmonary capillary
D. branch of a pulmonary artery

**Table 3-6**

| Parameter | Predicted | Actual | % Predicted |
|---|---|---|---|
| FVC | 4.65 L | 2.18 L | 47 |
| FEV$_1$ | 3.63 L | 1.95 L | 54 |
| FEV$_1$/FVC | | 89% | |
| FEF$_{25-75\%}$ | 4.05 L/sec. | 3.00 L/sec. | 74 |
| MVV | 126.0 L/min. | 88.5 L/min. | 70 |
| FRC | 2.65 L | 1.29 L | 49 |
| RV | 1.61 L | 0.81 L | 50 |
| TLC | 6.26 L | 2.99 L | 48 |
| DL$_{CO}$ (ml/min./mm Hg) | 22.0 | 15.2 | 69 |

136. Which of the following cardiac dysrhythmias illustrated in Figure 3-18 (A–D) can cause a decreased C.O.?

    A. I, II, III, IV
    B. I, IV only
    C. I, II, III only
    D. III, IV only

137. The presence of a radiolucent area between the visceral and parietal pleurae on a chest roentgenogram likely signifies the presence of a(n):

    A. pneumothorax.
    B. pleural effusion.
    C. atelectasis.
    D. hyperinflation.

138. Which of the following clinical aspects are used in compiling the Silverman score?

    I. heart sounds
    II. capillary refill
    III. expiratory grunting
    IV. amniocentesis
    V. xiphoid retractions

    A. I, II only
    B. II, IV only
    C. I, III, IV only
    D. III, V only

139. The lecithin/sphingomyelin (L/S) ratio is predictive of which disease condition?

    A. bronchiolitis
    B. retinopathy of prematurity
    C. infant respiratory distress syndrome
    D. Wilson–Mikity syndrome

140. Which of the following conditions would cause someone to hyperventilate via peripheral chemoreceptor stimulation?

    I. methemoglobinemia
    II. polycythemia
    III. a sea-level resident ascending to an altitude of 10,000 ft
    IV. cyanide poisoning
    V. carbon monoxide poisoning

    A. I, III, IV only
    B. I, II, III, IV only
    C. III, IV only
    D. II, V only

141. The mother of a 3-year-old child who has had recurrent pneumonia informs the pediatrician that when she kisses her child the infant's skin tastes salty. Which lab test would be indicated?

    A. complete blood count (CBC)
    B. sputum culture and sensitivity
    C. serum electrolytes
    D. sweat test

142. An RRT is requested to perform quality assessment on a patient who is receiving oxygen therapy. To satisfy Joint Commission on the Accreditation of Health Organizations (JCAHO) standards, the RRT should review and evaluate the care plan based on pre-established criteria. What should be some of the components of these criteria?

    I. goals or indications of therapy
    II. evaluation of the effectiveness of therapy
    III. identification of adverse effects of therapy
    IV. input from the medical director

    A. I, II, III only
    B. I, II, IV only
    C. III, IV only
    D. I, II, III, IV

143. Which combination of peak inspiratory pressure (PIP) and compressibility factor would cause the most volume "lost" in a ventilator circuit? Assume *no* PEEP is present.

    A. peak inspiratory pressure: 55 cm $H_2O$; compressibility factor: 3 cc/cm $H_2O$
    B. peak inspiratory pressure: 40 cm $H_2O$; compressibility factor: 5 cc/cm $H_2O$
    C. peak inspiratory pressure: 45 cm $H_2O$; compressibility factor: 4 cc/cm $H_2O$
    D. peak inspiratory pressure: 60 cm $H_2O$; compressibility factor: 2 cc/cm $H_2O$

144. Which of the following breathing patterns are associated with a decreased pulmonary compliance in a spontaneously breathing patient?

    I. rapid, shallow breathing
    II. slow, deep breathing
    III. accessory muscle usage
    IV. a prolonged expiratory time

    A. II, IV only
    B. II, III only
    C. III, IV only
    D. I, III only

145. Letter A on the ECG illustrated in Figure 3-19 on page 108 represents which cardiac activity?

    A. the absolute refractory period
    B. atrial depolarization
    C. ventricular repolarization
    D. atrial repolarization

**I.**

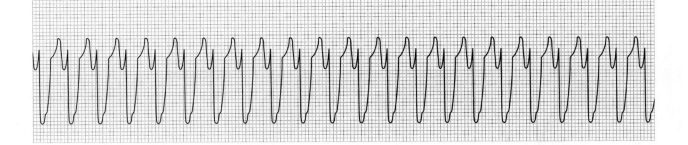

**II.**

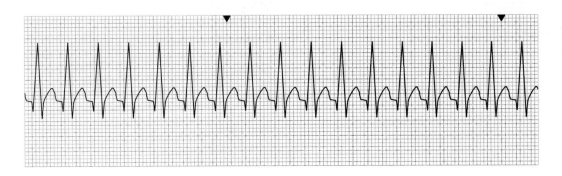

**III.**

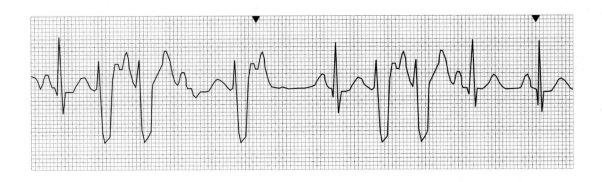

**IV.**

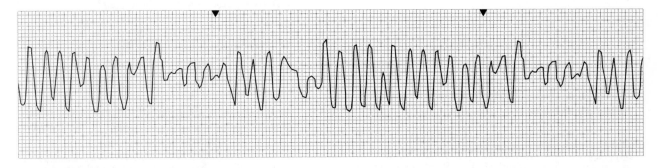

**Figure 3-18 (A–D)**

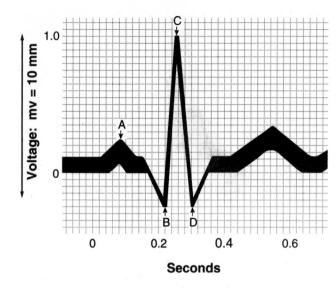

Voltage: mv = 10 mm

Seconds

**Figure 3-19:** Lead II ECG tracing.

146. Increased ventilatory rate, deviated trachea, unilaterally decreased vocal and tactile fremitus, hyperresonant percussion notes, and unilaterally decreased breath sounds might all be signs of which respiratory condition?

    A. tension pneumothorax
    B. pleural effusion
    C. consolidation
    D. atelectasis

147. Pulmonary stress testing is performed to evaluate all of the following EXCEPT:

    A. pulmonary disability
    B. exercise-induced asthma
    C. morbidity of lung resection
    D. dosage for bronchodilator

148. As the RRT auscultates directly over a patient's trachea, she hears loud, high-pitched sounds. What type of sounds is she hearing?

    A. crackles
    B. rhonchi
    C. bronchial
    D. bronchovesicular

149. A patient receiving mechanical ventilatory support with an $F_IO_2$ of 0.30 has been evaluated as having a 10% intrapulmonary shunt. What should the RRT recommend at this time?

    A. Do *nothing* because a 10% intrapulmonary shunt reflects little interference with gas exchange.
    B. Institute 5 to 10 cm $H_2O$ of PEEP to improve oxygenation.

    C. Increase the $F_IO_2$ to 0.80 to alleviate the shunt-effect component of the intrapulmonary shunt.
    D. Institute pressure-support ventilation (PSV) to decrease the work of breathing.

150. Which of the following sets of ABG and alveolar gas tension data are consistent with those of an asbestosis patient at rest and breathing room air?

    A. $PaO_2$ 85 torr; $PaCO_2$ 55 torr; $PaO_2$ 100 torr; $PaCO_2$ 40 torr
    B. $PaO_2$ 50 torr; $PaCO_2$ 40 torr; $PaO_2$ 100 torr; $PaCO_2$ 40 torr
    C. $PaO_2$ 95 torr; $PaCO_2$ 40 torr; $PaO_2$ 100 torr; $PaCO_2$ 40 torr
    D. $PaO_2$ 55 torr; $PaCO_2$ 30 torr; $PaO_2$ 100 torr; $PaCO_2$ 30 torr

151. Which disease entity is generally associated with the production of copious amounts of purulent, fetid, and sometimes bloody sputum that characteristically separates into three distinct layers when allowed to settle?

    A. tuberculosis
    B. bronchiectasis
    C. chronic bronchitis
    D. lung abscess

152. A 1,100-g, 31-week gestation neonate displays the following clinical signs:

ventilatory rate: 80 breaths/min.
breathing pattern: paradoxical with grunting, nasal flaring, and sternal retractions

ABG data at this time indicate the following:

$PO_2$ 45 torr
$PCO_2$ 65 torr
pH 7.20
$HCO_3^-$ 25 mEq/liter
B.E. 1 mEq/liter

Chest radiography shows reticulogranular densities, air bronchograms, a distinct cardiac shadow, and a "bell-shaped" thorax. What is the most likely diagnosis based on the review of these data?

    A. bronchopulmonary dysplasia
    B. respiratory distress syndrome
    C. meconium aspiration syndrome
    D. hiatal hernia

153. To differentially diagnose cardiogenic from noncardiogenic pulmonary edema, which of the following procedures and/or studies are essential?

    A. insertion of a pulmonary artery catheter
    B. insertion of a Carlens tube

C. plotting the patient's exhaled tidal volume over the plateau pressure on the patient's manometer

D. determining the patient's total oxygen content

154. Which of the following clinical conditions can cause pedal edema?

    I. left ventricular failure
    II. chronic hypoxemia
    III. right ventricular hypertrophy
    IV. systemic hypertension

    A. I, II only
    B. I, III only
    C. II, III only
    D. II, III, IV only

155. A patient who hyperventilates would be expected to have a(n) ___ $PCO_2$ in his ___ compared with a person who has a normal ventilatory pattern.

    I. decreased; cerebrospinal fluid
    II. decreased; arterial blood
    III. increased; cerebrospinal fluid
    IV. increased; arterial blood
    V. equivalent; cerebrospinal fluid

    A. III, IV only
    B. I, IV only
    C. I, II only
    D. II, III only

156. A mainstay in assessing the effectiveness of treatment for an asthmatic is the evaluation of:

    A. the $PaO_2$.
    B. before and after bronchodilator studies.
    C. cough production.
    D. a chest radiograph.

157. A 35-year-old female with a history of severe asthma is admitted to the emergency department. She appears agitated and is using her accessory muscles of ventilation. Her breath sounds are decreased with marked expiratory wheezes. Her peak flow rates on admission are 25% of predicted. An hour after aggressive bronchodilator therapy, her peak flow rate has increased to 35% of predicted. To further increase her peak flow rate, what should the RRT recommend the physician to do?

    I. Start antibiotic therapy.
    II. Initiate corticosteroid therapy.
    III. Continue aggressive bronchodilator therapy.
    IV. Administer a sedative.
    V. Administer a diuretic.

    A. I, II only
    B. II, III only
    C. III, IV only
    D. II, V only

158. A teenage drug-overdose victim was admitted to the emergency department. ABG data revealed the following:

$PO_2$ 59 torr
$PCO_2$ 82 torr
pH 7.13
$HCO_3^-$ 27 mEq/liter
B.E. 0 mEq/liter
$SO_2$ 70%

Which of the following acid-base interpretations and/or therapeutic interventions would be acceptable at this time?

    I. This patient has an uncompensated respiratory acidosis.
    II. Acute ventilatory failure is present.
    III. The patient should receive mechanical ventilation.
    IV. Pressure-control inverse-ratio ventilation (PC-IRV) should be initiated.

    A. I, II, III only
    B. I, II only
    C. III, IV only
    D. I, II, IV only

159. Where should the tip of a central venous pressure catheter be located when the catheter is properly positioned?

    A. left atrium
    B. left ventricle
    C. superior vena cava
    D. right ventricle

160. Which physiologic effect(s) is (are) characteristic of continuous mechanical ventilation?

    I. a potential decrease in urinary output
    II. a potential decrease in intracranial pressure
    III. a potential increase in C.O.
    IV. a decrease in the FRC

    A. I only
    B. I, II only
    C. II, III only
    D. III, IV only

161. An RRT auscultates a patient's blood pressure over the brachial artery with a stethoscope and blood pressure cuff during cardiopulmonary resuscitation (CPR). The blood pressure determined by this method might be

    I. accurate.
    II. lower than actual.
    III. higher than actual.

    A. I only
    B. II only
    C. I, II only
    D. I, III only

162. A young female patient is admitted to the emergency department. Her vital signs are as follows:

blood pressure: 130/90 torr
heart rate: 120 beats/min.
complaint: dyspnea

A CBC, room-air ABG, and chest X-ray have been ordered. The results are as follows:

chest X-ray: normal
ABG: $PO_2$ 95 torr; $PCO_2$ 30 torr; pH 7.48;
     $HCO_3^-$ 24 mEq/liter; B.E. 0 mEq/liter
CBC: RBC $3.5 \times 10^6/mm^3$; WBC 5,000/$mm^3$;
     hemoglobin 8 g/dL; HCT 30%

Which of the following conditions is she most likely experiencing?

- A. stagnant hypoxia
- B. histotoxic hypoxia
- C. hypoxic hypoxia
- D. anemic hypoxia

163. Which of the following chest radiographic findings are consistent with bronchiolitis?

  I. hyperinflation
  II. hyperlucency
  III. sternal bowing
  IV. patchy hilar infiltrates

- A. I, II only
- B. II, III, IV only
- C. I, II, III only
- D. II, IV only

164. What is the expected normal room air alveolar arterial oxygen tension difference for a 55-year-old person?

- A. 5 torr
- B. 9 torr
- C. 12 torr
- D. 16 torr

165. Which of the following clinical conditions would be associated with a higher than normal $C\bar{v}O_2$ value?

  I. cyanide poisoning
  II. carbon monoxide poisoning
  III. myocardial infarction
  IV. septic shock

- A. I, II, IV only
- B. I, III only
- C. I, IV only
- D. III, IV only

166. The RRT is asked to evaluate the placement of a chest tube that was inserted to treat a right-sided hemothorax. Assuming the patient is in the supine position, the RRT should observe the chest tube exiting from the:

- A. right posterior portion of the thorax.
- B. right lateral portion of the thorax.
- C. right anterior portion of the thorax.
- D. left anterior portion of the thorax.

167. Fluid balance (intake and output) is critical when weaning a patient from a mechanical ventilator to prevent which of the following pathophysiologic events from occurring?

  I. decrease mucociliary clearance
  II. decreased C.O.
  III. pulmonary edema
  IV. decreased blood pressure

- A. I, III only
- B. III, IV only
- C. II, IV only
- D. I, II, III, IV

168. Which of the following conditions might produce erroneous pulse oximeter results?

  I. hypothermia
  II. hypertension
  III. cardiac arrest
  IV. significant venous pulsation

- A. I, III only
- B. II, III, IV only
- C. I, III, IV only
- D. I, II, IV only

169. An RRT is asked to assist a physician in the placement of a central venous pressure (CVP) catheter. If the catheter is properly positioned and if the patient has *no* cardiopulmonary pathophysiology, which of the following statements are true?

  I. The CVP will read 5 to 15 cm $H_2O$.
  II. The catheter will be located at the junction of the superior vena cava and the right atrium.
  III. The CVP will reflect right ventricular preload.
  IV. The CVP will read 0 to 8 mm Hg.

- A. I, II only
- B. II, III, IV only
- C. I, III only
- D. I, II, III, IV

170. Which of the following conditions will be displayed by a ventilator-dependent patient who is overhydrated?

  I. decreased pulmonary compliance
  II. widened $P(A-a)O_2$ gradient
  III. evidence of congestive heart failure on chest radiograph
  IV. decreased PCWP
  V. decreased blood pressure

A. I, III, V only
B. I, II, IV only
C. II, III, IV only
D. I, II, III only

171. As the RRT palpates a patient's pulse, he observes that the heart rhythm is consistently irregular with a rate between 100 to 120 beats/min. The patient's blood pressure is normal and is *not* showing any signs of hemodynamic compromise. What common cardiac dysrhythmia would the RRT expect to see when looking at this patient's ECG?

    A. ventricular fibrillation
    B. ventricular tachycardia
    C. atrial fibrillation
    D. sinus bradycardia

172. The RRT is asked to evaluate a chest radiograph for the purpose of determining the presence of a right-sided tension pneumothorax. Which of the following radiographic findings would indicate the presence of this condition?

    A. blunted costophrenic angles
    B. an air bronchogram
    C. a mediastinal shift
    D. increased vascular markings on the right

173. Which of the following pulmonary pathologies are generally associated with an increase in intrapulmonary shunting?

    I. Klebsiella pneumonia
    II. pulmonary edema
    III. ARDS
    IV. pleural effusion

    A. I, II, III, IV
    B. II, III only
    C. III, IV only
    D. I, II only

174. A 1-year-old child who has been progressively more uncomfortable and irritable for the past 2 days presents with a low-grade fever, runny nose, hoarseness, and coarse bilateral breath sounds. The child is using accessory muscles for breathing and has a harsh, barking cough. The child is most likely experiencing:

    A. laryngotracheobronchitis.
    B. an acute asthma attack.
    C. foreign-body aspiration.
    D. epiglottitis.

175. Calculate the alveolar-arterial oxygen tension difference for a 35-year-old patient breathing supplemental oxygen via a simple mask operating at 10 L/min. This patient's ABG data reveal the following:

$PO_2$ 80 torr
$PCO_2$ 46 torr
pH 7.38
$HCO_3^-$ 26 mEq/liter
B.E. 2 mEq/liter

Assume a normal respiratory quotient and a normal barometric pressure.

    A. 10 to 15 torr
    B. 20 to 25 torr
    C. 25 to 30 torr
    D. This measurement *cannot* be calculated.

176. Which lung sounds might sometimes disappear as a result of an effective cough generated by the patient?

    A. crackles
    B. bronchovesicular
    C. vesicular
    D. rhonchi

177. The hemodynamic data shown here were obtained by way of pulmonary artery catheterization of an average-sized adult patient:

pulmonary artery systolic pressure: 41 mm Hg
pulmonary artery diastolic pressure: 31 mm Hg
pulmonary artery wedge pressure: 28 mm Hg
mean arterial pressure: 60 mm Hg
cardiac index: 2.0 L/min./m²

Which clinical condition(s) might account for the cardiac index value?

    I. right ventricular myocardial infarction
    II. hypovolemia
    III. hypervolemia
    IV. left ventricular myocardial infarction

    A. II, IV only
    B. II only
    C. IV only
    D. I, III only

178. The radiologic findings of reduced vascular lung markings in the right upper hemithorax and a linear opacity in the right lower hemithorax in a 4-year-old, ordinarily healthy boy who developed sudden shortness of breath while playing in the back seat of his parents' car suggest:

    I. left lower pneumonia.
    II. right lung atelectasis.
    III. foreign-object aspiration.

    A. I only
    B. II only
    C. I, II only
    D. II, III only

179. Upon routine evaluation of a ventilator patient in the ICU, the cuff pressure of a properly sized ET tube is

recorded as 40 mm Hg. What is the physiologic significance of that pressure?

   I.  Lymphatic flow will be obstructed.
  II.  Venous flow will be impaired.
 III.  Arterial capillary flow will occur.

  A.  I only
  B.  I, II only
  C.  II only
  D.  I, II, III

180. Which of the following measurements would best indicate whether the lungs of a mechanically ventilated patient were getting stiffer?

  A.  airway resistance
  B.  dynamic compliance
  C.  static compliance
  D.  arterial $PCO_2$

181. A patient who has a long history of COPD presents in the emergency department in marked distress. In addition to an increased work of breathing, what other observation would imply the presence of cardiac embarrassment?

  A.  cold extremeties
  B.  decreased heart rate
  C.  diaphoresis
  D.  bounding pulse

182. Which of the following conditions would be associated with a calculated shunt of 20%?

  A.  intrapulmonary abnormality of *no* clinical significance
  B.  the likelihood of successful weaning from mechanical ventilation
  C.  pulmonary disease incompatible with successful weaning from mechanical ventilation
  D.  life-threatening shunt requiring aggressive cardiopulmonary support

183. Which form of oxygen monitoring would be most appropriate for an adult patient who is believed to have *no* abnormal forms of hemoglobin?

  A.  co-oximetry
  B.  transcutaneous $O_2$ monitoring
  C.  pulse oximetry
  D.  ABG analysis

184. The evaluation of a 24-year-old febrile patient with tachycardia in the emergency department reveals the following information:

ABG data:
$PO_2$ 69 mm Hg

$PCO_2$ 33 mm Hg
pH 7.47
[Hb] 14 g%
HCT 45%

Which of the following laboratory analyses would be most appropriate to further evaluate this patient?

  A.  cardiac enzymes
  B.  serum electrolytes
  C.  CBC
  D.  urinalysis

185. Which physiologic alteration(s) would stimulate the peripheral chemoreceptors to send hyperventilation impulses to the medulla?

   I.  a decreased partial pressure of oxygen in arterial blood
  II.  an acute rise in dissolved arterial $CO_2$
 III.  an acute increase in arterial $[H^+]$
 IV.  an acute increase in arterial blood pH

  A.  I only
  B.  II, III, IV only
  C.  I, II only
  D.  I, II, III only

186. A 150-pound (IBW) male is receiving controlled mechanical ventilation with a $V_T$ of 500 ml at a rate of 12 breaths/min. Calculate his $\dot{V}_A/\dot{Q}_C$ given the following data:

$\dot{V}O_2$ 240 ml/minute
$CaO_2$ 20 vol%
$C\bar{v}O_2$ 14 vol%

  A.  0.90
  B.  1.05
  C.  1.45
  D.  2.08

187. A patient's chest X-ray reveals the trachea deviated to the left and mediastinal contents directed toward the unaffected lung. These findings are characteristic of a:

  A.  pneumopericardium.
  B.  pneumomediastinum.
  C.  mediastinal shift.
  D.  subcutaneous emphysema.

188. Which of the following statements are true regarding assessing apnea in premature newborns?

   I.  Most apneic incidents can be quickly terminated by gentle tactile stimulation.
  II.  Apnea is often associated with tachycardia.
 III.  Apnea of prematurity responds well to methylxanthines.

IV. CPAP is used to treat apnea of prematurity.

V. Apnea pauses of 30 seconds or less are normal for premature newborns.

A. I, II, V only
B. I, III, IV only
C. II, III, V only
D. I, II, III, IV, V

189. A 27-year-old male was fishing when his boat capsized. He was soon retrieved from the water by a passing Coast Guard vessel. Resuscitation was begun. He was air evacuated to the University of South Alabama Medical Center where he immediately received $O_2$ and $NaHCO_3$ and was placed on intermittent mandatory ventilation with the following settings:

$V_T$: 800 cc
$FiO_2$: 0.40
ventilatory rate: 5 breaths/min.

He had a spontaneous ventilatory rate of 12 breaths/min. and a spontaneous $V_T$ of 400 cc. When the ventilator cycled on to deliver the 800-cc tidal volume, the PIP consistently registered 30 cm $H_2O$. ABGs while on the ventilator were as follows:

$PaO_2$ 95 mm Hg
$PaCO_2$ 44 mm Hg
pH 7.38
$HCO_3^-$ 26 mEq/liter
B.E. 2 mEq/liter

Twenty-four hours after admission, the patient's ventilatory rate increased to 26 breaths/min., his heart rate increased to 130 beats/min., and he became cyanotic. Auscultation of the chest revealed normal breath sounds, and percussion revealed decreased resonance over the lung boundaries. The PIP during the mandatory breaths increased to 50 cm $H_2O$. ABGs at this time were:

$PaO_2$ 41 mm Hg
$PaCO_2$ 29 mm Hg
pH 7.50
$HCO_3^-$ 22 mEq/liter
B.E. −2 mEq/liter

The $FiO_2$ was increased to 0.80. The patient was sedated. The ventilator was changed to the control mode with a rate of 12 breaths/min. Twenty minutes after these changes were instituted, ABGs were:

$PaO_2$ 55 mm Hg
$PaCO_2$ 45 mm Hg
pH 7.38
$HCO_3^-$ 24 mEq/liter
B.E. 0 mEq/liter

What clinical condition is the probable cause of the patient's problems?

A. pulmonary embolism
B. ARDS
C. spontaneous pneumothorax
D. aspiration pneumonitis

190. A patient complains of wheezing during and after exercising in the winter. Her physician would most likely order which of the following pulmonary stress tests?

A. exercise-induced asthma test
B. quantitative methacholine challenge test
C. before and after bronchodilator spirometry
D. maximum voluntary ventilation

191. Evaluation of a patient in the emergency department reveals a patient who is tachypneic, tachycardic, and febrile. Which of the following laboratory tests would be the most appropriate to further evaluate this patient?

A. CBC
B. electrolytes
C. sputum culture and sensitivity
D. urine culture

## SITUATIONAL SETS

**Questions 192 and 193 refer to the same patient.**

The RRT has been asked to administer the $\beta_2$ agonist metaproterenol, to a wheezing chronic bronchitis patient.

Immediately before administering 0.5 ml of the drug diluted in 4 ml of normal saline via a hand-held nebulizer, she observes the following ECG tracing (Figure 3-20 on page 114) on the cardiac monitor. Five minutes into the treatment, she then notices the cardiac monitor displaying the ECG tracing also shown in Figure 3-21 on page 114.

192. Interpret the ECG tracing occurring during the treatment.

A. ventricular fibrillation
B. ventricular tachycardia
C. sinus tachycardia
D. premature ventricular contractions

193. What might have caused the ECG tracing to change during the aerosolized bronchodilator treatment?

A. The wrong diluent was used.
B. Too much diluent was used.
C. Too much metaproterenol was administered.
D. The wrong device was used to deliver the medication.

**Questions 194, 195, and 196 refer to the same patient.**

A 70-kg patient is about to be mechanically ventilated via a volume ventilator. Before establishing the initial ventilator settings, the RRT wishes to determine the

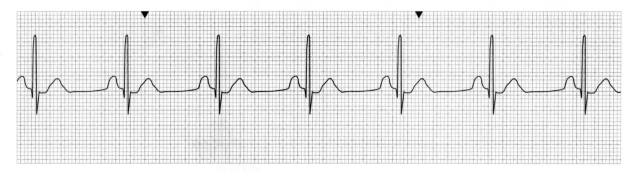

**Figure 3-20:** ECG tracing before the administration of metaproterenol.

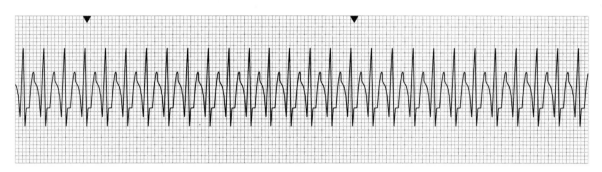

**Figure 3-21:** ECG tracing 5 minutes into the aerosol treatment.

system compliance for this ventilator. She sets the tidal volume to 200 ml and allows the machine to cycle to inspiration while occluding the patient connector. She then notes that the PIP is 65 cm $H_2O$.

194. Calculate the system compliance.

    A. 1.00 ml/cm $H_2O$
    B. 2.35 ml/cm $H_2O$
    C. 2.65 ml/cm $H_2O$
    D. 3.08 ml/cm $H_2O$

195. The RRT then establishes the following initial ventilator settings:

    $V_T$: 900 cc
    f: 12 breaths/min.
    $FIO_2$: 0.50
    peak flow rate: 45 L/min.
    PEEP: 10 cm $H_2O$
    inspiratory hold: 0.2 sec.

The patient is now receiving mechanical ventilation. It is noted that the PIP achieved is 45 cm $H_2O$. Calculate the patient's actual tidal volume.

    A. 808 cc
    B. 792 cc
    C. 781 cc
    D. 762 cc

196. When an inspiratory plateau of 0.5 sec. is activated, the static pressure noted is 35 cm $H_2O$. Determine the patient's static compliance.

    A. 31.68 cc/cm $H_2O$
    B. 31.24 cc/cm $H_2O$
    C. 30.48 cc/cm $H_2O$
    D. 22.65 cc/cm $H_2O$

**Questions 197, 198, and 199 refer to the following scenario:**

A 62-year-old female completed a 6-hour airplane flight. She immediately experienced pain in the calf of her left leg and noted that the area was slightly swollen and tender to the touch. That night she was awakened by a sudden pain in the left midlateral chest. The pain was sharp and became more intense during deep breathing and coughing. She also experienced an acute shortness of breath. A few hours later, she coughed up a small amount of clear, blood-tinged sputum. Examination by her physician revealed decreased thoracic movement and decreased breath sounds on the left side of the chest where friction rubs also were perceived. The ankle and calf were slightly swollen, with the calf warm and tender. A positive Homan's sign was observed. (This sign consists of pain in the calf when the foot is dorsiflexed.) The chest roentgenogram showed a triangular shadow in the left middle chest with its base along the pleural lining. A slight pleural effusion was also observed.

197. What is this patient's clinical problem?

    A. myocardial infarction
    B. pulmonary thromboembolism

C. coronary thrombosis

D. spontaneous pneumothorax

198. What does the triangular shadow in the left midchest with its base on the pleural lining signify?

A. acute pleuritis

B. atelectasis

C. pulmonary edema

D. pulmonary infarction

199. What was the significance of the painful legs?

A. atherosclerosis

B. thrombophlebitis

C. acute vasculitis

D. leg cramps

**Questions 200 and 201 are based on the following information.**

A neonate is observed at 1 minute after birth. Her heart rate is 110 beats/min. Her ventilatory rate is 40 breath/min. She is crying and exhibiting peripheral cyanosis. Some flexion of her extremities is displayed. The nurse has passed a suction catheter down the neonate's nose, causing the infant to sneeze.

200. What should the baby girl's Apgar score be?

A. 0

B. 4

C. 6

D. 8

201. Based on this 1-min. Apgar score, what action should be taken at this time?

A. Bag-mask ventilation and supplemental oxygen are indicated to alleviate the peripheral cyanosis.

B. Suctioning should precede the bag-mask ventilation and oxygen administration.

C. *No* resuscitative measures appear necessary.

D. CPR is indicated immediately.

**Questions 202, 203, and 204 refer to the following patient:**

A patient is being mechanically ventilated via the following settings:

mode: assist-control
tidal volume: 900 cc
peak flow rate: 60 L/min.
ventilatory rate: 12 breaths/min.
$FiO_2$: 0.60

202. Calculate this patient's minute ventilation.

A. 5.0 L/min.

B. 9.2 L/min.

C. 10.8 L/min.

D. 54.0 L/min.

203. Calculate the inspiratory time.

A. 0.9 sec.

B. 1.2 sec.

C. 1.6 sec.

D. 2.0 sec.

204. Calculate the inspiratory:expiratory (I:E) ratio.

A. 1.0:4.6

B. 1.0:3.4

C. 1.0:2.2

D. 1.0:1.7

**Questions 205 and 206 refer to the same patient.**

205. Calculate the maximum voluntary ventilation (MVV) for a 30-year-old male patient who exhaled 38 liters of air in 12 seconds.

A. 3.2 L/min.

B. 38 L/min.

C. 190 L/min.

D. 456 L/min.

206. Which of the following interpretations can be made from the data obtained from this MVV maneuver?

A. The subject will have difficulty sustaining adequate ventilation during exercise.

B. The subject failed to cooperate during the diagnostic procedure.

C. The subject is exhibiting air trapping and airflow limitation.

D. The subject has achieved a normal MVV value.

**Questions 207 and 208 refer to the same patient.**

207. A 22-year-old motor vehicle accident victim suffered massive blood loss, multiple contusions, lacerations, and two broken legs. She was admitted to the ICU and has been receiving mechanical ventilation for the last 20 hours. Her ventilator settings include:

mode: SIMV
$V_T$: 800 cc
SIMV rate: 12 breaths/min.
$FiO_2$: 0.40
PEEP: 5 cm $H_2O$
high-pressure limit: 40 cm $H_2O$

Her last ABG, performed 3 hours ago, revealed the following:

$PO_2$ 85 torr
$PCO_2$ 41 torr
pH 7.42

HCO$_3^-$ 26 mEq/liter
B.E. 2 mEq/liter

Suddenly, the ventilator's high-pressure alarm has begun sounding. ET suctioning was performed, resulting in insignificant secretions. Auscultation of the chest revealed bilateral breath sounds and fine crackles in both lungs. What should the RRT recommend at this time?

   I. performing an arterial puncture
  II. switching to control-mode ventilation
 III. increasing the high-pressure limit
 IV. ordering a STAT chest X-ray

  A. I, II only
  B. II, III only
  C. I, III, IV only
  D. I, II, III only

208. Current ABGs obtained from this patient reveal the following:

PO$_2$ 50 torr
PCO$_2$ 29 torr
pH 7.50
HCO$_3^-$ 22 mEq/liter
B.E. −2 mEq/liter

Ventilator settings at this time include the following:

mode: SIMV
V$_T$: 800 cc
SIMV rate: 12 breaths/min.
F$_I$O$_2$: 0.60
PEEP: 10 cm H$_2$O
high-pressure limit: 50 cm H$_2$O

The patient also has a spontaneous ventilatory rate of 12 breaths/min. Her chest radiograph revealed diffuse pulmonary infiltrates in all lung fields with areas of "whiteout" in the lower lobes. Which of the following pathophysiologic conditions is likely occurring in this patient?

  A. status asthmaticus
  B. pneumonia
  C. ARDS
  D. acute exacerbation of COPD

**Questions 209 and 210 refer to the same patient.**

209. Calculate the amount of reduced hemoglobin in a patient who has the following clinical data while breathing room air:

PaO$_2$ 30 torr
PaCO$_2$ 90 torr
pH 7.25
[Hb] 20 g%

SaO$_2$ 51%
S$\bar{v}$O$_2$ 45%

  A. 5.0 g%
  B. 8.5 g%
  C. 10.4 g%
  D. 12.0 g%

210. Based on the foregoing calculation, which of the following assessments can be made about this patient?

  A. The patient needs an infusion of packed cells.
  B. The patient is cyanotic.
  C. The patient is anemic.
  D. The patient's fluid volume is low.

**Questions 211 and 212 refer to the same patient.**

A 35-year-old, 80-kg woman who has thrombophlebitis displays the following signs and symptoms while spontaneously breathing:

dyspnea
chest pain
tachycardia
tachypnea
decreased breath sounds
slight wheezing

Her room air ABG and acid-base data reveal the following: PO$_2$ 80 torr; PCO$_2$ 30 torr; pH 7.51; HCO$_3^-$ 23 mEq/liter; and B.E. 0 mEq/liter. Analysis of this patient's exhaled gas indicates a P$\bar{E}$CO$_2$ of 10 torr.

211. Calculate this patient's V$_D$/V$_T$ ratio.

  A. 0.30
  B. 0.45
  C. 0.54
  D. 0.67

212. What likely is this patient's diagnosis?

  A. pulmonary infarction
  B. myocardial infarction
  C. pulmonary embolism
  D. acute pneumonia

213. During a patient interview, which of the following questions would provide useful information to the RRT about a patient's activities of daily living?

   I. "How many packs of cigarettes do you smoke per day?"
  II. "How does your breathlessness affect you?"
 III. "When did your cough start?"
 IV. "How much sputum or mucus do you cough up each day?"

  A. II only
  B. III, IV only

C. I, II only

D. II, III only

214. The RRT is asked to recommend bronchial hygiene therapy for a 9-year-old cystic fibrosis patient who will be visiting her 85-year-old grandmother for four weeks in the summer. Which of the following bronchial hygiene modalities would be appropriate for this patient?

I. percussion and vibration
II. flutter therapy
III. PEP therapy
IV. autogenic drainage

A. I, II only
B. II, IV only
C. II, III, IV only
D. I, II, IV only

215. An RRT is interviewing a patient in an attempt to determine information about the patient's complaint of "having a difficult time breathing." Which of the following questions would be appropriate for the RRT to ask to obtain more information about this symptom?

I. "What does it feel like?"
II. "How long does it last?"
III. "Where is it?"
IV. "What makes this sensation better?"

A. I, III only
B. II, III, IV only
C. I, II, IV only
D. I, II, III, IV

216. How can the RRT best determine whether a patient knows how to use a metered-dose inhaler (MDI)?

A. Ask the patient whether he knows what an actuator is.
B. Ask the patient to show you how to place the medication canister in the actuator.
C. Have the patient demonstrate the procedure to you.
D. Ask the patient how long he has been using an MDI and to estimate how many treatments he has taken.

217. A patient has been evaluated by an RRT who is preparing a respiratory care plan based on the following data obtained in the assessment:

- SpO$_2$/FiO$_2$: 98% while breathing room air
- respiratory pattern: regular pattern; rate of 12 breaths/min.
- mental status: confused; does not follow commands
- breath sounds: crackles in the bases, bilaterally
- cough: none
- activity level: ambulatory with assistance

The respiratory care plan written by the RRT is as follows:

1) albuterol QID and prn via a metered-dose inhaler
2) bronchial hygiene therapy via chest physiotherapy (postural drainage and percussion) applied to the basal segments of both lungs QID after each QID albuterol treatment

Which of the following statements accurately pertain to the respiratory care plan?

I. The albuterol treatment should be given three times per day while the patient is awake.
II. Incentive spirometry should be administered instead of postural drainage and percussion.
III. A bronchodilator does *not* appear to be indicated.
IV. The patient should be receiving oxygen therapy via a nasal cannula at 2 liters/min.

A. I, IV only
B. II, III only
C. III, IV only
D. I, II, IV only

218. A patient enters the pulmonary clinic complaining of dyspnea. The RRT begins to interview the patient. Which of the following questions would be useful in obtaining information about this symptom?

I. "Have you ever lived in or traveled near the San Joaquin Valley in California?"
II. "What type of work do you do?"
III. "How many stairs can you climb before you feel short of breath?"
IV. "How do people in your family feel about your shortness of breath?"

A. III only
B. II, IV only
C. I, II, III only
D. I, II, III, IV

219. A lateral neck X-ray obtained from a 3-year-old child experiencing respiratory distress demonstrates a steeple sign. Which of the following conditions does this child likely have?

A. epiglotittis
B. laryngotracheobronchitis
C. foreign body aspiration
D. tracheomalacia

220. A 4-year-old child is brought into the emergency department exhibiting respiratory distress, drooling, inspiratory stridor, and coughing. The patient is afebrile. The child's parents said that this condition occurred abruptly while the child was at play alone in her playroom. Lateral and anterioposterior neck radiographs do *not* reveal either the steeple or thumb sign.

Which of the following conditions does this child likely have?

A. laryngotracheobronchitis
B. epiglotittis
C. foreign body aspiration
D. tracheomalacia

221. A respiratory therapy department with a protocol system in place has found that one of the RRTs seldom makes changes in therapy. His assessments seem to always reflect a continuation of therapy at the same frequency, for example, QID. Which of the following actions would help resolve this situation?

   I. A supervisor should audit the care plans reviewed by the RRT in question to evaluate the correctness of the evaluations.
   II. The RRT should be reprimanded for sloppy work.
   III. The RRT should be asked to perform case-study exercises with defined assessment outcomes and care plans to see whether he develops a similar plan.
   IV. The situation could be overlooked because other RRTs will adjust the care plan at a later time.

   A. I only
   B. II, III only
   C. I, III only
   D. I, II, III, IV

222. A postoperative male patient was recently weaned from nasal oxygen. An RRT finds the patient displaying central cyanosis, disoriented, and having a heart rate of 120 beats per minute and a respiratory rate of 32 breaths per minute. A pulse oximeter check reveals an SpO$_2$ of 93%.

   Which of the following actions is warranted?

A. Monitoring and observing the patient carefully.
B. Providing oxygen via a nasal cannula at 4 liters per minute.
C. Calling a code.
D. Recommending that the patient be scheduled for a sleep study.

223. During an interview with an RRT, a patient states that she experiences a sudden onset of breathing difficulty when she sleeps in a recumbent position. She also states that the condition is accompanied by coughing and that the breathing difficulty is relieved when she assumes an upright position. She further informs the RRT that if she places two pillows behind her back before falling asleep, the breathing difficulty does *not* occur. Based on this information, which of the following conditions does this patient likely have?

A. nocturnal asthma
B. left ventricular failure
C. sleep apnea
D. pneumonia

224. The RRT performs percussion on a patient's thorax and hears decreased resonance. Which of the following conditions can cause this physical examination finding?

   I. pneumonia
   II. atelectasis
   III. pleural effusion
   IV. asthma

   A. II, III only
   B. I, II, III only
   C. I, II, IV only
   D. I, III, IV only

# Clinical Data Matrix Categories

| | | | |
|---|---|---|---|
| 1. IC2i | 47. IB10a | 93. IB1b | 139. IA1h |
| 2. IB9d | 48. IB8a | 94. IA1b | 140. IA1f(3) |
| 3. IB7b | 49. IB10c | 95. IB9b | 141. IA2a |
| 4. IA1a | 50. IB10c | 96. IB8c | 142. IC4 |
| 5. IB7a | 51. IA1c | 97. IA1h | 143. IA1f(4) |
| 6. IC2a | 52. IC2b | 98. IA1h | 144. IB1b |
| 7. IB9d | 53. IB9e | 99. IA1e | 145. IB10a |
| 8. IB1b | 54. IA1c | 100. IB10d | 146. IA1b |
| 9. IA1a | 55. IB4a | 101. IB10d | 147. IA2h |
| 10. IB10a | 56. IB10h | 102. 1IB3 | 148. IB4a |
| 11. IC1a | 57. IB9b | 103. IA1i | 149. IC2c |
| 12. IB7e | 58. IB10g | 104. IA1g(2) | 150. IB10c |
| 13. IB3 | 59. IB1b | 105. IA1f(3) | 151. IA1c |
| 14. IC2a | 60. IA1a | 106. IA1c | 152. IA1e |
| 15. IC2c | 61. IA1b | 107. IA1f(4) | 153. IA2e |
| 16. IB7c | 62. IA1b | 108. IA1b | 154. IA1g(2) |
| 17. IC1c | 63. IA1h | 109. IA1g(1) | 155. IB10c |
| 18. IC2c | 64. IB10d | 110. IB9d | 156. IC1a |
| 19. IA2d | 65. IC2a | 111. IB10a | 157. IC2a |
| 20. IA1g(1) | 66. IB10a | 112. IB6b | 158. IC2e |
| 21. IB10c | 67. IB9e | 113. IB9c | 159. IA1g(2) |
| 22. IA2b | 68. IB9d | 114. IC2a | 160. IA1f(1) |
| 23. IC2h | 69. IA1b | 115. IB2b | 161. IA1g(1) |
| 24. IB10c | 70. IB10c | 116. IC1c | 162. IA1c |
| 25. IB1a | 71. IC2e | 117. IA1h | 163. IA1e |
| 26. IB1b | 72. IA1f(3) | 118. IC2c | 164. IB10c |
| 27. IB10a | 73. IB4a | 119. IA1a | 165. IA1g(2) |
| 28. IB7e | 74. IC2c | 120. IA1e | 166. IB1c |
| 29. IC2c | 75. IA1b | 121. IB10d | 167. IA1f(1) |
| 30. IB9d | 76. IA1f(1) | 122. IB2b | 168. IB10a |
| 31. IB10g | 77. IA1b | 123. IC1e | 169. IA1g(2) |
| 32. IB9g | 78. IC2a | 124. IA1f(3) | 170. IC1d |
| 33. IC1c | 79. IB2b | 125. IB10c | 171. IB10a |
| 34. IC2e | 80. IA1f(3) | 126. IB8a | 172. IB7a |
| 35. IA1c | 81. IA1f(3) | 127. IA1c | 173. IC2c |
| 36. IB1a | 82. IC2c | 128. IA2a | 174. IA1b |
| 37. IB3 | 83. IA1c | 129. IA1e | 175. IB9c |
| 38. IC2i | 84. IA1b | 130. IA1c | 176. IB4a |
| 39. IB4b | 85. IA1g(2) | 131. IA1d | 177. IC1c |
| 40. IB10c | 86. IA1c | 132. IB1a | 178. IB7b |
| 41. IB9b | 87. IB9d | 133. IB1b | 179. IB10h |
| 42. IB2b | 88. IA2c | 134. IA1b | 180. IA1f(4) |
| 43. IC2a | 89. IA10c | 135. IA1g(2) | 181. IA1b |
| 44. IB10d | 90. IB9e | 136. IB10a | 182. IB10c |
| 45. IC2i | 91. IB10a | 137. IB7e | 183. IA1f(5) |
| 46. IB4a | 92. IB7a | 138. IA1h | 184. IA1c |

| 185. IA1d | 192. IB10a | 199. IA1b | 206. IC2a |
| 186. IA1i | 193. IC1b | 200. IB1c | 207. IA2b |
| 187. IB7e | 194. IC1g | 201. IIID1d | 208. IA1b |
| 188. IA1h | 195. IB9b | 202. IB9b | 209. IA1c |
| 189. IB10c | 196. IC1g | 203. IB9b | 210. IB1a |
| 190. IA2h | 197. IA1b | 204. IB9b | 211. IB9c |
| 191. IA1c | 198. IA1b | 205. IC1a | 212. IA1c |

# Chapter 3 Pretest Written Registry Examination Matrix Scoring Form

| CONTENT AREA | CLINICAL DATA ITEM NUMBER | CLINICAL DATA CONTENT AREA SCORE | |
|---|---|---|---|
| IA1. Review existing data in patient's record. | 4,9,20,35,51,54,60,61,62, 63,69,72,75,76,77,80,81, 83,84,85,86,89,94,97,98,99, 103,104,105,106,107,108, 109,117,119,120,124,127, 129,130,131,134,135,138, 139,140,143,146,151,152, 154,159,160,161,162,163, 165,167,169,174,180,181, 183, 184, 185, 186,188,191, 197,198,199,208,209,212 | $\frac{}{74} \times 100 =$ _____% | $\frac{}{83} \times 100 =$ _____% |
| IA2. Recommend procedures to obtain additional data. | 19,22,88,128,141, 147,153,190,207 | $\frac{}{9} \times 100 =$ _____% | |
| IB1. Assess patient's cardiopulmonary status by inspection. | 8,25,26,36,59,93,132, 133,144,166,200,210 | $\frac{}{12} \times 100 =$ _____% | $\frac{}{99} \times 100 =$ _____% |
| IB2. Assess patient's cardiopulmonary status by palpation. | 28,42,79,115,122 | $\frac{}{5} \times 100 =$ _____% | |
| IB3. Assess patient's cardiopulmonary status by percussion. | 13,37,73,102,224 | $\frac{}{5} \times 100 =$ _____% | |
| IB4. Assess patient's cardiopulmonary status by auscultation. | 39,46,55,148,176 | $\frac{}{5} \times 100 =$ _____% | |
| IB5. Assess patient's learning needs. | 216 | $\frac{}{1} \times 100 =$ _____% | |
| IB6. Interview patient. | 112,213,215,218,223 | $\frac{}{5} \times 100 =$ _____% | |
| IB7. Review chest radiograph. | 3,5,12,16,92, 137,172,178,187 | $\frac{}{9} \times 100 =$ _____% | |
| IB8. Review lateral neck radiograph. | 48,96,126,219,220 | $\frac{}{5} \times 100 =$ _____% | |

| CONTENT AREA | CLINICAL DATA ITEM NUMBER | CLINICAL DATA CONTENT AREA SCORE | |
|---|---|---|---|
| IB9. Perform bedside procedures. | 2,7,30,31,32,41,53,57,67, 87,90,95,110,113,150,175, 195,202,203,204,211 | $\dfrac{}{21} \times 100 = \underline{\hspace{1cm}}\%$ | |
| IB10. Interpret bedside procedures. | 10,21,24,27,40,44,47, 49,50,56,58,64,66,68,70, 91,100,101,111,121,125, 136,145,155,164,168,171, 179,182,189,192 | $\dfrac{}{31} \times 100 = \underline{\hspace{1cm}}\%$ | |
| IC1. Perform diagnostic procedures. | 6,11,14,17,18,29,33,116, 123,156,170,177,193, 194,196,205 | $\dfrac{}{16} \times 100 = \underline{\hspace{1cm}}\%$ | |
| IC2. Interpret results of diagnostic procedures. | 1,15,23,34,38,43,45,52,65, 71,74,78,82,114,118,149, 157,158,173,206 | $\dfrac{}{20} \times 100 = \underline{\hspace{1cm}}\%$ | $\dfrac{}{41} \times 100 = \underline{\hspace{1cm}}\%$ |
| IC3. Determine the appropriateness of prescribed respiratory care plan and recommend modifications. | 217,221,222 | $\dfrac{}{3} \times 100 = \underline{\hspace{1cm}}\%$ | |
| IC4. Participate in the development of the respiratory care plan. | 142,214 | $\dfrac{}{2} \times 100 = \underline{\hspace{1cm}}\%$ | |

Question 201 is part of a situational set and is categorized as matrix item IIID1d. Therefore, it is not included in this scoring form because it does not pertain to section I Clinical Data.

# NBRC Written Registry Examination for Advanced Respiratory Therapists (RRTs) Content Outline

## I. Select, Review, Obtain, and Interpret Data

**SETTING:** In any patient care setting, the advanced respiratory care therapist reviews existing clinical data and collects or recommends obtaining additional pertinent clinical data. The therapist evaluates all data to determine the appropriateness of the prescribed respiratory care plan, and participates in the development of the respiratory care plan.

| | RECALL | APPLICATION | ANALYSIS |
|---|---|---|---|
| | 3 | 3 | 11 |
| **A. Review patient records and recommend diagnostic procedures.** | 1* | 1 | 3 |
| 1. Review existing data in patient's record: | | | |
| a. patient history [e.g., present illness, admission notes, respiratory care orders, progress notes] | X** | | |
| b. physical examination [e.g., vital signs, physical findings] | X | | |
| c. lab data [e.g., CBC, chemistries/electrolytes, coagulation studies, Gram stain, culture and sensitivities, urinalysis] | X | X | |
| d. pulmonary function and blood gas results | X | X | |
| e. radiological studies [e.g., X-rays of chest/upper airway, CT, MRI] | X | X | |
| f. monitoring data | | | |
| (1) fluid balance (intake and output) | | | |
| (2) pulmonary mechanics [e.g., maximum inspiratory pressure (MIP), vital capacity] | X | X | |
| (3) respiratory monitoring [e.g., rate, tidal volume, minute volume, I:E, inspiratory and expiratory pressures; flow, volume and pressure waveforms] | X | X | |
| (4) lung compliance, airway resistance, work of breathing | X | X | |

| | RECALL | APPLICATION | ANALYSIS |
|---|---|---|---|
| (5) noninvasive monitoring [e.g., capnography, pulse oximetry, transcutaneous $O_2$/$CO_2$] | | X | X |
| g. results of cardiovascular monitoring | | | |
| (1) ECG, blood pressure, heart rate | | X | X |
| (2) hemodynamic monitoring [e.g., central venous pressure, cardiac output, pulmonary capillary wedge pressure, pulmonary artery pressures, mixed venous $O_2$, $C(a-\bar{v})O_2$, shunt studies ($\dot{Q}s/\dot{Q}t$)] | | X | X |
| h. maternal and perinatal/neonatal history and data [e.g., Apgar scores, gestational age, L/S ration, pre/post-ductal oxygenation studies] | | X | |
| i. other diagnostic studies [e.g., EEG, intracranial pressure monitoring, metabolic studies ($\dot{V}O_2$, $\dot{V}CO_2$, nutritional assessment), ventilation/perfusion scan, pulmonary angiography, sleep studies, other ultrasonography] | | | |
| 2. Recommend the following procedures to obtain additional data: | | | |
| a. CBC, electrolytes, other blood chemistries | | | |
| b. X-ray of chest and upper airway, CT scan, bronchoscopy, ventilation/perfusion lung scan, barium swallow | | X | X |
| c. Gram stain, culture and sensitivities | | X | X |
| d. Spirometry before and/or after bronchodilator, maximum voluntary ventilation, diffusing capacity, functional residual capacity, flow-volume loops, body plethysmography, nitrogen washout distribution test, total lung capacity, $CO_2$ response curve, closing volume, airway resistance, bronchoprovocation, maximum inspiratory pressure (MIP), maximum expiratory pressure (MEP) | | X | X |
| e. blood gas analysis, insertion of arterial, umbilical and/or central venous, pulmonary artery monitoring lines | | X | X |
| f. lung compliance, airway resistance, lung mechanics, work of breathing | | X | X |

*The number in each column is the number of items in that content area and cognitive level contained in each examination. For example, in category I.A., one item will be asked at the recall level, one item at the application level, and three items at the analysis level. The items could be asked relative to any tasks listed (1–2) under category I.A.

**Note: An "X" denotes the examination does NOT contain items for the given task at the cognitive level indicated in the respective column (Recall, Application, Analysis).

| | RECALL | APPLICATION | ANALYSIS |
|---|---|---|---|
| g. ECG, echocardiography, pulse oximetry, transcutaneous $O_2/CO_2$ monitoring | X | X | |
| h. $V_D/V_T$, $\dot{Q}s/\dot{Q}t$, cardiac output, cardiopulmonary stress testing | | | |
| **B. Collect and evaluate clinical information.** | **1** | **1** | **5** |
| 1. Assess patient's overall cardiopulmonary status by *inspection* to determine: | | | |
| a. general appearance, muscle wasting, venous distention, peripheral edema, diaphoresis, digital clubbing, cyanosis, capillary refill | X | X | |
| b. chest configuration, evidence of diaphragmatic movement, breathing pattern, accesory muscle activity, asymmetrical chest movement, intercostal and/or sternal retractions, nasal flaring, character of cough, amount and character of sputum | X | X | |
| c. transillumination of chest, Apgar score, gestational age | X | X | |
| 2. Assess patient's overall cardiopulmonary status by *palpation* to determine: | | | |
| a. heart rate, rhythm, force | X | X | |
| b. asymmetrical chest movements, tactile fremitus, crepitus, tenderness, secretions in the airway, tracheal deviation, endotracheal tube placement | X | X | |
| 3. Assess patient's overall cardiopulmonary status by *percussion* to determine diaphragmatic excursion and areas of altered resonance | X | X | |
| 4. Assess patient's overall cardiopulmonary status by *auscultation* to determine presence of: | | | |
| a. breath sounds [e.g., normal, bilateral, increased, decreased, absent, unequal, rhonchi or crackles (râles), wheezing, stridor, friction rub] | X | X | |
| b. heart sounds, dysrhythmias, murmurs, bruits | X | X | |
| c. blood pressure | X | X | |
| 5. Assess patient's learning needs [e.g., age and language appropriateness, education level, prior disease and medication knowledge] | X | X | |
| 6. Interview patient to determine: | | | |
| a. level of consciousness, orientation to time, place and person, emotional state, ability to cooperate | X | X | |
| b. presence of dyspnea and/or orthopnea, work of breathing, sputum | | | |

| | RECALL | APPLICATION | ANALYSIS |
|---|---|---|---|
| production, exercise tolerance and activities of daily living | X | X | |
| c. physical environment, social support systems, nutritional status | X | X | |
| 7. Review chest X-ray to determine: | | | |
| a. presence of, or changes in, pneumothorax or subcutaneous emphysema, other extra-pulmonary air, consolidation and/or atelectasis, pulmonary infiltrates | X | X | |
| b. presence and postion of foreign bodies | X | X | |
| c. position of endotracheal or tracheostomy tube, evidence of endotracheal or tracheostomy tube cuff hyperinflation | X | X | |
| d. position of chest tube(s), nasogastric and/or feeding tube, pulmonary artery catheter (Swan-Ganz), pacemaker, CVP, and other catheters | X | | |
| e. position of, or changes in, hemidiaphragms, hyperinflation, pleural fluid, pulmonary edema, mediastinal shift, patency and size of major airways | X | X | |
| 8. Review lateral neck X-ray to determine: | | | |
| a. presence of epiglottitis and subglottic edema | X | X | |
| b. presence or position of foreign bodies | X | X | |
| c. airway narrowing | X | X | |
| 9. Perform bedside procedures to determine: | | | |
| a. ECG, pulse oximetry, transcutaneous $O_2/CO_2$ monitoring, capnography, mass spectrometry | X | X | |
| b. tidal volume, minute volume, I:E | X | X | |
| c. blood gas analysis, $P(A\text{-}a)O_2$, alveolar ventilation, $V_D/V_T$, $\dot{Q}s/\dot{Q}t$, mixed venous sampling | X | X | |
| d. peak flow, maximum inspiratory pressure, maximum expiratory pressure, forced vital capacity, timed forced expiratory volumes [e.g., $FEV_1$], lung compliance, lung mechanics | X | X | |
| e. cardiac output, pulmonary capillary wedge pressure, central venous pressure, pulmonary artery pressures, fluid balance (intake and output) | | | |
| f. pulmonary vascular resistance and systemic vascular resistance | | | |
| g. apnea monitoring, sleep studies, respiratory impedance plethysmography | X | X | |
| h. tracheal tube cuff pressure, volume | X | X | |

| | RECALL | APPLICATION | ANALYSIS |
|---|---|---|---|
| 10. Interpret results of bedside procedures to determine: | | | |
| a. ECG, pulse oximetry, transcutaneous $O_2/CO_2$ monitoring, capnography, mass spectrometry | X | X | |
| b. tidal volume, minute volume, I:E | X | X | |
| c. blood gas analysis, P(A-a)$O_2$, alveolar ventilation, $V_D/V_T$, Qs/Qt, mixed venous sampling | X | X | |
| d. peak flow, maximum inspiratory pressure, maximum expiratory pressure, forced vital capacity, timed forced expiratory volumes [e.g., $FEV_1$], lung compliance, lung mechanics | X | X | |
| e. cardiac output, pulmonary capillary wedge pressure, central venous pressure, pulmonary artery pressures, fluid balance (intake and output) | | | |
| f. pulmonary vascular resistance and systematic vascular resistance | | | |
| g. apnea monitoring, sleep studies, respiratory impedance plethysmography | X | X | |
| h. tracheal tube cuff pressure, volume | X | X | |
| **C. Perform procedures and interpret results, determine appropriateness of and participate in developing and recommending modifications to respiratory care plan.** | 1 | 1 | 3 |
| 1. Perform and/or measure the following: | | | |
| a. spirometry before and/or after bronchodilator, maximum voluntary ventilation, diffusing capacity, functional residual capacity, flow-volume loops, body plethysmography, nitrogen washout distribution test, total lung capacity, $CO_2$ response curve, closing volume, airway resistance | X | X | |
| b. ECG, pulse oximetry, transcutaneous $O_2/CO_2$ monitoring | X | X | |
| c. $V_D/V_T$, Qs/Qt, mixed venous sampling, C(a-$\bar{v}$)$O_2$, cardiac output, pulmonary capillary wedge pressure, central venous pressure, pulmonary artery pressures, cardiopulmonary stress testing | | | |
| d. fluid balance (intake and output) | | | |

| | RECALL | APPLICATION | ANALYSIS |
|---|---|---|---|
| e. arterial sampling and blood gas analysis, co-oximetry, P(A-a)$O_2$ | X | X | |
| f. sleep studies, metabolic studies [e.g., indirect calorimetry] | | | |
| g. ventilator flow, volume, and pressure waveforms, lung compliance | X | X | |
| 2. Interpret results of the following: | | | |
| a. spirometry before and/or after bronchodilator, maximum voluntary ventilation, diffusing capacity, functional residual capacity, flow-volume loops, body plethysmography, nitrogen washout distribution test, total lung capacity, $CO_2$ response curve, closing volume, airway resistance, bronchoprovocation | X | X | |
| b. ECG, pulse oximetry, transcutaneous $O_2/CO_2$ monitoring | X | X | |
| c. $V_D/V_T$, Qs/Qt, mixed venous sampling, C(a-$\bar{v}$) $O_2$, cardiac output, pulmonary capillary wedge pressure, central venous pressure, pulmonary artery pressures, cardiopulmonary stress testing | | | |
| d. fluid balance (intake and output) | | | |
| e. arterial sampling and blood gas analysis, co-oximetry, P(A-a)$O_2$ | X | X | |
| f. peripheral venipuncture or insertion of intravenous line | | | |
| g. sleep studies, metabolic studies [e.g., indirect calorimetry] | | | |
| h. insertion of arterial and umbilical monitoring lines | | | |
| i. ventilator flow, volume, and pressure waveforms, lung compliance | X | X | |
| 3. Determine the appropriateness of the prescribed respiratory care plan and recommend modifications where indicated: | | | |
| a. perform respiratory care quality assurance | X | X | |
| b. develop quality improvement program | X | X | |
| c. review interdisciplinary patient and family care plan | X | X | |
| 4. Participate in development of respiratory care plan [e.g., case management, develop and apply protocols, disease management education] | X | X | |

# Clinical Data Answers and Analyses

**NOTE:** The references listed after each analysis are numbered and keyed to the reference list located at the end of this section. The first number indicates the text. The second number indicates the page where information about the question can be found. For example (1:14, 114) means that on pages 14 and 114 of reference number 1, you will find information about the question. Frequently, it will be necessary to read beyond the page number indicated to obtain complete information. Therefore, reference to the question will be found either on the page indicated or on subsequent pages.

## IC2i

1. A. Pressure-time tracing A depicts continuous positive pressure ventilation (CPPV) in the control mode with PEEP. There are no downward deflections, thus indicating the absence of spontaneous breathing efforts. Because of the presence of positive end-respiratory pressure PEEP, the pressure tracing remains above the baseline throughout the ventilatory cycle. This ventilation pattern is also called intermittent positive pressure ventilation (IPPV) with PEEP.

Tracing B illustrates CPPV in the assist-control mode with PEEP. The slight downward deflections that precede the large upward deflections represent patient-initiated efforts to which the ventilator responds by delivering a positive pressure breath. The pressure tracing remains above the baseline throughout the ventilatory cycle because of the PEEP.

Tracing C demonstrates intermittent mandatory ventilation (IMV) with continuous positive airway pressure (CPAP) or PEEP. The absence of a downward deflection preceding each larger upward deflection signifies that the breath delivered by the ventilator is not an assisted breath. Note that the mandatory breaths are equally spaced. This cycling pattern represents a preset rate that will deliver a mandatory breath at a regular interval, regardless of where in the spontaneous ventilatory cycle the patient's own breath happens to be. The sine wave-like deflections of smaller amplitude reflect the patient's spontaneous breathing efforts. The baseline does not return to zero; therefore, PEEP or CPAP is present.

Tracing D shows CPAP. The sine wave breathing pattern represents spontaneous ventilations. Note the absence of either patient "triggered" (assisted) or mandatory positive pressure breaths. The fact that the patient is spontaneously breathing at a pressure elevated above atmospheric pressure constitutes CPAP.

(1:846), (10:89, 265).

## IB9d

2. B. Transpulmonary pressure reflects the pressure across the lungs. It can be calculated by subtracting the intrapleural pressure from the intra-alveolar pressure:

$$\frac{\text{transpulmonary}}{\text{pressure}} = \frac{\text{intra-alveolar}}{\text{pressure}} - \frac{\text{intrapleural}}{\text{pressure}}$$

For example, if the intrapleural pressure in the lower lobes (upright position assumed) at functional residual capacity (FRC) was $-4$ cm $H_2O$, the transpulmonary pressure could be calculated as follows:

- intrapleural pressure = $-4$ cm $H_2O$
- intra-alveolar pressure = $0$ cm $H_2O$ (At FRC, the intra-alveolar pressure is $0$ cm $H_2O$—1 atm or 1,034 cm $H_2O$—throughout the lungs.)
- transpulmonary pressure = ??
- transpulmonary pressure = $0$ cm $H_2O - (-4$ cm $H_2O) = 4$ cm $H_2O$

Pulmonary compliance, in turn, can be calculated by dividing the transpulmonary pressure into the patient's tidal volume according to the following formula:

$$\text{lung compliance } (C_L) = \frac{\Delta V}{\Delta P} = \frac{\text{tidal volume}}{\text{transpulmonary pressure}}$$

A spirometer would provide for the measurement of the patient's tidal volume (i.e., volume change [$\Delta V$] from normal end-exhalation [FRC] to normal end-inspiration [$V_T$]). The intraesophageal pressure (which closely approximates the intrapleural pressure) can be measured via an intraesophageal balloon. Hemodynamic pressure deflections obtained from the proximal port of a pulmonary artery catheter or a central venous pressure (CVP) catheter (during ventilation) provide approximations of the intrapleural pressure. Therefore, once the tidal volume and the transpulmonary pressure have been measured, the pulmonary compliance can be determined.

(1:196, 200, 969), (10:30, 35, 111, 257).

## IB7b

3. D. An upper airway obstruction can be life threatening. If an aspirated foreign object is small enough to enter the tracheobronchial tree beyond the level of the mainstem bronchi, however, signs and symptoms of

this condition can overlap those of pneumonia, asthma, and sub- or supraglottic croup.

Chest radiography is sometimes helpful in determining the aspiration of a foreign object. Because airway obstructions produce more airway resistance during exhalation when the airways shorten and narrow, end-expiratory lung volumes tend to be increased. The reason is the partially obstructed region does not completely empty—exhalation is not complete in that area of the lung. Therefore, an expiratory chest film will often display unilateral hyperaeration, indicating the likelihood of unilateral bronchial obstruction (i.e., an aspirated foreign object).

Additionally, positioning the patient on his side results in the compression of the dependent lung under the weight of the mediastinal structures. In the absence of bronchial obstruction, a significant reduction of lung volume in the dependent lung will be apparent. If a foreign object is creating a partial obstruction, however, the volume loss in the dependent lung is less.

In this problem, an aspirated foreign object likely partially obstructed the left lower lobe bronchus, causing that area of the lung to become hyperaerated. This hyperinflation has shifted the mediastinum to the right. Furthermore, the left-lateral decubitus film demonstrates that air is being trapped in the left lower lobe, as evidenced by incomplete emptying of that lung region. If no foreign object were present there, the left lower lobe would empty more completely.

(9:178).

## IA1a

4. C. Myasthenia gravis is an autoimmune neuromuscular disease. The specific etiology and pathogenesis have not been completely identified, however.

Myasthenia gravis is most common in women in their 20s to 40s. The disease is characterized by general fatigability and striated muscle weakness, especially of the extremities. The patient frequently complains of double vision (diplopia), drooping eyelids (ptosis), difficult and slurred speech (dysphonia), and difficulty chewing and swallowing (dysphagia). Generally, these clinical manifestations are not present in the morning hours after a night's sleep or any time after the patient rests. They usually occur late in the day or when the patient undergoes physical or emotional stress.

The disease process results from the fact that the striated muscles ineffectively contract because of inadequate stimulation acetylcholine receptors at the neuromuscular junction. Under normal circumstances, acetylcholine is released from motor nerve endings and reacts with special receptors on the muscle end plate or the muscle cell membrane. After biochemical events, the striated muscle ultimately contracts. The enzyme acetylcholinesterase then inactivates the remaining acetylcholine at the neuromuscular junction to enable the muscle fibers to repolarize.

In the case of myasthenia gravis, it appears that there are antibodies against acetylcholine receptors on the muscle cell membrane, preventing normal neurotransmitter-receptor binding. In an effort to increase the stimulation of striated muscles, patients who have this disease are treated with anticholinesterase medication, such as neostigmine or Mestinon. Anticholinesterases inactivate acetylcholinesterase at the neuromuscular junction, thereby enabling the acetylcholine to remain longer in the synapse (causing increased muscle stimulation). Muscle stimulation is, however, not restored to normal.

Definitive diagnosis is made via the Tensilon (edrophonium chloride) test. Tensilon is a rapid-onset, short-duration anticholinesterase drug used for the diagnosis of myastenia gravis. Diagnosis is confirmed when the administration of Tensilon alleviates the signs and symptoms of the disease.

(1:543–544), (16:1049–1051, 1121–1122).

## IB7a

5. C. Subcutaneous emphysema is the presence of air beneath the skin. Subcutaneous emphysema characteristically occurs in the neck, shoulders, and face. Air can enter the area under the skin because of trauma, a surgical wound (recent tracheotomy), or a diagnostic procedure (transtracheal aspiration).

Palpation of the involved tissue produces a crackling-type sound resembling that of cellophane. This characteristic sound is referred to as *crepitus*. Radiograph-ically, subcutaneous emphysema demonstrates multiple linear lucencies within the subcutaneous adipose and muscle tissue of the involved regions.

(1:310, 483), (9:79, 274), (15:1082).

## IC2a

6. C. Response to bronchodilator administration is considered clinically significant when certain components of the forced vital capacity (FVC) increase more than 15% to 20%. In this situation, the FVC improved only 1.5%. The $FEV_1$ improved only 4.0%, whereas the $FEF_{25\%-75\%}$ increased just 4.2%. None of these percentages improved enough to reflect reversibility of airway obstruction.

Bronchodilator improvement is calculated according to the following formula:

$$\frac{\left(\begin{array}{c}\text{Postbron-}\\\text{chodilator}\\\text{value}\end{array}\right) - \left(\begin{array}{c}\text{Prebron-}\\\text{chodilator}\\\text{value}\end{array}\right)}{\left(\begin{array}{c}\text{Prebronchodilator}\\\text{value}\end{array}\right)} \times 100 = \begin{array}{c}\text{Percent}\\\text{improvement}\end{array}$$

(6:51), (11:176).

## IB9d

7. D. Note the labels on the three tracings shown in Figure 3-22 (A–C).

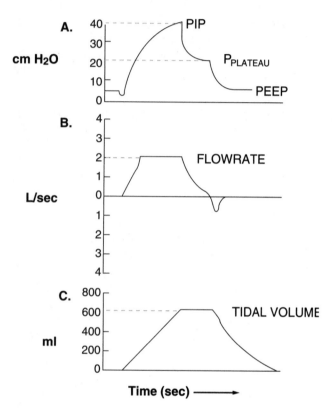

**Figure 3-22 (A–C):** Pressure-time tracing, (B) flow-time tracing, and (C) volume-time tracing.

The formula for static compliance ($C_{static}$) is

$$C_{static} = \frac{\text{tidal volume}}{\text{plateau pressure} - \text{PEEP}}$$

The tidal volume is obtained from the volume-time curve (C). The plateau pressure and PEEP are derived from the pressure-time curve (A).

Insert the values from the tracings into the $C_{static}$ formula.

$$C_{static} = \frac{600 \text{ cc}}{20 \text{ cm H}_2\text{O} - 5 \text{ cm H}_2\text{O}}$$

$$= 40 \text{ cc/cm H}_2\text{O}$$

The dynamic compliance ($C_{dynamic}$) can be calculated as follows:

$$C_{dynamic} = \frac{\text{tidal volume}}{\left(\begin{array}{c}\text{peak inspiratory}\\\text{pressure}\end{array}\right) - \text{PEEP}}$$

$$= \frac{600 \text{ cc}}{40 \text{ cm H}_2\text{O} - 5 \text{ cm H}_2\text{O}}$$

$$= 17.1 \text{ cc/cm H}_2\text{O}$$

The calculation for airway resistance ($R_{aw}$) is demonstrated below.

$$R_{aw} = \frac{\Delta P}{\dot{V}}$$

The flow rate can be obtained from the flow-time curve (B).

$$R_{aw} = \frac{\left(\begin{array}{c}\text{peak inspiratory}\\\text{pressure}\end{array}\right) - \left(\begin{array}{c}\text{plateau}\\\text{pressure}\end{array}\right)}{\text{flow rate}}$$

$$= \frac{40 \text{ cm H}_2\text{O} - 20 \text{ cm H}_2\text{O}}{2 \text{ L/sec.}}$$

$$= 10 \text{ cm H}_2\text{O/L/sec.}$$

(1:937–938), (9:285), (10:257–258).

## IB1b

8. A. In pulmonary emphysema, the lungs lose their elastic-recoil property, and air trapping or hyperaeration prevails. Because of the loss of the elastic-recoil property, exhalation is no longer passive for these patients. Exhalation occurs with the assistance of the accessory muscles of exhalation, which include the latissimus dorsi, rectus abdominus, external obliques, internal obliques, and transverse abdominus.

Because of deranged ventilatory mechanics, the pulmonary emphysema patient is at a mechanical disadvantage. In an effort to gain a mechanical advantage, this patient raises his upper chest (shoulders and clavicles) to help keep his airways open. In the process, his lungs become hyperaerated, and over time (years), his anteroposterior and transverse chest-wall diameters become equal. This configuration is described as "barrel chest." Ordinarily, the transverse chest diameter is twice that of the anteroposterior dimension.

Paradoxical chest-wall movement is associated with a flail chest. Paradoxical breathing refers to abdominal retractions during inspiration. Respiratory alternans describes the changes from a normal ventilatory pattern to paradoxical breathing. This occurrence is often the harbinger of diaphragmatic fatigue. Anterior protrusion of the sternum is called *pectus carinatum,* whereas a depressed sternum (funnel chest) is termed *pectus excavatum.*

(1:200, 414–416, 445), (9:37), (15:437), (16:1022).

## IA1a

9. C. Acute laryngotracheobronchitis (LTB), or croup, is an infection that produces mild to moderate airway obstruction in children 6 months to 3 years of age. Lateral radiographs of the neck ordinarily reveal a subglottic narrowing that is often described as the steeple sign, while the pharynx and epiglottis (supraglottic) appear normal. An anteroposterior (A–P) chest X-ray generally indicates subglottic narrowing as well. The barking cough and stridor manifest themselves a few days after the initial presentation of upper respiratory signs and symptoms (rhinorrhea, cough, and fever). As the barking cough and stridor develop, the child exhibits more apprehension, which in turn aggravates the dyspnea.

Table 3-7 outlines some of the salient differences between croup and epiglottitis.

(1:1038–1040), (9:231–232), (16:597–598).

## IB10a

10. A. Sinus bradycardia (Figure 3-23) has the following electrocardiogram (ECG) characteristics:

    • regular rhythm (the distance between QRS complexes is equal)
    • normal QRS complex
    • rate is less than 60 beats/min.
    • P wave precedes each QRS complex
    • normal and constant PR interval

Sinus bradycardia is a common finding in the early period of an acute myocardial infarction (AMI), especially on the inferior surface of the myocardium. An

**Table 3-7** Differentiation Between Croup (LTB) and Epiglottitis

|  | Croup (LTB) | Epiglottitis |
| --- | --- | --- |
| Etiologic factor | parainfluenza and other influenza viruses/ *Mycobacterium pneumoniae* | *Hemophilus influenzae* type B and *Streptococcus pneumoniae* |
| Pathophysiology | subglottic inflammation (larynx, trachea, bronchi) | supraglottic inflammation (epiglottis, aryepiglottic folds, arytenoid cartilages) |
| Clinical manifestations | low-grade fever hoarseness barking cough stridor | high fever hoarseness drooling stridor hyperextended head and neck |
| X-ray findings | subglottic narrowing steeple sign | supraglottic narrowing thumb sign obliterated vallecula |
| Treatment | mist tent nebulized racemic epinephrine oxygenation | artificial airway mechanical ventilation (likely) oxygenation antibiotics |

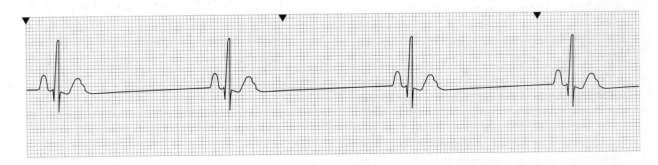

**Figure 3-23:** Lead II ECG tracing; sinus bradycardia.

AMI might decrease the cardiac output (C.O.) and might lead to congestive heart failure.

(1:326), (9:203), (16:858).

## IC1a

11. A. The maximum voluntary ventilation (MVV) is an extremely effort-dependent maneuver. The MVV is affected by the following factors:

    • ventilatory muscle status
    • respiratory system compliance
    • airway and tissue resistance
    • ventilatory control mechanisms

    Because of the wide variability among the normal population (150 to 200 L/min.), generally large decreases in the MVV are considered clinically significant.

    Because the MVV maneuver stresses the entire respiratory system, it is useful in approximating the degree of ventilation that can be anticipated during exercise. The MVV evaluates a person's ability to maintain a high level of ventilation for a period of time. Patients experiencing moderate to severe airway obstruction and having MVVs below 50 L/min. frequently display limited ventilation during exertion.

    (1:825, 941), (6:27, 47–49), (16:235).

## IB7e

12. C. High-pressure, or cardiogenic pulmonary, edema is associated with high pulmonary vascular-hydrostatic pressures. When the pulmonary vascular-hydrostatic pressure exceeds the capillary osmotic pressure, fluid leaves the pulmonary vasculature and enters the pulmonary interstitium. As the condition worsens and more fluid leaves the pulmonary vasculature, the alveoli then begin to fill.

    Radiographically, a number of characteristic findings appear. The heart enlarges, usually indicating congestive heart failure. Because fluid transudes out of the pulmonary vasculature, the pulmonary interstitium and alveoli become fluid-filled. This fluid is more radiopaque than air; consequently, these fluid-filled regions will present as whitened areas. Air-filled alveoli, of course, are dark because X-rays pass through air.

    Kerley B lines, generally viewed in the lateral aspects of the lower lobes, result from edema fluid accumulation in the subpleural septa throughout that region. These lines appear as short (1 to 2 cm), horizontal lines emanating from the pleural surface. The interstitial edema, likewise, causes peribronchial cuffing—the result of bronchial wall thickening.

    (1:411–412, 511, 513–514), (9:183, 359).

## IB3

13. D. Percussion of the thorax or abdomen is performed by tapping with the middle finger of one hand (dominant) against the distal joint of the other hand (nondominant), which is placed against the patient's thorax. Characteristic percussion notes help the RRT evaluate the relative degree of air, liquid, or solid matter in the underlying region of the lungs. The characteristic percussion notes are described as (1) normal, (2) resonant, (3) hyperresonant, (4) flat, and (5) dull.

    Resonant percussion notes are perceived over normal lung tissue. Hyperresonant percussion is heard over areas of the lungs where increased amounts of air are located (e.g., pneumothorax and air trapping). Tympanic percussion notes are produced by the presence of air in an enclosed chamber (i.e., the stomach) and are higher pitched than hyperresonant notes. Dull percussion notes indicate a decreased amount of air in the underlying lung tissue (e.g., pneumonia, atelectasis, and pleural effusion). Flat percussion sounds are generated in areas of extreme dullness (i.e., pneumonectomy).

    (1:310), (9:79–80).

## IC2a

14. B. A flow-volume loop is a graphic analysis of the expired and inspired flow and volume during an FVC maneuver. The flow rate is plotted on the $y$-axis, and the volume is plotted on the $x$-axis. The following illustration indicates some of the components of a normal flow-volume loop because of reduced lung volumes (Figure 3-24).

    If a patient has a restrictive lung disease, the effort-independent portion of this maneuver is generally more steep compared with a normal flow-volume loop.

    The following diagram provides a variety of flow-volume loops and their interpretations (Figure 3-25).

    (1:380–386, 397), (6:2, 41, 45).

## IC2c

15. C. All the vascular pressures are greatly reduced and the cardiac index (C.I.) reflecting the cardiac output (C.O.) is also extremely low. The heart rate is quite high in an attempt to maintain a circulating volume, however.

    This patient's problem is hypovolemia, which needs to be corrected with fluid administration. The CVP, a marker for intravascular fluid status, is normally 1 to 7 mm Hg (1 to 10 cm $H_2O$).

    (14:449–453, 465).

## IB7c

16. A. Both lungs should be auscultated after ET intubation to determine whether ventilation is going to both

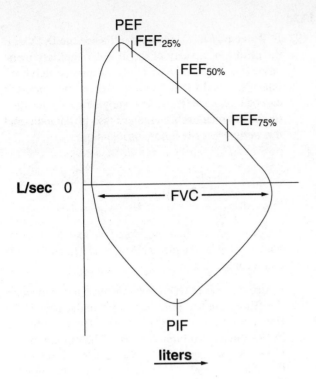

**Figure 3-24:** Components of a normal flow-volume loop.

17. A. In addition to alveolar hypoventilation, hypoxemia can be caused by diffusion impairments, ventilation-perfusion inequities, and intrapulmonary shunting.

Determining the extent of this patient's intrapulmonary shunting would be useful in assessing the cause of the hypoxemia. Administering 100% oxygen will generally decrease the $P(A-a)O_2$ if the hypoxemia is caused by a diffusion impairment or by ventilation-perfusion inequities. If the hypoxemia is caused by increased intrapulmonary shunting, however, the $P(A-a)O_2$ will widen with the administration of 100% oxygen. A shunt study performed on less than 100% oxygen will not help determine the nature of the hypoxemia. One hundred percent oxygen must be used.

The specific amount of intrapulmonary shunting present can be calculated by using the following formula:

$$\frac{\dot{Q}_S}{\dot{Q}_T} = \frac{C\dot{c}O_2 - CaO_2}{C\dot{c}O_2 - C\bar{v}O_2}$$

where

$\dot{Q}_S$ = shunted C.O. (L/min.)

$\dot{Q}_T$ = total C.O. (L/min.)

$C\dot{c}O_2$ = end-pulmonary capillary oxygen content (vol%)

$C\bar{v}O_2$ = total mixed venous oxygen content (vol%)

$CaO_2$ = total arterial oxygen content (vol%)

Normally, 2% to 5% of the C.O. is shunted (i.e., it does not participate in gas exchange). The 2% to 5% of normal shunting is accounted for by the bronchial veins,

lungs and to rule out inadvertent intubation of the esophagus and endobronchial intubation. Visual inspection of the chest wall helps determine air movement within the lungs. The portable chest X-ray film indicates the position of the tube in relationship to the carina. The radiopaque line that extends down to the distal tip assists in locating the tube's position. Measuring exhaled $CO_2$ is also an excellent method to determine whether the ET tube is in the trachea.

(1:597–601), (9:165), (15:833–835), (16:590–591).

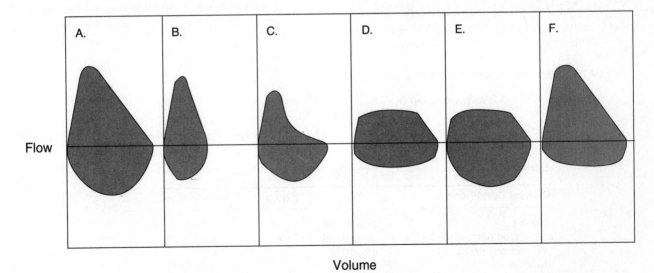

**Figure 3-25:** Interpretation of select flow-volume loops: (A) Normal, (B) Restrictive disorder, (C) Small Airway Obstruction, (D) Fixed large airway obstruction, (E) Variable intrathoracic obstruction, and (F) Variable extrathoracic obstruction.

pleural veins, and thebesian veins. Alveolar hypoventilation can ordinarily be corrected with mechanical ventilatory support.

(1:930), (10:272), (17:46–51).

## IC2c

18. D. The normal arterial-venous oxygen content difference ($CaO_2$-$C\bar{v}O_2$) or the arterial-venous difference, is 5 vol%. This value represents the amount of oxygen removed from the arterial blood by the tissues. Normally, this oxygen need is easily fulfilled by both oxygen-transport mechanisms; that is, $HbO_2$ (combined $O_2$) and $PaO_2$ (dissolved $O_2$). With a 35% COHb% in this situation, the ability of the hemoglobin to transport oxygen to the tissues is greatly impaired. Therefore, the plasma must be used to transport more oxygen (i.e., increasing the amount of oxygen in the dissolved state [$PaO_2$]).

Administering 100% $O_2$ at 1 ATA (atmosphere absolute—normobaric conditions) can *theoretically* elevate the $PaO_2$ only to 673 torr.

$[P_B - (PaCo_2 + P_{H_2O})]F_IO_2$

$\times 0.003$ ml $O_2$/ml plasma/torr $PO_2$ = vol% (dissolved $O_2$)

(For the derivation of the conversion factor 0.003 volumes %/torr, refer to Wojciechowski, W., *Respiratory Care Sciences: An Integrated Approach 3rd,* Delmar Publishers, Inc., Albany, NY, 2000, pp. 162–163.)

For example,

$[760$ torr $- (40$ torr $+ 47$ torr$)]1.0$

$\times 0.003$ vol%/torr = 2.01 vol% (dissolved $O_2$)

This amount of $O_2$ administration falls short of the tissue's needs. An $FIO_2$ of 0.80 at 3 ATA is sufficient to provide the tissue $O_2$ needs of 5 vol%, however.

$[(3$ ATA $\times 760$ torr$) - (40$ torr $+ 47$ torr$)]0.8$

$\times 0.003$ vol%/torr = 5.2 vol% dissolved $O_2$.

(1:763–765), (15:940, 1108–1109), (17:131–132).

## IA2d

19. D. Three physiologic factors influence the $D_LCO$: (1) the diffusion capacity of the alveolar capillary membrane ($D_MCO$), (2) the pulmonary capillary blood volume ($V_C$), and (3) the rate of the reaction between carbon monoxide (CO) and hemoglobin ($\theta$). Quantitatively, the relationship among these physiologic factors is shown in the following equation:

$$\frac{1}{D_LCO} = \frac{1}{D_M} + \frac{1}{V_C \times \theta}$$

The factor $D_M$ is often considered the membrane component, whereas the factor ($V_C \times \theta$) is described as the blood component.

Notice that the $D_LCO$ measurement is a conductance (i.e., the reciprocal of resistance). Conductance is the flow rate of a gas/pressure change. The units for the $D_LCO$ value are ml/min./mm Hg. The ml/min. represents the flow rate (actually, the transfer of CO across the alveolar capillary membrane), and the mm Hg refers to the pressure gradient across the alveolar capillary membrane. Resistance is the pressure change/flow rate (volume/time), the units of which would be mm Hg/ml/min.

The clinical application of these theoretical considerations are illustrated in Table 3-8 below.

In the situations of anemia and decreased hematocrit, the $D_LCO$ is reduced because of the reduced rate of the reaction between CO and hemoglobin ($\theta$). Regarding supine body position and exercise, the $D_LCO$ value increases because of the increase in pulmonary capillary blood volume ($V_C$). Finally, diffuse pulmonary fibrosis and granulomatosis are associated with a decreased $D_LCO$ because of impeding movement (reduced diffusion) of CO across the alveolar capillary membrane ($D_MCO$).

(6:111–125), (15:509–511), (17:86–87).

## IA1g(1)

20. C. The chest or precordial lead uses the left arm, right arm, and left leg as negative terminals and uses a pos-

### Table 3-8

| Clinical Conditions | $D_LCO$ | Equation Component Influenced |
|---|---|---|
| anemia | decreased | $\theta$ |
| decreased hematocrit (HCT) | decreased | $\theta$ |
| supine body position | increased | $V_C$ |
| exercise | increased | $V_C$ |
| diffuse pulmonary fibrosis | decreased | $D_M$ |
| granulomatosis | decreased | $D_M$ |

itive chest lead placed in six different sites located over the anterior and lateral chest walls. Table 3-9 shows the positive precordial electrode and its different locations.

**Table 3-9** Precordial Leads

| Lead | Location of Positive Electrode |
| --- | --- |
| $V_1$ | 4th intercostal space to right of sternum |
| $V_2$ | 4th intercostal space to left of sternum |
| $V_3$ | between 4th and 5th intercostal spaces left of sternum |
| $V_4$ | 5th intercostal space (left midclavicular) |
| $V_5$ | 5th intercostal space (left anterior axillary) |
| $V_6$ | 5th intercostal space (left mid-axillary) |

The chest leads $V_4$, $V_5$, and $V_6$ display a positive ECG tracing because the depolarization wave travels toward the positive chest electrode. Whenever a depolarization wave travels toward a positive electrode, an upward or positive deflection occurs on an ECG tracing. On the contrary, a wave of depolarization moving away from a positive electrode results in a downward deflection (an inverted tracing).

The chest leads $V_1$ and $V_2$ provide a negative or downward ECG tracing because they are placed above and to the right of the heart. As a result of their location, the wave of depolarization moves in the opposite direction of the positive electrode. The $V_3$ lead renders an ECG that has both upward and downward deflections (each having similar amplitudes).

(9:190, 198–201), (16:849–851).

**IB10c**

21. D. The normal dead space–tidal volume ratio ranges between 0.20 to 0.40. The normal dead space is composed of the conducting airways where no gas exchange occurs. The physiologic dead space is the sum of the anatomic dead space and the alveolar dead space. Alveolar dead space results from alveoli that are ventilated but not perfused. The $V_D/V_T$ ratio increases with mechanical ventilation. The Enghoff modification of the Bohr equation is as shown:

$$V_D/V_T = \frac{PaCO_2 - P\bar{E}CO_2}{PaCO_2}$$

where

$V_D$ = dead space ventilation (cc)
$V_T$ = tidal volume (cc)

$PaCO_2$ = arterial carbon dioxide tension (torr or mm Hg); end-tidal $CO_2$ tension can also be used

$P\bar{E}CO_2$ = mean exhaled carbon dioxide tension (torr or mm Hg) enables the calculation of the dead space–tidal volume ratio.

The end-tidal carbon dioxide tension can substitute for the $PaCO_2$ because the end-tidal $PCO_2$ represents the carbon dioxide from the alveoli and actually is the $PACO_2$. The $PaCO_2$ and $PACO_2$ are considered to be in equilibrium.

end-tidal $PCO_2$ = 44 mm Hg

mean exhaled $PCO_2$ = 33 mm Hg

$$\frac{44 \text{ mm Hg} - 33 \text{ mm Hg}}{44 \text{ mm Hg}} = 0.25$$

or $100 \times 0.25 = 25\%$

(1:927, 935), (9:290–292), (10:434), (17:25–29).

**IA2b**

22. B. The clinical presentation described here indicates the strong possibility of a right-sided pneumothorax. Before any further action is taken, a STAT chest radiograph should be obtained because it would provide the best diagnostic information.

If the patient was rapidly deteriorating, an immediate therapeutic intervention would be necessary (e.g., rapid decompression via the insertion of a 19-gauge needle into the second or third anterior intercostal space at the nipple line). The scenario here does not suggest this condition, however. Once the presence of a pneumothorax is confirmed by chest X-ray, a chest tube must be inserted through the anterior chest wall into the affected area.

(1:408–410), (9:92–93, 178–179, 260), (15:974, 1081–1083).

**IC2h**

23. D. The tracing represents a normal intra-arterial pressure tracing. The highest point of the pressure waveform is the systolic pressure (Point A). As the pressure in the ventricle drops below the aortic pressure, the aortic valve closes. This sudden closure of the aortic valve produces a notch on the down slope of the tracing, as the pressure decreases, and is called the *dicrotic notch* (Point B). Diastole appears as the lowest point of pressure on the tracing (Point C). Figure 3-26 on page 134 illustrates these events.

(1:942), (9:336), (14:94, 191).

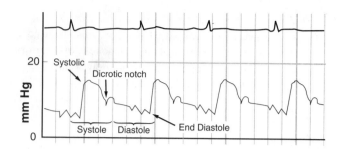

**Figure 3-26:** A normal intra-arterial pressure tracing showing systolic pressure, dicrotic notch, and diastolic pressure.

### IB10c

24. B. The mixed venous oxygen saturation ($S\bar{v}O_2$) represents the degree to which hemoglobin in the pulmonary artery is carrying oxygen. The $S\bar{v}O_2$ represents the average saturation of hemoglobin in venous circulation. The normal $S\bar{v}O_2$ ranges between 70% to 75%.

The $S\bar{v}O_2$ is often used to reflect the C.O. and tissue oxygen delivery. A number of factors affect the $S\bar{v}O_2$ measurement, making its interpretation rather complex. These factors include (1) the C.O., (2) the tissue oxygen consumption ($\dot{V}O_2$), and (3) the arterial oxygen content ($CaO_2$).

When the $\dot{V}O_2$ is normal (250 ml/min.), the $S\bar{v}O_2$ will decrease if the C.O. decreases. Furthermore, if the $CaO_2$ is low while the C.O. and $\dot{V}O_2$ remain constant, a lower $S\bar{v}O_2$ value will likewise be obtained. A fall in the $S\bar{v}O_2$ does not always signify a decreased C.O., however. For example, during exercise, the C.O. increases. Tissue oxygen consumption increases, however, rendering a lower $S\bar{v}O_2$. On the other hand, the $S\bar{v}O_2$ might increase. If the $\dot{V}O_2$ and the $CaO_2$ remain constant, an excessive C.O. will result in a high (greater than 75%) $S\bar{v}O_2$ value.

In addition to an excessive C.O., there are a number of specific clinical conditions that are generally associated with an increased $S\bar{v}O_2$ value. Sepsis is associated with peripheral vascular shunting, which causes tissue oxygen deprivation. The $\dot{V}O_2$ is probably elevated. Because of the peripheral vascular shunting, however, less oxygen would be extracted from the blood in the systemic capillaries. Consequently, a higher-than-normal $S\bar{v}O_2$ is generally obtained. Similarly, patients who are hypothermic experience a decreased $\dot{V}O_2$, hence, their $S\bar{v}O_2$ would increase as less oxygen is required by the tissues.

In the case of cyanide poisoning, the mitochondria of the tissue cells cannot use the oxygen available to them via the highly oxygenated arterial blood. This condition is tantamount to a decreased $\dot{V}O_2$; therefore, the $S\bar{v}O_2$ measurement will increase.

In a situation where a mixed venous blood sample is being withdrawn from a pulmonary artery catheter that is in the wedge position, the likelihood of aspirating pulmonary capillary blood is great. The result of obtaining blood that has been arterialized is sampling blood with a high oxygen saturation. Similarly, the clinician must also be mindful of the rate of aspirating the blood sample from the pulmonary artery catheter. If the rate of aspiration is too fast, arterial blood might end up in the sample, causing a falsely high $S\bar{v}O_2$ value.

The $S\bar{v}O_2$ measurement functions as a sensitive indicator of the patient's C.O. and tissue oxygenation (perfusion) when the $\dot{V}O_2$ remains relatively constant.

(1:225), (4:214), (14:347–365).

### IB1a

25. A. Patients who have either pulmonary emphysema or cystic fibrosis experience muscle wasting. The high work of breathing performed by these two types of patients contributes significantly to the muscle wasting that they experience. Pulmonary emphysema and cystic fibrosis patients expend an increased amount of energy to maintain their ventilation.

Ordinarily, between 1% to 2% of the body's total oxygen consumption (250 ml/min.) is needed to fuel a person's work of breathing. In certain pulmonary disease conditions, the amount of energy and oxygen required to support the muscles of ventilation increases dramatically as minute ventilation increases. This increased demand to operate the respiratory system represents increased caloric consumption, which in turn contributes to muscle wasting. A patient who has chronic bronchitis is generally slightly overweight.

(1:445, 459, 1040, 1079), (9:378), (16:423, 990, 1020).

### IB1b

26. B. Paradoxical abdominal movement is characterized by an inward movement of the abdomen during inspiration and an outward movement of the abdomen during exhalation. The significance of this occurrence is that it reflects the presence of dyspnea or diaphragmatic paralysis.

In the course of normal breathing, the external intercostal muscles contract along with the diaphragm. Diaphragmatic contraction results in the downward movement of the diaphragm, causing pressure changes in both the thoracic and abdominal cavities. The pressure in the thoracic cavity decreases, whereas the pressure in the abdominal cavity increases. The increased abdominal cavity pressure causes the abdomen to move outward during inspiration.

During normal exhalation, the diaphragm relaxes and moves upward, thereby reversing the pressure changes in these two cavities. Therefore, the subatmospheric abdominal pressure results in the inward movement of the abdomen at this point in the ventilatory cycle.

When the diaphragm becomes fatigued or paralyzed, the external intercostals and accessory inspiratory muscles of ventilation become more active. As these muscles contract and create a subatmospheric intrathoracic pressure, the flaccid diaphragm rises. Consequently, the abdominal wall moves inward.

Conversely, as the external intercostals and the accessory inspiratory muscles relax at end inspiration, the intrathoracic pressure becomes supra-atmospheric, causing the diaphragm to descend and the abdomen to push out.

Pendulluft breathing refers to the theoretical, to-and-fro movement of air from one lung to the other that occurs during the ventilatory cycle in patients who have flail chest or pneumothorax. Again, this paradoxical abdominal movement signifies dyspnea (diaphragmatic fatigue) or diaphragmatic paralysis.

(1:308), (9:76–77), (15:45–49, 780, 1142).

### IB10a

27. C. On an ECG, the T wave follows the QRS complex and represents ventricular repolarization. The QRS complex represents ventricular depolarization. The following diagram depicts the various electrophysiologic events of the normal cardiac cycle (Figure 3-27).

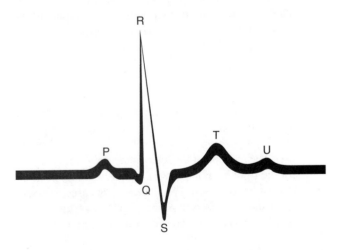

**Figure 3-27:** Lead II normal ECG associating electrophysiologic event with ECG representation.

(1:324), (9:197), (16:856).

### IB7e

28. D. The end-expiratory intrapleural pressure determines the side toward which the mediastinum will shift. If the end-expiratory intrapleural pressure becomes more subatmospheric (negative) on the affected side, as in atelectasis and pulmonary fibrosis, the mediastinum will shift in that direction. If fluid or air collects in the intrapleural space, end-expiratory pressure is increased on that side. Therefore, the mediastinum shifts to the uninvolved side in a pleural effusion and pneumothorax.

(9:92–94).

### IC2c

29. C. As with any cardiopulmonary condition, the major concern is ultimately tissue hypoxia. The $PaO_2$ and $CaO_2$ are best reflective of oxygen delivery. The static compliance will reflect the stiffness of the lungs and will provide valuable noninvasive information regarding the condition of the lungs. With the exception of dysoxia and ARDS, however, the $P\overline{v}O_2$ best reflects the presence or absence of hypoxia.

(10:286, 292–294, 324), (15:534).

### IB9d

30. B. The $FEF_{25\%–75\%}$ represents the flow rate during the middle 50% of an FVC maneuver. The expiratory flow rate during the initial 25%–last 25% of the FVC are ignored. The $FEF_{25\%–75\%}$ represents the flow rate of air from the medium to small airways and is expressed in L/min. or L/sec.

The $FEF_{25\%–75\%}$ will be erroneously high (above normal) if the patient terminates her forced exhalation before achieving residual volume.

(1:384, 387), (6:39), (10:149–150).

### IB10g

31. B. Brief periods of apnea are normal during sleep. The sleep apnea syndrome, however, is defined as the occurrence of five or more apneic periods per hour, each lasting at least 10 seconds. There must be at least five episodes per hour.

(1:554), (9:408).

### IB9g

32. C. When a mixed venous blood sample is needed, the sample must be obtained via a pulmonary artery catheter. The right atrium and right ventricle serve as mixing chambers receiving venous blood of differing $PO_2$, $PCO_2$, pH, and saturation values from the entire body. Obtaining a venous blood sample from an isolated organ or from a specific limb often renders data

that vary considerably with time and the metabolism of the area sampled.

Therefore, to accumulate information about mixed venous blood because it reflects the adequacy of tissue oxygen delivery, the blood sample must be obtained from a pulmonary artery catheter. Data derived from such a sample render information about (1) the C.O., (2) overall tissue metabolism, and (3) peripheral circulation.

(1:345–346), (9:352), (15:534–535).

## IC1c

33. B. The formula for determining the C.I. can be rearranged to solve for the body surface area (BSA) when the C.I. and the C.O. are given:

$$BSA = \frac{C.O.}{C.I.}$$

$$= \frac{6.7 \text{ L/min}}{3.4 \text{ L/min/m}^2}$$

$$= 1.97 \text{ m}^2$$

(1:949), (9:309, 311), (10:119, 136).

## IC2e

34. C. Cyanosis will appear if a person has 5.0 g% (5.0 g/dl) or more of unsaturated hemoglobin in total circulation (arterial and venous). The degree of unsaturation can be calculated as follows:

STEP 1: Calculate the percentage of unsaturated arterial hemoglobin (Hb).

$$
\begin{array}{r}
100\% \\
-51\% \text{ SaO}_2 \\
\hline
49\% \text{ unsaturated arterial Hb}
\end{array}
$$

STEP 2: Determine the percentage of unsaturated venous hemoglobin.

$$
\begin{array}{r}
100\% \\
-45\% \text{ S}\bar{\text{v}}\text{O}_2 \\
\hline
55\% \text{ unsaturated venous Hb}
\end{array}
$$

STEP 3: Compute the amount of reduced hemoglobin in arterial blood.

20 g% [Hb] × 0.49 = 9.8 g% reduced Hb (arterial)

STEP 4: Obtain the amount of reduced hemoglobin in venous blood.

20 g% [Hb] × 0.55 = 11.0 g% reduced Hb (venous)

STEP 5: Calculate the amount of reduced hemoglobin in total circulation (average of that in arterial and venous blood).

$$\frac{9.8 \text{g}\% + 11.0 \text{g}\%}{2} = \frac{20.8\%}{2}$$

$$= 10.4 \text{g}\% \text{ reduced Hb in total circulation}$$

Because the amount of total unsaturated (reduced) hemoglobin in this example is greater than 5.0 g%, this person will display cyanosis.

(1:318), (9:16), (15:437, 668).

## IA1c

35. A. The diagnostic procedure associated with cystic fibrosis is the sweat test. Pilocarpine iontophoresis stimulates the sweat glands in a local area, enabling the collection and measurement of sweat chloride. A sweat chloride concentration of greater than 60 mEq/liter is diagnostic of cystic fibrosis. Therefore, because the chloride concentration was found to be only 28 mEq/liter, the test results are normal. The normal sweat chloride concentration is 28 mEq/liter.

(9:107), (15:121).

## IB1a

36. B. Jugular venous distention provides information relating to the volume and pressure of the venous blood in the right heart. Normally, when a person lies flat, supine neck vein distention occurs. When venous pressure is normal, and when the head of the bed is elevated 45°, the level of venous distention of the internal jugular vein falls to about 3 to 4 cm above the clavicle. The level of venous distention in this position will increase in the event of right-ventricular failure.

(9:70–71, 276–277), (14:551).

## IB3

37. D. As a normal person breathes tidally, the right and left hemidiaphragms come to rest at the posterior T-9 and T-10 positions, respectively, at end-tidal exhalation. The location of the liver on the right side accounts for the right hemidiaphragm's slightly higher position in relation to the left. Percussion is also used to assess the inspiratory descent of the diaphragm. This evaluation is likewise performed over the posterior thorax.

(1:310), (9:79–80).

## IC2i

38. B. A constant-flow generator ordinarily is characterized as a ventilator that creates high internal pressures. In so doing, a constant-flow generator would create a

square-flow waveform and a rectilinear pressure flow curve. The high internal pressure essentially overcomes lung compliance and airway resistance changes in the patient. Therefore, alterations in these lung characteristics will not interfere with the flow waveform. It remains unchanged (square).

The pressure waveforms will respond to these pulmonary characteristics when they change. For example, if lung compliance decreases, the steepness and amplitude of the pressure curve will increase. Similarly, if the airway resistance increases, the amplitude of the pressure curve would increase, although the steepness of the curve would be less. Both of these changes in the pressure waveform would occur in response to the back pressure developed in the ventilator–patient system caused by the decreased lung compliance and increased airway resistance.

Some mechanical ventilators (e.g., Nelcor Puritan Bennett 7200, the Siemens Servo 900 series, and the Bear 1) are classified as constant-flow generators. These ventilators develop only moderately high internal pressures, however. Therefore, when these machines are used in clinical situations associated with low to moderate airway pressures, they truly are constant-flow generators. When these ventilators encounter high airway pressures, however (e.g., markedly decreased pulmonary compliance or increased airway resistance), the inspiratory flow rate decreases and the flow waveform is altered. The decrease in the flow during inspiration results in a change between the generated pressure and the applied pressure.

The following diagram compares the flow waveforms developed by a constant-flow generator that develops only moderately high internal pressures for (A) normal lungs and (B) markedly decreased compliance or markedly increased airway resistance (Figure 3-28).

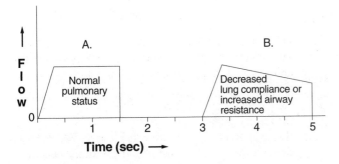

**Figure 3-28:** Flow-time waveforms developed by a constant-flow generator with moderately high internal pressures for (A) normal lungs and (B) markedly decreased pulmonary compliance or markedly increased airway resistance.

In the case where the lungs are normal (A), the inspiratory flow rate remains constant for the entire 1.5 sec-

onds of inspiration. Observe what happens, however, when either lung compliance decreases or airway resistance increases markedly (B). The inspiratory flow rate progressively diminishes, and the inspiratory time increases (2 seconds). As long as the ventilator does not achieve its pressure limit, higher pressures will develop in the upper airway and in the patient's alveoli in (B). The flow waveform in (B) is sometimes called a modified square or a tapered square waveform.

(1:840, 852), (10:45–46, 53–56, 196).

**IB4b**

39. D. The first heart sound ($S_1$) is created by the closure of the mitral and tricuspid valves. The second heart sound ($S_2$) is created by the closure of the aortic and pulmonic valves.

(9:89–90), (14:134–135).

**IB10c**

40. C. After performing a slow vital capacity maneuver, the subject inspires 100% $O_2$ to total lung capacity (TLC). At that point, he begins to exhale as slowly and as evenly as possible once again to residual volume. When exhalation proceeds in that manner, the tracing (normal) shown is obtained.

The tracing presents four phases: Phase I, the first part of the exhaled volume containing only 100% $O_2$ (anatomic dead space gas); Phase II, increasing amounts of $N_2$ exhaled as alveolar gas mixes with anatomic dead space gas; Phase III, gas from alveolar units of the basal and middle lung zones; and Phase IV, alveolar gas from the apices.

This test helps identify the manner in which air flows through the tracheobronchial tree. When airflow is uniform, a normal single-breath nitrogen-washout curve is displayed. In the presence of airway obstruction (nonuniform distribution of ventilation), the tracing will become distorted. The extent of distortion depends on the degree of the obstructive disease.

(1:388), (6:83–86).

**IB9b**

41. A. The inspiratory:expiratory (I:E) ratio can be determined as follows:

STEP 1: Determine the total cycle time (TCT).

$$TCT = \frac{60 \text{ sec./min.}}{f}$$

$$= \frac{60 \text{ sec./min.}}{60 \text{ breaths/min.}}$$

$$= 1 \text{ sec./breath}$$

**STEP 2:** Obtain the expiratory time ($T_E$) by subtracting the inspiratory ($T_I$) from the TCT.

$$T_E = TCT - T_I$$
$$= 1 \text{ sec.} - 0.5 \text{ sec.}$$
$$= 0.5 \text{ sec.}$$

**STEP 3:** Calculate the I:E ratio by dividing the $T_I$ and the $T_E$ by the $T_I$.

$$\text{I:E ratio} = \frac{T_I}{T_I} : \frac{T_E}{T_I}$$
$$= \frac{0.5 \text{ sec}}{0.5 \text{ sec}} : \frac{0.5 \text{ sec}}{0.5 \text{ sec}}$$
$$= 1:1$$

(1:860), (10:205–206).

### IB2b

42. C. Characteristically, a pleural effusion renders the following findings during physical assessment of the chest. Depending on the size of the effusion, inspection of the chest wall will reveal either reduced or absent movement. Tracheal deviation, along with mediastinal shift, occurs in the direction of the unaffected lung because the end-expiratory intrapleural pressure increases on the affected side (Figure 3-29).

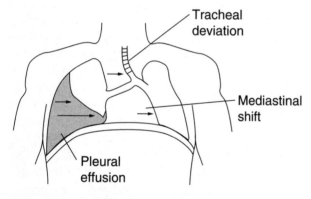

**Figure 3-29:** Pleural effusion causing tracheal deviation and mediastinal shift toward the unaffected lung.

Sound waves transmitted through the chest wall during patient phonation (vocal fremitus) and perceived by the RRT's palm against the patient's thorax refer to the term *tactile fremitus*. In a pleural effusion, tactile fremitus is either diminished or absent, as determined via palpation.

During percussion, the notes produced over a pleural effusion sound dull or flat. Auscultation reveals diminished or absent breath sounds over the affected area. Occasionally, a high-pitched bronchial sound is heard. In some instances, a pleural rub can be detected over the pleural effusion.

All of the chest physical assessment (inspection, palpation, percussion, and auscultation) signs lend evidence to the fact that this patient has a left-sided pleural effusion.

(1:308–311), (9:79–83, 93).

### IC2a

43. C. Because of the vast cross-sectional area provided by the small airways (equal to or greater than 2 mm in diameter), a small airway obstruction generally does not prove as symptomatic as an obstruction in a large airway (greater than 2 mm in diameter) unless, of course, the small airway obstruction is diffuse and extensive. An upper-airway obstruction can be more immediately life-threatening if no air can reach any of the gas exchange units.

Overdistention (air trapping) can occur in the presence of a partial airway obstruction. During inspiration, the airways elongate and widen; on exhalation, they contract and narrow. Consequently, air might move beyond an obstruction during inspiration and get trapped during exhalation. Such an obstruction is termed a *check-valve obstruction* (Figure 3-30).

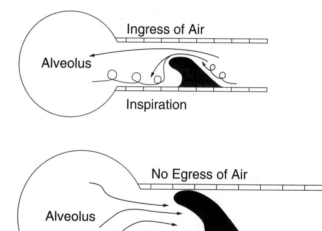

**Figure 3-30:** A check-valve obstruction depicting the ingress of air during inspiration and the prevention of egress of air during exhalation.

When airway obstruction (small or large) becomes symptomatic, the work of breathing increases. This situation can be clinically illustrated when the patient displays nasal flaring (alae nasi), uses accessory ventilatory muscles, and/or exhibits chest-wall retractions.

An airway obstruction can adversely affect both the patient's acid-base and oxygenation status. As the severity of the obstruction increases, the more impaired alveolar ventilation becomes. Consequently, carbon dioxide levels in the blood elevate, causing the blood's pH to fall. Over time, the kidneys respond by retaining bicarbonate to compensate for the increased blood carbon dioxide levels and to normalize the pH. Similarly, the decreased alveolar ventilation reduces the amount of oxygen that enters the gas-exchange regions of the lungs, thereby compromising the blood oxygen levels and causing hypoxemia.

(1:643).

## IB10d

44. A. Mixed venous blood can be sampled through the distal port on a pulmonary artery catheter while the balloon is inflated and located in the pulmonary artery. Blood found in the right ventricle and pulmonary arteries is described as mixed venous blood because these structures contain venous blood that has come from all parts of the body. The blood in the right ventricle and pulmonary arteries does not predominantly reflect the venous values from a specific body region or organ system. Rather, it represents an amalgamation of venous blood from the entire body.

Table 3-10 outlines the normal, mixed venous blood measurements and values.

**Table 3-10** Normal, Mixed Venous Blood Gas Data

| Measurement | Value |
| --- | --- |
| $P\bar{v}O_2$ | 40 torr |
| $P\bar{v}CO_2$ | 44 to 48 torr |
| pH | 7.34 to 7.38 |
| $S\bar{v}O_2$ | 70% to 75% |

(1:225, 345), (4:25, 29, 215), (9:120).

## IC2i

45. D. Tracing D demonstrates synchronized intermittent mandatory ventilation (SIMV) without PEEP or CPAP. The patient's spontaneous inspiratory and expiratory breathing efforts can be observed as the slight upward and downward deflections, respectively. The ventilator "senses" the patient's breathing efforts and therefore provides a mandatory breath only at a point in the spontaneous ventilatory pattern corresponding with inspiration. Breath "stacking," characteristic of IMV, is then avoided. At the end of each mandatory breath, the pressure returns to baseline (atmosphere).

Tracing A exhibits IMV with CPAP or PEEP. The absence of a downward deflection preceding each larger upward deflection signifies that the breath delivered by the ventilator is not an assisted (patient-"triggered") breath. Note that the mandatory breaths are equally spaced. This cycling represents a preset rate that will de-

liver a mandatory breath at a regular interval regardless of where the patient is during his own spontaneous ventilatory cycle. This random (nonsynchronized) interaction between the patient's spontaneous breathing and the ventilator's mandatory delivered breaths occasionally result in breath "stacking." Breath "stacking" refers to the situation that occurs when a mandatory breath is delivered when the patient is somewhere in his spontaneous inspiratory cycle. The sine-wave-like deflections of smaller amplitude indicate the patient's spontaneous breathing efforts. The baseline does not return to zero, therefore PEEP or CPAP is present.

Tracing B illustrates IMV without PEEP or CPAP. This mode of ventilation is characterized by periodically controlled ventilator breaths delivered at a preset rate and volume. Again, the sine-wave-like undulations reflect the patient's spontaneous breathing efforts. Breath stacking occurs in this mode of ventilation. Because the pressure returns to baseline, neither PEEP nor CPAP is present.

Tracing C depicts continuous positive pressure breathing (CPPB) in the control mode. The patient is making no spontaneous efforts. The ventilator is providing the patient with a fixed tidal volume at a preset rate. PEEP is absent because the pressure at the end of exhalation returns to baseline.

(1:861), (10:265).

## IB4a

46. C. Ordinarily, vesicular breath sounds are heard over the lung periphery, whereas bronchial breath sounds are perceived over the larger airways. Vesicular sounds can be replaced by bronchial sounds in peripheral lung regions when the underlying lung tissue becomes more dense. Lung tissue density increases when atelectasis or pneumonia are present. Breath sounds associated with a pleural effusion are either diminshed or absent based on the size of the pleural effusion. Harsh vesicular sounds are heard over areas of the lung that have become fibrotic.

(1:313, 315), (9:81–86).

## IB10a

47. D. In most patients, the $PtcO_2$ and the $PaO_2$ correlate well. The fact that these two measurements "correlate well" does not mean that the values are the same, however. What is meant by correlating well is that when the $PtcO_2$ increases, the arterial $PO_2$ likewise increases.

For infants with a normal C.O. and normal fluid balance, the $PtcO_2$ and the $PaO_2$ will be similar but not the same. In normal infants, the $PtcO_2$–$PaO_2$ gradient is approximately 10 torr. A 20-torr difference between these two measurements signifies the likelihood of the presence of right-to-left shunting through the patent ductus arteriosus. Any time a preductal (right upper arm: $PtcO_2$) and postductal (umbilical artery catheter: $PaO_2$) oxygen tension gradient of greater than 15 torr exists, the suspicion should be a right-to-left shunting through a patent ductus arteriosus.

Air bubbles between the skin and the electrode would cause the $PtcO_2$ value to remain high. Tissue edema would result in a $PtcO_2$ lower than the $PaO_2$. Increased skin temperature produces burns and elevated $PtcO_2$ values. Anemia would likely have no effect on the $PtcO_2$ measurement.

(1:353–354), (10:227, 301), (13:265–269).

## IB8a

48. C. Epiglottitis is caused by the microorganism *Hemophilus influenzae* type B. In the process, the supraglottic region becomes edematous, interfering with breathing and swallowing. Specifically, the structures involved are the epiglottis, aryepiglottic folds, and arytenoid cartilages.

The diagnosis of this condition is confirmed by lateral neck X-rays, which reveal the following presentations: (1) a ballooned hypopharynx (laryngopharynx), (2) an obliterated vallecula, (3) thickened aryepiglottic folds, and (4) a broadened and flattened epiglottis. The broadened and flattened epiglottis is described as the thumb sign.

(1:1039), (9:232).

## IB10c

49. B. The arterial blood gas (ABG) and acid-base data are consistent with acute ventilatory failure. The patient is experiencing moderate to severe hypoxemia, hypercapnia, and acidemia. The hypoxemia and hypercapnia result from a decreased alveolar ventilation. Generally, acute ventilatory failure is associated with an arterial $PO_2$ less than 60 torr, an arterial $PCO_2$ greater than 50 torr, and a pH less than 7.30.

A patient who is experiencing an asthmatic episode in its early stage would tend to display mild to moderate hypoxemia, hypocapnia, and alkalemia. Diabetic ketoacidosis is associated with an arterial $PCO_2$ in the teens or single digits, a normal to high arterial $PO_2$, and severe acidosis. Chronic ventilatory failure is characterized by mild to moderate hypoxemia, hypercapnia (approximately 50 torr), and a compensated pH. Massive doses of steroids produce a metabolic alkalosis.

(1:267, 270–271, 273–276), (16:1008).

## IB10c

50. B. The increased mean intrathoracic pressure impedes venous return, which ultimately reduces left ventricular output. Mechanically assisted ventilation generally

increases alveolar ventilation ($\dot{V}_A$). Therefore, a decreased C.O. or a decreased capillary perfusion ($\dot{Q}_C$) and an increase in $\dot{V}_A$ results in an increased $\dot{V}_A/\dot{Q}_C$.

(1:885–886), (10:142–143).

## IA1c

51. B. An empyema is an accumulation of pus in a body cavity. Because the pleural cavity is the most common site, the body fluid or specimen to be collected will be pleural fluid.

(1:436–437, 479–480), (16:214).

## IC2b

52. B. Ventricular fibrillation indicates numerous ectopic foci, resulting in an inadequate C.O. No pulse can be palpated when this dysrhythmia occurs. It can be considered a form of cardiac arrest. Defibrillation is immediately indicated.

(1:652–653), (16:853).

## IB9e

53. D. The following diagram depicting the waveforms generated from floating a Swan–Ganz, or pulmonary artery catheter, into position corresponds with the pressures generated within the anatomic structures through which the catheter passes (Figure 3-31). The diagram also shows the location of the tip of a Swan–Ganz catheter and its corresponding waveform as the catheter is being advanced to the wedged position.

Section A represents pressures in the right atrium; Section B demonstrates pressures in the right ventricle; Section C depicts pressures in the pulmonary artery; and Section D illustrates pressure in a branch of the pulmonary artery with the catheter "wedged."

(1:947), (9:347), (10:125).

## IA1c

54. D. Small amounts of meconium can be passed by the fetus well in advance of parturition. The infant appears discolored without visible particulate meconium. No special resuscitative measures are indicated for these infants because they are described as *vigorous*.

Infants presenting with thick meconium, however, require pharyngeal suctioning upon presentation of the head. Then, immediately after delivery, the infant must be intubated and thoroughly suctioned for the removal of residual meconium.

(1:1028–1029), (16:924), (18:36, 67, 419–420, 422).

## IB4a

55. D. Stridor is produced by the rapid flow of air through an obstructed airway. In such a situation, the stridor

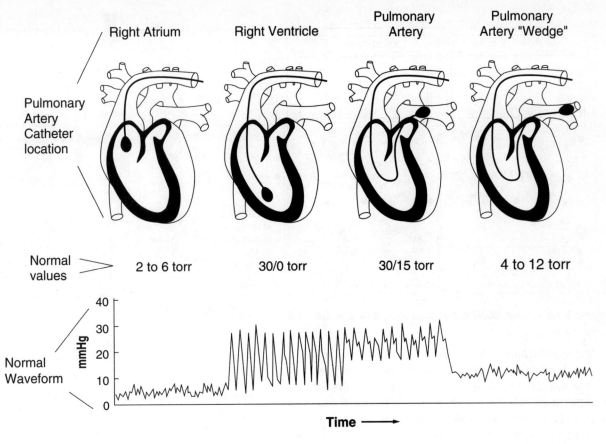

Right Atrium     Right Ventricle     Pulmonary Artery     Pulmonary Artery "Wedge"

Pulmonary Artery Catheter location

Normal values: 2 to 6 torr    30/0 torr    30/15 torr    4 to 12 torr

Normal Waveform

Time →

**Figure 3-31:** Pulmonary artery catheter location indicating corresponding normal values and normal waveforms.

can be associated with an inflammation of the upper respiratory tract.

The potential causes of the airway inflammation include croup, epiglottitis, or post-extubation edema.

(1:312–313), (9:38, 83, 257), (18:95).

## IA10h

56. D. Intracuff pressures exceeding 18 mm Hg restrict the flow of tracheal venous blood in the region of the trachea in contact with the cuff. Intracuff pressures exceeding 30 mm Hg cause tracheal arterial blood flow to be obstructed. Ideally, intracuff pressure should seal the airway by means of the least amount of pressure possible. An intracuff pressure of less than 20 mm Hg is recommended.

(1:609–610), (16:575–576).

## IA9b

57. C. The inspiratory time percent control establishes how much of the total cycle time (TCT) will be devoted to inspiration. The inspiratory time percent control settings available on the Siemens Servo 900C are 20%, 25%, 33%, 50%, 67%, and 80%.

STEP 1: Determine the TCT according to the following expression:

$$TCT = \frac{60 \text{ sec./min.}}{f}$$

$$= \frac{60 \text{ sec/min.}}{12 \text{ breaths/min.}}$$

$$= 5 \text{ sec./breath}$$

STEP 2: Divide the TCT into the inspiratory time ($T_I$) to determine the inspiratory time percent.

$$\text{inspiratory time \%} = \frac{T_I}{TCT} \times 100$$

$$= \frac{1.65 \text{ sec.}}{5.00 \text{ sec.}} \times 100$$

$$= 33\%$$

The inspiratory time percent that will achieve an inspiratory time of 1.65 seconds is 33%. The Servo 900C panel illustrated in Figure 3-32 on page 142 indicates the inspiratory time percent setting (note arrow).

(5:478), (13:517–518).

## IA10g

58. A. Sleep apnea is classified into three categories: (1) central apnea, (2) obstructive apnea, and (3) mixed apnea. In central apnea, the termination of airflow

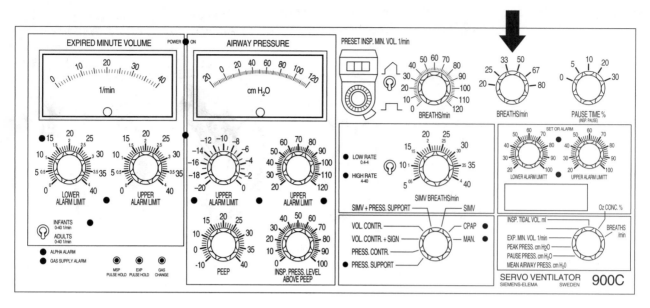

**Figure 3-32:** Servo 900C panel: inspiratory time percent control (note arrow).

through the lungs results from a lack of ventilatory effort. In obstructive apnea, the termination of airflow into and out of the lungs results from an upper airway obstruction (relaxation of the genioglossus muscle and pharyngeal muscles during sleep). Both abdominal and thoracic movements are present. The mixed variety is a combination of the other two. Signs and symptoms of sleep apnea include the following:

- hypersomnalence (excessive daytime sleepiness)
- personality changes
- sexual problems
- nocturnal enuresis (bed wetting)
- snoring
- abnormal motor activity (thrashing) during sleep
- hypertension
- deteriorating intellectual capacity (cognitive dysfunction)
- morning headaches
- sudden death during sleep

An apneic episode is defined as the cessation of airflow through the nose and mouth for at least 10 seconds. Sleep apnea is defined as the occurrence of at least 30 apneic episodes during 7 hours of sleep.

(1:554–557), (10:408–410).

**IB1b**

59. C. During normal breathing, the diaphragm moves outward on inspiration and inward during expiration. When the diaphragm is dysfunctional or fatigued, accessory muscles of ventilation become active. As a result of accessory ventilatory muscle use, greater than normal subatmospheric pressure is generated in the intrapleural space. The increased subatmospheric pressure during inspiration pulls the diaphragm upward

and causes the abdomen to move inward. This movement of the diaphragm is termed *abdominal paradox.*

Respiratory alternans is characterized by the periodic usage of chest-wall muscles for inspiration alternating with diaphragmatic contractions. Paradoxical chest-wall movement occurs when the integrity and stability of the chest wall are compromised. This situation develops in the presence of flail chest, which manifests when three or more adjacent ribs are fractured in two or more places. Paradoxical abdominal movement is associated with dyspnea or paralysis of one of the hemidiaphragms.

Pendulluft breathing describes the theoretical movement of air from one lung into the other. It is thought to occur in conjunction with an open pneumothorax as the mediastinum shifts from side to side during breathing or with a flail chest as the unstable chest wall segment moves paradoxically.

(1:308), (9:76–77), (15:307–308), (16:935–936).

**IA1a**

60. A. Myasthenia gravis is an autoimmune, neuromuscular disease treated with anticholinesterase medications. Long-term anticholinesterase medications include neostigmine methylsulfate, pyridostigmine (Mestinon), and ambernomium (Mytelase). During the course of treatment, these patients sometimes experience a myasthenic or cholinergic crisis. A myasthenic crisis takes place if the patient is either delinquent in taking her medication or is receiving an inadequate dosage. A cholinergic crisis occurs when the muscle cell membrane essentially becomes desensitized to acetylcholine. In either crisis, the signs and symptoms are the same (i.e., muscle weakness and ventilatory failure).

The Tensilon test distinguishes between these two crises. Tensilon (edrophonium chloride) is a fast-acting, short-duration (5 minute) anticholinesterase medication used only for diagnostic purposes. When Tensilon is administered and the patient improves, the patient is having a myasthenic crisis. If the patient does not improve after the Tensilon administration, the crisis is a cholinergic one.

Once the type of crisis has been identified, appropriate treatment can be instituted. A myasthenic crisis usually can be terminated by increasing the patient's dosage of anticholinesterase medication or by urging the patient to be more diligent in taking her medication. A cholinergic crisis often requires mechanically ventilating the patient and withholding her anticholinesterase medication for some time to allow the muscle cell membranes at the neuromuscular junctions to again become responsive to acetylcholine.

(1:543–544), (15:230, 710), (16:1049–1050).

## IA1b

61.  A. Hyperdynamic septic shock often occurs before the hypodynamic state. Typical signs include (1) fever, (2) markedly increased C.O., (3) low systemic vascular resistance, (4) tachypnea, (5) bounding pulses, (6) normal or slightly decreased blood pressure, (7) adequate urinary output, and (8) warm and dry skin.

(9:354), (16:871–1126).

## IA1b

62.  D. The early clinical presentation of lung abscess resembles that of pneumonia: cough, pleuritic pain, leukocytosis (increased white blood cell count), fever, chills, and general malaise. An abscess often produces large amounts of foul-smelling, foul-tasting, blood-tinged sputum. The sputum produced in bronchiectasis generally is foul smelling and separates into three distinct layers upon settling. Weight loss and anorexia are usually associated with pulmonary neoplasms. Amphoric breath sounds are characteristic of cavitations associated with lung abscesses. Amphoric breath sounds resemble the sound produced as air is blown over the mouth of an empty pop bottle.

(15:351).

## IA1h

63.  B. The Silverman score provides a means of assessing the degree of respiratory distress of a neonate. Scores range from 0 to 10. Scores of 0 to 3 indicate little or no respiratory distress. Scores of 4 to 6 indicate moderate respiratory distress. Scores of 7 to 10 represent severe respiratory distress. The clinical signs evaluated and the points assigned are shown in Table 3-11 below.

(1:1006), (18:51–52).

## IB10d

64.  A. Guillain-Barré syndrome is a neuromuscular disease that generally afflicts the muscles of the hands and feet before proceeding centrally. Therefore, the signs and symptoms of ventilatory failure occur only when the muscles of inspiration (diaphragm and external intercostals) are affected.

Such patients must be closely monitored in terms of their ventilatory function. Specifically, physiologic measurements such as maximum inspiratory pressure (MIP) and forced vital capacity (FVC) must be obtained. As soon as the patient's ventilatory status deteriorates to the level where the MIP is less than $-20$ to $-25$ cm $H_2O$, and the FVC falls below 10 to 15 ml/kg, the patient should be intubated and mechanically ventilated.

In the course of 4 hours, this patient's MIP decreased from $-45$ cm $H_2O$ to $-15$ cm $H_2O$, and his FVC fell from 60 ml/kg to 10 ml/kg.

$$\left(4{,}500 \text{ ml}/\frac{165 \text{ lbs}}{2.2 \text{ lbs/kg}}\right) = 60 \text{ ml/kg}$$

$$\left(750 \text{ ml}/\frac{165 \text{ lbs}}{2.2 \text{ lbs/kg}}\right) = 10 \text{ ml/kg}$$

Both measurements indicate the progression of muscle paralysis and impending ventilatory failure.

(1:545), (15:230, 306, 709–710, 1065).

## IC2a

65.  B. The carbon monoxide lung-diffusion study ($D_L CO$) provides a measure of the amount of functioning pulmonary capillary bed that is in contact with functioning alveoli. In pulmonary emphysema, the $D_L CO$ will be reduced because of a loss of the alveolar capillary

**Table 3-11** Silverman Score

| Sign | 0 | 1 | 2 |
| --- | --- | --- | --- |
| Upper chest movement | Synchronized movement | Lag of upper chest or inspiration | Asynchronized movement |
| Lower chest movement | No retractions | Occasional retractions | Many retractions |
| Xiphoid retractions | No retractions | Occasional retractions | Many retractions |
| Dilatation of nares | Absent | Minimal dilatation | Maximal dilatation |
| Expiratory | Absent | Perceived only with aid of stethoscope | Perceived with unaided ear |

bed. The destructive disease process reduces the surface area available for gas exchange.

Three physiologic factors influence the $D_LCO$: (1) the diffusion capacity of the alveolar capillary membrane ($D_MCO$), (2) the pulmonary capillary blood volume ($V_C$), and (3) the rate of the reaction between carbon monoxide and hemoglobin ($\theta$). Quantitatively, the relationship is as follows:

$$\frac{1}{D_LCO} = \frac{1}{D_M} + \frac{1}{V_C \times \theta}$$

The factor $D_M$ is often considered the membrane component, whereas the factor ($V_C \times \theta$) is called the *blood component*. Notice that the $D_LCO$ is a conductance, or a reciprocal of resistance. The clinical applications of these theoretical considerations are shown in Table 3-12.

Table 3-12

| Clinical Conditions | $D_LCO$ | Equation Component Influenced |
|---|---|---|
| Anemia | decreased | $\theta$ |
| Decreased hematocrit | decreased | $\theta$ |
| Supine body position | increased | $V_C$ |
| Exercise | increased | $V_C$ |
| Diffuse pulmonary fibrosis | decreased | $D_MCO$ |
| Granulomatosis | decreased | $D_MCO$ |

In the cases of anemia and decreased hematocrit, the $D_LCO$ is reduced because of the reduced rate of reaction between CO and Hb ($\theta$). In the situations involving supine body position and exercise, the $D_LCO$ is increased because of an increased pulmonary capillary blood volume ($V_C$). Last, diffuse pulmonary fibrosis and granulomatosis both decrease the $D_LCO$ because of impeding the movement (diffusion) of CO across the alveolar capillary membrane ($D_MCO$).

(6:111–125), (15:235, 510–512), (17:85–87).

**IB10a**

66. C. The slow-speed capnograph waveform illustrated as follows indicates five normal breaths (A) followed by seven breaths (B), where the inspiratory limb of the tracing did not return to the baseline (Figure 3-33). During those seven breaths, the patient was rebreathing a portion of her own exhaled $CO_2$ (i.e., the inspired $CO_2$ was greater than zero). Area B on the tracing represents the time when mechanical dead space was added to the ventilator circuit.

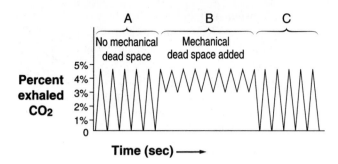

**Figure 3-33:** Slow-speed capnography showing (A) and (C) breaths without mechanical dead space and (B) breaths with mechanical dead space added to the ventilator circuit.

(1:363–365), (10:99, 101–102), (15:501–503).

**IB9e**

67. D. The Fick equation (as follows) can be used to calculate the C.O. in this situation:

$$\dot{Q}_T = \frac{\dot{V}O_2}{(CaCO_2 - C\bar{v}O_2)}$$

where

$\dot{Q}_T$ = C.O. (L/min.)

$\dot{V}O_2$ = oxygen consumption (ml/min.)

$CaO_2 - C\bar{v}O_2$ = arterial–venous $O_2$ content difference (vol%)

Therefore,

$$\dot{Q}_T = \frac{250 \text{ ml } O_2/\text{min.}}{5 \text{ ml } O_2/100 \text{ ml blood}}$$

$$= \frac{250 \text{ ml } O_2/\text{min.}}{0.05 \text{ ml } O_2/\text{ml blood}}$$

$$= 5{,}000 \text{ ml/min. or } 5 \text{ L/min.}$$

Remember, the unit volumes percent, or vol%, in this equation represents milliliters of $O_2$/100 ml of blood. Therefore, whenever the $CaO_2 - C\bar{v}O_2$ is used in the Fick equation, one must take into account the aspect of 100 ml of blood.

(1:225–226, 930), (9:323), (15:530), (17:135, 163).

**IB9d**

68. C. The ventilation time constant is the product of the airway resistance and the pulmonary compliance, as the following expression illustrates:

time constant = airway resistance × pulmonary compliance

second = (cm $H_2O$/L/sec.)(L/cm $H_2O$)

The ventilation time constant indicates the time required to empty or fill the lungs. Quantitatively, one time constant represents the time required for the lungs to exhale 63% of the tidal volume. Two time constants refer to the time needed to exhale 84% of the tidal volume. The time required for the lungs to empty 95% of the tidal volume is represented by three time constants as shown in Figure 3-34.

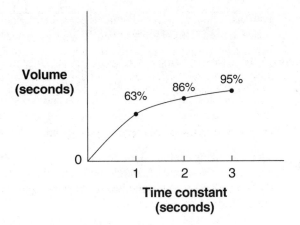

**Figure 3-34:** Ventilation time constants.

The following two steps outline how to calculate the time needed to provide for exhalation based on knowing the ventilation time constant:

STEP 1: Determine the ventilation time constant.

$$\text{time constant} = \left(\begin{array}{c}\text{airway} \\ \text{resistance}\end{array}\right)\left(\begin{array}{c}\text{pulmonary} \\ \text{resistance}\end{array}\right)$$
$$= (30 \text{ cmH}_2\text{O/L/sec.})(0.02 \text{ L/cmH}_2\text{O})$$
$$= 0.6 \text{ second}$$

One time constant, given the airway resistance and pulmonary compliance values here, is 0.6 second.

STEP 2: Calculate the expiratory time ($T_E$) required to enable the lungs to empty.

$$T_E = \left(\begin{array}{c}\text{time} \\ \text{constant}\end{array}\right)\left(\begin{array}{c}\text{number of time constants in} \\ \text{which 95\% of } V_T \text{ is emptied}\end{array}\right)$$
$$= (0.6 \text{ sec.})(3)$$
$$= 1.8 \text{ seconds}$$

(10:37–38, 358), (17:58, 115, 320–325).

**IB4a**

69. B. Chest hair can interfere with auscultation of the chest. Chest hairs moving against the stethoscope's diaphragm can produce a sound resembling crackles. To avoid this potential source of misinterpretation of breath sounds, the RRT should moisten the area of the chest to be auscultated. The wet hair should eliminate the misinterpretation of chest hair sounds as adventitious lung sounds.

(1:310), (9:81), (16:171).

**IB10c**

70. C. The dead space–tidal volume ratio ($V_D/V_T$) represents the portion of the tidal volume that does not participate in gas exchange (i.e., wasted ventilation). As intrapulmonary gas exchange improves, the $V_D/V_T$ ratio is generally reduced. Anatomic dead space volume is approximately equal to 1 cc/lb of ideal body weight (IBW) and comprises about 25% to 40% of the normal $V_T$.

The $V_D/V_T$ ratio is a useful measurement for evaluating the effectiveness of ventilation. Consequently, it is often determined when a patient is being weaned from mechanical ventilation. A $V_D/V_T$ ratio of less than 0.60 is considered acceptable for supporting spontaneous breathing.

The Enghoff-modified Bohr equation is used to calculate the $V_D/V_T$ ratio:

$$\frac{V_D}{V_T} = \frac{PaCO_2 - P\bar{E}CO_2}{PaCO_2}$$

where,

$V_D$ = dead space volume (ml)
$V_T$ = tidal volume (ml)
$PaCO_2$ = arterial partial pressure of $CO_2$ (torr)
$P\bar{E}CO_2$ = mean exhaled partial pressure of $CO_2$ (torr)

(1:927, 935), (9:290–292), (10:248, 434), (15:99–100, 489).

**IC2e**

71. A. These ABG values are considered acceptable for a normal 1-hour-old preterm infant. Generally, ABGs obtained soon after birth indicate a metabolic acidosis and a low arterial oxygen tension. These values normalize in a relatively short time.

(1:1007), (18:107–108).

**IA1f(3)**

72. A. A number of evaluation procedures are useful to determine whether a mechanically ventilated patient is ready to be weaned. The evaluation procedures and their accepted values are shown in Table 3-13.

**Table 3-13** Weaning Evaluation

| Evaluation Procedure | Accepted Value |
|---|---|
| vital capacity | > 15 cc/kg (IBW) |
| maximum inspiratory capacity (MIP) | < −20 cm $H_2O$ |
| $V_D/V_T$ | < 0.60 |
| sensorium | awake; alert |
| $\dot{Q}_S/\dot{Q}_T$ | ≤ 0.15 |
| $\dot{V}_E$ | < 10 L/min. |

Other criteria include ABGs, $F_IO_2$, ventilatory rate, PEEP level, and peak inspiratory pressure (PIP).

(1:971), (10:325).

## IB3a

73. D. Stridor is a high-pitched sound heard most often during inspiration. It is associated with the reduction of the airway diameter of large airways.

(1:312–313), (9:38, 83), (16:982).

## IB4a

74. B. Alveolar dead space represents alveoli that are ventilated but not perfused (Figure 3-35). These alveoli do not participate in gas exchange. The gas composition of such alveolar units should closely approximate that of tracheal air.

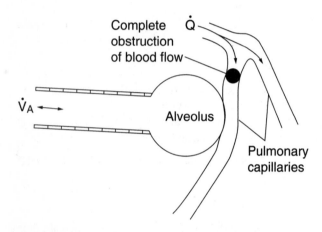

**Figure 3-35:** Alveolar dead space characterized by a ventilated alveolus devoid of perfusion.

The predominant source of alveolar $CO_2$ is the person's metabolic functions (atmospheric $CO_2$ is 0.04% of 760 torr, or 0.3 torr). If blood flow to certain alveolar units is prevented, $P_ACO_2$ levels will decrease in those regions.

In this situation, the alveolar $PCO_2$ will decrease because none of the $CO_2$-laden (venous) blood can come into contact with the ventilated alveolus. Similarly, the alveolar $PO_2$ will be higher than usual because venous blood, which has a $PO_2$ of about 40 torr, cannot participate in gas exchange.

(1:211, 212), (9:128, 290–291), (15:102–103).

## IA1b

75. A. Cyanosis is the bluish discoloration of the skin and mucous membranes caused by 5 grams percent (g%) or more of desaturated hemoglobin in total circulation. Cyanosis generally appears at the ends of the digits (fingers and toes) through the translucent fin-

gernails. It is also perceptible on the lips, earlobes, and conjunctiva.

*Peripheral cyanosis* or acrocyanosis describes this bluish discoloration when it is confined to the extremities. The term *central cyanosis* refers to this feature when the arterial and venous desaturations are extremely high, affecting the upper torso.

Patients who are polycythemic (i.e., a hemoglobin concentration [Hb] of greater than 16 g%) are prone to exhibit cyanosis more easily than anemic patients ([Hb] less than 12g%). Polycythemic patients are chronically hypoxemic. In fact, it is the hypoxemia that stimulates red blood cell production and produces the polycythemia. These patients have difficulty sufficiently saturating an adequate amount of hemoglobin.

The following calculations demonstrate how the amount of desaturated hemoglobin is calculated. The arterial and venous saturations used here represent normal values.

STEP 1: Determine the percent of desaturated hemoglobin in arterial circulation given an arterial saturation ($SaO_2$) of 97.5%.

$$\begin{array}{r} 100\% \text{ maximum saturation possible} \\ -97.5\% \text{ arterial saturation} \\ \hline 2.5\% \text{ arterial } \textit{desaturation} \end{array}$$

STEP 2: Determine the percent of desaturated hemoglobin in venous circulation given a mixed venous saturation ($S\bar{v}O_2$) of 75%.

$$\begin{array}{r} 100\% \text{ maximum saturation possible} \\ -75\% \text{ mixed venous saturation} \\ \hline 25\% \text{ venous } \textit{desaturation} \end{array}$$

STEP 3: Calculate the amount of desaturated hemoglobin in arterial circulation. Assume a normal hemoglobin concentration of 15 g%.

$$[Hb] \times \frac{\% \text{ arterial}}{\text{desaturation}} = \frac{\text{amount of}}{\text{desaturated arterial Hb}}$$

15 g% × 2.5% = 0.375 g% desaturated arterial Hb

STEP 4: Calculate the amount of desaturated hemoglobin in venous circulation. Assume a normal [Hb] of 15 g%.

$$[Hb] \times \frac{\% \text{ venous}}{\text{desaturation}} = \frac{\text{amount of}}{\text{desaturated venous Hb}}$$

15 g% × 25% = 3.75 g% desaturated venous Hb

STEP 5: Compute the average amount of desaturated Hb in total circulation.

$$\frac{\text{arterial desat.} + \text{venous desat.}}{2} = \left(\begin{array}{c}\text{average amount}\\ \text{desaturated Hb in}\\ \text{total circulation}\end{array}\right)$$

$$\frac{0.375 \text{ g\%} + 3.75\% \text{ g\%}}{2} = 2.06 \text{ g\%}$$

Because the value obtained for the average amount of desaturated Hb in total circulation is less than 5 g%, cyanosis will not be exhibited.

(1:318), (9:16, 69, 77), (15:437, 668).

## IA1f(1)

76. C. The transpulmonary pressure gradient (intra-alveolar pressure minus intrapleural pressure) varies vertically throughout the tracheobronchial tree. At FRC, that gradient is greater in the apices than in the bases. Therefore, at FRC, the apical alveoli are more distended than the basal alveoli. This is one of the reasons why gas on inspiration goes preferentially to the basal segments and why, over the course of time, the bases experience a greater minute ventilation ($\dot{V}_E$) than the apices. Elastance (E) is the reciprocal of compliance (C).

Because

$$C = \frac{\Delta V}{\Delta P} = \frac{L}{cm \ H_2O}$$

and

$$E = \frac{\Delta P}{\Delta V} = \frac{cm \ H_2O}{L}$$

Therefore,

$$C = \frac{1}{E} \quad \text{and} \quad E = \frac{1}{C}$$

The pulmonary elastance is greater in the apices than in the bases of an upright, normal lung.

(1:200–201), (10:35–48), (17:97, 141, 316).

## IA1b

77. B. An abnormally high hemidiaphragm generally implies either total relaxation, such as in paralysis, or stiffness, which is preventing normal expansion of the lung. Contraction of the diaphragmatic muscle results in flattening. Any damage to the phrenic nerve, which controls this muscle, will leave the muscle paralyzed and arched upward. Fibrosis or scar tissue will create a stiffness of the lung and prevent normal vertical expansion, which appears as an elevated diaphragm on the affected side. The diaphragm elevates in this case

because the intrapleural pressure decreases in the region of the fibrosis. The more subatmospheric pressure causes the hemidiaphragm to rise.

(1:545–546), (9:76–77, 80), (16:1047).

## IC2a

78. C. A patient who has pulmonary emphysema possesses blebs and bullae on his lungs. These regions represent areas of trapped air (i.e., they do not participate in gas exchange).

The closed-circuit helium dilution and open-circuit nitrogen washout tests are methods that can provide for the determination of the functional residual capacity (FRC). In a patient who has obstructive airway disease (i.e., pulmonary emphysema), however, the flow of gas throughout the tracheobronchial tree is maldistributed. Therefore, areas that are characterized by low $\dot{V}/\dot{Q}_S$ (perfusion in excess of ventilation) will receive varying degrees of the gas used in either method of FRC determination. Consequently, all of the air (volume) in the lungs will not be measured, and the FRC will be less than actual.

Body plethysmography, however, employs an enclosed system that does not depend on the distribution of gas flow through the lungs to measure the FRC. Consequently, a patient who has pulmonary emphysema with blebs and bullae and maldistribution of ventilation will have a larger FRC value measured via body plethysmography than by either of the other two methods. The body box, based on Boyle's law, uses a pressure-volume relationship to determine the FRC. Poorly ventilated lung regions where air is trapped are taken into account.

(1:377–380), (6:78–86).

## IB2b

79. B. Palpation of the trachea to determine its position is generally performed while the patient is recumbent or sitting upright. Also, the patient's neck should be slightly flexed.

Right upper lobe atelectasis is often associated with tracheal deviation to the right. The retraction of the collapsed lung tissue in that region causes the intrapleural pressure there to become more subatmospheric. Consequently, the lung tissue and adjacent structures, including the trachea, are pulled to the right. Fibrosis of the right lung will also cause a rightward shift of the trachea. If either of these conditions (atelectasis or fibrosis) occurs on the left side, the tracheal deviation will be to the left. If extensive enough, conditions such as a pneumothorax and a pleural effusion cause tracheal deviation to the unaffected side. For example, a left-sided pneumothorax, or a left-sided pleural effusion, can cause the mediastinum to shift to the right. Similarly, hyperinflation of a lung, as in the case of inadvertent right mainstem bronchus intubation, will cause the mediastinum to shift to the unaffected side. Consolidation does not cause tracheal deviation.

(9:91–94), (15:441).

## IA1f(3)

80. C. The inspiratory flow rate for a time-cycled, volume-limited, constant-flow generator can be calculated according to the following formula:

$$V_T = T_I \times \dot{V}_I$$

where

$V_T$ = delivered volume (ml)
$T_I$ = inspiratory time (sec.)
$\dot{V}_I$ = inspiratory flow rate (L/min.)

STEP 1:  Rearrange the equation to solve for the inspiratory flow rate ($\dot{V}_I$).

$$\dot{V}_I = \frac{V_T}{T_I}$$

$$= \frac{800 \text{ cc}}{1.2 \text{ sec.}}$$

$$= 666.57 \text{ cc/sec.}$$

STEP 2:  Convert the inspiratory $\dot{V}_I$ to L/sec.

$$= \frac{666.67 \text{ cc/sec.}}{1,000 \text{ L/cc}}$$

$$= 0.667 \text{ L/sec.}$$

STEP 3:  Convert 0.667 L/sec. to L/min.

$$\dot{V}_I = (0.667 \text{ L/sec.})(60 \text{ sec/min.})$$
$$= 40 \text{ L/min.}$$

(1:899–901), (10:206, 210).

## IA1f(3)

81. A. An inspiratory hold is a maneuver that delays the onset of the expiratory phase. Other terms used to describe this maneuver include *inflation hold* and *end-inspiratory pause*. This maneuver is instituted immediately following inspiration. For example, immediately after a preset pressure has been achieved or a preset volume has been delivered, the exhalation valve remains closed for a brief time, thereby momentarily holding the delivered volume in the patient's lungs.

During this time, gas flow has stopped. No airway resistance is manifested. The needle on the ventilator's pressure manometer falls to a lower reading. In other words, the needle on the pressure gauge will deflect from the PIP to a lower point. The point to which the needle moves is called the *plateau* or *static pressure*. It represents the pressure that is maintaining the lungs in their inflated state, or the alveolar distending pressure. This plateau pressure (minus any PEEP) is used to calculate the patient's effective static compliance. The difference between the PIP and the plateau (static) pressure represents the pressure generated to overcome airway resistance during inspiration.

In addition to allowing for these clinical measurements, the inspiratory hold maneuver is intended to provide better gas distribution throughout the tracheobronchial tree. Similarly, it enhances the delivery and deposition of in-line nebulized medications, such as bronchodilators.

The pressure tracing obtained when the maneuver is used is characterized by a downward deflection of the tracing from the peak inspiratory level to the plateau level where the tracing levels off. When the inflation hold ends, the tracing descends to the baseline. Note the following diagram (Figure 3-36).

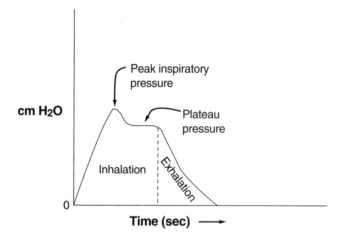

**Figure 3-36:** Intermittent positive pressure ventilation with inspiratory hold.

(1:845, 879), (10:85, 145).

## IC2c

82. D. Because positive pressure ventilation elevates the mean intrathoracic pressure, hemodynamic measurements such as central venous pressure (CVP) and pulmonary artery pressure (PAP) are likewise increased. The extent to which hemodynamic measurements are increased during positive pressure ventilation depends on (1) the ventilatory frequency, (2) the tidal volume, (3) the pulmonary compliance, (4) the mean airway pressure, and (5) the presence of PEEP.

Elevation of the CVP and the PAP causes venous return to the right side of the heart to decrease, which results in a reduced right ventricular preload and stroke volume.

(1:886–888), (10:141–143).

## IA1c

83. B. The Gram's stain is a staining method that is utilized to classify bacteria. By taking advantage of chemical composition variations of bacterial cell walls, the Gram's stain demonstrates bacterial morphology and staining characteristics.

   Table 3-14 below outlines the Gram's stain results of some of the more common bacteria encountered in the clinical setting.

   *Streptococcus pneumoniae* is also known as *Diplococcus pneumoniae.*

   (1:432), (9:112–113), (17:514).

## IA1b

84. D. Percussion, palpation, tactile fremitus, and auscultation are all assessment techniques that are used to evaluate normal or abnormal function of the airways and/or lung parenchyma.

   (1:306–314), (9:74–80).

## IA1g(2)

85. D. The Fick equation can be used to calculate the C.O. The equation is shown as follows:

$$\dot{Q}_T = \frac{\dot{V}O_2}{CaO_2 - C\bar{v}O_2}$$

   where

   $\dot{Q}_T$ = total C.O. (L/min. or ml/min.)

   $\dot{V}O_2$ = oxygen consumption (ml/min.)

   $CaO_2 - C\bar{v}O_2$ = arterial-venous oxygen content difference (vol%)

Therefore,

$$\dot{Q}_T = \frac{250 \ ml \ O_2/min.}{\dfrac{19.5 \ ml \ O_2}{100 \ ml \ blood} - \dfrac{14.5 \ ml \ O_2}{100 \ ml \ blood}}$$

$$= \frac{250 \ ml/min.}{0.195 \ ml \ blood - 0.145 \ ml \ blood}$$

$$= \frac{250 \ ml \ O_2/min.}{0.05 \ ml \ blood}$$

$$= 5,000 \ ml/min. \ or \ 5 \ L/min.$$

When performing calculations by using the Fick equation, one must know how to work with the unit volumes %. The unit volumes % refers to a number of milliliters of gas transported in 100 ml of blood. For example, the $CaO_2$ in this problem was 19.5 vol%, which means that 19.5 ml of $O_2$ are transported in each 100 ml of blood, or 19.5 ml $O_2/100$ ml blood (19.5 vol%).

Consequently, in the equation, the arterial and mixed venous oxygen contents must be divided by 100 ml of blood. Then, the $CaO_2$ of 19.5 ml of $O_2/100$ ml of blood becomes 0.195 ml of $O_2/ml$ of blood, and the mixed venous oxygen content ($C\bar{v}O_2$) of 14.5 ml of $O_2/100$ ml of blood becomes 0.145 ml of $O_2/ml$ of blood.

Because the C.O., the oxygen consumption, and arterial–venous oxygen content difference are all normal, the patient does not seemingly require any cardiac medication.

(1:225–226, 930), (10:323), (14:327).

## IA1c

86. B. *Mycobacterium avium-intracellulare,* for which there is no known treatment, often appears among HIV-positive patients who develop AIDS. This microorganism is an atypical form of tuberculosis and is resistant to the usual regimen of tuberculosis therapy (i.e., isoniazid [INH], rifampin, and pyrazinamide).

   (15:769, 773).

## IB9d

87. D. The MIP maneuver evaluates the adequacy of inspiratory muscle function. The patient is instructed to exhale to residual volume and then perform a rapid and

**Table 3-14** Gram Stain Results of Certain Common Bacteria

| Bacterium | Gram's Stain Results |
| --- | --- |
| *Streptococcus pneumoniae* | encapsulated, lancet-shaped, gram-positive diplococci |
| *Klebsiella pneumoniae* | encapsulated, short, fat, gram-negative rods |
| *Staphylococcus aureus* | clustered, gram-positive cocci |
| *Pseudomonas aeruginosa* | long, thin, gram-negative rods |
| *Haemophilus influenzae* | encapsulated or nonencapsulated, gram-negative coccobacilli |

forceful inspiratory maneuver for about 20 seconds. The mouthpiece is connected to a pressure manometer to record the negative pressure generated throughout the effort. The mouthpiece also contains one-way valves that prevent air from entering the patient's lungs but enable exhalation. An MIP of less than $-20$ cm $H_2O$ generally indicates that the patient cannot support his own ventilations and needs mechanical ventilatory support.

(1:825, 971), (9:287–288), (1:155–156).

## IA2c

88. C. The presence of fever and tachycardia suggest the possibility of infection. The probability of infection is further suggested by the white blood cell count, which is elevated above 10,000/mm³. The mild hypoxemia suggests a pulmonary infection, which can be further defined by a sputum culture and sensitivity.

(1:331–332), (9:46–47).

## IA10c

89. D. Both pulmonary perfusion and ventilation are influenced by gravity. The effect of gravity on ventilation, however, is more profound than the straightforward impact it has on pulmonary blood flow. The vertical transpulmonary pressure and intrapleural pressure differences are a direct result of the effect of gravity on the tracheobronchial tree in its normal, upright position. With positional changes, these two (transpulmonary and intrapleural) pressure gradients change; therefore, the distribution of ventilation changes. The following diagram depicts the transpulmonary and intrapleural pressures ranging from the bases to the apices in an upright lung at FRC (Figure 3-37).

In a normal, erect person, the perfusion in the lung bases exceeds the ventilation in that area. In the apices, however, ventilation exceeds perfusion.

(1:232–236), (9:123, 171, 173).

## IB9e

90. C. The Fick equation is shown as follows:

$$\dot{V}_{O_2} = C.O. \times C(a - \bar{v})O_2$$

where

$\dot{V}_{O_2}$ = oxygen consumption (ml/min.)

C.O. = cardiac output (L/min.)

$C(a-\bar{v})O_2$ = arterial–venous oxygen content difference (vol %)

According to the Fick equation, oxygen consumption is equal to the C.O. multiplied by the difference of the total oxygen content in the arterial blood minus the total oxygen content in the venous system. The equation can be rearranged to solve for the C.O.,

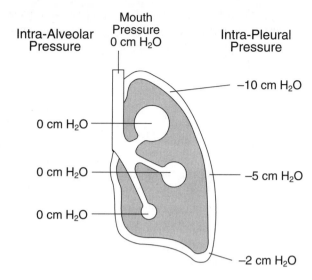

**Figure 3-37:** An upright lung at FRC showing vertical intra-pleural and transpulmonary pressures. The vertical intrapleural pressure (Ppl) differences are indicated on the right. The numbers used are arbitrary, but the Ppl is greater in the apex than at the base. This Ppl difference results from gravity's effect on the lungs when they are upright. The $P_{transpul.}$ is obtained by subtracting the intra-alveolar pressure ($P_{alv}$) from the Ppl.

however. When the equation is rearranged, the relationship becomes:

$$C.O. = \frac{\dot{V}_{O_2}}{C(a - \bar{v})O_2}$$

(1:225–226, 930), (9:323), (15:530), (17:135, 163).

## IB10a

91. C. The ECG depicts a third-degree atrioventricular (AV) block, or complete heart block. The P waves and QRS complexes occur independently (i.e., the P waves are unrelated to the QRS complexes). The QRS complex in this situation originates from a junctional or ventricular pacemaker site.

An AV block occurs when the AV node is diseased and has difficulty conducting atrial impulses (P waves) to the ventricles. Common causes are myocardial infarction and arteriosclerosis. Atrioventricular blocks are classified as first-, second-, and third-degree blocks. In first-degree AV blocks, the PR-interval is increased over 0.20 second. Wenckebach (Mobitz I) and Mobitz II are both types of second-degree AV blocks. The Mobitz I pattern shows a progressively lengthening PR interval from one beat to the next until finally the AV node cannot conduct the impulse and a beat fails. The "rested" AV node then is able to fire on the next beat, but the cycle (progressively lengthening PR interval) repeats. In Mobitz II, some beats are conducted and others are not. The PR interval is consistent for conducted beats. Failed beats are identified by the presence of a P wave without an ensuing QRS complex.

(1:326–328), (9:207).

**IB7a**

92. C. In a normal chest radiograph, the right and left heart borders are distinct. The distinction arises from the density differences between the air-filled lungs and the fluid-filled heart. Specifically, the right middle lobe of the lung and the right side of the heart share a common border. Therefore, the fluid-filled heart appears lighter than the air-filled right middle lobe on a normal chest radiograph. This distinction disappears when the right middle lobe becomes fluid-filled (pneumonia) or atelectatic. The right heart border becomes obscured in this situation because the contrast between these two structures has disappeared. This loss of distinction of a common border is termed the *silhouette sign*. The right hemidiaphragm remains apparent when right middle-lobe atelectasis or a pneumonia occurs.

In the case of a right lower-lobe pneumonia or atelectasis, the right heart border remains distinct. The right hemidiaphragm becomes indistinct. The right heart border will always remain visible no matter how extensive the right lower-lobe pneumonia or atelectasis becomes because these two structures do not share a common border.

(1:411–412), (9:176–177), (15:604–605).

**IB1b**

93. C. During respiratory distress or during increased work of breathing, an adult patient generates a much greater negative intrapleural pressure than during normal spontaneous breathing. In so doing, the skin and subcutaneous soft tissue covering the thorax retract inward at specific locations on the chest wall during inspiration. These retractions are generally described as intercostal retractions (between the ribs), subcostal retractions (below the lower margin of the ribs), and supraclavicular retractions (above the clavicles). Newborns frequently exhibit sternal retractions because the chest wall is not as rigid as that of an adult.

(1:307), (9:76, 219), (15:436–437).

**IA1b**

94. B. Hyaline membrane disease (HMD), or respiratory distress syndrome (RDS), occurs commonly in premature infants whose mothers either experience bleeding or are diabetic. Clinical manifestations of this disease include (1) expiratory grunting, (2) nasal flaring, (3) sternal and intercostal retractions, (4) cyanosis, (5) diminished breath sounds, and (6) rapid or slow ventilatory rates. Chest X-rays often show a ground-glass or reticulogranular appearance with decreased lung volume.

At 33 weeks' gestation, it would be expected that the infant would have an adequate production of pulmonary surfactant to sustain extrauterine life. In the presence of maternal diabetes, however, surfactant production is sometimes delayed.

Ordinarily, pulmonary surfactant begins at approximately 22 to 24 weeks of intrauterine life. The biochemical synthesis of this phospholipid molecule (dipalmitoyl lecithin) relies on the presence of two metabolic pathways—the methyltransferase system (22 to 24 weeks) and the phosphocholine transferase system (35 weeks).

(1:1030–1031), (15:29–30), (18:5, 31, 147–152).

**IB9b**

95. A. The ventilation time constant is a function of local airway resistance and lung-compliance characteristics. The lung, as an entire organ, is composed of millions of ventilation–perfusion ($\dot{V}_A/\dot{Q}_C$) ratios, rendering a composite $\dot{V}_A/\dot{Q}_C$ (0.8 to 1.0) for the lung. It is also composed of millions of time constants. Each lung region has its own ventilation time constant based on regional airway resistance and lung-compliance qualities. Therefore, the time constant for the lungs *en toto* is the average of all the individual time constants.

The ventilation time constant represents the time it takes for the lungs to fill or empty. The calculations are outlined as follows:

STEP 1: Calculate the effective static compliance according to the following formula:

$$\text{effective static compliance} = \frac{\text{tidal volume}}{\text{plateau pressure} - \text{PEEP}}$$

$$= \frac{0.8 \text{ L}}{20 \text{ cm H}_2\text{O} - 5 \text{ cm H}_2\text{O}}$$

$$= 0.053 \text{ L/cm H}_2\text{O}$$

STEP 2: Compute the airway resistance ($R_{aw}$) according to the following relationship:

$$R_{aw} = \frac{\text{pressure gradient}}{\text{gas flow rate}}$$

A) Convert the inspiratory flow rate ($\dot{V}_I$) of 50 L/min. to L/sec. Because 1 min. = 60 sec.,

$$\dot{V}_I = \frac{50 \text{ L/min.}}{60 \text{ sec./min.}}$$

$$= 0.83 \text{ L/sec.}$$

B) Obtain the pressure generated to overcome the airway resistance ($\Delta P$) by subtracting the plateau pressure from the PIP.

$$\Delta P = PIP - \text{plateau pressure}$$
$$= 40 \text{ cm } H_2O - 20 \text{ cm } H_2O$$
$$= 20 \text{ cm } H_2O$$

C) $R_{aw} = \dfrac{\Delta P}{\dot{V}_I}$

$$= \dfrac{20 \text{ cm } H_2O}{0.83 \text{ L/sec.}}$$

$$= 24 \text{ cm } H_2O/\text{L/sec.}$$

STEP 3: Calculate the time constant by multiplying the *compliance* (C) by the airway resistance ($R_{aw}$).

time constant = $C \times R_{aw}$
 = 0.053 L/cmH₂O × 24 cmH₂O/L/sec
 = 1.27 sec.

(1:210), (10:37–39, 358), (17:320–324).

**IA8c**

96. B. The overinflation of endotracheal ET and tracheostomy tube cuffs might result in tracheal chasing and tracheal dilatation visible on a chest X-ray.

(1:609–610), (16:570, 832).

**IA1h**

97. C. Infants who are born with persistent pulmonary hypertension of the newborn (PPHN) are ordinarily severely hypoxemic and cyanotic just hours after birth. Right-to-left shunting through the ductus arteriosus occurs secondary to the pulmonary hypertension.

When other causes of right-to-left shunting, such as cardiac abnormalities, meconium aspiration, septicemia, and intraventricular hemorrhage, are ruled out, PPHN is strongly suspected.

The appropriate diagnostic procedure in this case would be to measure pre- and postductal blood oxygen levels. Therefore, simultaneous transcutaneous oxygen monitoring of preductal blood (right arm) and postductal blood (lower extremity) should be performed in order to ascertain the presence or absence of a lowered oxygen level across the ductus arteriosus. A preductal and postductal $PO_2$ difference of 15 torr or more indicates the presence of right-to-left shunting through the patent ductus arteriosus. Failure to demonstrate this shunt does not rule out PPHN with right-to-left shunting through a patent foramen ovale.

(1:1034), (16:940–943), (18:225–227).

**IA1h**

98. C. Blood drawn from an umbilical artery catheter in neonates who have a patent ductus arteriosus sometimes reflects a low arterial saturation because the arterial catheter is located distal to the patent ductus arteriosus. The blood at the catheter site is sometimes less oxygenated because of the venous admixture caused by a patent ductus arteriosus that is associated with right-to-left shunting.

When a patent ductus arteriosus is present, blood from the pulmonary artery mixes with blood leaving the left ventricle through the aorta. Generally, pulmonary vasoconstriction causes the pulmonary artery pressure to exceed pressure in the aorta. Therefore, venous blood from the pulmonary artery enters arterial circulation through the patent ductus arteriosus, which connects the pulmonary artery to the aorta. As a result of the patent ductus arteriosus, blood obtained from an umbilical artery catheter will have a lower oxygen saturation and $PO_2$ than blood from the right upper quadrant, which reflects preductal blood.

The following diagram illustrates the heart of a newborn with a patent ductus arteriosus as it appears in PPHN (Figure 3-38).

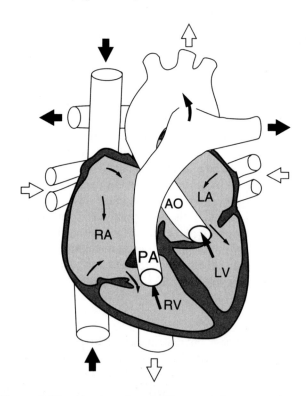

**Figure 3-38:** Newborn heart with patent ductus arteriosus, as it appears in persistent pulmonary hypertension of the newborn (PPHN).

(1:1034), (16:940–943), (18:225–227).

## IA1e

99. A. Once a patient has been determined to come from a high-risk group for HIV infection, evidence of pneumonia must lead to suspicion of *Pneumocystis carinii*. This microorganism is not easily identified through routine means. Definitive diagnosis usually requires acquiring a biopsy of the involved tissue.

   (1:429–434), (16:492, 1084).

## IB10d

100. A. Normally, the static pressure and dynamic pressure curves are parallel, as illustrated in Figure 3-39.

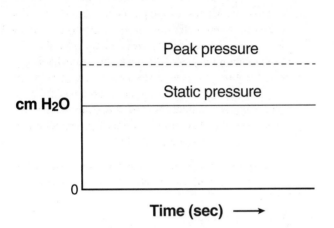

**Figure 3-39:** Peak and static pressures representing no changes in either effective dynamic compliance or effective static compliance over time. Therefore, tracings are parallel.

The static pressure curve will always reside below the peak pressure curve.

In the presence of pulmonary pathologies and changing airway conditions, however, the PIP and static (plateau) pressure will change accordingly. The PIP will increase when either lung compliance decreases (chest wall and ventilator tubing compliances are assumed to be constant) or when airway resistance increases.

The static (plateau) pressure, however, will increase only when the lung compliance decreases (becomes stiffer). When airway resistance increases (e.g., in the presence of increased secretions or bronchospasm), the static pressure does not increase. However, the PIP does.

Therefore, when airway resistance increases, the difference between the static pressure and the PIP becomes greater. At the same time, the static pressure remains constant. Consequently, the dynamic compliance decreases whereas the static compliance does not change.

   (1:199–200), (9:152), (10:259).

## IB10d

101. B. A forced vital capacity (FVC) maneuver, plotting flow against volume, provides a variety of flow rates. For example, $Vmax_{25}$, $Vmax_{50}$, and $Vmax_{75}$, representing the flow rates at 25%, 50%, and 75% of FVC, respectively, are obtained.

The configuration of the flow-volume loop is also diagnostically significant. The six flow-volume loops illustrated as follows represent patterns (shaded portion) derived from general types of pulmonary impairments (Figure 3-40).

Patients who experience hyperinflation and varying degrees of airway obstruction will commonly demonstrate

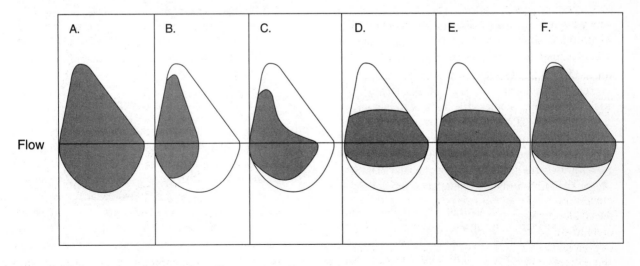

**Figure 3-40:** Interpretation of frequently encountered pulmonary impairments: (A) normal, (B) restrictive disorder, (C) small airway obstruction, (D) fixed large airway obstruction, (E) intrathoracic variable large airway obstruction, and (F) extrathoracic variable large airway obstruction.

a flow-volume loop with a "scooped out," effort-independent limb, as opposed to the normal (outlined) linear decreasing appearance.

Performing a flow-volume loop on a patient provides generalized information on the nature of his pulmonary impairment. Other pulmonary function tests would help supply other useful diagnostic data.

(1:396–397), (6:2, 41, 61), (16:227).

## IB3

102.  C. Resonant notes on percussion are heard over areas containing air, whereas a dull note is heard over dense tissue. Determining the distance the resonant note can vary between maximal inspiration and exhalation implies the range of excursion of the diaphragm.

(1:310), (9:79–80), (16:170–171).

## IA1i

103.  C. Continuous positive airway pressure (CPAP) is a nonsurgical approach to treating obstructive apnea. In obstructive apnea, the muscles of the pharynx lose their tone, become flaccid, and narrow the patient's upper airway, impairing the flow of air into and out of the lungs. Similarly, the genioglossus muscle of the tongue lies against the posterior pharyngeal wall to contribute to the upper airway obstruction during sleep.

The use of nasal CPAP effectively splints open the upper airway by creating a positive intrapharyngeal pressure. The negative pressure generated in this region during normal breathing contributes substantially to the obstructive apnea. The upper airway often becomes patent with the use of CPAP, which causes the elimination of this subatmospheric upper airway pressure.

The level of nasal CPAP needed to create and maintain a patent airway in the treatment of sleep apnea has been shown to range between 5 cm $H_2O$ and 17 cm $H_2O$. The appropriate amount needed to provide airway patency is usually determined by subjecting the patient to CPAP trials during sleep studies. The mask used in conjunction with nasal CPAP fits tightly over only the nose. The mouth remains uncovered. Patient compliance with this mode of therapy is sometimes problematic. The rushing of air, the sensation of pressure, and a claustrophobic feeling contribute to compliance problems.

Interestingly, if CPAP is used for several nights, there will be a reduction in apneic episodes for several nights even after CPAP is stopped. This beneficial effect is temporary, however. If the lapse in CPAP usage extends beyond 2 to 3 nights, a return to the previous symptomatic state is inevitable.

(1:557–559), (9:408–415), (15:752).

## IA1g(2)

104.  C. Pathophysiologic conditions that can cause high-pressure pulmonary edema generally are associated with an elevated pulmonary capillary wedge pressure (PCWP). High-pressure pulmonary edema occurs when the pulmonary capillary hydrostatic pressure rises above the oncotic (colloid osmotic) pressure in the pulmonary vasculature. Plasma proteins, primarily albumin, are responsible for the oncotic or colloid osmotic pressure in the vasculature. The Starling forces are disrupted, resulting in fluid transudation from the pulmonary capillary bed into the pulmonary interstitium and ultimately into the alveoli. Hypervolemia and left ventricular infarction can cause high-pressure pulmonary edema.

Adult respiratory distress syndrome (ARDS), which causes permeability pulmonary edema as the alveolar capillary membrane loses its integrity and fluid exudes from the vasculature into the pulmonary interstitium and alveolar spaces, is not associated with an increased PCWP unless the patient is fluid overloaded. Right ventricular infarction causes the central venous pressure to rise, but not the PCWP.

(1:513–514, 948), (10:135), (15:530–532).

## IA1f(3)

105.  A. The compressible volume, or volume that is "lost" in the ventilator circuit during the inspiratory phase of the ventilatory cycle, is the product of the PIP and the tubing-ventilator compressibility factor (compliance of the system). The more pliable and distensible the tubing, the higher the tubing compressibility factor or compliance factor. Conversely, the more rigid or stiff the tubing, the lower the tubing compressibility factor.

A number of other factors influence the compressible volume. These factors include (1) the preset tidal volume, (2) inspiratory flow rate, (3) PIP, and (4) temperature of the ventilator circuit.

(1:874–875), (10:209).

## IA1c

106.  D. Chronic bronchitis, cystic fibrosis, bronchiectasis, and pneumonia are diseases associated with the production of purulent sputum. Each of these pulmonary pathologies is associated with bacterial infections. Bacterial infections generally involve the presence of white blood cells (WBCs), or leukocytes, in the area of the infection. Sputum resulting from the presence of WBCs is termed *purulent* and is generally yellow or green.

Staining the sputum will help identify the type of WBCs present. For example, an allergic patient (extrinsic asthma) will show a preponderance of eosinophils in the sample, whereas in a bacterial pneumonia patient, neutrophils (polymorphonuclear leukocytes or PMNs) will predominate.

(1:299, 332, 795), (9:29, 100, 112–113).

## IA1f(4)

107. A. Anatomic dead space is composed of the conducting airways of the tracheobronchial tree. These structures do not participate in gas exchange. The oral and nasal cavities and generations 0 (trachea) through 16 (terminal bronchioles), inclusively, constitute the anatomic dead space. Alveolar dead space results from clinical conditions characterized by ventilation–perfusion abnormalities, wherein ventilation occurs in unperfused alveoli. Physiologic dead space includes both anatomic and alveolar dead space (i.e., anatomic dead space plus alveolar dead space). Therefore, subtracting the alveolar dead space from the physiologic dead space equals the anatomic dead space.

(1:203, 211), (15:489), (16:132, 329–330).

## IA1b

108. A. Persons who experience bone fractures are prone to the development of fat embolization. The clinical features of this condition include acute onset, refractory hypoxemia, diaphoresis, dyspnea, tachypnea, tachycardia, cyanosis, diminished sensorium and petechiae, and pulmonary infiltrates.

This syndrome develops when fat globules from the fracture site enter circulation for the purpose of lipid mobilization to increase energy for healing. What follows is an inflammatory response to the enzymatic degradation of triglycerides to free fatty acids by lipases. After free fatty-acid formation, diffuse vasculitis and pulmonary capillary leakage develop. This characteristic development usually occurs 24 to 48 hours posttraumatically. This condition can progress to ARDS.

Massive doses of steroids have been shown to reduce the inflammation and reduce mortality. This intervention must occur relatively early, however—in fact, be-

fore the onset of the syndrome. Once the fat embolism syndrome manifests itself, ET intubation and mechanical ventilation are indicated.

(15:239), (16:210, 822), (20:308–310).

## IA1g(1)

109. C. During the insertion of a pulmonary artery catheter, it is not uncommon for the patient to experience transient premature ventricular contractions (PVCs). The PVCs on the ECG tracing in Figure 3-41 below are labeled. Note the compensatory pause following each PVC.

If the PVCs become more numerous, it might be necessary to withdraw the catheter immediately. Therefore, it is imperative to monitor pulmonary artery catheterization via continuous electrocardiography. Ventricular tachycardia is also another cardiac dysrhythmia that can take place during this procedure.

(1:943–944), (10:127–128), (14:313–319).

## IB9d

110. B. The relationship shown here

$$FEV_{T\%} = \frac{FEV_T}{FVC} \times 100$$

is the general equation used to obtain the percent of any of the $FEV_T$s ($FEV_{0.5}$, $FEV_1$, $FEV_2$, and $FEV_3$) expressed as a percentage of the FVC. For example,

$$FEV_{1\%} = \frac{FEV_1}{FVC} \times 100$$

$$= \frac{5.64 \text{ L}}{7.60 \text{ L}} \times 100$$

$$= 74\%$$

(6:37–38), (11:32), (15:459–460).

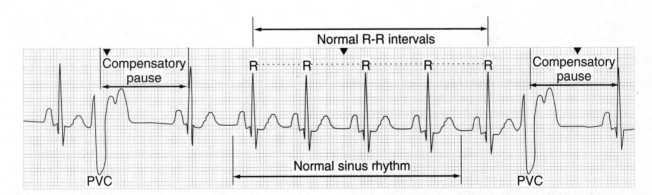

**Figure 3-41:** Premature ventricular contractions (PVCs) followed by a compensatory pause.

111. B. Adequate perfusion is required for transcutaneous monitoring to be effective and to correlate with the arterial PO$_2$. These monitors rely on the diffusion of gases (oxygen and carbon dioxide) from the capillary blood through the patient's skin to the sensor.

Because the PtcO$_2$ electrode measures the partial pressure of oxygen diffusing through the skin, neither carboxyhemoglobin levels nor methemoglobinemia affects the PtcO$_2$ values. Similarly, anemia does not adversely influence this measurement. Irregular ventilatory patterns would produce a certain arterial PCO$_2$ level that would be sensed by the PtcCO$_2$ electrode.

(1:354–356), (10:102–104), (11:261–263).

**IB6b**

112. D. Dyspnea is based on physical limitations, with Grade I being short of breath on severe exertion and Grade V being the most severe (i.e., shortness of breath without exertion).

(6:87, 199), (11:161).

**IB9c**

113. D. The Bohr equation is used to determine the dead space/tidal volume (V$_D$/V$_T$) ratio. When the dissolved arterial carbon dioxide tension (PaCO$_2$) and the mean exhaled carbon dioxide tension (PĒCO$_2$) are given, the (V$_D$/V$_T$) can be calculated as follows:

$$\frac{V_D}{V_T} = \frac{PaCO_2 - P\bar{E}CO_2}{PaCO_2}$$

$$\frac{V_D}{V_T} = \frac{40 \text{ mm Hg} - 28 \text{ mm Hg}}{40 \text{ mm Hg}}$$

$$\frac{V_D}{V_T} = \frac{12 \text{ mm Hg}}{40 \text{ mm Hg}}$$

$$\frac{V_D}{V_T} = 0.30$$

(1:212), (10:434), (11:112–115).

**IC2a**

114. D. The single-breath nitrogen (SBN$_2$)-elimination test is performed by having the patient exhale slowly to residual volume. At that point, the patient inhales 100% O$_2$ to total lung capacity. The patient is then instructed to exhale slowly and evenly once again to residual volume. Throughout this expiratory maneuver, the percent of the patient's exhaled nitrogen is measured by a nitrogen analyzer, and the exhaled volume is measured by a spirometer. A normal SBN$_2$ curve is illustrated in Figure 3-42.

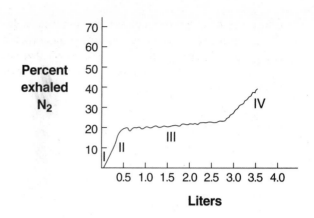

**Figure 3-42:** Normal single-breath nitrogen-elimination curve: (I) anatomic dead space gas, (II) anatomic dead space and alveolar gas, (III) alveolar plateau, and (IV) apical alveolar gas.

This test is useful in assessing the degree of nonuniformity of ventilation throughout the tracheobronchial tree. As the degree of nonuniformity worsens, the greater the tracing becomes distorted. It becomes difficult to distinguish Phase III from Phase IV. At times, Phase III loses its horizontal appearance and instead gradually rises obliquely. The $\Delta N_{2_{750-1250}}$ is the measurement that is made to quantify the degree of uniformity of gas distribution. The lower the $\Delta N_{2_{750-1250}}$, the more uniform the gas distribution. There is a gradual increase in the $\Delta N_{2_{750-1250}}$ with age. This gradual increase is normal.

The diffusing capacity (D$_L$CO) assesses the transfer of carbon monoxide gas (CO) across the alveolarcapillary membrane. The volume of isoflow (VisoV) is useful in determining small airways disease. The maximum voluntary ventilation (MVV) is used to evaluate the integrity and function of the lung-thorax system. The MVV is affected by the status of the muscles of ventilation, the compliance of the respiratory system, and airway resistance and is useful for assessing a person's ability to maintain ventilation during exercise.

(6:83), (11:118–122).

**IB2b**

115. A. The transmission of sound waves produced during phonation can be perceived on the chest wall. The vibrations produced during phonation are called *vocal fremitus*. The vibrations that are felt on the chest wall are termed *tactile fremitus*.

During the examination, the subject repeatedly states the number 99 while the practitioner palpates the thorax, feeling for the intensity of the sound waves passing through the lungs and chest wall in the form of vibrations. The vibrations are either increased, decreased, or absent.

A consolidation, as occurs sometimes with pneumonia, results in an increased transmission of sound waves and therefore an increased tactile fremitus.

Obese or muscular patients can demonstrate a decreased tactile fremitus. In the case of a pneumothorax or a pleural effusion, tactile fremitus can be either decreased or absent, depending on the amount of air or fluid in the intrapleural space.

(1:308), (15:440–441), (16:169–170).

## IC1c

116. D. The Fick equation is as follows:

$$\dot{Q}_T = \frac{\dot{V}o_2}{CaCO_2 - C\bar{v}O_2}$$

where

$\dot{Q}_T$ = C.O. (L/min.)

$\dot{V}o_2$ = oxygen consumption (ml/min.)

$CaO_2$ = arterial oxygen content (vol%)

$C\bar{v}O_2$ = mixed venous oxygen content (vol%)

In the equation, if the $\dot{V}o_2$ is constant, $\dot{Q}_T$ and $CaO_2 - C\bar{v}O_2$ (arterial–mixed venous oxygen content difference) are inversely related. Therefore, if the $\dot{Q}_T$ increases, the $CaO_2 - C\bar{v}O_2$ (a-v difference) decreases. The converse is also true.

(1:225–226, 930), (9:323), (7:135–136).

## IA1h

117. B. Amniotic fluid is derived from fetal lung fluid and urine. Other lesser components are also present, such as vernix caseosa, hair, cells, and blood. Meconium, which is fetal intestinal tract fluid, frequently enters the amniotic fluid. This condition often occurs in infants who are older than 36 to 40 weeks' gestation. When a neonate is born meconium stained, it usually indicates that the fetus has experienced an episode of asphyxia in utero. The degree of meconium staining on the infant appears to correlate with the severity of the aspiration syndrome.

In-utero ventilatory efforts are made by the baby as term approaches. These efforts stop if fetal asphyxia occurs. As the episode of asphyxia continues, the infant gasps deeply, resulting in the likely aspiration of amniotic fluid along with the meconium. Postterm infants are at greater risk of meconium aspiration.

(16:924), (18:34, 37)

## IC2c

118. A. The tracing being displayed for this patient represents a normal pulmonary artery waveform. Therefore, nothing needs to be done. The four characteristic waveforms associated with pulmonary artery catheterization are illustrated in Figure 3-43.

Waveform A represents the catheter in the right atrium. Tracing B shows the catheter in the right ventricle. Note the larger amplitude because the pressure is

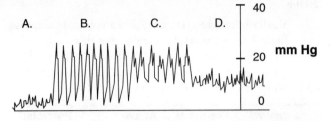

**Figure 3-43:** Pulmonary artery catheter location indicating corresponding normal values and normal waveforms.

higher here when the right ventricle contracts. Tracing C indicates that the Swan–Ganz catheter is located in the pulmonary artery, which is its normal position between wedge-pressure recordings. Finally, Waveform D shows the wedge position as the balloon tip is inflated with air (1.5 cc) to "view" the left side of the heart and obtain a left ventricular end-diastolic pressure (LVEDP) reading. To reduce the risk of pulmonary infarction, the balloon tip should not remain inflated for more than 15 seconds.

(1:947), (10:125), (15:530–533).

## IA1a

119. C. Cromolyn sodium has been used to successfully treat patients who have allergic (extrinsic) asthma or exercise-induced asthma. Cromolyn helps maintain the integrity of the mast cells by inhibiting antigen–antibody reactions on the surface of these cells. By blocking the antigen–antibody reactions, cromolyn (Intal) maintains mast cell membrane integrity, thereby preventing the release of the mediators (histamine, leukotrienes, ECF-A, bradykinins, serotonin, etc.), which lead to inflammation and bronchospasm. Cromolyn has also demonstrated its effectiveness in these types of asthmatics by reducing their steroid dependency. Steroid reduction in these patients must proceed in a tapered manner.

The other drugs listed are described as follows: (1) racemic epinephrine, primarily a vasoconstrictor; (2) procainamide, which reduces the excitability of the myocardium; (3) bretylium, which prolongs repolarization of myocardial tissue; and (4) n-acetylcysteine (Mucomyst), which reduces the viscosity of mucoid sputum.

(8:215–216, 218–219), (15:188).

## IA1e

120. C. Both a chest X-ray and an ECG can assist in the diagnosis of a pulmonary embolism. A definitive diagnosis would require an assessment of perfusion, however, as well as ventilation to the lungs. Prothrombin time (PT) deals with clotting times and might be valuable in assessing treatment. It would not aid in the diagnosis of pulmonary embolism, however.

(1:495–497), (9:36, 40, 173), (15:240).

121.  B. All of the actual/predicted (% predicted) values in Table 3-15 are normal except for the $FEF_{25\%-75\%}$.

**Table 3-15**

| Measurement | Predicted | Actual | % Predicted |
| --- | --- | --- | --- |
| FVC | 2.10 L | 1.97 L | 94% |
| $FEV_1$ | 1.81 L | 1.76 L | 97% |
| PEFR | 3.41 L/sec. | 3.10 L/sec. | 91% |
| $FEV_1/FVC$ | 83% | 89.3% | |
| $FEF_{200-1200}$ | 3.03 L/sec. | 2.66 L/sec. | 88% |
| $FEF_{25\%-75\%}$ | 2.89 L/sec. | 1.85 L/sec. | 64% |
| $FEV_T$ | | 6.51 sec. | |

The $FEF_{25\%-75\%}$ represents the average flow rate during the middle 50% of the forced vital capacity (FVC). This measurement reflects the status of the medium-sized and small airways. When airway obstruction is present in the these airways, the $FEF_{25\%-75\%}$ is lower than normal. Comparatively, the $FEF_{25\%-75\%}$ is much less dependent on patient effort than the $FEF_{200-1200}$.

It is not uncommon for asymptomatic asthmatics to exhibit a low $FEF_{25\%-75\%}$ while having most, if not all, the other FVC components measure as normal. When other spirometric values are normal and the $FEF_{25\%-75\%}$ is low, early small airways disease is often suggested.

Some authorities believe that $FEF_{25\%-75\%}$ values as low as 60% should be considered normal. However, measurements below 80% predicted are generally held to be abnormal by most authorities.

(1:387), (6:34), (11:38), (15:461).

**IB2b**

122.  C. Palpation to determine tracheal position is accomplished by inserting the tip of a fully extended finger into the suprasternal notch immediately medial to the sternoclavicular joint. The examiner should gently press or push her finger inward and move her finger from one side of the suprasternal notch to the other. This area of the suprasternal notch represents the most mobile region of the trachea. If a tracheal shift has occurred in either direction, it can be readily discerned in this region. While this evaluation is being conducted, the patient can assume either a sitting or recumbent position with the neck slightly flexed and the chin midline.

The condition that would cause a leftward tracheal shift is left upper lobe atelectasis. The mediastinum shifts to the affected side in the case of either atelectasis or fibrosis because the affected lung tissue is withdrawn from the intrapleural space in that area and

causes the intrapleural pressure at end exhalation to become more subatmospheric.

This subatmospheric pressure causes the mediastinum to be pulled toward the affected side. Consequently, the trachea will deviate in the same direction. A pleural effusion, a tension pneumothorax, and a non-tension pneumothorax, however, cause mediastinal shift and tracheal deviation toward the unaffected lung. Consolidation and air trapping do not result in mediastinal shift and tracheal deviation.

(9:93–94, 262, 264), (15:441).

**IC1e**

123.  A. The fact that this patient was described as a mechanic who was found unconscious in a garage should lead one to immediately suspect carbon monoxide (CO) poisoning. Hemoglobin has an affinity for CO 210 times greater than that for oxygen. Therefore, the presence of even small amounts of CO in the atmosphere can severely diminish the arterial oxygen saturation ($SaO_2$).

Pulse oximeters essentially use two wavelengths of light (red and infrared) to measure the $SaO_2$. In fact, the device does not sense the presence of carboxyhemoglobin (HbCO) in the blood. Therefore, the pulse oximeter value for the $SaO_2$ will be erroneously high if HbCO is present.

The instrument that measures HbCO blood levels is the co-oximeter. This device uses monochromatic light at four different wavelengths. The light passes through an analytical cuvette, which contains the blood sample. Four types of hemoglobin can be detected by the co-oximeter: oxyhemoglobin, deoxyhemoglobin, methemoglobin, and carboxyhemoglobin.

Consequently, it is inappropriate to use pulse oximetry to evaluate the arterial oxygen saturation in a patient who is suspected of having had CO exposure. The instrument that is to be used in such a situation is the co-oximeter.

(1:928–929), (10:97–98), (11:226–228, 229–232).

**IA1f(3)**

124.  A. During pressure-controlled ventilation, the pressure is maintained constant regardless of changes in lung compliance and airway resistance. Therefore, if the compliance and/or airway resistance change during pressure-controlled ventilation, the volume and flow waveforms become altered, not the pressure waveform.

During volume-controlled ventilation, the volume waveform remains constant and the pressure and flow waveforms change when either or both lung compliance and airway resistance change.

(1:836–839).

125. C. A small percentage of chronic obstructive pulmonary disease (COPD) patients having $CO_2$ retention are at risk of having their hypoxic drive eliminated by the administration of high oxygen ($O_2$) concentrations. Chronic $CO_2$ retainers sometimes lose their ventilatory responsiveness to $CO_2$ and rely entirely on their hypoxic drive for the continuation of their spontaneous ventilations. The hypoxic drive results from the hyperventilatory signals sent from the aortic and carotid bodies (peripheral chemoreceptors) to the medulla. The peripheral chemoreceptors sense the low arterial partial pressure of oxygen in the plasma. Therefore, the administration of excessively high $FIO_2$s can raise the level of arterial $PO_2$ and eliminate the hyperventilatory impulses sent from the aortic and carotid bodies to the medulla, resulting in the cessation of breathing.

The appropriate $O_2$-therapy device to use on COPD patients who are experiencing an acute exacerbation of their lung disease is a Venturi mask at a low $FIO_2$ (less than 0.30). A Venturi mask is appropriate because it ordinarily provides inspiratory flow rates high enough to meet the patient's inspiratory demands. The $FIO_2$ delivered by this high-flow oxygen-delivery device is thereby unaffected if the patient's minute ventilation ($V_T$ and f) and ventilatory pattern change.

Low oxygen concentrations are generally sufficient to overcome the patient's hypoxemia because COPD is characterized by lung units having perfusion in excess of ventilation. These regions of shunt effect or venous admixture usually are quite amenable to oxygen therapy.

(1:742), (16:375,1124).

126. C. Epiglottitis, an acute and life-threatening infection of the upper airway, is caused by *Haemophilus influenzae* type B. It does not characteristically present with a "barky" cough nor a "steeple sign" on a chest radiograph. A lateral neck X-ray of the upper airway assists in the differential diagnosis, with the "thumb sign" indicating a markedly thickened and flattened epiglottis.

(1:1039), (9:83, 232), (18:200).

127. D. In chronic bronchitis, the sputum might range from mucoid to mucopurulent. If the bronchitic has no superimposed infection, the sputum is mucoid, or clear and somewhat viscid. When a pulmonary infection is present, the mucus becomes mucopurulent (i.e., thick, viscous, and green to yellow). In asthma, the sputum is usually mucoid unless the patient has an underlying infection or a complicating disease state.

The sputum of cystic fibrosis patients is characteristically mucopurulent and fetid (foul smelling). Sputum

associated with lung abscess is frequently purulent (yellow or green) and fetid. Bronchogenic carcinoma is often associated with blood-tinged sputum.

(1:299), (9:29, 112–113), (20:6–7, 25–27).

128. B. This child matches the clinical presentation of cystic fibrosis, including the following characteristics:

- frequent pulmonary infections
- abnormal stools (steatorrhea)
- productive cough
- thick, greenish mucus (*Pseudomonas aeruginosa* infections)
- failure to thrive (malnourished appearance)

The diagnostic test needed to confirm this disease, however, is a sweat chloride test. Sweat glands are stimulated by pilocarpine iontophoresis. The sweat is collected from the sweat glands of the patient's arm or thigh, and the sodium concentration of the sweat is measured. Values higher than 60 mEq/liter are considered diagnostic. The normal sodium concentration in the sweat is 28 mEq/liter.

(1:459–460, 794), (18:91, 184–185), (20:187–189).

129. B. Because of the destruction of alveolar septa, the formation of blebs and bullae, and air trapping, the lungs of an emphysematous patient become hyperinflated. This condition manifests itself on a chest X-ray as increased lung volumes, flattened diaphragms, and increased retrosternal air space (lateral chest radiographic view). The increased lung volumes (hyperaeration) cause the intercostal spaces to widen.

(1:148, 414–416).

130. D. The sodium and chloride content of sweat in children with cystic fibrosis is two to five times greater than that of normal children and occurs in 98% of affected children. For diagnostic purposes, the quantitative test is performed on sweat obtained by iontophoresis of pilocarpine, in which a small electric current that carries the cholinergic drug pilocarpine into a small patch of skin to stimulate the local sweat glands.

Normally, the sweat chloride content ranges between about 10 to 40 mEq/liter. A chloride concentration greater than 60 mEq/liter is diagnostic of cystic fibrosis.

(1:460, 794), (9:107), (20:184).

131. B. Kyphoscoliosis and asbestosis (pneumoconiosis) are classified as restrictive lung diseases. Such lung

abnormalities are generally characterized by reduced lung volumes and capacities and sometimes normal flow rates. The data here show a decreased FVC, residual volume (RV), FRC, TLC, and a normal peak expiratory flow rate (PEF).

The forced expiratory volume in one second ($FEV_1$) might be low because the lung volumes are low. Therefore, the $FEV_1$/FVC ratio will be either normal if both the $FEV_1$ and FVC decrease proportionately or increased if the FVC decreases disproportionately compared with the $FEV_1$.

(1:391), (9:144, 156), (11:101–103).

## IB1a

132. A. Applying direct pressure to the nailbed of a patient's finger and relieving that pressure to determine the time to restore circulation (blanch to pink) constitutes assessing capillary refill. Capillary refill is performed to evaluate peripheral perfusion and the adequacy of the C.O.

When the C.O. is low, the time that it takes for circulation to re-establish itself in the nailbed generally exceeds 3 seconds. Normally, capillary refill is almost immediate. Refill time of 3 seconds or less indicates sufficient peripheral perfusion.

(1:318), (9:91, 269), (15:441).

## IB1b

133. B. Table 3-16 lists both the inspiratory and expiratory accessory muscles of ventilation.

**Table 3-16** Accessory Muscles of Ventilation

| Inspiratory | Expiratory |
| --- | --- |
| sternocleidomastoids | latissimus dorsi |
| scalenes | internal intercostals |
| pectoralis minor | rectus abdominis |
| pectoralis major | obliquus externus abdominus |
| trapezius | obliquus internus abdominus |
| serratus anterior | transversus abdominus |
| serratus posterior | |
| levatores costarum | |
| sacrospinalis | |

These muscles do not participate in normal, tidal breathing. They do become active to varying degrees during cardiopulmonary disease, however. For example, if a patient experiences airway inflammation and partial obstructions because of retained secretions, the resistance encountered by the flowing air will increase. Likewise, air will be nonuniformly distributed throughout the tracheobronchial tree, resulting in shunt effect (venous admixture) and hypoxemia. The hypoxemia and increased airway resistance lead to an increased work of breathing. The increased work of breathing is accomplished by the accessory muscles of ventilation.

Similarly, complete airway obstruction from retained secretions can result in absorption atelectasis. Significant atelectasis causes lung compliance to decrease, which in turn increases the work of breathing. Again, the accessory muscles of ventilation produce the increased work of breathing.

An increased pulmonary compliance can also cause the accessory muscles of ventilation to operate. The accessory muscles used are generally those of expiration, however. For example, a pulmonary emphysema patient has to use accessory muscles to attempt to overcome the mechanical disadvantage resulting from the increased lung compliance and loss of elastic recoil. Exhalation becomes quite active.

Patients who are grossly obese (e.g., those with alveolar hypoventilation syndrome) experience a decreased chest-wall compliance because of the tremendous amount of adipose tissue opposing thoracic movements during inspiration. To overcome this restrictive effect, the patient must use accessory inspiratory muscles of ventilation to get air into the lungs.

(1:149), (15:45–50, 558).

## IA1b

134. A. Sarcoidosis is a systemic, granulomatous disease of unknown etiology. The disease is prevalent among Blacks in the Southeast. Although clinical manifestations of sarcoidosis are varied because this disease is a multisystem disorder, pulmonary signs and symptoms are frequent.

Ordinarily, the patient will have an unremarkable physical examination. Breath and voice sounds are usually normal. If advanced fibrosis is present, however, bronchial breath sounds will predominate. Coughing is a common complaint, but sputum production is uncommon. The patient also expresses being fatigued and having general malaise. Dyspnea at rest and on exertion might occur. Radiologically, bilateral hilar adenopathy with or without alveolar or pulmonary interstitial infiltrates are observed. Pulmonary function studies in sarcoidosis patients ordinarily reflect a restrictive abnormality.

(1:465), (15:224–226), (20:199–215).

## IA1g(2)

135. D. When properly placed, the pulmonary artery catheter tip should be positioned in a branch (pulmonary arteriole) of the pulmonary artery. The balloon should be inflated to completely occlude the proximal blood flow through that branch, as shown in the diagram in Figure 3-44 on page 161. The recorded pressure measurement

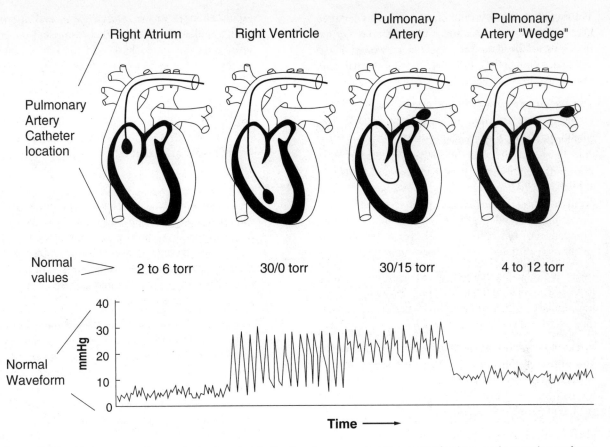

| Right Atrium | Right Ventricle | Pulmonary Artery | Pulmonary Artery "Wedge" |
|---|---|---|---|

Pulmonary Artery Catheter location

Normal values: 2 to 6 torr | 30/0 torr | 30/15 torr | 4 to 12 torr

Normal Waveform

**Figure 3-44:** Pulmonary artery catheter location indicating the corresponding normal values and normal waveforms.

is referred to as the pulmonary capillary wedge pressure (PCWP), or pulmonary artery occluding pressure (PAOP). The normal mean range of the PCWP is 4 to 12 mm Hg.

Once the PCWP has been obtained, the balloon tip needs to be deflated so that blood flow through the pulmonary arteriole, in which the catheter resides, can resume.

(1:493–494), (10:127–128), (15:532).

**IB10a**

136.   A. The four ECG patterns are identified as follows:

I.   ventricular tachycardia
II.   nodal or junctional tachycardia
III.   premature ventricular contractions (PVCs)
IV.   ventricular fibrillation

Each of the dysrhythmias shown can cause a decreased C.O. During ventricular tachycardia, nodal (junctional) tachycardia, ventricular fibrillation, and ventricular diastole time might be insufficient to provide an adequate preload, thereby reducing the stroke volume and ultimately the C.O. If PVCs frequently occur, their presence can adversely influence the C.O. PVCs can cause the heart pattern to degenerate to ventricular fibrillation.

(1:330–331), (16:857, 858, 864).

**IB7e**

137.   A. A pneumothorax develops when air invades the intrapleural space. The presence of air between the visceral and parietal pleurae will present itself as a radiolucent area. The two pleurae will be visible while the lung on the affected side retracts toward the hilum. If no pleural adhesions are present and if the amount of air is small, the air will be visible apically. Pleural adhesions sometimes result in a loculated pneumothorax by preventing the air from ascending to the apex within the intrapleural space.

Other physical features that accompany a pneumothorax include (1) unilateral reduction of chest-wall excursion, (2) unilateral absence or reduction of breath sounds, and (3) unilateral hyperresonance to percussion.

(1:405–408), (9:92–93, 178–179, 260).

**IA1h**

138.   D. The Silverman score is a method whereby a neonate's ventilatory status is assessed. The scale ranges from 0 to 10, with 0 being the best score. The clinical signs evaluated are as follows:

• upper chest movements
• lower chest movements

- xiphoid retractions
- dilatation of nares
- expiratory grunting

(1:1006), (18:51).

## IA1h

139. C. Assessing the lecithin/sphingomyelin (L/S) ratio via amniocentesis provides a measure of lung maturity. Before 35 weeks' gestation, sphingomyelin (another phospholipid) predominates, thus rendering an L/S ratio of less than 2. At approximately 35 weeks' gestation, lecithin production increases, and its concentration in the amniotic fluid begins to exceed that of sphingomyelin. An L/S ratio of 2:1 or greater reflects lung maturation sufficient to support extrauterine life. Such an L/S ratio indicates less than a 5% risk for the development of infant respiratory distress syndrome (RDS), whereas a ratio of 1:1 or less is associated with a greater than 90% risk. A transitional L/S ratio (1.5:1) indicates a 50% probability of risk. The L/S ratio becomes less reliable when the mother is a diabetic. The risk of the development of RDS is still present in such a situation even when the L/S ratio is 2:1.

Another phospholipid used in assessing fetal lung maturity during intrauterine life is phosphatidylglycerol (PG). PG begins to appear in the amniotic fluid at about 36 weeks' gestation. Its concentration continues to rise until term.

(1:1001), (18:6–7).

## IA1f(3)

140. C. Any situation that causes a reduced arterial $PO_2$ supply to the aortic and carotid bodies (peripheral chemoreceptors) results in an increase in the minute ventilation; for example, ascending to a higher altitude (hypoxic hypoxia) and cyanide poisoning (histotoxic hypoxia).

Certain conditions that do not reduce the $PaO_2$ will not stimulate the peripheral chemoreceptors to emit hyperventilatory signals to the medulla. These include methemoglobinemia ($Fe^{+3}$ instead of $Fe^{+2}$ in the center of the heme structure) and CO poisoning (CO binds 210 times stronger to Hb than $O_2$ does).

In cyanide poisoning, oxygen transport in the blood can be normal ($PaO_2$ 100 mm Hg and $SaO_2$ 97.5%). The tissues, however, including the peripheral chemoreceptors, are unable to use the oxygen because of the presence of hydrocyanic acid in the cells. Therefore, regardless of a normal $PaO_2$, the peripheral chemoreceptors would send hyperventilatory signals to the medulla. In the case of ascending to a higher altitude, fewer oxygen molecules diffuse across the alveolar capillary membrane. Hence, the $PaO_2$ decreases and the peripheral chemoreceptors are stimulated.

Acute changes in the arterial $PCO_2$ and arterial pH also stimulate the peripheral chemoreceptors. For example, the increased hydrogen ion concentration in the arterial blood causes the hyperventilation that is associated with diabetic ketoacidosis by stimulating the aortic and carotid bodies. The arterial $PO_2$ in this condition is either normal or increased (not greater than 120 mm Hg).

(1:287–289), (15:129–132).

## IA2a

141. D. Cystic fibrosis is a disease affecting the exocrine glands. The sweat produced by the sweat glands has an unusually high sodium and chloride concentration. Quite often, parents of cystic fibrosis children report to their physicians that their children's skin has a salty taste. This salty taste is commonly perceived whenever these parents kiss their children.

The sweat test that is used to evaluate the chloride concentration of sweat is an important diagnostic measure in cystic fibrosis. The sweat test is conducted by pilocarpine iontophoresis. The process stimulates the sweat glands, enabling the measurement of sweat electrolyte concentration. Normally, the sweat chloride concentration is about 28 mEq/liter. Chloride concentrations greater than 60 mEq/liter are diagnostic of cystic fibrosis.

(1:459–460, 1040), (15:121), (18:183–188).

## IC4

142. D. According to the Joint Commission on the Accreditation of Health Organizations (JCAHO) standards, the following criteria must be met to achieve quality assurance: (1) quality and appropriateness of care should be reviewed and evaluated in accordance with the hospital plan; (2) the review should involve the medical record; (3) the review should be based on preestablished criteria to include indications, effectiveness, and adverse effects of therapy; (4) the review should include input from the medical community; (5) the review should be done within the hospital quality-assurance program; and (6) particular attention should be given to services of highest utilization rates.

(1:4, 12, 1107), (16:73).

## IA1f(4)

143. B. During positive pressure ventilation, not all of the preset volume is delivered to the patient's lungs. Some of that preset volume is compressed or "lost" in the ventilator tubing.

Knowing the compressibility factor and the peak inspiratory pressure (PIP), one can determine the amount of the preset volume that remains in the ventilator tubing and in the ventilator's internal circuitry. The volume compressed in the tubing-ventilator system is obtained by multiplying the compressibility factor by the PIP, shown as follows:

$$\left(\begin{array}{c}\text{compressed}\\\text{volume}\end{array}\right) = \left(\begin{array}{c}\text{compressibility}\\\text{factor}\end{array}\right)(\text{PIP})$$

$$= (5 \text{ cc/cmH}_2\text{O})(40 \text{ cmH}_2\text{O})$$

$$= 200 \text{ cc}$$

Ventilators, such as the Nellcor Puritan Bennett 7200, are capable of automatically compensating for volume lost because of compression.

(1:874–875), (10:209).

**IB1b**

144.   D. The four components of chest physical assessment are (1) inspection, (2) palpation, (3) percussion, and (4) auscultation. Inspection entails the evaluation of the patient's position or posture, chest configuration, ventilatory pattern, mental status, and skin color.

When a person experiences a decreased lung compliance, she generally breathes in a rapid, shallow manner and uses the accessory muscles of ventilation. The breathing pattern is often associated with restrictive lung disease. Obstructive lung disease is characterized by prolonged exhalation and slow, deep breathing. For example, upper airway obstruction, the larynx in epiglottitis, is associated with a prolonged inspiratory time.

(1:306–313), (9:69–87), (15:436–438).

**IB10a**

145.   B. The letter shown on the ECG tracing (Lead II) designates atrial depolarization (i.e., atrial contraction). The letters BCD represent ventricular depolarization. The letter E signifies ventricular repolarization.

(1:324–325), (16:855–856).

**IA1b**

146.   A. A pneumothorax takes on a variety of clinical forms: (1) tension pneumothorax, (2) spontaneous pneumothorax, (3) iatrogenic pneumothorax, and (4) traumatic pneumothorax. A tension pneumothorax exists if air trapped in the intrapleural space rises above atmospheric pressure. A spontaneous pneumothorax is often seen in young, tall, and otherwise healthy persons. This form of pneumothorax is usually associated with a subpleural bleb rupture. A spontaneous pneumothorax frequently requires no direct medical intervention aside from monitoring the patient, because the intrapleural air ultimately becomes reabsorbed. An iatrogenic pneumothorax is either intentionally or accidentally induced for or during medical treatment. Before

antituberculosis medications, a pneumothorax was frequently induced to treat pulmonary tuberculosis. Inadvertent creation of a pneumothorax can occur in conjunction with thoracentesis, Swan–Ganz catheter insertion, mechanical ventilation (barotrauma), and so on. A traumatic pneumothorax can result from a penetrating or nonpenetrating chest-wall injury.

With a tension pneumothorax, the patient is usually dyspneic and expresses chest pain. Chest-wall movement on the affected side is decreased. Tactile and vocal fremitus and breath sounds, likewise, decrease on the affected side. Percussion over a pneumothorax produces hyperresonance. The trachea is deviated from midline toward the unaffected lung.

A pleural effusion, if large enough, will also produce tracheal deviation toward the unaffected lung. It is, likewise, associated with decreased tactile fremitus. Percussion over a pleural effusion produces a dull sound, however.

Lung or lobar consolidation does not cause tracheal deviation. It causes increased tactile fremitus and a dull percussion note. Atelectasis, if extensively unilateral, produces tracheal deviation toward the affected lung, increased tactile fremitus, and dull percussion sounds.

(1:310, 313, 405, 485), (9:41, 92–93, 178–179, 260).

**IA2h**

147.   D. Pulmonary disability evaluation, exercise-induced asthma (EIA), and determining the morbidity of lung resection are all indications for pulmonary stress testing, where the patient's response to physical stress must be evaluated.

(1:168, 457).

**IB4a**

148.   C. The normal sounds heard when auscultating the trachea are loud and high pitched. The expiratory sounds are about the same duration or slightly longer than those heard during inspiration. The normal sounds perceived over the trachea are called bronchial or tracheal breath sounds.

(1:312), (9:81–82), (15:442–443).

**IC2c**

149.   A. A 10% intrapulmonary shunt ($\dot{Q}_S/\dot{Q}_T$) represents no clinical significant impairment in the gas-exchange mechanism. This degree of shunting, while the patient is receiving mechanically assisted ventilation, is thought to be comparable to normal pulmonary physiology in a spontaneously breathing person. Therefore, no immediate intervention is needed at the moment.

Of course, the patient should be closely monitored for changes in his condition. Again, a 10% $\dot{Q}_S/\dot{Q}_T$ poses no immediate threat to the patient's well-being.

Clinical practice has shown that the greater the $\dot{Q}_S/\dot{Q}_T$, the less effect increasing the $FIO_2$ has on the patient's arterial $PO_2$. Some clinicians believe that if the $\dot{Q}_S/\dot{Q}_T$ exceeds 30%, an $FIO_2$ of 1.0 cannot be expected to appreciably elevate the arterial $PO_2$.

Table 3-17 below outlines guidelines for the interpretation of intrapulmonary shunt (capillary shunt plus shunt effect) measurements for mechanically ventilated patients.

(1:221–222, 234), (15:487–488), (16:257, 1098).

## IB10c

150. D. Asbestosis (white lung) is a pneumoconiosis caused by chronic pulmonary exposure to asbestos fibers, which frequently causes bilateral basilar pleural fibrosis. The diffuse, bilateral, basilar pulmonary fibrosis causes thickening of the alveolar capillary membrane and decreases the diffusion of oxygen from the alveoli to the pulmonary capillary blood.

The decreased lung-diffusing capacity results in a widened alveolar arterial oxygen tension gradient [i.e., $P(A\text{-}a)O_2$]. Carbon dioxide, however, maintains its relative ease of diffusibility across the alveolar-capillary membrane, and the alveolar and arterial $PCO_2$ tensions generally remain in equilibrium.

Therefore, Dataset D, which reflects a $P(A\text{-}a)O_2$ of 45 torr (100 torr − 55 torr = 45 torr) and a low arterial $PCO_2$ (30 torr), is consistent with this condition. The low arterial and alveolar carbon dioxide tensions result from the hyperventilation caused by the hypoxemia. Peripheral chemoreceptor (carotid and aortic bodies) stimulation by the low arterial $PO_2$ is responsible for the hyperventilation.

(1:217, 234–235), (9:125), (15:227, 367–368).

## IA1c

151. B. Bronchiectasis is an obstructive lung disease characterized by abnormal and irreversible dilatation of the bronchi and bronchioles. Its etiology is unknown; however, it is frequently associated with chronic obstructive lung conditions such as cystic fibrosis, and it has congenital links (e.g., Kartagener's syndrome).

In bronchiectasis, the sputum produced by a chronic, loose cough is characteristically copious, purulent (yellow or green), fetid (foul smelling), and sometimes bloody (hemoptysis). When the sputum is allowed to settle, it separates into three distinct layers (i.e., a top cloudy, mucous layer; a clear saliva middle layer; and a purulent to mucopurulent bottom layer sometimes containing Dittrich's plugs [small particles in fetid sputum composed of pus, detritus, or bacteria]).

(1:459, 794), (9:29), (20:177–183).

## IA1e

152. B. Respiratory distress syndrome (RDS), or hyaline membrane disease (HMD), is caused by an inadequate amount or the absence of pulmonary surfactant at birth. Neonates born before 34 weeks' gestation usually are low birth weight, and have an inadequate amount of surfactant to reduce the surface tension forces in the lungs. Little to no functional residual capacity (FRC) develops. Consequently, each breath is equivalent to the infant's first breath (i.e., high energy expenditure and high intrapleural pressure). In a relatively short time, the newborn fatigues and develops respiratory failure because of the increased work of breathing and fluid-filled alveoli. These two pathophysiologic conditions result in (1) decreased pulmonary compliance, (2) refractory hypoxemia, and (3) mixed acidemia.

Clinical manifestations of RDS include tachypnea (ventilatory rate greater than 60 breaths/min.), sternal retractions, grunting, nasal flaring, and paradoxical breathing. Radiologic features related to RDS are classified in four stages representing degrees of disease severity. Typical radiographic findings include a "bell-shaped" thorax, clear to indistinct cardiac shadows, bilateral, diffuse reticulogranular densities, and air bronchograms. The severity of the RDS depends on the degree of these presentations. Normal preterm ABG data for 1 to 5 hours following parturition are as follows:

$PO_2$ 60 torr
$PCO_2$ 47 torr

**Table 3-17** $\dot{Q}_S/\dot{Q}_T$ Interpretation Guidelines for Mechanically Ventilated Patients

| $\dot{Q}_S/\dot{Q}_T$ | Interpretation |
| --- | --- |
| 10% | Essentially normal pulmonary physiology allowing patient to assume and maintain spontaneous ventilation |
| 11% to 19% | Signifies pulmonary derangement that would likely not prevent spontaneous breathing |
| 20% to 29% | Implies abnormal lung physiology that would likely prevent patient from maintaining spontaneous ventilation, especially regarding patients with cardiovascular instability and central nervous system (CNS) disorders |
| 30% | Reflects severe compromise of cardiopulmonary homeostasis, demanding immediate intervention directed toward cardiopulmonary stabilization |

pH 7.33

$HCO_3^-$ 25 mEq/lier

(1:1030–1031), (20:417–422).

## IA2e

153. A. A Carlens tube is used for independent lung ventilation. Plotting the exhaled tidal volume over the
plateau pressure would provide static compliance.
Neither of these two actions, nor the determination of
the total oxygen content, would aid in the diagnosis of
cardiogenic versus noncardiogenic pulmonary edema.
To differentially diagnose this condition, the RRT
would suggest the insertion of a Swan–Ganz (pulmonary artery) catheter to assess the PCWP.

In cardiogenic or high-pressure pulmonary edema,
pulmonary vascular pressures ordinarily rise to levels
exceeding the protein osmotic (oncotic) pressure in the
blood. The protein osmotic pressure generally ranges
between 25 torr and 32 torr. A pulmonary artery
catheter enables the monitoring of the pulmonary vascular pressures. When the PCWP exceeds the protein
osmotic pressure, pulmonary edema (cardiogenic or
high pressure) occurs.

Noncardiogenic or permeability pulmonary edema develops when the pulmonary capillary endothelium
loses its integrity and vascular fluid floods the pulmonary interstitium. This condition, associated with
ARDS, is generally not characterized by high pulmonary vascular pressures. Therefore, a pulmonary
artery catheter is useful in differentiating between cardiogenic and noncardiogenic pulmonary edema.

(1:375, 1098), (10:240, 259, 270, 309), (15:525–532).

## IA1g(2)

154. C. Peripheral or pedal edema occurs when blood flow to
the right side of the heart (i.e., venous return) diminishes. The pooling of blood in the gravity-dependent,
peripheral venous circulation alters the pressures involved in the Starling equation. Pooling of blood in
the venous circulation elevates the capillary hydrostatic pressure. The Starling-factor change is consistent
with an increased transudation of vascular fluid into
the peripheral interstitium. Clinical conditions that are
associated with peripheral edema include (1) right-
ventricular failure, (2) chronic hypoxemia (causing
pulmonary vasoconstriction), and (3) right-ventricular
hypertrophy.

(1:318), (9:44–45, 277), (15:117–118).

## IB10c

155. C. As a person hyperventilates, the amount of $CO_2$ dissolved in arterial blood decreases. Subsequently, the
amount of $CO_2$ in the cerebrospinal fluid (CSF) will

also decrease because $CO_2$ passively moves across the
blood–brain barrier out the CSF. For a given metabolic
rate, the $PaCO_2$ and $P_{CSF}CO_2$ are inversely related to
the ventilatory rate.

(1:287–289), (16:129–130, 1044).

## IC1a

156. B. Virtually every definition provided for asthma specifies the need for reversibility of the airflow obstruction. Thus, to assess the effectiveness of bronchodilator
therapy, the RRT has to perform pre- and postspirom-
etry studies.

(1:450), (15:683), (16:1002).

## IC2a

157. B. Bronchodilator therapy can proceed with continuous patient monitoring. Systemic corticosteroid therapy will treat the edema and mucous plugging that is
present when bronchodilator therapy alone does not
improve after 60 to 90 minutes of aggressive beta-two
agonist administration.

(American Association for Respiratory Care, Aerosol
Consensus Statement—1991, *Respiratory Care,* September 1991, Vol. 36, No. 9, p. 918).

## IC2e

158. A. This condition can be deceiving. The absorption of
more drug might worsen the situation quickly. Therefore, mechanical ventilation is indicated. ABGs reveal
that this patient is experiencing uncompensated respiratory acidosis (i.e., acute ventilatory failure). The
blood gas and acid-base condition resulted from CNS
depression caused by the drug overdose. Ventilatory
support would be expected to improve the patient's
oxygenation status.

Intermittent mandatory ventilation (IMV) would not
be necessary in this situation because the patient appears to be having difficulty breathing spontaneously.
Therefore, IMV as an initial mode of ventilation
would not be considered important because this patient's condition might worsen, and the patient will not
be ready for weaning.

(1:863), (15:946–948).

## IA1g(2)

159. C. The tip of a central venous pressure (CVP) catheter
is positioned in either the superior vena cava or in the
right atrium. The CVP measurement is an excellent index for fluid administration and vasoactive medications. The CVP reflects the end-diastolic pressure in the
right ventricle immediately preceding ventricular systole (i.e., the right ventricular end-diastole pressure or

RVEDP). The RVEDP indicates right ventricular pre-load. Normal CVP is generally less than 12 cm $H_2O$.

(1:190, 416, 946), (10:135, 249), (15:77, 119).

## IA1f(1)

160.  A. Physiologic effects of continuous mechanical ventilation include a potential decrease in the C.O. and a potential increase in intracranial pressure. The functional residual capacity (FRC) is not necessarily affected by continuous mechanical ventilation unless PEEP is instituted. In the presence of PEEP, the FRC increases. Continuous mechanical ventilation can potentially decrease urinary output, however. This physiologic effect can occur by decreasing blood flow to the kidneys, potentially compromising kidney function. The potential decrease in venous return can be interpreted as a state of relative hypovolemia. Actually, this physiologic effect results from an increase in the production of antidiuretic hormone and other factors, such as a decreased renal perfusion.

(1:886–888), (10:141–145).

## IA1g(1)

161.  C. In patients who have a compromised hemodynamic status, as occurs during cardiopulmonary resuscitation (CPR), the systolic blood pressure values determined by the arm cuff method might either be normal or substantially underestimated.

(15:537).

## IA1c

162.  D. Based on the data presented, the indices for oxygen-carrying capacity are the most likely sources for this patient's dyspnea. Subnormal values were obtained for red blood cell concentration, hemoglobin concentration, and hematocrit. Table 3-18 outlines the normal concentrations of these blood components.

Because this patient has a low hemoglobin concentration (less than 12 g%, or 12 g/dL), erythrocyte concentration (less than $4.5 \times 10^6/mm^3$), and hematocrit (less than 37%), she is likely experiencing anemic hypoxia. Compensation for anemic hypoxia is an increased C.O. Hypoxemia is not reflected in the ABG

data because it is measured by dissolved oxygen rather than the arterial oxygen content. Further analysis by co-oximetry would be helpful under this circumstance because it would yield direct information about the oxygen carrying capacity of the blood.

(1:232–233).

## IA1e

163.  C. Bronchiolitis is an obstructive disease that affects the small airways. It is an infectious process usually (~75%) caused by the respiratory syncytial virus (RSV). Other pathogens responsible for causing bronchiolitis include the parainfluenza virus, adenovirus, rhinovirus, and *Myobacterium pneumoniae.*

The obstructive process results from inflammation of the bronchioles caused by bronchiolar wall edema, spasm, and mucus production. Roentgenographically, bronchiolitis is characterized by hyperinflation, flattened hemidiaphragms, increased anteroposterior (A–P) chest-wall diameter (sternal bowing), and generalized hyperlucency.

(1:1037–1038), (15:398–401), (16:987–990).

## IB10c

164.  D. The room-air alveolar-arterial oxygen tension difference [i.e., $P(A-a)O_2$] increases (widens) with advancing age. The cause of the $P(A-a)O_2$ changes with age is deterioration of ventilation–perfusion ratios.

At age 20, the $P(A-a)O_2$ on room air is about 4 to 5 torr. The gradient widens by approximately 4 torr for each decade after 20. Therefore, by the fifth decade of life, the room air $P(A-a)O_2$ is expected to be around 16 torr. This degree of widening peaks by 80 years of age.

The $P(A-a)O_2$ is sometimes used to estimate the degree of shunting. One estimate used indicates that while a person breathes 100% oxygen, a 5% shunt exists for every 100 torr $P(A-a)O_2$. The $P(A-a)O_2$ is also sometimes used in the assessment of a patient for weaning from a mechanical ventilator. For example, a $P(A-a)O_2$ of less than 300 to 350 torr is acceptable if the person is breathing 100% $O_2$. The estimated shunt for this situation would be less than 15% to 15.5%.

(1:217, 234–235), (15:170, 946–947), (16:256–257).

**Table 3-18** Normal Range of Concentrations for RBCS, WBCS, HB, and HCT

| Blood Component | Normal Range |
| --- | --- |
| RED BLOOD CELLS (RBCs, erythrocytes) | 4.5 to 5.0 $\times$ 106/mm³ |
| WHITE BLOOD CELLS (WBCs, leukocytes) | 5,000 to 9,000/mm³ |
| HEMOGLOBIN CONCENTRATION (Hb) | 12 to 16 g%, or 12 to 16 g/dL |
| HEMATOCRIT (HCT) | females 37% to 47% |
| | males 40% to 54% |

165. C. The total amount of oxygen remaining in the right atrial blood after gas exchange at the tissue level takes place is the mixed venous oxygen content ($C\overline{v}O_2$). The $C\overline{v}O_2$ is the sum of the oxygen dissolved in the right atrial venous blood ($P\overline{v}O_2$) and the oxygen combined with hemoglobin in venous circulation. The $C\overline{v}O_2$ is calculated as follows:

$$C\overline{v}O_2 = (P\overline{v}O_2)(0.003\ vol\%/torr) + (1.34 \times [Hb] \times S\overline{v}O_2)$$

Clinically, oxygen delivery and tissue oxygen uptake are sometimes evaluated on the basis of either the mixed venous oxygen tension ($P\overline{v}O_2$) or the mixed venous oxygen saturation ($S\overline{v}O_2$). The normal $P\overline{v}O_2$ range is 33 to 53 torr, and the normal range for the $S\overline{v}O_2$ is 67% to 88%. When these measured values are below their normal limit, oxygen delivery to the tissues is ordinarily considered inadequate.

Because different organ systems have different oxygen requirements, the RRT must be mindful that a normal $CaO_2 - C\overline{v}O_2$ (4.0 to 6.0 vol%) might not reflect adequate tissue oxygenation for all organ systems.

Furthermore, the RRT must be cognizant of two particular clinical conditions that render higher-than-normal mixed venous oxygen measurements but actually are associated with reduced tissue oxygen extraction: cyanide poisoning (histotoxic hypoxia) and ARDS caused by septicemia. In cyanide poisoning, the oxygen-transport mechanisms in the blood are normal. The mitochondria in the cells of the tissues cannot utilize the oxygen delivered there, however. Hence, the blood returning to the heart in the venous circulation has a higher than normal oxygen content. Similarly, in ARDS, particularly from septicemia, oxygen delivery ($\dot{Q}_T$) and tissue oxygen consumption ($\dot{V}o_2$) sometimes decrease. Therefore, based on the following Fick equation,

$$\dot{Q}_T = \frac{\dot{V}o_2}{CaO_2 - C\overline{v}O_2}$$

the $C\overline{v}O_2$ will remain relatively constant. Additionally, blood can be shunted past the tissue vascular beds, causing the $C\overline{v}O_2$ to increase.

(1:225, 232), (9:120), (15:301, 329–300).

**IBc**

166. B. When attempting to drain a hemothorax, the chest tube would likely be exiting laterally on the affected side because blood occupying the affected area will generally settle at the gravity-dependent portion of the anatomy. Anterior placement on the affected side is appropriate for a pneumothorax.

(1:480), (9:260), (15:1092).

**IA1f(1)**

167. D. Dehydration, as exemplified by a decreased urinary output, might decrease mucociliary clearance, decrease the C.O., and lower the blood pressure. Overhydration might produce pulmonary edema.

(15:119, 286).

**IB10a**

168. C. The accuracy of a pulse oximeter requires pulsatile arterial blood flow. If the arterial pulse diminishes or becomes imperceptible, data from a pulse oximeter will be erroneous. Examples of clinical conditions with which inaccurate pulse oximetry ($SaO_2$) is associated include (1) hypothermia, (2) hypotension, (3) cardiac arrest, and (4) significant venous pulsation. Hypothermia, hypotension, and cardiac arrest are associated with sluggish blood flow, which diminishes arterial blood pulsation.

Significant venous blood pulsations can interfere with arterial blood pulsations, however, producing unreliable data. Conditions such as right-ventricular failure, reduced venous return, highly elevated intrathoracic pressures, and tricuspid regurgitation can significantly increase venous blood pulsations.

(1:361–363, 923, 925, 928), (9:245, 295), (10:98–99).

**IA1g(2)**

169. D. Normally, a central venous pressure (CVP) catheter is placed at the junction of the superior vena cava and the right atrium. The tip of the catheter generally resides in the superior vena cava or rests in the right atrium. CVP measurements reflect right ventricular preload (i.e., the volume of blood in the right ventricle immediately before systole). The measurement that reflects right ventricular preload is called the right ventricular end-diastolic pressure (RVEDP). Normal CVP pressure readings are 5 to 15 cm $H_2O$, or 1 to 16 mm Hg.

(1:416, 946), (9:313, 338–339), (15:76–78).

**IC1d**

170. D. If a ventilator patient is overhydrated, he could develop congestive heart failure that could result in high pressure pulmonary edema. This condition would result in a decreased pulmonary compliance. Fluid in the alveoli would result in intrapulmonary shunting (capillary shunting plus venous admixture) and a widened P(A-a)$O_2$ gradient. A PCWP greater than 6 to 12 mm Hg

would be measured. In fact, with cardiogenic or high-pressure pulmonary edema, the pulmonary capillary hydrostatic pressure exceeds the capillary osmotic pressure. The patient would be hypertensive, not hypotensive.

(1:513–514), (10:135, 241–242).

## IB10a

171. C. Atrial fibrillation is the most common ECG disturbance. In atrial fibrillation, the P waves (atrial contractions) are not distinguishable and are associated with rates higher than 350 beats/min. The atrial contractions are followed by irregular, slower ventricular contractions, often with a rate between 100 to 200 beats/min.

The atria are in a state of chaos and are incapable of any pumping ability. Consequently, the ventricles are not sufficiently filled, and C.O. is compromised. The C.O. does not plummet, however. Generally, the patient can move about but experiences some degree of interference with normal activities of daily living.

(1:329–330), (9:204–205).

## IB7a

172. C. Blunted costophrenic angles are indicative of poor aeration, pleural effusions, and/or a pneumonic process. Vascular markings might indicate pulmonary hypertension. An air bronchogram could indicate a pneumonia, interstitial edema, atelectasis, or hemorrhage. A mediastinal shift can occur as a result of a tension pneumothorax or a significant collapse of a lung.

(1:144, 306, 410), (9:70, 177), (15:1089–1090).

## IC2c

173. A. Frequently, the presence of hypoxemia is associated with varying degrees of shunting. There are a number of different types of shunting. For example, an anatomic shunt includes blood that does not enter the pulmonary capillary network (normally 2% to 5%). Intrapulmonary shunting is composed of two components: capillary shunting (perfusion of nonventilated alveoli) and venous admixture or shunt effect (perfusion in excess of ventilation). Physiologic or total shunt represents the portion of the C.O. that does not participate in gas exchange. It is the sum of the (1) anatomic shunt, (2) capillary shunt, and (3) shunt effect (venous admixture or perfusion in excess of ventilation).

A number of pulmonary diseases are associated with increased intrapulmonary shunting. Any pneumonia increases intrapulmonary shunting because of the presence of secretions impeding airflow, causing either partial or complete airway obstruction. The increased intrapulmonary shunting caused by pulmonary edema results from vascular fluid-occupying alveoli.

Adult respiratory distress syndrome (ARDS) produces an exudation of vascular fluid into the pulmonary interstitium and alveolar spaces. A pleural effusion can compress the alveoli and prevent air from entering the alveoli, thereby depriving venous blood from becoming oxygenated.

(1:220–222, 234), (10:272), (15:487).

## IA1b

174. A. Although several pediatric disorders might share low-grade fevers and runny noses, the hallmark sign of croup, or laryngotracheobronchitis (LTB), is a harsh, barking cough. This distressed cough is the result of a narrowed airway from subglottic swelling secondary to infection. A lateral neck radiograph will confirm this suspicion, especially if the steeple sign is viewed.

(1:1038–1039), (9:231), (18:196–199).

## IB9c

175. D. The difference between the oxygen gas tensions in the alveoli and in the pulmonary capillaries is referred to as the $P(A-a)O_2$. This measurement is useful in differentiating between hypoventilation as a cause of hypoxemia and other causes. Because hypoventilation does not change the $P(A-a)O_2$, a distinction can be made in terms of conditions that do affect the $P(A-a)O_2$. Increases in capillary shunting and ventilation–perfusion abnormalities are associated with an increased $P(A-a)O_2$.

To calculate the $P(A-a)O_2$, which normally is less than 15 torr for room air breathing, both the arterial and alveolar $PO_2$ values must be known. The arterial $PO_2$ is obtained via an arterial puncture, whereas the alveolar $PO_2$ requires knowing the arterial $PO_2$, the $F_IO_2$, and the respiratory quotient (R).

In this situation, because the patient was breathing oxygen from a low-flow system (simple mask), the $F_IO_2$ could not be obtained. A low-flow device does not provide a constant, precise oxygen concentration. Therefore, the alveolar air equation, which requires knowing the $F_IO_2$, cannot be used to calculate the alveolar $PO_2$ in this case.

(1:217, 234), (15:101, 946), (16:256, 369).

## IB4a

176. D. Rhonchi are caused by the rapid flow of air through airways that are partially obstructed, causing a continuous, low-pitched sound. The causes of the partial obstruction include (1) aspirated foreign objects, (2) bronchospasm, (3) mucous plugs, and (4) mucosal edema.

If rhonchi are produced by a mucous plug, an effective cough generated by the patient can sometimes eliminate the rhonchi. Wheezing (a continuous high-pitched sound) resulting from bronchospasm is often relieved by the administration of a bronchodilator.

(1:312), (9:82, 243), (15:443), (16:173).

## IC1c

177. C. When the left ventricle fails, it cannot keep pace with the output of the right ventricle. Blood then accumulates in the pulmonary vasculature, causing increased pulmonary vascular resistance (PVR) and pulmonary hypertension. An excellent diagnostic indicator of left-ventricular function is the PCWP. This measurement usually reflects the status of the left ventricle, because it measures the left ventricular end-diastolic pressure (LVEDP). The LVEDP reflects the left ventricular preload and helps determine the stroke volume.

In this case, a PCWP of 28 mm Hg is high (normal PCWP = 6 to 12 mm Hg), which reflects an inordinately high LVEDP. Hypervolemia also causes a high PCWP, however. Consequently, a diagnosis cannot be made solely on the PCWP value.

Other measurements requiring attention include the central venous pressure (CVP), mean arterial pressure (MAP), and cardiac index (C.I.) values. The CVP indicates right ventricle status and is often a guide to fluid management. The CVP can remain normal when the left ventricle infarcts. Therefore, it is not a reliable indicator of left ventricular function. In hypervolemic states, the CVP will be high; in hypovolemia, the CVP will be low. The MAP will be low in left ventricular failure and high in hypervolemia.

The C.I. (normal = 2.5 to 4.0 L/min./m$^2$) serves a useful purpose in determining the presence of left ventricular function. Because the C.I. is calculated by dividing the body surface area (BSA) into the C.O., it will be low in left ventricular failure. The low C.O. in left heart failure renders a low C.I. In hypervolemia, the C.I. will be high because of a higher C.O.

(1:943–950), (9:339–353), (10:122–127, 135–136), (15:535–537).

## IB7b

178. D. These findings are consistent with right lung atelectasis, which, under the circumstances, could be the result of obstruction of the right mainstem bronchus by an aspirated foreign object.

The lung tissue beyond the obstruction has collapsed because ventilation could not move beyond the obstruction. Ultimately, the trapped air was absorbed by the pulmonary capillary blood. The massive atelectasis can also cause a mediastinal shift to the affected side.

(1:772–773), (9:94), (15:604).

## IB10h

179. D. Airway cuffs should be inflated minimally to achieve an adequate seal of the airway for positive pressure mechanical ventilation. The effects of high lateral wall pressure in the trachea can be prevented by using the lowest possible pressure. Lymphatic flow will be inhibited at intracuff pressures greater than 5 mm Hg, venous flow at 18 mm Hg, and arterial flow at 30 mm Hg. If 40 mm Hg is measured in a patient's cuff, mucosal ischemia will ensue if the pressure inside the cuff is not reduced. An intracuff pressure of 40 mm Hg will obstruct (1) arterial blood flow, (2) venous blood flow, and (3) lymphatic drainage. Generally, the intracuff pressure range that is sought is 20 to 25 mm Hg. Intracuff pressure manometers are ordinarily calibrated in centimeters of water, however. Therefore, a range of 27 to 33 cm $H_2O$ is considered suitable for intracuff pressures.

(1:609–610), (16:575, 832–833).

## IA1f(4)

180. C. The static compliance, which is measured by dividing the plateau pressure minus the total PEEP (auto-PEEP plus therapeutic PEEP) into the corrected tidal volume will reflect changes in the pulmonary compliance. This measurement reflects the compliance of the lung-thorax system (i.e., total compliance). With this measurement, however, the usual assumption made is that the chest-wall compliance is constant and that any change in the calculated static compliance value is attributed to a change in the lung status.

The dynamic compliance measurement incorporates the pressure generated by the flowing gas to overcome airway resistance. Therefore, changes that occur relative to the dynamic compliance calculation prohibits one from determining the reason for any altered values.

(1:937), (9:285), (10:256–257).

## IA1b

181. A. A decrease in peripheral skin temperature and a "clammy" surface is an indication of perfusion deficit. Vital organ perfusion is favored over peripheral perfusion as hypoxia worsens.

(1:304, 924), (9:44, 61), (15:432).

## IB10c

182. C. An intrapulmonary shunt of 20% is indicative that a patient might not be successfully weaned from mechanical ventilation. A shunt of less than 15% is compatible with weaning a patient from mechanical ventilation.

(1:971), (10:327).

183. C. Pulse oximetry makes no distinction between oxygen bound to hemoglobin and certain forms of abnormal hemoglobin (e.g., carboxyhemoglobin [COHb] and methemoglobin [MetHb]). This distinction is prevented because pulse oximeters employ only two wavelengths of light (i.e., 805 nm [infrared] and 650 nm [red]). The 805-nm wavelength is the isobestic point, which means that at that wavelength, both oxy- and deoxyhemoglobin absorb infrared light equally. At the 650-nm wavelength, however, a wide difference exists between these two forms of hemoglobin in terms of red light absorbance. Therefore, the difference in red and infrared light absorption at 805 nm and 650 nm enables the calculation of the oxygen saturation ($SO_2$).

The method of $SO_2$ measurement just described provides what is termed the *functional* $SO_2$, as opposed to the *fractional* $SO_2$. A pulse oximeter does not differentiate between normal and abnormal hemoglobin. For example, if a patient has a COHb level of 30% and an $O_2$Hb saturation of 65%, a pulse oximeter will indicate an oxygen saturation of 95%. This situation can have hazardous consequences, especially if it is unsuspected that the patient is a CO-poisoning victim. The pulse oximeter in this case would render an erroneously high $SO_2$ value. Again, this measurement represents the functional $SO_2$ because no differentiation between normal and dysfunctional forms of hemoglobin has been made. In such a situation, a co-oximeter must be used so that the fractional $SO_2$ can be obtained. The fractional $SO_2$ represents the percentage of $O_2$Hb compared to all other forms of hemoglobin in circulation at that time. A co-oximeter can measure methemoglobin, carboxyhemoglobin, oxyhemoglobin, and deoxyhemoglobin.

The following relationships represent the operational differences between a pulse oximeter (functional saturation measurement) and a co-oximeter (fractional saturation measurement).

**Pulse Oximeter (Functional $SO_2$)**

$$SpO_2 = \frac{\text{saturated Hb}}{\text{saturated Hb + desaturated Hb}}$$

**Co-oximeter (Fractional $SO_2$)**

$$\text{co-oximeter } SO_2 = \frac{\text{saturated Hb}}{\underset{\text{Hb}}{\text{saturated}} + \underset{\text{Hb}}{\text{desaturated}} + \underset{\text{globins}}{\text{dyshemo-}}}$$

The dyshemoglobins measured by a co-oximeter are carboxyhemoglobin (COHb) and methemoglobin (MetHb).

(1:359), (9:295–296), (10:97).

**IA1c**

184. C. The presence of fever and tachycardia suggest the possibility of infection. This probability could be fur-ther defined by the evaluation of the white blood cell (WBC) component of the complete blood count (CBC). A total WBC count greater than 10,000/mm³ suggests infection.

(1:331–332), (9:102–104), (16:178).

**IA1d**

185. D. The peripheral chemoreceptors are essentially the oxygen ($PaO_2$) sensors in the blood. Hyperventilation occurs when arterial blood acutely high in carbon dioxide or acutely high in $H^+$ ions flows through the carotid and aortic bodies, however. This response to stimuli other than low oxygen dissolved in the plasma is evidenced by the hyperventilation that occurs in patients who have diabetic ketoacidosis. The acute increase in the arterial blood hydrogen ion concentration stimulates the carotid and aortic bodies despite the normal-to-high arterial $PO_2$ exhibited by these patients.

(1:287–288), (16:130, 1044).

**IA1i**

186. B. A normal $\dot{V}_A/\dot{Q}_C$ ratio ranges between 0.8 and 1.0. The two extremes of the $\dot{V}_A/\dot{Q}_C$ spectrum are capillary shunt ($\dot{V}_A/\dot{Q}_C = 0$) and alveolar dead space ($\dot{V}_A/\dot{Q}_C = \infty$). $\dot{V}_A/\dot{Q}_C$ ratios that are less than 0.8 but greater than 0 are described as perfusion in excess of ventilation, shunt effect, or venous admixture. $\dot{V}_A/\dot{Q}_C$ ratios that are greater than 1 but less than $\infty$ (infinity) constitute ventilation in excess of perfusion.

The first four steps will provide for the calculation of the alveolar minute ventilation ($\dot{V}_A$):

STEP 1: One pound of IBW approximately equals 1 cc of anatomic dead space.

150 lb of IBW $\simeq$ 150 cc if anatomic dead space

STEP 2: Calculate the dead space ventilation ($\dot{V}_D$).

$$V_D \times f = \dot{V}_D$$
150 cc $\times$ 12 breaths/min. = 1,800 cc/min.

STEP 3: Calculate the minute ventilation ($\dot{V}_E$).

$$V_T \times f = \dot{V}_D$$
500 cc/breath $\times$ 12 breaths/min. = 6,000 cc/min.

STEP 4: Calculate the alveolar ventilation ($\dot{V}_A$).

$$\dot{V}_E - \dot{V}_D = \dot{V}_A$$
6,000 cc/min. $-$ 1,800 cc/min. = 4,200 cc/min.

The C.O. can be determined by using the Fick equation.

$$\dot{Q}_T = \frac{\dot{V}O_2}{CaO_2 - C\bar{v}O_2}$$

where

$$\dot{Q}_T = \text{C.O. (ml/min.)}$$

$\dot{V}O_2$ = oxygen consumption (ml/min.)

$CaO_2$ = arterial oxygen content (vol%)

$C\bar{v}O_2$ = mixed venous oxygen content (vol%)

(Recall that the $CaO_2 - C\bar{v}O_2$ is the a–v oxygen content difference expressed in vol%.)

STEP 5:  Insert the known values into the Fick equation to calculate the C.O. $(\dot{Q}_T)$.

$$\dot{Q}_T = \frac{240 \text{ ml/min.}}{20 \text{ vol}\% - 14 \text{ vol}\%}$$

$$= \frac{240 \text{ cc/min.}}{\left(\dfrac{20 \text{ cc } O_2}{100 \text{ cc blood}}\right) - \left(\dfrac{14 \text{ cc } O_2}{100 \text{ cc blood}}\right)}$$

$$= \frac{240 \text{ cc/min.}}{\left(\dfrac{6 \text{ cc } O_2}{100 \text{ cc blood}}\right)}$$

$$= 4,000 \text{ cc/min., or } 4.0 \text{ L/min.}$$

STEP 6:  Calculate the $\dot{V}_A/\dot{Q}_C$ ratio.

$$\frac{\dot{V}_A}{\dot{Q}_C} = \frac{4,200 \text{ ml/min}}{4,000 \text{ ml/min}}$$

$$= 1.05$$

(1:233, 930), (9:123, 171), (10:100).

## IB7e

187. C. A number of clinical conditions (e.g., pneumothorax, pleural effusion, and atelectasis) can cause the mediastinum to shift. Mediastinal shifting is generally readily observable on a chest radiograph. It is characterized by either a rightward or a leftward deviation of the mediastinal contents (esophagus, heart, and great vessels) from midline.

In the presence of a large-volume pleural effusion or a tension pneumothorax, the patient's trachea is deviated away from the affected lung. Likewise, the mediastinal contents (esophagus, heart, and great vessels) are shifted toward the unaffected (contralateral) lung. On the contrary, massive, unilateral atelectasis will cause the mediastinum to shift to the affected side because the intrapleural pressure in that region of the lung becomes more subatmospheric. The greater negative pressure at that site pulls the mediastinum to that side. These findings are readily observable on a chest X-ray.

(1:306), (9:92–94), (15:601–602).

## IA1h

188. B. Apnea is often associated with bradycardia, not tachycardia. Apnea pauses of 15 seconds or less are normal occurrences. Apneic periods exceeding 20 seconds and those causing hypotonia, pallor, cyanosis, or bradycardia are deemed abnormal. Gentle, tactile stimulation (i.e., flicking the soles of the feet) often causes breathing to resume. Methylxanthines (caffeine and theophylline) are used to stimulate breathing via the central nervous system. Continuous positive airway pressure (CPAP) is used to treat apnea of prematurity. CPAP probably stimulates vagal receptors in the lungs, thereby reflexly increasing the output of respiratory centers in the brain stem.

(1:258, 968), (9:35, 60), (10:158, 284).

## IB10c

189. B. Adult respiratory distress syndrome (ARDS) is a common sequelae of near drowning. It is not uncommon for such a patient to be stabile for 24 to 48 hours then deteriorate suddenly. The abrupt deterioration is actually the early stage of ARDS. The patient experiences refractory hypoxemia, decreased lung compliance, tachypnea, and chest X-rays showing bilateral alveolar infiltrates (honeycomb effect).

Near-drowning victims must be watched very closely during this 24 to 48 hour latent period because the onset of ARDS is rapid. The usual primary concern when initially treating near-drowning victims is the correction of hypoxemia and acidemia. Obviously, oxygen should be administered. The mixed acidemia—respiratory and metabolic—is ordinarily treated with mechanical ventilation and sodium bicarbonate ($NaHCO_3$) administration.

(15:331–338), (16:993–994).

## IA2h

190. A. Exercise-induced asthma is typified by bronchospasm during or immediately following vigorous exercise. It is thought to be related to heat loss from the upper airway accompanying the increased minute ventilation during exercise, and it is more often seen in the colder winter months. The heat loss results from evaporation as high flow rates of air pass over the epithelial surface of the airways. Cromolyn sodium is sometimes useful in prophylactically preventing exercise-induced asthma.

(1:168, 457), (15:216, 515–516, 589, 795).

## IA1c

191. A. A complete blood count (CBC) is a routine test used to determine the absence or presence of infections. The symptoms of tachypnea, tachycardia, and fever are indicative of infection.

(1:331–333), (9:99–102).

## Situational Sets

### IB10a

192. C. The ECG tracing now appearing on the cardiac monitor represents sinus tachycardia. As the sino-atrial (SA) node discharges over 100 times per minute, the term *sinus tachycardia* applies. The approximate heart rate indicated in this situation is 140 beats/minute.

To determine the heart rate, count the number of R waves present within a 6-second interval and multiply that total by 10. Each of the time tics above the ECG tracing represents 3 seconds. Sinus tachycardia is shown in the tracing in Figure 3-45.

As the SA node discharge rate increases, the P wave of a cardiac cycle appears closer to the T wave of the previous beat. At rapid rates, the P wave becomes more difficult to distinguish. There are 14 R waves within the 6-second interval shown. Therefore, $14 \times 10 = 140$ beats/min.

The ECG tracings of the other cardiac dysrhythmias listed are illustrated in Figures 3-46, 3-47, and 3-48).

(1:326, 330–331), (9:203, 205–207).

### IC1b

193. C. Metaproterenol sulfate is a $\beta_2$ agonist. $\beta_2$ agonists produce bronchodilatation. The usual dosage for nebulized metaproterenol is 0.3 ml in 4 ml of normal saline. The amount of metaproterenol administered to this patient was 0.5 ml diluted in 4 ml of normal saline. Therefore, too much of the beta-adrenergic drug was given, and the patient experienced one of the potential side ef-

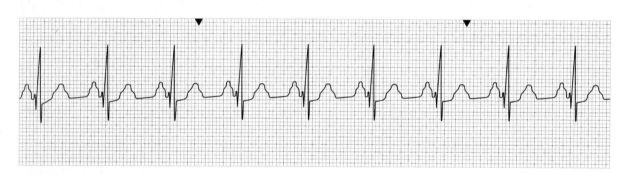

**Figure 3-45:** Lead II ECG tracing; sinus tachycardia.

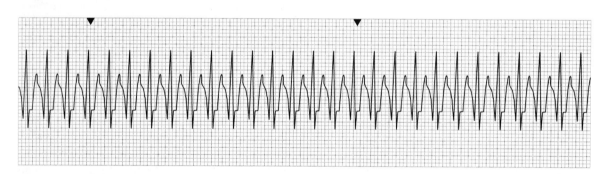

**Figure 3-46:** Lead II ECG tracing; ventricular fibrillation.

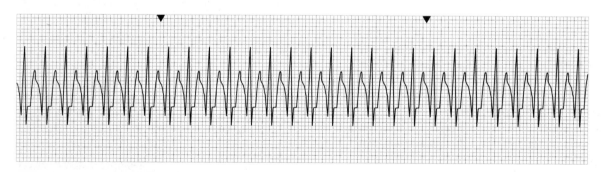

**Figure 3-47:** Lead II ECG tracing; ventricular tachycardia.

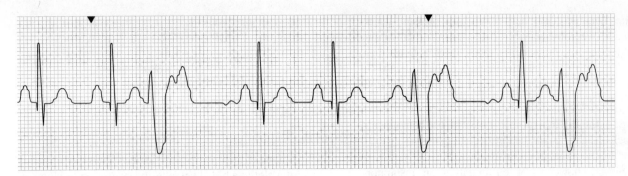

**Figure 3-48:** Lead II ECG tracing; premature ventricular contraction (PVC).

fects of the medication—tachycardia. His heart rate increased from about 60 beats/min. to 140 beats/min.

Under these circumstances, the treatment must be terminated, and the patient's heart rate must be allowed to normalize. After an appropriate amount of time elapses, the patient should be given the proper dosage of medication.

(1:455, 475), (16:482–484).

IC1g

194. D. The term *system compliance* refers to the compliance (volume/pressure) of the ventilator-tubing system. The patient's pulmonary, chest-wall, and total compliance measurements are not included in this value. Knowing the system compliance enables the RRT to determine the actual tidal volume the patient is receiving. System compliance is obtained as follows:

STEP 1: Set a tidal volume (e.g., 200 cc).

STEP 2: Set the pressure limit to its maximum limit.

STEP 3: Cycle the ventilator to inspiration, occlude the patient wye, and note the peak inspiratory pressure (PIP). In this example, the PIP is 65 cm $H_2O$.

STEP 4: Divide the $V_T$ (200 cc) by the PIP (65 cm $H_2O$) to calculate the system compliance factor.

$$\frac{200 \text{ cc}}{65 \text{ cm } H_2O} = 3.08 \text{ cc/cm } H_2O$$

This value means that for each cm $H_2O$ indicated on the pressure manometer during the patient's inspiration, 3.08 ml of gas are compressed ("lost") in the ventilator-tubing system.

(15:643–644).

IB9b

195. B. By multiplying the difference between the PIP and PEEP by the system compliance factor, the RRT can compute the amount of the preset tidal volume lost in the ventilator-tubing system. The patient's actual tidal volume can then be obtained by subtracting the compressed volume from the preset tidal volume. The following three steps describe this procedure:

STEP 1: Subtract the amount of PEEP from the PIP to determine the pressure generated to deliver the preset $V_T$.

$$PIP - PEEP = \frac{\text{pressure generated to}}{\text{deliver the preset } V_T}$$

$$45 \text{ cm } H_2O - 10 \text{ cm } H_2O = 35 \text{ cm } H_2O$$

STEP 2: Multiply the pressure generated to deliver the preset $V_T$ by the system compliance factor to compute the volume compressed in the ventilator-tubing system.

$$PIP \times \text{tubing compliance factor} = \text{compressed volume}$$
$$(35 \text{ cmH}_2\text{O})(3.08 \text{ cc/cmH}_2\text{O}) = 107.8 \text{ cc}$$

STEP 3: Subtract the compressed volume from the $V_T$ set on the ventilator to calculate the patient's actual tidal volume.

$$\text{set } V_T - \text{compressed volume} = \text{actual } V_T$$
$$900 \text{ cc} - 108 \text{ cc} = 792 \text{ cc}$$

(10:209), (15:643–644).

IC1g

196. A. The PIP registered on the pressure manometer has two components: a static component and a dynamic component. The static component refers to the pressure caused by the compliance of the patient–ventilatory system. It represents the pressure generated to effect the volume change in that system.

The dynamic component reflects the pressure generated to overcome airway resistance as the tidal volume is flowing into the patient's lungs. It refers to the pressure resulting from the interaction of the molecules of the flowing gas and the molecules and the walls (tubing and airways) of the patient–ventilator system.

Again, the PIP incorporates both of these components. Each one can be obtained by occluding the tubing leading to the exhalation valve when the PIP has been achieved, however, or by initiating an inspiratory pause. In either case, the pressure manometer needle will fall to a reading termed the *plateau pressure,* or *static pressure.* It is from this point that the static and dynamic components of the PIP can be isolated. Note the diagram of a pressure manometer shown as follows (Figure 3-49).

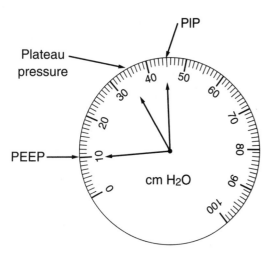

**Figure 3-49** Pressure manometer indicating PIP, plateau pressure, and PEEP.

The static pressure is the pressure that is required to effect the volume change in the patient's lungs during inspiration. It is the pressure being exerted by the 792 ml of gas residing in the lungs at end inspiration.

The pressure that was generated to overcome the resistance of the patient–ventilator system while the volume was being delivered to the lungs is represented by the difference between the plateau pressure and the PIP. The static compliance can be calculated as follows:

STEP 1: Subtract the PEEP from the plateau pressure to obtain the pressure inflating the lungs (distending pressure).

plateau pressure − PEEP = ΔP
$$35 \text{ cm } H_2O - 10 \text{ cm } H_2O = 25 \text{ cm } H_2O$$

STEP 2: Calculate the static compliance by dividing the patient's actual tidal volume by the ΔP, or plateau pressure minus PEEP.

$$\frac{\text{actual } V_T}{\Delta P} = \text{static compliance}$$

$$\frac{792 \text{ cc}}{25 \text{ cm } H_2O} = 31.68 \text{ cc/cm } H_2O$$

(1:937), (10:257), (15:643–644).

**IA1b**

197. B. One of the three factors that facilitates the formation of a clot in a blood vessel is the stagnation of blood, or venous stasis. This elderly woman was confined to an airplane seat for six hours. This amount of immobility can place an elderly person, such as this woman, at risk for developing a thromboembolism. The clinical manifestations of pulmonary thromboembolism are nonspecific. Generally, dyspnea and the angina-like chest pain are the most common symptoms. The sudden onset of this clinical disorder is also noteworthy.

The other clues to suspecting this diagnosis are the presence of pain, tenderness, and swelling of the extremities. Approximately 50% of patients who have deep venous thrombosis have the physical signs of thrombophlebitis, which include swelling, warmth, tenderness, and redness of the calf. Decreased breath sounds, reduced chest movement, and friction rubs on the affected side are important signs. Chest roentgenograms commonly reveal a pleural effusion. Hemoptysis, although uncommon, is important to the diagnosis when present.

It should be mentioned here that pulmonary thromboembolism (PTE) can only be definitively diagnosed via a positive pulmonary angiogram. It can be suspected by a positive ventilation–perfusion scan. Clinical signs and symptoms alone are not definitively diagnostic.

(1:497, 500–501), (10:135, 309), (15:240–241).

**IA1b**

198. D. Pulmonary infarction is a rare occurrence following thromboembolic events. Approximately 10% of the patients who experience a pulmonary embolism have a pulmonary infarction. The presence of a pulmonary infarction on a chest roentgenogram characteristically reveals an opacity that takes on a triangular, conical, or wedge shape. The apex of the triangle is directed toward the hilum, and the base lies along the pleural lining. A pleural effusion is a common radiographic finding associated with a pulmonary embolism.

(1:497, 500–501), (10:135, 309), (15:240–241).

**IA1b**

199. B. The vast majority of pulmonary emboli originate from the deep veins of the lower extremities. Three factors are involved in the formation of a thrombus: (1)

vessel-wall damage or abnormality, (2) stasis or stagnation of blood, and (3) a state of hypercoagulability.

The positive Homan's sign, along with the tender, warm, swollen calf and ankle, all indicate that the pathogenesis of the pulmonary embolism was the dislodgement of a deep leg vein thrombus or thromboembolism.

(1:493–497, 500–501), (10:135, 309), (15:240–241).

## IB1c

200. D. The Apgar score is used to evaluate the clinical status of neonates at 1 and 5 minutes after birth. The highest possible score is 10, and the lowest is 0. The score obtained helps determine the need for resuscitative measures. The Apgar rating scale is shown in Table 3-19 below. Based on the clinical information presented in the question, the Apgar score is determined as follows:

- heart rate of 110 beats/min.: 2 points
- a good ventilatory effort accompanied by crying: 2 points
- color reflected peripheral cyanosis; central color assumed to be good because not mentioned: 1 point
- muscle tone indicated by some flexion of the extremities: 1 point
- reflex irritability represented by the sneeze caused by passage of suction catheter into nose: 2 points

Apgar score: 8

(1:1002), (9:215), (18:43–44).

## IIID1d

201. C. There appears to be no need to perform any resuscitative measures at this time because an Apgar score in the range of 7 to 10 generally indicates that the infant has a stable cardiopulmonary status. However, the Apgar score at 5 minutes after birth might indicate otherwise. The infant can deteriorate between Apgar evaluations.

To summarize, Apgar scores ranging from 7 to 10 indicate no immediate need to resuscitate; 4 to 6 suggest that the infant needs to be suctioned, oxygenated, and possibly ventilated; and 0 to 3 indicate the need for CPR.

(1:1002), (9:215), (18:43–44).

## IA9b

202. C. The minute ventilation can be determined in the following manner:

$$\dot{V}_E = V_T \times f$$

where

$\dot{V}_E$ = minute ventilation (L/min.)
$V_T$ = tidal volume (L)
$f$ = ventilatory rate (breaths/min.)

STEP 1: Convert the tidal volume (900 cc) to L.

$$V_T = \frac{900 \text{ cc}}{1,000 \text{ cc/L}}$$

$$= 0.9 \text{ L}$$

STEP 2: Solve for $\dot{V}_E$.

$$\dot{V}_E = 0.9 \text{ L/breath} \times 12 \text{ breaths/min.}$$
$$= 10.8 \text{ L/min.}$$

(1:211), (9:145), (15:136).

## IA9b

203. A.

STEP 1: Convert the peak inspiratory flow rate (60 L/min.) to L/sec.

$$\dot{V} = \frac{60 \text{ L/min.}}{60 \text{ sec./min.}}$$

$$= 1 \text{ L/sec.}$$

STEP 2: Convert the peak inspiratory flow rate to cc/sec.

$$\dot{V} = (1 \text{ L/sec.})(1,000 \text{ cc/L})$$
$$= 1,000 \text{ cc/sec.}$$

STEP 3: Calculate the inspiratory time ($T_I$).

$$T_I = \frac{V_T}{\dot{V}} = \frac{900 \text{ cc}}{1,000 \text{ cc/sec.}}$$

$$= 0.9 \text{ sec.}$$

(1:860), (10:205–206), (15:977).

**Table 3-19** Ratings and Signs for Apgar Score

| SIGN | 0 | 1 | 2 |
|---|---|---|---|
| Heart rate | Absent | Less than 100 beats/min. | Greater than 100 beats/min. |
| Ventilatory effort | Absent | Slow, irregular | Good, crying |
| Muscle tone | Limp | Some flexion | Active motion |
| Reflex irritability | No response | Grimace | Cough or sneeze |
| Color | Central and peripheral cyanosis | Peripheral cyanosis | Completely pink |

**IA9b**

204.  A. STEP 1: Obtain the total cycle time (TCT).

A ventilatory rate of 12 breaths/min. is equivalent to 12 breaths/60 sec. Therefore, TCT equals:

$$TCT = \frac{60 \text{ sec./min.}}{12 \text{ breaths/min.}}$$

$$= 5 \text{ sec./breath}$$

STEP 2:  Subtract the $T_I$ from the TCT to determine the $T_E$.

$$T_E = 5.0 \text{ sec.} - 0.9 \text{ sec.}$$
$$= 4.1 \text{ sec.}$$

STEP 3:  Determine the I:E ratio.

$$I{:}E = \frac{T_I}{T_I} : \frac{T_E}{T_I}$$

$$= \frac{0.9 \text{ sec.}}{0.9 \text{ sec.}} : \frac{4.1 \text{ sec.}}{0.9 \text{ sec.}}$$

$$= 1{:}4.6$$

(1:860), (10:205–206).

**IC1a**

205.  C. The MVV is performed by having the patient breathe as rapidly and as deeply as she can for either 10, 12, or 15 seconds. The actual MVV is obtained by extrapolating the volume exhaled within the time interval (10, 12, or 15 seconds) used and is expressed in liters per minute. For example, if a subject exhaled 38 liters of air in 12 seconds, the MVV would be calculated as follows:

STEP 1:  Determine how many 12-sec. intervals are in one minute. Because one minute equals 60 sec.,

$$\frac{60 \text{ sec/min}}{12 \text{ sec.}} = 5 \text{ intervals/min.}$$

STEP 2:  Extrapolate the MVV value.

$$38 \text{ L} \times 5 \text{ intervals/min.} = 190 \text{ L/min.}$$

(1:386–387), (6:47–49), (15:463–464).

**IC2a**

206.  D. The normal range for MVV values in healthy, young males is between 150 to 200 liters/min. The following conditions are associated with a decreased MVV:

- ventilatory muscle weakness or fatigue
- increased airway resistance
- moderate to severe obstructive pulmonary disease
- decreased pulmonary and/or thoracic compliance

A high degree of variability exists for the MVV among the normal healthy population. The degree of variability is said to be as large as 25% to 30%. Therefore, to be clinically significant, the MVV value obtained must be considerably reduced. The MVV value determined for the subject described here is acceptable and considered normal.

(1:386–387), (6:47–49), (15:463–464).

**IA2b**

207.  C. Because the last ABG was performed 3 hours ago, and because the patient's clinical condition has apparently deteriorated, obtaining another ABG would be useful. With the high-pressure alarm sounding with each inspiration, the patient might not be receiving an adequate tidal volume. Therefore, it would be necessary to increase the high-pressure limit to enable the patient to receive the full tidal volume.

Last, ordering a STAT chest X-ray is imperative to help diagnose this problem. Changing the mode of ventilation from synchronized intermittent mandatory ventilation (SIMV) to control is unwarranted because of the lack of information indicating that alteration.

(1:854, 903–904), (10:311–312), (15:331–338).

**IA1b**

208.  C. Adult respiratory distress syndrome (ARDS) is a condition characterized by a constellation of signs and symptoms brought about by a variety of etiologic factors. Frequently occurring etiologic factors include (1) sepsis, (2) aspiration, (3) drug overdose, (4) near drowning, (5) multiple transfusions, (6) pulmonary contusions, and (7) multiple fractures. The patient in this problem was at great risk for developing ARDS because she experienced massive blood loss and had multiple long bone trauma.

ARDS frequently follows a 12- to 24-hour latent period (sometimes as long as 72 hours) wherein the patient might appear relatively normal and seemingly make a recovery from the condition that caused the hospitalization in the first place. Suddenly, and usually within the 12- to 24-hour period, the patient rapidly deteriorates, developing refractory hypoxemia and decreased lung compliance.

These pathophysiologic events manifest themselves in terms of higher $F_IO_2$ requirements in the face of plummeting arterial $PO_2$ values, increased spontaneous minute ventilation, high PIPs for those who are receiving mechanical ventilation, and chest X-rays showing generalized lung infiltrates sometimes to the extent of complete "whiteout."

In association with this patient's etiologic factors, she developed refractory hypoxemia—demanding a greater $F_IO_2$ and a higher PEEP value. Her spontaneous minute ventilation increased along with her PIP. Her chest roentgenogram exhibited pulmonary infiltrates and areas of "whiteout."

(1:508, 512, 904), (10:239, 259, 279), (15:331–338).

## IA1c

209. C. The amount of reduced (unoxygenated) hemoglobin in total circulation can be determined as follows:

STEP 1: Calculate the percentage of desaturated arterial hemoglobin.

$$
\begin{array}{r}
100\% \\
-51\%\ SaO_2 \\
\hline
49\%\ \text{desaturated arterial hemoglobin}
\end{array}
$$

STEP 2: Calculate the percentage of desaturated venous hemoglobin.

$$
\begin{array}{r}
100\% \\
-45\%\ S\bar{v}O_2 \\
\hline
55\%\ \text{desaturated venous hemoglobin}
\end{array}
$$

STEP 3: Determine the amount of reduced hemoglobin in arterial blood.

$$
\begin{aligned}
\%\ \text{reduced arterial Hb} &= [Hb] \times \%\ \text{arterial desaturation} \\
&= 20\ g\% \times 0.49 \\
&= 9.8\ g\%
\end{aligned}
$$

STEP 4: Determine the amount of reduced hemoglobin in venous blood.

$$
\begin{aligned}
\%\ \text{reduced venous Hb} &= [Hb] \times \%\ \text{venous desaturation} \\
&= 20\ g\% \times 0.55 \\
&= 11.0\ g\%
\end{aligned}
$$

STEP 5: Calculate the average of reduced Hb in total circulation (average of that in arterial and venous blood).

$$
\frac{9.8\ g\% + 11.0\ g\%}{2} = \text{average of reduced Hb in total circulation}
$$

$$
\frac{20.8\ g\%}{2} = 10.4\ g\%
$$

(1:318), (9:69, 77, 90, 269), (15:437, 668).

## IB1a

210. B. Cyanosis will appear if a person has an average of 5.0 g% (5.0 g/dl) or more of desaturated hemoglobin in total circulation (arterial and venous). The degree of desaturation was calculated in the previous problem. Because the average amount of desaturated (reduced) hemoglobin in this example is greater than 5.0 g%, this person will display cyanosis.

(1:318), (9:69, 77, 90, 269), (15:437, 668).

## IA9c

211. D. The Enghoff modification of the Bohr equation is used to calculate the dead space–tidal volume ($V_D/V_T$) ratio. The equation is shown as follows:

$$
\frac{V_D}{V_T} = \frac{PaCO_2 - P\bar{E}CO_2}{PaCO_2}
$$

$$
= \frac{30\ torr - 10\ torr}{30\ torr}
$$

$$
= \frac{20\ torr}{30\ torr}
$$

$$
= 0.67
$$

(1:212), (9:290–292), (15:489), (17:25–29).

## IA1c

212. C. Pulmonary embolism is a dead space-producing disease. Thrombophlebitis is frequently the cause of pulmonary embolism. Deep leg vein blood clots can dislodge, become an embolus (or emboli), and depending on the size lodge in a pulmonary vessel. This situation can significantly disrupt the flow of blood distal to the embolus.

If the embolus lodges in a relatively large pulmonary artery, it prevents blood from reaching the distal alveoli. Consequently, those alveoli will be characterized by a ventilation–perfusion relationship, wherein the affected alveoli will receive ventilation but no perfusion. Such a $\dot{V}_A/\dot{Q}_C$ match is described as alveolar dead space.

The Bohr equation used in the previous problem indicated that the $V_D/V_T$ ratio was extremely high for a spontaneously breathing patient. Normally, the $V_D/V_T$ ratio is about 0.30. Positive pressure ventilation causes the $V_D/V_T$ ratio to increase because of the greater distribution of air to less perfused (nongravity-dependent) lung regions. A $V_D/V_T$ ratio between 0.40 and 0.60 is considered acceptable for patients who are receiving positive pressure ventilation.

Furthermore, the signs and symptoms presented here support the diagnosis of pulmonary embolism. If this patient was experiencing a myocardial infarction, her ABG and acid-base status would show greater deterioration. Because the signs and symptoms of a pulmonary embolism resemble those of myocardial infarction, however, pulmonary embolism is sometimes misdiagnosed as a myocardial infarction.

Pneumonia and ARDS are shunt-producing diseases. They would be associated with an obvious hypoxemic condition. A pulmonary infarction sometimes is associated with a pulmonary embolism. In fact, only approximately 10% of pulmonary embolism patients have an associated pulmonary infarction.

(1:428, 497, 500–501, 508, 904), (10:135, 309), (15:240–241, 489).

## IB6b

213. A. Because the RRT is attempting to ascertain the patient's ability to perform activities of daily living, asking the question, "How does your breathlessness affect you?" would be useful. Inquiring about how many packs of cigarettes the patient smokes per day or when the patient's cough began or determining the quantity of sputum coughed up each day does not provide information about the patient's ability to perform activities of daily living.

The question, "How does your breathlessness affect you?" likely will result in the patient identifying activities that cannot be performed or those that are performed to a limited degree.

(9:27–36), (15:430).

## IC4

214. C. A number of combinations of bronchial hygiene therapies can be given to this patient. Percussion and vibration would not be appropriate, however, because the patient's grandmother is likely too elderly to maintain a rigorous therapeutic schedule and the demands of the therapy. The patient needs to be prescribed modalities that can be performed independently of someone else. Her respiratory care plan for the four weeks she will be staying at her grandmother's house needs to be modified to incorporate modalities that do not involve the girl's grandmother.

Therefore, flutter therapy, PEP therapy, and autogenic drainage are viable alternatives in this situation. The patient can be prescribed PEP therapy and flutter therapy or PEP therapy and autogenic drainage.

(1:812).

## IB6b

215. C. A symptom is a subjective complaint expressed by the patient. A sign is an objective measurement or observation made by the practitioner. Dyspnea and pain are symptoms; hyperventilation and bradycardia are signs.

Any time a patient complains about a symptom such as dyspnea, the RRT should be concerned with ques-

tions that ask (1) what, (2) where, (3) when, and (4) how regarding the symptom, for example, (1) "How does it feel?" (2) "Where is it?" (3) "When does it occur?" and (4) "What makes it better?"

(9:18), (15:429–430).

## IB5

216. C. The best way to assess a patient's ability to perform a procedure or to use a piece of equipment is to have the patient demonstrate the psychomotor activity. The only method to evaluate how well a patient can perform any task is to observe the patient's performance. The patient can either perform the skill or not. If the patient performs the overall activity, including its subtasks, then no patient education is likely necessary. On the other hand, if the patient fails to perform component steps in the overall procedure or appears uncoordinated, further instruction and practice are warranted.

(1:777).

## IC3

217. B. This patient was oxygenating well because the $SpO_2$ was 98% while the patient breathed room air. A bronchodilator does not appear to be warranted. Auscultation does not reveal wheezing, nor is the patient in respiratory distress. This patient has a regular respiratory pattern and a respiratory rate of 12 breaths/min.

Because auscultation has identified crackles in the lower lobe of each lung, incentive spirometry might be useful to treat the possible atelectasis. A chest radiograph would be beneficial to help evaluate the status of the basal segments of the lungs.

(1:9–10).

## IB6b

218. C. Dyspnea, or shortness of breath, is generally associated with lung or heart disease. Nonpulmonary and noncardiac causes also exist, including (1) hematologic, (2) metabolic, (3) chemical, (4) neurologic, (5) psychogenic, and (6) mechanical.

Because of these numerous causes of dyspnea, and because dyspnea can occur any time of day and under many conditions, questions used to ascertain information about dyspnea or shortness of breath must be carefully worded.

Some questions to obtain useful information about this symptom include:

- Have you ever lived in or traveled near the San Joaquin Valley in California?

—Ascertains whether the patient has been exposed to *Coccidiodes immitis*, the fungus that causes coccidioidomycosis

- Have you ever lived in or traveled to the midwestern or southeastern United States?
  —Determines whether the patient has had exposure to fungus *H. capsulatum,* known to cause histoplasmosis

- What type of work do you do?
  —Establishes a link between this patient's dyspnea and any occupational lung disease (pneumoconiosis), such as asbestosis, silicosis, and coal worker's pneumoconiosis
  —Demonstrates a relationship between this symptom and any type of hypersensitivity pneumonitis such as farmer's lung, bagassosis, and pigeon breeder's disease

- How many stairs can you climb before you become short of breath?
  —Finds out whether the dyspnea is related to activity suggesting inefficient mechanics of breathing, inadequate ventilation, or blood flow

(1:297–298), (9:30–36).

## IB8

219. B. Laryngotracheobronchitis (croup) is a viral condition characterized by subglottic swelling, two to three days of nasal congestion, fever, and a barking cough. When this condition is fully manisfested, inspiratory and expiratory stridor are present.

Epiglotittis is a supraglottic inflammatory condition causing sore throat stridor and labored breathing. It is caused by the bacterium *Hemophilus influenzae*, type B.

Croup and epiglotittis are often difficult to differentiate based on the patient's clinical presentations. A lateral neck radiograph frequently provides the differential diagnosis, however. The narrowing occurring with laryngotracheobronchitis is located below the glottis (subglottic edema) and often reveals the steeple sign in that area of the neck.

Epiglotittis, on the other hand, demonstrates airway narrowing above the glottis (supraglottic edema) and generally displays the thumb sign. The swollen epiglottis appears as a thumb on the lateral neck radiograph.

Tracheomalacia is the softening of the trachea's cartilaginous rings, causing some degree of upper airway obstruction.

(1:1038–1040), (9:232), (16:597–598), (16:395–396).

## IB8b

220. C. This child has likely aspirated a small object that is obstructing his upper airway. Epiglotittis generally produces a swollen, inflamed epiglottis that resembles a thumb on a lateral neck X-ray. This radiographic appearance is called the thumb sign.

Laryngotracheobronchitis often demonstrates a steeple sign, a steeple-shaped shadow located below the glottis.

The absence of either of these radiographic features and the afebrile state of the patient helps lead to the diagnosis of foreign body obstruction. The abruptness of the respiratory distress further points to this diagnosis.

(20:201–202).

## IC3a

221. C. Monitoring the quality of respiratory care protocol programs and the abilities of the therapists to perform evaluations and develop respiratory care plans is imperative for effective patient care. One method is an audit system where a therapist (or therapists) is skilled in providing respiratory care and in assessing patients. In the audit system, the auditor visits a selected patient who has been evaluated. If the auditor develops a respiratory care plan different from the original evaluator, then feedback must be provided to the original evaluator.

Alternately, case-study exercises with sets of patient scenarios can be provided to the evaluator. The evaluator will complete assessment sheets and develop care plans based on the assessment. These results can be compared to the "correct" assessments and care plans developed for these exercises.

(1:12–13).

## IC3c

222. B. The clinical signs displayed by this patient are consistent with hypoxemia. The pulse oximeter seems to indicate adequate oxygenation (SpO$_2$ 93%). The best clinical judgement to follow is to respond to the interpretation of these clinical signs. Pulse oximeters have limited accuracy, and considering that this patient was recently weaned from oxygen, restoration of his previous oxygen therapy might likely resolve this situation. The patient will require continued monitoring to make sure he improves clinically, however. He might not require 4 liters of oxygen per minute. The oxygen flow rate can be decreased once his status has improved. The physician must be notified of the situation.

(1:740).

223. B. What this patient is describing are classic features of paroxysmal nocturnal dyspnea. Paroxysmal nocturnal dyspnea is a sudden onset of dyspnea while sleeping in the recumbent position. The patient achieves relief when assuming an upright position. Patients with this symptom often find relief when they prop one or more pillows behind their back. The pillows prevent the patient from becoming completely supine.

Paroxysmal nocturnal dyspnea occurs in patients who have congestive heart failure (right or left ventricular failure). Patients who have primary cardiac disease causing left heart failure and patients with COPD and cor pulmonale can experience this symptom.

Orthopnea, dyspnea resulting from assuming a recumbent position, tends to occur when the faltering left ventricle fails to accommodate the increased venous blood flow associated with that body position. Pulmonary vascular congestion develops, leading to dyspnea.

(1:297), (9:34–35).

224. B. Percussion sounds are evaluated for their intensity and pitch. Whenever percussion is performed over airless lung regions, the normal resonance is lost. The percussion note described in this situation is dull or flat. Conditions associated with a dull or flat percussion note include pneumonia, atelectasis, and pleural effusion.

When percussion is performed over lung regions that are characterized by overinflation or air trapping, the note heard is hyperresonant. This note is heard in pulmonary emphysema and pneumothorax, for example.

(1:310), (9:79–80).

# References

1. Scanlan, C., Spearman, C., and Sheldon, R., *Egan's Fundamentals of Respiratory Care*, 7th ed., Mosby-Year Book, Inc., St. Louis, MO, 1999.

2. Kacmarek, R., Mack, C., and Dimas, S., *The Essentials of Respiratory Care*, 3rd ed., Mosby-Year Book, Inc., St. Louis, MO, 1990.

3. Shapiro B., Peruzzi, W., and Kozlowska-Templin, R., *Clinical Applications of Blood Gases*, 5th ed., Mosby-Year Book, Inc., St. Louis, MO, 1994.

4. Malley, W., *Clinical Blood Gases: Application and Noninvasive Alternatives*, W.B. Saunders Co., Philadelphia, PA, 1990.

5. White, G., *Equipment Theory for Respiratory Care*, 3rd ed., Delmar, Albany, NY, 1999.

6. Ruppel, G., *Manual of Pulmonary Function Testing*, 7th ed., Mosby-Year Book, Inc., St. Louis, MO, 1998.

7. Barnes, T., *Core Textbook of Respiratory Care Practice*, 2nd ed., Mosby-Year Book, Inc., St. Louis, MO, 1994.

8. Rau, J., *Respiratory Care Pharmacology*, 5th ed., Mosby-Year Book, Inc., St. Louis, MO, 1998.

9. Wilkins, R., Sheldon, R., and Krider, S., *Clinical Assessment in Respiratory Care*, 4th ed., Mosby-Year Book, Inc., St. Louis, MO, 2000.

10. Pilbeam, S., *Mechanical Ventilation: Physiological and Clinical Applications*, 3rd ed., Mosby-Year Book, Inc., St. Louis, MO, 1998.

11. Madama, V., *Pulmonary Function Testing and Cardiopulmonary Stress Testing*, 2nd ed., Delmar, Albany, NY, 1998.

12. Koff, P., Eitzman, D., and New, J., *Neonatal and Pediatric Respiratory Care*, 2nd ed., Mosby-Year Book, Inc., St. Louis, MO, 1993.

13. Branson, R., Hess, D., and Chatburn, R., *Respiratory Care Equipment*, J.B. Lippincott, Co., Philadelphia, PA, 1995.

14. Darovic, G., *Hemodynamic Monitoring: Invasive and Noninvasive Clinical Application*, 2nd ed., W.B. Saunders Company, Philadelphia, PA, 1995.

15. Pierson, D, and Kacmarek, R., *Foundations of Respiratory Care*, Churchill Livingston, Inc., New York, NY, 1992.

16. Burton, et al., *Respiratory Care: A Guide to Clinical Practice*, 4th ed., Lippincott-Raven Publishers, Philadelphia, PA, 1997.

17. Wojciechowski, W., *Respiratory Care Sciences: An Integrated Approach*, 3rd ed., Delmar, Albany, NY, 2000.

18. Aloan, C., *Respiratory Care of the Newborn and Child*, 2nd ed., Lippincott-Raven Publishers, Philadelphia, PA, 1997.

19. Dantzker, D., MacIntyre, N., and Bakow, E., *Comprehensive Respiratory Care*, W.B. Saunders Company, Philadelphia, PA, 1998.

20. Farzan, S., and Farzan, D., *A Concise Handbook of Respiratory Diseases*, 4th ed., Appleton & Lange, Stamford, CT, 1997.

# CHAPTER 4 ———————————————— EQUIPMENT

**PURPOSE:** This chapter consists of 130 items intended to assess your understanding and comprehension of subject matter contained in the equipment portion of the Written Registry Examination for Advanced Respiratory Therapy Practitioners. In this chapter, you are required to answer questions regarding the following activities:

A. Selecting and obtaining equipment and assuring equipment cleanliness
B. Assembling and checking equipment function, identifying and correcting equipment malfunctions, and performing quality control

> **NOTE:** Please refer to the examination matrix key located at the end of this chapter. This examination matrix key will enable you to identify the specific areas on the Written Registry Examination Matrix that require remediation, based on your performance on the test items in this chapter. Use the answer sheet located at the front of this chapter to record your answers as you work through questions relating to equipment. Remember to study the analyses that follow the questions in this chapter. The purpose of each analysis is to present you with the rationale for the correct answer, and in many instances, reasons are given for why the distractors are incorrect. The references at the end of each analysis provide you with resources to seek more information regarding each question and its associated Written Registry Examination Matrix item. Proceed at your own pace. You are not expected to complete this chapter in one sitting. Perhaps consider working on this chapter in three sessions to avoid fatigue. For example, you might elect to use the following approach:

SESSION 1: 1 to 50 questions, analyses, and matrix items
SESSION 2: 51 to 90 questions, analyses, and matrix items
SESSION 3: 91 to 130 questions, analyses, and matrix items

# Equipment Answer Sheet

**DIRECTIONS:** Darken the space under the selected answer.

| | A | B | C | D |   | | A | B | C | D |
|---|---|---|---|---|---|---|---|---|---|---|
| 1. | ❏ | ❏ | ❏ | ❏ | | 25. | ❏ | ❏ | ❏ | ❏ |
| 2. | ❏ | ❏ | ❏ | ❏ | | 26. | ❏ | ❏ | ❏ | ❏ |
| 3. | ❏ | ❏ | ❏ | ❏ | | 27. | ❏ | ❏ | ❏ | ❏ |
| 4. | ❏ | ❏ | ❏ | ❏ | | 28. | ❏ | ❏ | ❏ | ❏ |
| 5. | ❏ | ❏ | ❏ | ❏ | | 29. | ❏ | ❏ | ❏ | ❏ |
| 6. | ❏ | ❏ | ❏ | ❏ | | 30. | ❏ | ❏ | ❏ | ❏ |
| 7. | ❏ | ❏ | ❏ | ❏ | | 31. | ❏ | ❏ | ❏ | ❏ |
| 8. | ❏ | ❏ | ❏ | ❏ | | 32. | ❏ | ❏ | ❏ | ❏ |
| 9. | ❏ | ❏ | ❏ | ❏ | | 33. | ❏ | ❏ | ❏ | ❏ |
| 10. | ❏ | ❏ | ❏ | ❏ | | 34. | ❏ | ❏ | ❏ | ❏ |
| 11. | ❏ | ❏ | ❏ | ❏ | | 35. | ❏ | ❏ | ❏ | ❏ |
| 12. | ❏ | ❏ | ❏ | ❏ | | 36. | ❏ | ❏ | ❏ | ❏ |
| 13. | ❏ | ❏ | ❏ | ❏ | | 37. | ❏ | ❏ | ❏ | ❏ |
| 14. | ❏ | ❏ | ❏ | ❏ | | 38. | ❏ | ❏ | ❏ | ❏ |
| 15. | ❏ | ❏ | ❏ | ❏ | | 39. | ❏ | ❏ | ❏ | ❏ |
| 16. | ❏ | ❏ | ❏ | ❏ | | 40. | ❏ | ❏ | ❏ | ❏ |
| 17. | ❏ | ❏ | ❏ | ❏ | | 41. | ❏ | ❏ | ❏ | ❏ |
| 18. | ❏ | ❏ | ❏ | ❏ | | 42. | ❏ | ❏ | ❏ | ❏ |
| 19. | ❏ | ❏ | ❏ | ❏ | | 43. | ❏ | ❏ | ❏ | ❏ |
| 20. | ❏ | ❏ | ❏ | ❏ | | 44. | ❏ | ❏ | ❏ | ❏ |
| 21. | ❏ | ❏ | ❏ | ❏ | | 45. | ❏ | ❏ | ❏ | ❏ |
| 22. | ❏ | ❏ | ❏ | ❏ | | 46. | ❏ | ❏ | ❏ | ❏ |
| 23. | ❏ | ❏ | ❏ | ❏ | | 47. | ❏ | ❏ | ❏ | ❏ |
| 24. | ❏ | ❏ | ❏ | ❏ | | 48. | ❏ | ❏ | ❏ | ❏ |

|      | A | B | C | D |      | A | B | C | D |
|------|---|---|---|---|------|---|---|---|---|
| 49.  | ❏ | ❏ | ❏ | ❏ | 77.  | ❏ | ❏ | ❏ | ❏ |
| 50.  | ❏ | ❏ | ❏ | ❏ | 78.  | ❏ | ❏ | ❏ | ❏ |
| 51.  | ❏ | ❏ | ❏ | ❏ | 79.  | ❏ | ❏ | ❏ | ❏ |
| 52.  | ❏ | ❏ | ❏ | ❏ | 80.  | ❏ | ❏ | ❏ | ❏ |
| 53.  | ❏ | ❏ | ❏ | ❏ | 81.  | ❏ | ❏ | ❏ | ❏ |
| 54.  | ❏ | ❏ | ❏ | ❏ | 82.  | ❏ | ❏ | ❏ | ❏ |
| 55.  | ❏ | ❏ | ❏ | ❏ | 83.  | ❏ | ❏ | ❏ | ❏ |
| 56.  | ❏ | ❏ | ❏ | ❏ | 84.  | ❏ | ❏ | ❏ | ❏ |
| 57.  | ❏ | ❏ | ❏ | ❏ | 85.  | ❏ | ❏ | ❏ | ❏ |
| 58.  | ❏ | ❏ | ❏ | ❏ | 86.  | ❏ | ❏ | ❏ | ❏ |
| 59.  | ❏ | ❏ | ❏ | ❏ | 87.  | ❏ | ❏ | ❏ | ❏ |
| 60.  | ❏ | ❏ | ❏ | ❏ | 88.  | ❏ | ❏ | ❏ | ❏ |
| 61.  | ❏ | ❏ | ❏ | ❏ | 89.  | ❏ | ❏ | ❏ | ❏ |
| 62.  | ❏ | ❏ | ❏ | ❏ | 90.  | ❏ | ❏ | ❏ | ❏ |
| 63.  | ❏ | ❏ | ❏ | ❏ | 91.  | ❏ | ❏ | ❏ | ❏ |
| 64.  | ❏ | ❏ | ❏ | ❏ | 92.  | ❏ | ❏ | ❏ | ❏ |
| 65.  | ❏ | ❏ | ❏ | ❏ | 93.  | ❏ | ❏ | ❏ | ❏ |
| 66.  | ❏ | ❏ | ❏ | ❏ | 94.  | ❏ | ❏ | ❏ | ❏ |
| 67.  | ❏ | ❏ | ❏ | ❏ | 95.  | ❏ | ❏ | ❏ | ❏ |
| 68.  | ❏ | ❏ | ❏ | ❏ | 96.  | ❏ | ❏ | ❏ | ❏ |
| 69.  | ❏ | ❏ | ❏ | ❏ | 97.  | ❏ | ❏ | ❏ | ❏ |
| 70.  | ❏ | ❏ | ❏ | ❏ | 98.  | ❏ | ❏ | ❏ | ❏ |
| 71.  | ❏ | ❏ | ❏ | ❏ | 99.  | ❏ | ❏ | ❏ | ❏ |
| 72.  | ❏ | ❏ | ❏ | ❏ | 100. | ❏ | ❏ | ❏ | ❏ |
| 73.  | ❏ | ❏ | ❏ | ❏ | 101. | ❏ | ❏ | ❏ | ❏ |
| 74.  | ❏ | ❏ | ❏ | ❏ | 102. | ❏ | ❏ | ❏ | ❏ |
| 75.  | ❏ | ❏ | ❏ | ❏ | 103. | ❏ | ❏ | ❏ | ❏ |
| 76.  | ❏ | ❏ | ❏ | ❏ | 104. | ❏ | ❏ | ❏ | ❏ |

|      | A | B | C | D |      | A | B | C | D |
|------|---|---|---|---|------|---|---|---|---|
| 105. | ❑ | ❑ | ❑ | ❑ | 118. | ❑ | ❑ | ❑ | ❑ |
| 106. | ❑ | ❑ | ❑ | ❑ | 119. | ❑ | ❑ | ❑ | ❑ |
| 107. | ❑ | ❑ | ❑ | ❑ | 120. | ❑ | ❑ | ❑ | ❑ |
| 108. | ❑ | ❑ | ❑ | ❑ | 121. | ❑ | ❑ | ❑ | ❑ |
| 109. | ❑ | ❑ | ❑ | ❑ | 122. | ❑ | ❑ | ❑ | ❑ |
| 110. | ❑ | ❑ | ❑ | ❑ | 123. | ❑ | ❑ | ❑ | ❑ |
| 111. | ❑ | ❑ | ❑ | ❑ | 124. | ❑ | ❑ | ❑ | ❑ |
| 112. | ❑ | ❑ | ❑ | ❑ | 125. | ❑ | ❑ | ❑ | ❑ |
| 113. | ❑ | ❑ | ❑ | ❑ | 126. | ❑ | ❑ | ❑ | ❑ |
| 114. | ❑ | ❑ | ❑ | ❑ | 127. | ❑ | ❑ | ❑ | ❑ |
| 115. | ❑ | ❑ | ❑ | ❑ | 128. | ❑ | ❑ | ❑ | ❑ |
| 116. | ❑ | ❑ | ❑ | ❑ | 129. | ❑ | ❑ | ❑ | ❑ |
| 117. | ❑ | ❑ | ❑ | ❑ | 130. | ❑ | ❑ | ❑ | ❑ |

# Equipment Assessment

**DIRECTIONS:** Each of the questions or incomplete statements below is followed by four suggested answers or completions. Select the one that is best in each case and then blacken the corresponding space on the answer sheet found in the front of this chapter. Good luck.

1. The RRT is monitoring a patient who is receiving BiPAP® when suddenly the estimated, exhaled tidal volume display light begins flashing. Which of the following system checks should the RRT perform?

   I. Check the integrity of the circuitry.
   II. Check the fitting of the mask.
   III. Observe for the presence of mouth breathing if a nasal mask is used.
   IV. Check for leaks through the exhalation ports.

   A. I, II, III, IV
   B. III, IV only
   C. I, II, IV only
   D. I, II, III only

2. While obtaining a central venous pressure (CVP) measurement, the RRT observes that the dome of the strain gauge appears to be at the level of the patient's phlebostatic axis. What should she do at this time?

   A. Lower the pressure transducer by 5 cm.
   B. Zero the pressure transducer.
   C. Recalibrate the pressure transducer.
   D. Accept the CVP reading obtained.

3. A metal laryngoscope handle and blade have just been removed from an ethylene oxide sterilizer. How long do these materials need to aerate before they can be used clinically?

   A. They must aerate at least 24 hours.
   B. A minimum of 4 hours aeration time is necessary.
   C. *No* less than 30 minutes aeration time is required.
   D. *No* aeration time is necessary.

4. How can the RRT determine whether a pleural drainage system is *not* functioning properly?

   A. by noting the absence of constant bubbling in the suction control bottle.
   B. by observing a steady rise of the water level in the water-seal bottle.
   C. by observing the absence of constant bubbling in the drainage-collection bottle.
   D. by noticing increased fluid in the drainage-collection bottle.

5. During resuscitation, a patient is receiving ventilation from a demand-valve, gas-powered resuscitator. The patient has been triggering the device but suddenly stops. Which of the following malfunctions might have occurred?

   I. The exhalation leaf diaphragm developed a tear.
   II. The sensing line is obstructed.
   III. The sensing diaphragm developed a leak.

   A. I only
   B. II, III only
   C. II only
   D. I, II, III

6. Criteria for ideal patient selection for home ventilation include which of the following features?

   I. whether the patient is receiving an $FIO_2$ of 1.0.
   II. whether the patient is cardiovascularly stable.
   III. a diagnosis of a neuromuscular disorder.
   IV. a diagnosis of sleep apnea.

   A. I, IV only
   B. II, III, IV only
   C. I, II, III only
   D. III, IV only

7. Which of the following statements accurately refer to continuous-flow intermittent mandatory ventilation (IMV), H-valve assembly?

   I. The reservoir bag must have an adjustable screw clamp.
   II. The one-way valve, separating mandatory breathing from spontaneous breathing, should be situated between the humidifier and the patient.
   III. This system does not require the use of a demand valve.
   IV. The reservoir bag must not be allowed to completely collapse on inspiration.

   A. I, III, IV only
   B. I, II, III only
   C. II, IV only
   D. III, IV only

8. A home care patient calls to inform the RRT that his transtracheal catheter accidentally fell out last night and that he was unable to reinsert it. The patient should be told to

A. continue attempts to reinsert the catheter.

B. insert a dilating or stenting device.

C. use a nasal cannula until another transtracheal catheter is brought to the home.

D. use a nasal cannula and call his physician as soon as possible.

9. An RRT is initiating mechanical ventilation with the Puritan-Bennett Companion 2801 ventilator in a patient's home. The patient has been prescribed to receive an $FIO_2$ of 0.30. The $FIO_2$ is analyzed and found to be 0.24. What intervention would be most appropriate at this time?

A. readjusting the $FIO_2$ control dial to 0.30

B. reconnecting the oxygen bleed-in tube

C. increasing the oxygen flow rate to correspond to an $FIO_2$ of 0.30

D. replacing the ventilator

10. With a patient committed to mechanical ventilation, assume there are *no* provisions available for the continuous measurement of volume and flow rates. Which of the following devices would provide the RRT with the most accurate volume and flow rate measurements?

A. Wright Respirometer

B. Fleisch pneumotachometer

C. Dräger Volumeter

D. Tissot spirometer

11. The RRT is preparing to affix a transcutaneous $PO_2$/$PCO_2$ electrode to a cardiac arrest victim who is being resuscitated. Where should the electrode be located to best evaluate the efficacy of cardiopulmonary resuscitation (CPR)?

A. on the abdomen

B. on either shoulder

- C. on the mid-sternum

D. on either thigh

12. A pediatric patient is being transported and is receiving continuous flow nasal CPAP at 15 cm $H_2O$ via a Bio-Med MVP-10 ventilator. The RRT notices that the pressure manometer indicates 10 cm $H_2O$ each time the patient inspires. What is the possible cause of this situation?

A. The inspiratory time control is set too low.

B. The maximum pressure-control valve might be only partially open.

C. The continuous flow in the system is too low.

D. The CPAP level is set beyond the capability of the delivery device.

13. The RRT is measuring the volume output of an adult volume ventilator that has recently been decontami-

nated. After he securely attaches all components of the ventilator circuit to the machine, he sets the tidal volume on the ventilator at 800 cc. He then affixes a Wright Respirometer to the breathing circuit and notes that a reading of 740 cc registers on the dial. What should be done at this time?

A. Have the defective Wright Respirometer sent away for repair.

B. Decrease the high-pressure limit on the ventilator.

C. Accept the measured volume as accurate.

D. Increase the sensitivity adjustment.

14. A tracheotomized patient is receiving an $FIO_2$ of 0.40 via a Briggs adaptor. As the RRT enters the room, she observes *no* aerosol mist exiting the distal end of the Briggs adaptor. The patient is *not* cyanotic, but does complain of shortness of breath. In proper sequence, what steps should the RRT take to correct this situation?

I. Check the flow meter for an adequate flow rate setting.

II. Manually ventilate the patient with a resuscitation bag.

III. Check the nebulizer water level.

IV. Inspect the tubing for disconnections, occlusions, or kinks.

A. II, IV, III only

B. II, III, IV only

C. IV, II, III, I

D. IV, I, III only

15. While performing a procedure with a co-oximeter, the RRT notices consistently high hemoglobin readings. What appropriate action(s) need(s) to be taken to correct this problem?

I. Assure that the correct diluent is being used.

II. Assure that the specimen is well mixed.

III. Assure the patency of the diluent feed line.

A. II only

B. I, II only

C. I, III only

D. I, II, III

16. The RRT is summoned to the bedside of a patient whose brachial arterial line catheter shows a backup of blood flow in the intravenous (I.V.) tubing. The most appropriate action would be to:

A. check all connections.

B. maintain constant and continuous fluid flow of 12 to 14 ml/hour.

C. ensure that I.V. bag pressure is greater than the patient's arterial pressure.

D. have nursing personnel periodically flush the system.

17. A patient is receiving oxygen from a home liquid oxygen system weighing 100 pounds. The gauge indicates that the system is $\frac{3}{4}$ full. Calculate the duration of flow for this system delivering oxygen at 3 L/min. via a nasal cannula.

   A. 1.0 day
   B. 2.0 days
   C. 4.5 days
   D. 6.0 days

18. Which limb lead(s) normally display(s) a(n) inverted electrocardiagram(s)?

   I. aVR
   II. lead III
   III. lead I
   IV. aVF

   A. I only
   B. IV only
   C. I, III only
   D. I, IV only

19. Gas-powered resuscitators are sometimes used in resuscitation situations. The only real advantage for their use is they provide:

   A. an $F_{IO_2}$ of 1.00.
   B. adequate volumes.
   C. adequate pressure.
   D. adequate flow rates.

20. The RRT has assembled suctioning equipment by using a wall outlet and regulator for adult application. Upon occluding the orifice of the suction tubing, she notices that the gauge pressure indicates $-200$ mm Hg. Adjustments made with the control knob do *not* change the gauge reading. What is the likely cause of this situation?

   A. The gauge is measuring line vacuum, so the regulator should be switched to adjustable vacuum.
   B. *No* adjustments need to be made because this pressure is normal.
   C. Occluding the suction tubing orifice is *unnecessary* because the suction gauge should be read when the orifice is unoccluded.
   D. The collection chamber is probably leaking.

21. A mechanically ventilated patient is scheduled for a magnetic resonance imaging (MRI) of the thorax. Continuous mechanical ventilation *cannot* be interrupted. Which of the following ventilators would be acceptable to use in the environment of the MRI unit?

   A. Siemens Servo 900C
   B. Bird Mark 14

   C. Bear 5
   D. Monaghan 225/SIMV

22. While performing intensive care unit (ICU) rounds, the RRT notices that the low exhaled volume monitor on a Bear 1 ventilator is indicating zero. She quickly assesses that the patient is alert, stable, has normal bilateral breath sounds, and is *not* in respiratory distress. What should she do to correct this problem?

   A. Reconnect the inspiratory limb.
   B. Reconnect the tubing between the patient and the expiratory diaphragm.
   C. Remove the condensation that has accumulated on the ultrasonic transducer.
   D. Remove the obstruction in the flow tube of the vortex-shedding ultrasonic flow transducer.

23. The RRT is setting up a pneumatically powered mechanical ventilator in the home of an oxygen-dependent chronic obstructive pulmonary disease (COPD) patient. After adjusting the ventilator settings, the RRT connects the patient's liquid oxygen system to the ventilator. Despite the connection to this pressure source, the ventilator's low-pressure alarm continuously sounds. What might be the cause of this situation?

   A. The liquid oxygen system is an inappropriate supply source for the ventilator.
   B. The low pressure alarm is set too low.
   C. The liquid oxygen system's flow-control valve needs to be opened further.
   D. The liquid oxygen system's pressure-release valve is stuck in the open position.

24. Which of the following statements refer to internal quality-control programs?

   I. Another name for internal quality control is proficiency testing.
   II. Data are obtained from quality-control samples and are then sent to a distribution center.
   III. Internal quality-control mechanisms are intended to detect discrepancies in instrumentation performance.
   IV. The purpose of such programs is to ascertain the precision of laboratory instrumentation.

   A. I, II, IV only
   B. II, III, IV only
   C. III, IV only
   D. I, II, III only

25. Which of the following conditions can cause blood gas analyzer electrode data to shift?

   I. protein contamination of the membrane
   II. contamination of the calibration standards

III. air bubbles under the electrode membrane

IV. an aging mercury battery

A. II, III only
B. II, IV only
C. III, IV only
D. I, II, III only

26. Which statement best describes the operation of the exhalation valve and/or gas flow through ventilator tubing?

A. The exhalation valve opens during inspiration.
B. During exhalation, the patient's expirate follows the path of least resistance.
C. Gas from the patient operates the exhalation valve.
D. The gas in the expiratory limb is rebreathed by the patient.

27. The RRT is requested to measure the total work of breathing of a patient who is being mechanically ventilated. Which device would she use to make this measurement?

A. Wright Respirometer
B. body plethysmograph
C. differential pressure pneumotachometer
D. positive displacement meter

28. Into what channel is the injectate inserted for a thermodilution cardiac output (C.O.) determination via a four-lumen pulmonary artery catheter (PAC)?

A. thermistor channel
B. distal channel
C. balloon inflation channel
D. proximal channel

29. How will condensation accumulating in the capillary tubes of the Fleisch pneumotachometer affect the flow measurements?

A. The measured flow rate will be less than actual.
B. The measured flow rate will be higher than actual.
C. The measured flow rate will be accurate.
D. The flow rate will require atmospheric temperature and pressure saturated (ATPS) to body temperature and pressure saturated (BTPS) correction.

30. The RRT is about to disinfect the exterior surfaces of an ECG machine that has been splattered with blood. She locates a container labeled 50% isopropyl alcohol. What should she do at this time?

A. Use this solution to disinfect the ECG machine.
B. Dilute the solution to 30% isopropyl alcohol.
C. Administer two applications of the 50% isopropyl alcohol solution.
D. Do *not* use the 50% isopropyl alcohol solution.

31. An RRT enters the ICU to assist in the assessment of the endotracheal (ET) tube of a patient receiving continuous mechanical ventilation. Radiologic assessment demonstrates that the tube is 3 cm above the carina. Physical assessment demonstrates bilateral breath sounds. The patient is alert and verbally communicative. The needle on the ET tube cuff pressure manometer is reading 15 cm $H_2O$, and upon disconnection from the pilot balloon it returns very slowly to a baseline of 2 cm $H_2O$. What should the RRT do at this time?

A. Record a cuff pressure of 13 cm $H_2O$ on the flow sheet.
B. Reposition the ET tube and repeat the X-ray.
C. Add 3 cc of air to the cuff.
D. Replace the manometer and send it for calibration.

32. An RRT is changing an intermittent positive pressure breathing (IPPB) circuit. He removes the new circuit from the package and notes three separate tubes. The instructions indicate that one is for the main flow, a second for the expiratory valve assembly, and the third for the nebulizer. As he removes the old circuit from the Bird Mark VII, he observes only two tubes. The most appropriate explanation is:

A. This situation is normal because one line is needed to power both the nebulizer and the exhalation valve.
B. One tube has obviously been inadvertently omitted, thus either the nebulizer or the exhalation valve is not functioning properly.
C. The third line is only required when continuous mechanical ventilation is employed.
D. This setup is normal because exhalation is passive and an expiratory tube is not required.

33. While checking the fiberoptic bronchoscope before a bronchoscopic procedure, the RRT notices that *no* light is being emitted from the tip of the bronchoscope. How should the RRT troubleshoot this condition?

I. Pass a cytology brush through the accessory port in the bronchoscope.
II. Wipe the tip of the bronchoscope with sterile gauze to remove possible residue.
III. Check to see that the power source is plugged into the wall.
IV. Reseat the bronchoscope to the light source connection.

A. II, IV only
B. I, III only
C. II, III, IV only
D. I, II, III, IV

34. Why is fluoroscopy generally *not* used for Swan–Ganz catheter insertion?

I. The prolonged exposure to radiation during catheter insertion would damage myocardial tissue.

II. The catheter has flow-directed capabilities provided by the inflatable balloon at the catheter tip.

III. Each cardiac chamber and associated vessels generate characteristic pressure waveforms enabling the discernment of the catheter position.

IV. The catheter is not radiopaque; consequently, fluoroscopy would *not* be useful.

A. IV only
B. I, II, III only
C. II, III only
D. I, III only

35. When is troubleshooting a blood gas electrode indicated?

I. when data have been out of control for two daily shifts

II. any time a random error occurs

III. when the data consistently lie within $\pm 2$ standard deviations from the mean

IV. any time a single value is greater than $\pm 3$ standard deviations from the mean

A. II, IV only
B. I, II, IV only
C. I, II, III only
D. I, IV only

36. The RRT is ventilating a patient with 100% oxygen via bag-mask ventilation. Despite the proper application of this intervention, the patient remains cyanotic. Which of the following mechanical aspects affecting oxygen delivery should the RRT troubleshoot?

I. Determine whether the reservoir on the bag inlet is properly attached.

II. Ensure that the oxygen supply tubing is attached to the flow meter.

III. Check the flow meter to ensure a flow rate of 10 to 15 L/min.

IV. Remove the bag from the patient to determine whether the pop-off valve works.

A. I, II, III only
B. I, II only
C. II, III, IV only
D. III, IV only

37. While being summoned to the bedside of a patient ventilated with a fluidic ventilator, the RRT is informed that, although the patient is alert, communicative, and obviously in *no* respiratory distress, the ventilator is exceedingly noisy and is consuming a sizable supply of source gas. What is the likely cause of this occurrence?

A. A tubing disconnection has occurred.
B. The exhalation valve has a faulty expiratory diaphragm.
C. An internal system leak has developed.
D. The condition described is normal.

38. The RRT is about to analyze an arterial blood gas (ABG) sample in the emergency department. She notices that the co-oximeter is flashing "check cuvette." In the proper sequence, how would the RRT troubleshoot the co-oximeter?

I. Aspirate cleaning solution through the cuvette and window.
II. Ice the sample.
III. Attempt to auto-zero.
IV. Clean the tubing and cuvette.
V. Call the manufacturer to obtain technical assistance.

A. II, I, III, IV, V
B. III, II, V, I, IV
C. V, II, III, IV, I
D. I, V, III, II, IV

39. An RRT is called to the ICU to assist with the intubation of a patient. The anesthesiologist is inserting a double-lumen ET tube. Which of the following conditions is most likely to warrant the insertion of this type of artificial airway?

A. severe adult respiratory distress syndrome (ARDS)
B. tracheal malacia
C. unilateral interstitial fibrosis
D. diffuse idiopathic consolidated pneumonia

40. Which of the Levey-Jennings charts shown in Figure 4-1 (A-D) indicates the phenomenon of dispersion?

A. A
B. B
C. C
D. D

41. Co-oximetry is performed on a 1-week-old neonate. The data obtained indicate a high carboxyhemoglobin concentration and a low arterial oxygen saturation. What condition might have accounted for these data?

A. An air bubble was probably introduced into the sample.
B. Venous blood was probably obtained and analyzed.
C. The co-oximeter views fetal hemoglobin as carboxyhemoglobin.
D. The sample was inserted too quickly, reducing the contact time between the sample and the photodetector.

**A.**

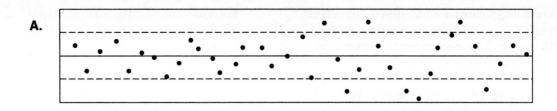

**B.**

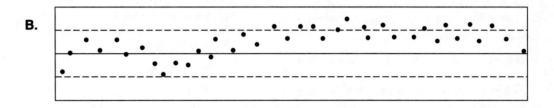

**C.**

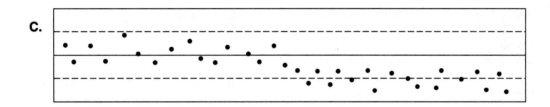

**D.**

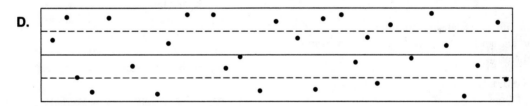

**Figure 4-1**

42. In establishing a respiratory care plan for a cystic fibrosis patient, which of the following types of equipment would be the most therapeutically useful?

    A. incentive spirometer
    B. positive expiratory pressure (PEP) mask
    C. pneumotachometer
    D. ultrasonic nebulizer

43. The pressure-time tracing depicted in Figure 4-2 represents the pressure changes during a ventilatory cycle of a patient receiving 8 cm $H_2O$ demand flow mask CPAP.

Which of the following situations might have produced this tracing?

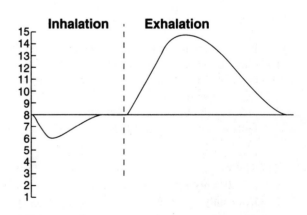

**Figure 4-2:** CPAP system pressure-time tracing.

A. The demand valve requires a large patient effort.
B. The flow rate through the system is inadequate.
C. The patient experienced a forceful exhalation.
D. A threshold resistor is being used.

44. A home care patient has called to complain of discomfort stemming from receiving oxygen via a nasal cannula connected to an oxygen concentrator. Upon arrival at the home, the RRT notes that the concentrator flow rate is set at 4 L/min. when the original order required 2 L/min. Which of the following statements is true regarding the changed flow rate?

   A. The patient was receiving an $FIO_2$ greater than that prescribed in original order.
   B. The patient was receiving an $FIO_2$ less than the original order intended.
   C. The patient was receiving the intended $FIO_2$ at the time of the RRT's arrival at the home.
   D. The influence of the patient having changed the original flow rate cannot be ascertained.

45. A patient who is receiving transtracheal oxygen complains of a persistent cough. The RRT notes that wheezes are heard upon auscultation. Which of the following conditions might be responsible for this situation?

   I. A mucous plug has formed at the tip of the catheter.
   II. The patient has coughed the catheter into a cephalad position.
   III. The catheter is causing irritation.
   IV. The patient has developed an infection from the catheter.

   A. I, II, III only
   B. III, IV only
   C. I, II only
   D. I, II, III, IV

46. Identify desirable characteristics associated with infant mechanical ventilators.

   I. low compressibility factor for the breathing circuit
   II. rapid response time to patient-initiated breaths
   III. positive end-respiratory pressure (PEEP) and CPAP capabilities
   IV. pressure-limited, time-cycled capabilities for infants with noncompliant lungs

   A. I, II, III, IV
   B. III only
   C. I, II, III only
   D. II, IV only

47. During ventilation of a neonate with the Life Pulse high-frequency jet ventilator, the RRT observes condensation in the circuit near the high–low jet tube and

fluctuation of the pressure readings. What action should be taken *first*?

   A. Replace the bacterial filter in the jet line.
   B. Decrease the cartridge temperature setting.
   C. Flush the monitor line with 10 cc of air.
   D. Suction the patient.

48. The RRT is preparing to place into an ethylene oxide chamber the valve assembly of a manual resuscitator that became covered with vomitus during CPR. How should the valve assembly be prepared *before* ethylene oxide sterilization?

   I. The valve assembly should be surgically clean.
   II. The valve assembly needs to be wet.
   III. The equipment should be wrapped in muslin.
   IV. The equipment should be rinsed in hot water before being placed in the sterilizer.

   A. II, III, IV only
   B. I, IV only
   C. I, III only
   D. I, II, III only

49. What will be the effect of nitrous oxide on the analysis of oxygen via a polarographic oxygen analyzer?

   A. *No* prediction can be made.
   B. It will cause the analyzer to fluctuate above and below the patient's actual $O_2\%$.
   C. The analyzer will indicate an $O_2\%$ less than the patient is actually receiving.
   D. The analyzer will indicate an $O_2\%$ greater than the patient is actually receiving.

50. Which of the following measurements is(are) available from an indwelling arterial catheter?

   I. mean arterial pressure
   II. systemic vascular resistance
   III. pulse pressure
   IV. ventricular afterload

   A. I only
   B. I, III only
   C. II, IV only
   D. I, II, III only

51. What would be the effect on an $FIO_2$ of greater than 0.40 from a jet nebulizer if an additional 6 feet of aerosol tubing was connected to 6 feet of large-bore tubing already in place in the system?

   A. The influence on the $FIO_2$ *cannot* be predicted.
   B. The $FIO_2$ would increase above 0.40.
   C. The $FIO_2$ would remain at 0.40.
   D. The $FIO_2$ would fluctuate above and below 0.40.

52. If a fluidic logic circuit in a fluidic ventilator fails to control a component of mechanical ventilation, this failure results from the loss of which aspect of the mechanical ventilator?

    A. pressure
    B. electrical power
    C. volume
    D. $F_IO_2$

53. A patient is being ventilated with a high-frequency jet ventilator by means of a standard ET tube and angiocath. Initial ABGs showed a stable and normal acid-base balance. One hour after returning from a computerized axial tomography (CAT) scan, however, another ABG indicates an abnormal respiratory acid-base condition. The RRT is assured that the ventilator and patient's condition have *not* changed. This situation is most likely the result of:

    A. improper calibration of the blood gas analyzer.
    B. movement and improper location of the angiocath in the ET tube.
    C. fluctuations in oxygen outlet pressure.
    D. variations in the barometric pressure.

54. When a CO analyzer is "zeroed," what must the RRT do at this time?

    A. Flush the device with gas containing 0% carbon monoxide.
    B. Flush the analyzer with room air.
    C. Calibrate the device to the low-value test signal.
    D. Calibrate the analyzer to the high-value test signal.

55. What pressure reading(s) is(are) normally made when the balloon tip of a PAC is deflated?

    I. pulmonary capillary wedge pressure (PCWP)
    II. pulmonary artery diastolic pressure
    III. right ventricular pressure
    IV. pulmonary artery systolic pressure

    A. I only
    B. II, IV only
    C. IV only
    D. I, III only

56. Which of the following equipment is necessary during fiberoptic bronchoscopy?

    I. pulse oximeter
    II. maximum inspiratory pressure meter
    III. peak flow meter
    IV. single-lead ECG monitor

    A. I, IV only
    B. I only
    C. II, IV only
    D. I, II, III only

57. How will the accumulation of condensate in the large-bore tubing of an air-entrainment aerosol-delivery device, with oxygen as the source gas, affect the operation of the system?

    I. It will cause the $F_IO_2$ to decrease.
    II. It will result in an increased delivered flow rate.
    III. It will produce a higher $F_IO_2$.
    IV. It will cause the production of a more dense mist.

    A. III only
    B. II, IV only
    C. III, IV only
    D. I only

58. While administering ribavirin via a SPAG-2 unit to an infant who has bronchiolitis, the RRT notices that the pressure gauge is registering 50 psig. What should he do at this time?

    A. *nothing* because the unit is functioning normally
    B. increase the pressure setting to 60 psig
    C. decrease the pressure setting to 26 psig
    D. decrease the pressure setting to 14.7 psig

59. A molecular sieve-type oxygen concentrator is operating at 3 L/min. and is analyzed as delivering 88% oxygen. At what flow setting would the concentrator likely deliver greater than 90% oxygen?

    A. 1 L/min.
    B. 4 L/min.
    C. 7 L/min.
    D. 8 L/min.

60. A sudden decrease in a mechanically ventilated patient's end-tidal $CO_2$ has just occurred. A repeated analysis yields the same results. Which of the following situations might have accounted for these readings?

    I. The ventilator has become disconnected.
    II. There is a leak around the ET tube.
    III. There is an increase in alveolar dead space.
    IV. The carbon dioxide absorber is exhausted.

    A. III, IV only
    B. I, II, III only
    C. I, II, IV only
    D. I, II, III, IV

61. The RRT is about to place the sensor of a polarographic oxygen analyzer in the circuitry of a mechanical ventilator. Where along the ventilator tubing is the best location to place this sensor?

    A. as close as possible to the patient Y adaptor on the inspiratory limb
    B. anywhere along the length of the inspiratory limb
    C. between the ventilator and the humidifier
    D. near the exhalation port

62. The RRT is preparing to perform PEP therapy on a cystic fibrosis patient. Where in the system should the line attached to the pressure manometer be inserted?

   I. between the one-way valve and the mask
   II. between the one-way valve and the opening of the inspiratory port
   III. along the expiratory limb between the resistor and the mask
   IV. at the opening of the resistor

   A. I, IV only
   B. I, III only
   C. II, III, IV only
   D. I, II, IV only

63. Assuming that a cardiac monitor is *not* available, what other device would be useful to help determine the restoration of circulation in a cardiac arrest victim?

   A. capnometer
   B. spectrophotometer
   C. pulse oximeter
   D. co-oximeter

64. Regarding instrumentation quality control, balancing a device refers to:

   A. zeroing the instrument.
   B. calibrating the instrument while it is exposed to the low-value test signal.
   C. calibrating the instrument while it is exposed to the high-value test signal.
   D. performing a one-point calibration.

65. An RRT observes that a $PtcO_2$ electrode set at 44.0°C on an adult patient is indicating a value fluctuating 5 torr above and below the arterial $PO_2$ value. What should the RRT do at this time?

   A. Increase the temperature of the electrode by 2°C.
   B. Discontinue using the transcutaneous oxygen monitor.
   C. Change the electrode application site.
   D. Use both the transcutaneous and arterial $PO_2$ data for trending purposes only.

66. How will hemodynamic measurements be affected if the PAC transducer, after having been zeroed, is placed above the phlebostatic axis?

   A. The pressure readings will be accurate.
   B. The pressure readings will be erroneously high.
   C. The pressure readings will be erroneously low.
   D. The pressure readings will fluctuate.

67. The RRT enters the room of a patient who is receiving nasal oxygen at 2 L/min. humidified via a bubble-diffusion humidifier. Upon entering the room, the RRT hears a chirping, whistling, clattering sound coming from the humidifier. What is the cause of this noise?

   A. a low water level in the humidifier
   B. a loose connection at the humidifier
   C. kinked oxygen tubing
   D. a low oxygen liter flow

68. An eccentrically inflated cuff causing the tip of an ET tube to impinge against the anterior tracheal wall might cause ___.

   A. a tracheoesophageal fistula
   B. brachiocephalic artery erosion
   C. ventilation of the right mainstem bronchus
   D. otitis media

69. What is the recommended minimum positive pressure that is to be used in conjunction with PEP mask therapy?

   A. 5 cm $H_2O$
   B. 10 cm $H_2O$
   C. 15 cm $H_2O$
   D. 20 cm $H_2O$

70. How can the RRT assure that a patient who is receiving BiPAP® is being adequately oxygenated?

   A. employing a pulse oximeter to monitor the patient's $SpO_2$
   B. making certain that the liter flow on the oxygen flow meter is at least 5 L/min.
   C. analyzing the $FiO_2$ with an oxygen analyzer
   D. ensuring that the oxygen line is connected at the mask

71. While performing an ABG analysis, an RRT encounters a relatively abrupt change in measurement outcome, followed by a clustering or plateauing of data. Which of the following conditions is most likely responsible for this response?

   A. an aging electrode
   B. an aging mercury battery
   C. protein contamination of the electrode
   D. air bubbles beneath the electrode membrane

72. An RRT is serving as a member of the transport team and is ventilating a patient with the Aequitron LP-10 ventilator. After 1.5 hours of flight, the RRT observes inconsistencies in ventilator control function and performance. The problem is most likely related to:

   A. air turbulence and in-flight variables.
   B. depletion of the electrical energy source.
   C. variations in altitude and decreases in atmospheric pressure.
   D. increases in cabin pressure, hence excessive pressures in the ventilator-control regulator.

73. A patient has been prescribed to receive an $F_IO_2$ of 0.50 via an aerosol face mask provided by a blender. While performing rounds, the RRT analyzes the $F_IO_2$ to be 0.35 with the flow meter dialed to 15 L/min. The air entrainment port of the nebulizer is set at an $F_IO_2$ of 0.60, whereas the blender is set to deliver 50% oxygen. How can the RRT resolve this problem?

A. Change blenders.
B. Administer mask CPAP at 5 cm $H_2O$ with 50% oxygen.
C. Administer an $F_IO_2$ of 0.60 via a Venturi mask.
D. Set the nebulizer to 100% oxygen.

74. What hemodynamic equipment is needed to monitor left-ventricular preload in the presence of left heart failure or pulmonary disease?

A. central venous pressure (CVP) monitor
B. PAC
C. arterial pressure measurements
D. electrocardiography

75. Which technique(s) is(are) useful for obtaining sputum specimens *not* contaminated by upper airway microorganisms?

I. passing a suction catheter through a nasal or oral ET tube
II. fiberoptic bronchoscopy
III. passing a suction catheter through a tracheostomy tube
IV. performing transtracheal aspiration

A. I, III only
B. II, III, IV only
C. II only
D. II, IV only

76. The RRT is performing a quality-control check on a Bennett 7200 mechanical ventilator. While evaluating the ventilator's maximum flow rate, he is using a Wright Respirometer and obtains a readout of 120 L/min. How useful is this value?

A. Disregard it because it exceeds the maximum flow capabilities of the Wright Respirometer.
B. Disregard it because it falls below the minimum flow rate capabilities of the Wright Respirometer.
C. Accept the value as accurate.
D. Remeasure the ventilator's maximum flow rate because the value is too low.

77. Which of the following modes of oxygen delivery would be most appropriate for a home care oxygen patient who is self-conscious of the cosmetics of the device?

A. the reservoir cannula
B. transtracheal oxygen

C. simple mask
D. nasal catheter

78. The recyclable ventilator tubing last used on a patient who succumbed to *Clostridium botulinum* is about to be placed in a pasteurizer. Which of the following considerations should be taken into account by the RRT?

A. This process will routinely kill *Clostridium botulinum* spores.
B. The flash process must be employed.
C. *Clostridium botulinum* spores are not a concern in this process.
D. Equipment contaminated by this microorganism must be exposed to the batch process.

79. The RRT is checking a transcutaneous monitor attached to a 36-week-old newborn in the neonatal ICU. She observes that the $PtcO_2$ is performing erratically and that the electrode power needed to stabilize the temperature to the probe is very low. What steps should the RRT take to correct the problem?

A. Remove and reposition the electrode adding a new drop of sterile water.
B. Leave the electrode where it is and replace the transcutaneous monitor.
C. Obtain an ABG to see whether there is a correlation.
D. Remembrane the electrode.

80. A patient has been intubated with a double-lumen ET tube for the purpose of independent lung ventilation. The patient has a right middle-lobe and right lower lobe pneumonia. Ventilation of the left lung will occur via a Briggs adaptor with room air, whereas the right lung will receive synchronized intermittent mandatory ventilation (SIMV) with pressure-support ventilation. When both modes are connected to their respective lumens, the low-pressure alarm on the ventilator continuously sounds. What might be the cause of this situation?

A. The double-lumen ET tube has not been advanced sufficiently down the trachea.
B. The double-lumen ET tube has been inserted too far into the tracheobronchial tree.
C. The cuff of the lumen connected to the Briggs adaptor is deflated.
D. The cuff of the lumen connected to the ventilator is overinflated.

81. An RRT is performing mouth-to-mouth ventilation while noting chest excursions. A nurse has given the RRT a mouth-to-valve mask resuscitator. When he attempts to deliver a breath through the valve, he encounters high resistance and notices that *no* air is entering the victim's lungs. What action should he take at this time?

A. Reverse the valve and attempt to ventilate.
B. Adjust the seal around the mask and face.
C. Resume mouth-to-mouth ventilation.
D. Stop ventilating and request another mouth-to-valve resuscitator.

82. A home care patient has a portable liquid oxygen system that holds 3 pounds of liquid oxygen. How long will this supply of oxygen last if the patient uses the oxygen intermittently at 2 L/min.?

A. 6.5 hours
B. 8.5 hours
C. 9.0 hours
D. The duration of flow *cannot* be determined.

83. The RRT has just inserted a double-lumen ET tube for the purpose of applying independent lung ventilation to a patient. How can she determine whether the ET tube is properly positioned?

A. Alternately clamp each lumen and listen for air movement on the contralateral side.
B. Insert a suction catheter through each lumen to determine the degree of resistance.
C. Encourage the patient to cough while each lumen is clamped.
D. Manually resuscitate each lumen and observe the rise and fall of the chest wall.

84. A 2.8-kg neonate is being ventilated with the SensorMedics 3100 high-frequency oscillatory ventilator at a rate of 15 Hz with a 2.5 mm I.D. ET tube. Despite an oscillatory pressure amplitude of 80 cm $H_2O$ at the proximal airway, the patient's $PaCO_2$ remains high. Which of the following is the most likely cause?

A. The amplitude reading is erroneous.
B. The ET tube is too small.
C. Inadequate humidification has damaged the trachea.
D. The frequency is too low.

85. An RRT is performing a quality-control procedure on a gas metering device. She plotted the procedure on an *x–y* axis and obtained the data illustrated in Figure 4-3.

What quality-control characteristic has she measured?

A. hysteresis
B. slewing
C. linearity
D. drift

86. A COPD patient is receiving 24% oxygen from an air-entrainment mask. The RRT analyzes the $FIO_2$ inside

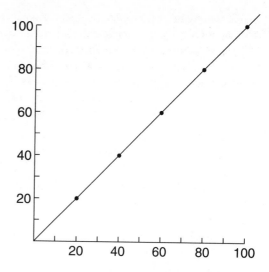

**Figure 4-3:** Gas metering device quality-control data.

the mask and finds it to be 0.35. The accuracy of the analyzer is ±0.02. What is the possible cause of this situation?

A. The patient's tidal volume decreased.
B. The patient's inspiratory flow rate increased.
C. The patient's ventilatory rate increased.
D. The air entrainment port is partially obstructed.

87. Which of the following factors are associated with falsely low transcutaneous $PO_2$ electrode readings?

I. hyperthermia
II. alkalemia
III. air leak around the electrode
IV. low capillary perfusion

A. II, IV only
B. I, II, IV only
C. III, IV only
D. I, II, III only

88. Which of the following sources of oxygen would be able to operate a device that required a minimum pressure of 50 psig?

I. an H tank of oxygen
II. an oxygen concentrator
III. a liquid oxygen system

A. I, II only
B. III only
C. I only
D. II, III only

89. The RRT analyzes the $FIO_2$ delivered by a home care ventilator and determines that the $FIO_2$ is much less than that prescribed. Which of the following conditions might have accounted for this situation?

A. The continuous flow system has failed.
B. The 50-psig oxygen source has failed.
C. The PEEP valve has malfunctioned.
D. The oxygen accumulating device has become disconnected.

90. The RRT is summoned to the emergency department to prepare to intubate a cardiac arrest victim en route to the hospital. While preparing for the procedure, the RRT discovers that the light on the laryngoscope blade will *not* illuminate. In proper sequence, how should she troubleshoot the laryngoscope to prepare for the victim's arrival?

    I. Attach another laryngoscope blade.
    II. Remove and reattach the original blade to see whether it will light.
    III. Replace the batteries in the handle.

    A. II, III, I
    B. III, I, II
    C. II, I, III
    D. III, II, I

91. Which device(s) incorporate(s) a Wheatstone bridge?

    I. strain gauge pressure transducer
    II. polarographic oxygen analyzer
    III. ABG analyzer
    IV. thermoconductivity oxygen analyzer

    A. II, IV only
    B. II, III only
    C. III only
    D. I, IV only

92. A 1-week-old infant who appears to be in respiratory distress while receiving nasal CPAP reveals the fol-
lowing radiographic results: small cysts of air bilaterally in the lung periphery linearly aligned and perpendicular to the lateral aspect of the pleura. Which of the following therapeutic interventions would be most appropriate at this time?

    A. insertion of chest tubes
    B. increased CPAP level
    C. high-frequency jet ventilation
    D. removal of the umbilical artery catheter

93. As the RRT approaches a patient's bedside to obtain a central venous pressure (CVP) measurement, she observes the situation depicted in Figure 4-4.

What should she do at this time?

    A. Obtain the CVP measurement.
    B. Raise the level of the pressure transducer.
    C. Lower the level of the pressure transducer so the stopcocks are at the level of the right atrium.
    D. Level the dome of the transducer with the patient's mid-chest.

94. While performing electrocardiography on a patient, the RRT obtains the ECG shown in Figure 4-5 on page 198.

What should he do at this time?

    A. Increase the paper speed.
    B. Continue with the procedure.
    C. Calibrate the ECG.
    D. Have the unit inspected by the electrical safety engineer.

95. While performing hemodynamic monitoring, the RRT notices the patient's arterial pressure waveform displaying:

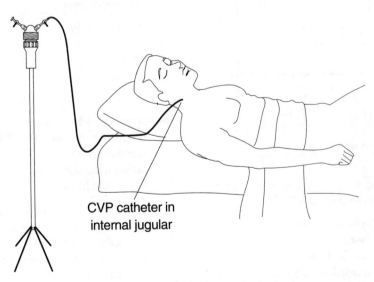

CVP catheter in
internal jugular

**Figure 4-4:** Patient with CVP catheter in place.

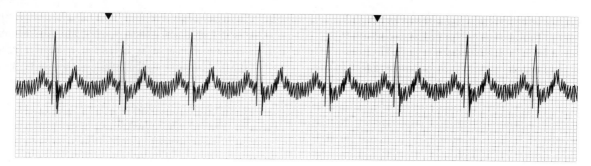

**Figure 4-5:** ECG tracing.

- an overshoot of the systolic pressures
- an undershoot of the diastolic pressure
- numerous small oscillations throughout the tracing

Note the arterial pressure waveform in Figure 4-6.

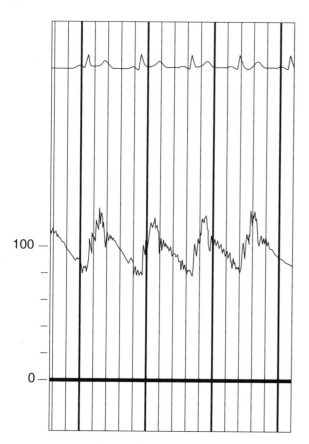

**Figure 4-6:** Arterial pressure waveform.

Which of the following factors can cause this type of arterial pressure waveform distortion?

I. air bubbles in the system
II. blood clots in the system
III. soft, compliant tubing in the system
IV. a small diameter catheter ($<7$ Fr)

A. III, IV only
B. I, II, III only
C. I, IV only
D. I, II, III, IV

96. Which of the following situations/conditions are associated with a decreased correlation between transcutaneous $PO_2$ electrode readings and ABG $PO_2$ values?

I. halothane
II. hypothermia
III. severe acidemia

A. I, III only
B. II, III only
C. II only
D. I, II, III

97. For which of the following disease entities would slow-speed capnography be beneficial?

I. apnea
II. cardiac arrest
III. pulmonary edema
IV. pneumonia

A. I, IV only
B. II, III, IV only
C. I, II only
D. II, III only

98. A patient who is receiving PEP mask therapy is *not* producing mucus. The RRT notices the pressure manometer is reading 5 cm $H_2O$. The most appropriate action needed to obtain the desired effect of PEP therapy would be to:

A. correct for the loss of mask pressure.
B. increase the flow rate.
C. sedate the patient.
D. do *nothing* because the desired effect is being achieved.

99. Which of the following equipment malfunction conditions can be suspected with the use of a capnometer?

    I.   a leak around the cuff of an artificial airway
    II.  a ruptured balloon on a PAC
    III. a ventilator disconnection
    IV.  a co-oximeter out of calibration

    A. II, III, IV only
    B. I, II, III only
    C. I, III only
    D. I, II only

100. A patient receiving mechanical ventilation has a capnometer in-line at the Y-connector of the ventilator circuit for continuous exhaled $CO_2$ monitoring. The capnogram suddenly indicates an abrupt decrease in the $P_{ET}CO_2$ from 5.3% to 0.0%. What situation might have occurred?

    A. The exhalation valve has malfunctioned.
    B. The heated wire in the ventilator circuit might be overheating.
    C. A bronchodilator might have been administered in-line to the patient.
    D. A circuit disconnection might have taken place.

101. A patient who has recently been extubated has become tachypneic and is using accessory muscles of ventilation. Ventilatory muscle fatigue appears imminent. Which form of therapeutic intervention would be most appropriate at this time?

    A. high-frequency jet ventilation
    B. BiPAP®
    C. mask CPAP
    D. PEP mask therapy

102. While performing ventilator rounds in the ICU, the RRT observes a tidal volume that is 250 ml lower than the machine set volume. The patient is stable as the RRT begins to troubleshoot the problem. Two different spirometers confirm the 250-ml reading, as does measuring the volume on the inspiratory limb before the humidifier. What action is most appropriate at this time?

    A. Note the discrepancy and recommend a 250-ml adjustment when the machine is monitored.
    B. Loosen the hex screw on the volume-control dial and readjust it to correspond with the correct reading.
    C. Disregard the problem because it is *not* presenting any problems to the patient.
    D. Discontinue using the ventilator and contact the manufacturer.

103. A patient is receiving intermittent mandatory ventilation (IMV) via an H-valve assembly operating with a nebulizer. How can the RRT ensure that the flow rate through the spontaneous breathing circuit is adequate?

    I.   if mist is being continuously emitted from the exhalation port
    II.  if the pressure manometer deflects *no* more than $-2$ cm $H_2O$ with each patient inspiratory effort
    III. if condensate is *not* accumulating in the tubing
    IV.  if the patient's $PaCO_2$ is 40 mm Hg or less

    A. I, II, IV only
    B. II, III only
    C. I, II only
    D. I, IV only

104. While performing ICU ventilator rounds, the RRT is alerted by a low pressure alarm sounding on a ventilator. What corrective action would be appropriate?

    A. Increasing the low pressure alarm limit.
    B. Inspecting the ventilator circuitry for a disconnection.
    C. Administering an in-line bronchodilator.
    D. Increasing the high-pressure limit.

105. Which statement(s) represent(s) a disadvantage of gas-powered resuscitators?

    I.   They are unable to administer 100% oxygen.
    II.  They are usually pressure limited.
    III. Rupture of the diaphragm exposes the patient to a pressure of 50 psig.
    IV.  Many units do *not* contain a pressure-relief valve.

    A. I, IV only
    B. III only
    C. I, II, IV only
    D. I, III only

106. As a physician inserts a fiberoptic bronchoscope through a patient's oral ET tube, the patient becomes agitated and bites against the ET tube. The fiberoptic bronchoscope has remained in position, and the physician begins viewing. He observes numerous black dots in the field of vision. What might have accounted for this occurrence?

    A. a blood clot on the tip of the fiberoptic bronchoscope
    B. a number of broken fiber bundles
    C. dirt on the lens of the fiberoptic bronchoscope
    D. a light source that is not adequately plugged into the outlet

107. The RRT is calibrating a spirometer by using a 3-liter calibration syringe. The data that she obtained are listed in Table 4-1.

**Table 4-1** Spirometer Calibration Data

| Attempt # | Predicted Volume | Mearured Volume |
|-----------|------------------|-----------------|
| 1 | 3.00 liters | 2.59 liters |
| 2 | 3.00 liters | 2.56 liters |
| 3 | 3.00 liters | 2.58 liters |

What should she do?

A. Perform testing with this device but add 3.00 liters to the volume measured.
B. Conduct testing with the spirometer because it has been satisfactorily calibrated.
C. Conduct testing with this device but add 10% to all volumes measured.
D. Recalibrate the spirometer and look for system leaks.

108. During PAC insertion through the subclavian vein, the following waveform is observed on the monitor (Figure 4-7).

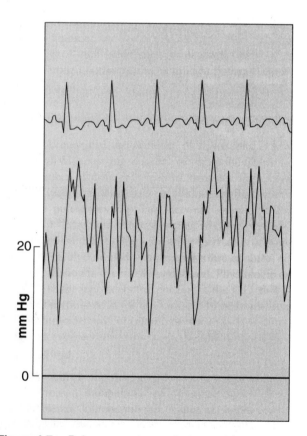

**Figure 4-7:** Pulmonary artery catheter waveform.

This waveform persists as the 80-cm mark of the catheter have been inserted. Which of the following conditions might account for this situation?

A. The catheter is coiling in the right ventricle.
B. The balloon tip is *not* inflated.
C. The catheter tip has migrated into Zone 2 of the lungs.
D. The catheter tip has entered the pericardium.

109. A chest tube placed in the third or fourth anterior intercostal space along the midaxillary line is suited for drainage of ___ from the intrapleural space.

A. fluid
B. blood
C. air
D. pus

110. What action should be taken if arterial blood samples with values beyond the electrode's calibration limits are to be frequently measured?

A. Prior to the introduction of the sample, perform a two-point calibration on the electrode by using the same standards to ensure linearity within the normal operating range.
B. Before the sample is introduced, perform a one-point calibration on the electrode by using the limit of the range that will be exceeded.
C. Before the introduction of the sample, perform a two-point calibration by using standards beyond the calibration limit that is expected to be exceeded.
D. *No* action is necessary as long as usual calibration and quality-control measures have been applied.

111. A manual resuscitation bag that has been used on an active tuberculosis patient is about to be immersed in a 2% alkaline glutaraldehyde solution. How long must the resuscitator be immersed for tuberculocidal activity to occur?

A. Ten minutes immersion is minimally necessary.
B. The bag must be immersed for at least 30 minutes.
C. Tuberculocidal activity will occur after one hour of immersion.
D. Two percent alkaline glutaraldehyde is *not* tuberculocidal.

112. A COPD patient experiencing angina pectoris has been prescribed Isordil. The use of which of the following clinical analyzing devices would be most helpful?

A. co-oximeter
B. transcutaneous oxygen monitor
C. capnograph
D. pulse oximeter

113. A patient is being monitored with a combined transcutaneous $PO_2/PCO_2$ electrode. The most recent ABG data (shown as follows) indicate that the $PtcCO_2$ and the $PaCO_2$ no longer correlate:

$PO_2$ 85 torr
$PCO_2$ 34 torr
pH 7.32
$HCO_3^-$ 17 mEq/liter
B.E. $-$ 7 mEq/liter

Which of the following conditions might have accounted for this situation?

A. hyperventilation
B. hypoxemia
C. metabolic acidosis
D. hypoxia

114. A mechanically ventilated patient with a peak inspiratory pressure (PIP) of 55 cm $H_2O$ is being monitored via a sidestream capnometer that has a 30-ml water trap attached just before the gas enters the analyzing chamber. The RRT notices a brief expiratory (upward) deflection during the mechanical ventilator's inspiratory cycle. What condition might have caused this occurrence?

A. Cardiac oscillations produce such aberrations.
B. Premature ventricular contractions cause this artifact.
C. The size of the water trap causes this deflection.
D. The deflection coincides with an inspiratory pause.

115. The RRT is monitoring the ventilator of a home care patient and notices that the patient's PIP suddenly falls from 33 cm $H_2O$ to 0 cm $H_2O$. Which of the following factors might have accounted for this change?

I. The patient's compliance increased.
II. The patient Y became disconnected from the ET tube.
III. The patient's airway resistance decreased.
IV. The exhalation valve is stuck in the inspiratory position.

A. I, III only
B. II, III, IV only
C. I, IV only
D. II only

116. An RRT has received an order to administer positive expiratory pressure (PEP) mask therapy to a cystic fibrosis patient in the outpatient clinic. Upon entering the room to instruct the patient, she notices that there is *no* gas pressure source in the room. What should she do?

A. Proceed as ordered because PEP mask therapy requires no positive pressure source.
B. Obtain an E cylinder of oxygen from the supply room.
C. Describe the modality first, then return to the department for an air compressor.
D. Immerse the expiratory limb of the device 2 to 3 cm below the level of water placed in a cup.

117. A patient has a unilateral lung infection. Which of the following devices might be useful to help prevent infection of the contralateral lung?

A. Kamen–Wilkenson tube
B. Jackson–Reese tube
C. double-lumen ET tube
D. esophageal obturator

118. The RRT is preparing to deliver high-frequency ventilation to a neonatal patient. This patient must receive adequate humidification. Which of the following high-frequency ventilators would provide the easiest form of humidification?

I. high-frequency jet ventilation
II. high-frequency oscillation
III. high-frequency positive pressure ventilation

A. I only
B. II only
C. I, III only
D. I, II, III

119. A vortex-shedding, flow-sensing device is being used to measure a patient's vital capacity. The device has a high flow rate limit of 250 L/min. What should the RRT do in this situation?

A. Use the instrument only for measuring the vital capacity of a pediatric patient.
B. The device can be used to measure the vital capacity of pediatric and adult patients.
C. Use the device to measure only the slow vital capacity.
D. Make sure that the device is heated to body temperature.

120. While performing mouth-to-valve mask ventilation, the RRT observes that the patient's chest is *not* rising with each inspiration. Which of the following conditions may be the cause of this problem?

I. The one-way valve is *not* functioning properly.
II. The one-way valve is positioned backward.
III. The mask might *not* be sealing adequately on the patient's face.
IV. The patient might have vomited into the mask.

A. I, III only
B. II, IV only
C. I, II, III only
D. I, II, III, IV

121. A pediatric patient requiring mechanical ventilation is about to be transported to another health-care institution that has magnetic resonance imaging (MRI) capabilities. Which of the following ventilators would be able to accommodate the transport and the MRI exposure?

I. Newport E100i
II. Bio-Med MVP 10
III. Omni-Vent D
IV. Monaghan 225

A. I, II, IV only
B. III, IV only
C. III only
D. I only

122. The CANNOT-MEET-PIP alarm on the Life Plus high-frequency jet ventilator has been activated. Which of the following situations can cause this condition?

I. The pinch valve in the patient box might *not* be opening enough.
II. The purge solenoid in the patient box has malfunctioned.
III. The patient might be too large.
IV. The patient box is located too close to the monitoring lumen of the Hi-Lo Jet tracheal tube.

A. II, IV only
B. I, III only
C. I, III, IV only
D. I, II, III, IV

123. Upon entering the Neonatal Intensive Care Unit (NICU), the RRT notices that the SensorMedics 3100 high-frequency oscillatory ventilator is situated alongside a conventional mechanical ventilator. What should be her consideration at this time?

A. that the conventional ventilator is being used to humidify the gas delivered by the SensorMedics 3100
B. that the pressure gauges on the SensorMedics 3100 have malfunctioned and those on the conventional ventilator are being used
C. that the patient might be about to be weaned from high-frequency oscillatory ventilation
D. that periodic hyperinflations are being delivered by the conventional ventilator

SITUATIONAL SETS

**Questions 124 and 125 refer to the same patient.**

124. A 65-year-old patient is brought to the emergency department complaining of chest pains but displaying *no* signs of respiratory distress. The RRT immediately obtains an ECG that indicates ST-segment deviation and T-wave flattening. What form of oxygen therapy should the RRT institute?

A. Briggs adaptor at 40%
B. aerosol mask at 60%
C. trach collar at 50%
D. nasal cannula at 2 to 4 L/min.

125. Thirty minutes later, this patient begins coughing pink, frothy sputum. ABGs at this time reveal the following:

PO$_2$ 55 torr
PCO$_2$ 29 torr
pH 7.50
HCO$_3^-$ 22 mEq/liter
B.E. 0 mEq/liter

His ventilatory pattern is regular with a ventilatory rate of 20 breaths/min. and a tidal volume of 500 cc. The chest radiograph indicates pulmonary infiltrates and Kerley B lines. What type of oxygen-delivery device should the RRT now recommend?

A. nasal cannula at 6 L/min.
B. non-rebreathing mask at 10 L/min.
C. simple oxygen mask at 10 L/min.
D. aerosol mask at 40%

**Questions 126, 127, and 128 refer to the same patient.**

The RRT is preparing to ventilate a 145-pound (ideal body weight), 16-year-old patient with a Siemens Servo 900C ventilator. Before connecting the patient to the ventilator, the RRT sets the machine in the volume-control mode with a minute ventilation of 2 L/min. and a ventilatory rate of 10 breaths/min. She occludes the Y connector while the ventilator cycles on to inspiration. She observes the PIP reaching 55 cm H$_2$O in the presence of a PEEP of 5 cm H$_2$O.

126. Calculate the tubing compliance factor for this ventilator.

A. 3.00 cc/cm H$_2$O
B. 3.33 cc/cm H$_2$O
C. 4.00 cc/cm H$_2$O
D. 25.50 cc/cm H$_2$O

127. The RRT establishes the following settings on the Siemens Servo 900C:

minute ventilation: 8 L/min.
ventilatory rate: 10 breaths/min.
$F_{I}O_2$: 0.30
inspiratory time %: 33%
PEEP: 5 cm $H_2O$
mode: SIMV
SIMV rate: 8 breaths/min.

When the ventilator cycles to inspiration, the PIP achieved is 40 cm $H_2O$. Calculate this patient's actual tidal volume.

A. 500 cc
B. 615 cc
C. 660 cc
D. 800 cc

128. The physician's order indicates that the patient's tidal volume must equal 10 cc/kg of IBW. What ventilator setting adjustment must the RRT make?

A. Increase the minute ventilation to 10 L/min.
B. Decrease the minute ventilation to 6.5 L/min.
C. Decrease the ventilatory rate to 8 breaths/min.
D. *No* change is necessary.

**Questions 129 and 130 refer to the same patient.**

A 340-pound, 5-ft. 4-in, 38-year-old female was admitted to the hospital lethargic and somnolent. The following ABG data were obtained:

$PO_2$ 49 mm Hg
$PCO_2$ 76 mm Hg
pH 7.33

129. Which condition is this patient most likely experiencing?

A. sleep apnea syndrome
B. emotional stress or anxiety
C. pulmonary embolism
D. pulmonary fibrosis

130. Which therapeutic procedure would you institute immediately?

A. an air-entrainment mask at 24% $O_2$
B. ultrasonic nebulization with normal saline prn
C. q4h IPPB with Albuterol
D. q4h postural drainage

# Equipment Matrix Categories

1. IIB2e(3)
2. IIB2n(2)
3. IIA2
4. IIB1r
5. IIB1d
6. IIA1e(1)
7. IIA1i(3)
8. IIB1a(1)
9. IIB1e(1)
10. IIA1o
11. IIB1h(4)
12. IIB1e(1)
13. IIB2o
14. IIB2a(2)
15. IIB2h(4)
16. IIB2q(2)
17. IIB1h(2)
18. IIB1p
19. IIA1d
20. IIB1r
21. IIA1e(1)
22. IIB2e(1)
23. IIB1e(1)
24. IIB3b
25. IIB3a
26. IIA1i(1)
27. IIA1o
28. IIA1q(1)
29. IIB1o
30. IIA2
31. IIB1n(1)
32. IIB1i(1)
33. IIB1s

34. IIA1q(1)
35. IIB1h(4)
36. IIB2d
37. IIB1e(1)
38. IIB2h(4)
39. IIA1f(2)
40. IIB3
41. IIB1h(4)
42. IIA1k
43. IIB1i(2)
44. IIA1h(2)
45. IIB1a(1)
46. IIA1e(2)
47. IIB1e(2)
48. IIA2
49. IIB1h(5)
50. IIA1q(1)
51. IIB1c
52. IIB1e(1)
53. IIB1i(1)
54. IIB1h(5)
55. IIA1q(1)
56. IIA1u
57. IIB1c
58. IIB2s
59. IIA1h(2)
60. IIB1h(4)
61. IIA1h(5)
62. IIA1k
63. IIA1h(4)
64. IIB3b
65. IIB1h(4)
66. IIB1n(2)

67. IIB1a(1)
68. IIB1f(2)
69. IIA1k
70. IIA1h(4)
71. IIB3a
72. IIB1e(1)
73. IIB2c
74. IIA1q(1)
75. IIA1u
76. IIB3c
77. IIA1a(1)
78. IIA2
79. IIB2h(4)
80. IIB1f(2)
81. IIB2d
82. IIA1h(2)
83. IIB1f(2)
84. IIB2e(2)
85. IIB3c
86. IIB1a(2)
87. IIB1h(4)
88. IIA1h(3)
89. IIB1e(1)
90. IIB1f(4)
91. IIA1h(5)
92. IIA1e(2)
93. IIB1q(1)
94. IIB1p
95. IIB1q(1)
96. IIB1h(4)
97. IIA1h(4)
98. IIB2k
99. IIA1h(4)

100. IIB1h(4)
101. IIA1e(3)
102. IIB1e(1)
103. IIA1i(3)
104. IIB2e(1)
105. IIA1d
106. IIB1s
107. IIB3b
108. IIB1q(1)
109. IIA1r
110. IIB3a
111. IIA2
112. IIA1h(4)
113. IIB1h(4)
114. IIB1h(4)
115. IIB1e(1)
116. IIB1k
117. IIA1f(2)
118. IIA1e(2)
119. IIA1o
120. IIB1d
121. IIA1e(1)
122. IIB2e(2)
123. IIB1e(2)
124. IIA1a(1)
125. IIA1a(1)
126. IA1f
127. IB9b
128. IB10b
129. IA1a
130. IIA1a(1)

# Chapter 4 Equipment: Written Registry Examination Matrix Scoring Form

| Content Area | Equipment Item Number | Equipment Content Area Score | |
|---|---|---|---|
| IIA1. Select and obtain equipment. | 6,7,10,19,21,26,27,28, 34,39,42,46,50,55,56,59, 61,62,63,69,70,74,75,77, 82,88,91,92,97,99,101, 103,105,109,112,117,118, 119,121,124,125,130 | $\frac{}{42} \times 100 = \underline{\hspace{1cm}}\%$ | $\frac{}{48} \times 100 = \underline{\hspace{1cm}}\%$ |
| IIA2. Assure selected equipment cleanliness. | 3,30,44,48,78,111 | $\frac{}{6} \times 100 = \underline{\hspace{1cm}}\%$ | |
| IIB1. Assemble, check for proper function, and identify malfunctions of equipment. | 4,5,8,9,11,12,17,18,20, 23,29,31,32,33,35,37,41, 43,45,47,49,51,52,53,54, 57,60,65,66,67,68,72,80, 83,86,87,89,90,93,94,95, 96,100,102,106,108,113, 115,116,120,123 | $\frac{}{51} \times 100 = \underline{\hspace{1cm}}\%$ | $\frac{}{78} \times 100 = \underline{\hspace{1cm}}\%$ |
| IIB2. Take action to correct malfunctions of equipment. | 1,2,13,14,15,16, 22, 36,38,58,73,79,81,84, 98,104,114,122 | $\frac{}{18} \times 100 = \underline{\hspace{1cm}}\%$ | |
| IIB3. Perform quality control procedures. | 24,25,40,64,71, 76,85,107,110 | $\frac{}{9} \times 100 = \underline{\hspace{1cm}}\%$ | |

The following questions were part of situational sets and are not located on this scoring form because they do not pertain to section II, Equipment:

- 126 IA1f
- 127 IB9b
- 128 IB10b
- 129 IA1a

# NBRC Written Registry Examination for Advanced Respiratory Therapists (RRTs) Content Outline

This content outline is reprinted with permission of the copyright holder, the National Board For Respiratory Care, Inc., 8310 Nieman Rd, Lenexa, KS 66214. All rights reserved. Effective July 1999

| | RECALL | APPLICATION | ANALYSIS |
|---|---|---|---|
| **II. Select, Assemble, and Check Equipment for Proper Function, Operation, and Cleanliness** **SETTING:** In any patient care setting, the advanced respiratory therapist selects, assembles, and assures cleanliness of all equipment used in providing respiratory care. The therapist checks all equipment and corrects malfunctions. | **3** | **4** | **13** |
| **A. Select and obtain equipment and assure equipment cleanliness.** | **1** | **2** | **5** |
| 1. Select and obtain equipment appropriate to the respiratory care plan: | | | |
| a. oxygen administration devices | | | |
| (1) nasal cannula, mask, reservior mask (partial rebreathing, nonrebreathing), face tents, transtracheal oxygen catheter, oxygen conserving cannulas | X | X | |
| (2) air-entrainment devices, tracheostomy collar and T-piece, oxygen hoods and tents | X | X | |
| (3) CPAP devices | X | X | |
| b. humidifiers [e.g., bubble, passover, cascade, wick, heat moisture exchanger] | X | X | |
| c. aerosol generators [e.g., pneumatic nebulizer, ultrasonic nebulizer] | X | X | |
| d. resuscitation devices [e.g, manual resuscitator (bag-valve), pneumatic (demand-valve), mouth-to-valve mask resuscitator] | X | X | |
| e. ventilators | | | |
| (1) pneumatic, electric, microprocessor, fluidic | X | X | |
| (2) high frequency | | | |
| (3) noninvasive positive pressure | X | X | |
| f. artificial airways | | | |
| (1) oro- and nasopharyngeal airways | X | X | |
| (2) oral, nasal and double-lumen endotracheal tubes | X | X | |
| (3) tracheostomy tubes and buttons | X | X | |

| | RECALL | APPLICATION | ANALYSIS |
|---|---|---|---|
| (4) intubation equipment [e.g., laryngoscope and blades, exhaled $CO_2$ detection devices] | X | X | |
| (5) other airways [e.g., laryngeal mask airway (LMA), Esophageal Tracheal Combitube® (ETC)] | | | |
| g. suctioning devices [e.g., suction catheters, specimen collectors, oropharyngeal suction devices] | X | X | |
| h. gas delivery, metering and clinical analyzing devices | | | |
| (1) regulators, reducing valves, connectors and flowmeters, air/oxygen blenders, pulse-dose systems | X | X | |
| (2) oxygen concentrators, air compressors, liquid oxygen systems | X | X | |
| (3) gas cylinders, bulk systems and manifolds | X | X | |
| (4) capnograph, blood gas analyzer and sampling devices, co-oximeter, transcutaneous $O_2/CO_2$ monitor, pulse oximeter | X | X | |
| (5) CO, He, $O_2$ and specialty gas analyzers | X | X | |
| i. patient breathing circuits | | | |
| (1) IPPB, continuous mechanical ventilation | X | X | |
| (2) CPAP, PEEP valve assembly | X | X | |
| (3) H-valve assembly | | | X |
| j. environmental devices | | | |
| (1) incubators, radiant warmers | | | |
| (2) aerosol (mist) tents | X | X | |
| (3) scavenging systems | | X | X |
| k. positive expiratory pressure device (PEP) | | | |
| l. Flutter® mucous clearance device | | | X |
| m. other therapeutic gases [e.g., $O_2/CO_2$, He/$O_2$] | | | |
| n. manometers and gauges | | | |
| (1) manometers—water, mercury and aneroid, inspiratory/expiratory pressure meters, cuff pressure manometers | X | X | |
| (2) pressure transducers | X | X | |
| o. respirometers [e.g., flow-sensing devices (pneumotachometer), volume displacement] | X | X | |

| | RECALL | APPLICATION | ANALYSIS |
|---|:---:|:---:|:---:|
| p. electrocardiography devices [e.g., ECG oscilloscope monitors, ECG machines (12-lead), Holter monitors] | X | X | |
| q. hemodynamic monitoring devices | | | |
|   (1) central venous catheters, pulmonary artery catheters [e.g., Swan-Ganz], cardiac output, continuous $S\bar{v}O_2$ monitors | | | |
|   (2) arterial catheters | | | |
| r. vacuum systems [e.g., pumps, regulators, collection bottles, pleural drainage devices] | X | X | |
| s. metered dose inhalers (MDI), MDI spacers | X | X | |
| t. Small Particle Aerosol Generators (SPAG) | X | X | |
| u. bronchoscopes | X | X | |
| 2. Assure selected equipment cleanliness [e.g., select or determine appropriate agent and technique for disinfection and/or sterilization, perform procedures for disinfection and/or sterilization, monitor effectiveness of sterilization procedures] | X | X | |
| **B. Assemble and check equipment function, identify and correct equipment malfunctions, and perform quality control.** | **2** | **2** | **8** |
| 1. Assemble, check for proper function, and identify malfunctions of equipment: | | | |
| a. oxygen administration devices | | | |
|   (1) nasal cannula, mask, reservoir mask (partial rebreathing, nonrebreathing), face tents, transtracheal oxygen catheter, oxygen conserving cannulas | X | X | |
|   (2) air-entrainment devices, tracheostomy collar and T-piece, oxygen hoods and tents | X | X | |
|   (3) CPAP devices | X | X | |
| b. humidifiers [e.g., bubble, passover, cascade, wick, heat moisture exchanger] | X | X | |
| c. aerosol generators [e.g., pneumatic nebulizer, ultrasonic nebulizer] | X | X | |
| d. resuscitation devices [e.g., manual resuscitator (bag-valve), pneumatic (demand-valve), mouth-to-valve mask resuscitator] | X | X | |
| e. ventilators | | | |
|   (1) pneumatic, electric, microprocessor, fluidic | X | X | |
|   (2) high frequency | | | |
|   (3) noninvasive positive pressure | X | X | |

| | RECALL | APPLICATION | ANALYSIS |
|---|:---:|:---:|:---:|
| f. artificial airways | | | |
|   (1) oro- and nasopharyngeal airways | X | X | |
|   (2) oral, nasal and double-lumen endotracheal tubes | X | X | |
|   (3) tracheostomy tubes and buttons | X | X | |
|   (4) intubation equipment [e.g., laryngoscope and blades, exhaled $CO_2$ detection devices] | X | X | |
| g. suctioning devices [e.g., suction catheters, speciment collectors, oropharyngeal suction devices] | X | X | |
| h. gas delivery, metering and clinical analyzing devices | | | |
|   (1) regulators, reducing valves, connectors and flowmeters, air/oxygen blenders, pulse-dose systems | X | X | |
|   (2) oxygen concentrators, air compressors, liquid oxygen systems | X | X | |
|   (3) gas cylinders, bulk, systems and manifolds | X | X | |
|   (4) capnograph, blood gas analyzer and sampling devices, co-oximeter, transcutaneous $O_2/CO_2$ monitor, pulse oximeter | X | X | |
|   (5) CO, He, $O_2$ and specialty gas analyzers | X | X | |
| i. patient breathing circuits | | | |
|   (1) IPPB, continuous mechanical ventilation | X | X | |
|   (2) CPAP, PEEP valve assembly | X | X | |
|   (3) H-valve assembly | | X | X |
| j. environmental devices | | | |
|   (1) incubators, radiant warmers | | | |
|   (2) aerosol (mist) tents | X | X | |
| k. positive expiratory pressure (PEP) device | | | |
| l. Flutter® mucous clearance device | | | X |
| m. other therapeutic gases [e.g., $O_2/CO_2$, He/$O_2$] | | | |
| n. manometers and gauges | | | |
|   (1) manometers—water, mercury and aneroid, inspiratory/expiratory pressure meters, cuff pressure manometers | X | X | |
|   (2) pressure transducers | | | |
| o. respirometers [e.g., flow-sensing devices (pneumotachometer), volume displacement] | X | X | |
| p. electrocardiography devices [e.g., ECG oscilloscope monitors, ECG machines (12-lead), Holter monitors] | X | X | |

| | RECALL | APPLICATION | ANALYSIS |
|---|:---:|:---:|:---:|
| q. hemodynamic monitoring devices | | | |
|   (1) central venous catheters, pulmonary artery catheters [e.g., Swan-Ganz], cardiac output, continuous $s\bar{v}O_2$ monitors | | | |
|   (2) arterial catheters | | | |
| r. vacuum systems [e.g., pumps, regulators, collection bottles, pleural drainage devices] | X | X | |
| s. bronchoscopes | | | X |
| 2. Take action to correct malfunctions of equipment: | | | |
|   a. oxygen administration devices | | | |
|     (1) nasal cannula, mask, reservoir mask (partial rebreathing, nonrebreathing), face tents, transtracheal oxygen catheter, oxygen conserving cannulas | X | X | |
|     (2) air-entrainment devices, tracheostomy collar and T-piece, oxygen hoods and tents | X | X | |
|     (3) CPAP devices | X | X | |
|   b. humidifiers [e.g., bubble, passover, cascade, wick, heat moisture exchanger] | X | X | |
|   c. aerosol generators [e.g., pneumatic nebulizer, ultrasonic nebulizer] | X | X | |
|   d. resuscitation devices [e.g., manual resuscitator (bag-valve), pneumatic (demand-valve), mouth-to-valve mask resuscitator] | X | X | |
|   e. ventilators | | | |
|     (1) pneumatic, electric, microprocessor, fluidic | X | X | |
|     (2) high frequency | | | |
|     (3) noninvasive positive pressure | X | X | |
|   f. artificial airways | | | |
|     (1) oro- and nasopharyngeal airways | X | X | |
|     (2) oral, nasal and double-lumen endotracheal tubes | X | X | |
|     (3) tracheostomy tubes and buttons | X | X | |
|     (4) intubation equipment [e.g., laryngoscope and blades, exhaled $CO_2$ detection devices] | X | X | |
|   g. suctioning devices [e.g., suction catheters, specimen collectors, oropharyngeal suction devices] | X | X | |
|   h. gas delivery, metering and clinical analyzing devices | | | |
|     (1) regulators, reducing valves, connectors and flowmeters, air/oxygen blenders, pulse-dose systems | X | X | |
|     (2) oxygen concentrators, air compressors, liquid oxygen systems | X | X | |

| | RECALL | APPLICATION | ANALYSIS |
|---|:---:|:---:|:---:|
|     (3) gas cylinders, bulk systems and manifolds | X | X | |
|     (4) capnograph, blood gas analyzer and sampling devices, co-oximeter, transcutaneous $O_2/CO_2$ monitor, pulse oximeter | X | X | |
|     (5) CO, He, $O_2$ and specialty gas analyzers | | | |
|   i. patient breathing circuits | | | |
|     (1) IPPB, continuous mechanical ventilation | X | X | |
|     (2) CPAP, PEEP valve assembly | X | X | |
|     (3) H-valve assembly | | | X |
|   j. environmental devices | | | |
|     (1) incubators, radiant warmers | | | X |
|     (2) aerosol (mist) tents | X | X | |
|   k. positive expiratory pressure (PEP) device | | | |
|   l. Flutter® mucous clearance device | | | X |
|   m. other therapeutic gases [e.g., $O_2/CO_2$, $He/O_2$] | | | |
|   n. manometers and gauges | | | |
|     (1) manometers—water, mercury and aneroid, inspiratory/expiratory pressure meters, cuff pressure manometers | X | X | |
|     (2) pressure transducers | | | |
|   o. respirometers [e.g., flow-sensing devices (pneumotachometer), volume displacement] | X | X | |
|   p. electrocardiography devices [e.g., ECG oscilloscope monitors, ECG machines (12-lead), Holter monitors] | | | |
|   q. hemodynamic monitoring devices | | | |
|     (1) central venous catheters, pulmonary artery catheters [e.g., Swan-Ganz], cardiac output, continuous $S\bar{v}O_2$ monitors | | | |
|     (2) arterial catheters | | | |
|   r. vacuum systems [e.g., pumps, regulators, collection bottles, pleural drainage devices] | X | X | |
|   s. Small Particle Aerosol Generators (SPAG) | | X | X |
|   t. bronchoscopes | | | X |
| 3. Perform quality control procedures for: | | | |
|   a. blood gas analyzers and sampling devices, co-oximeters | X | X | |
|   b. pulmonary function equipment, ventilator volume/flow/pressure calibration | X | X | |
|   c. gas metering devices | X | X | |
|   d. noninvasive monitors [e.g., transcutaneous] | | | |

# Equipment Answers and Analyses

**NOTE:** The references listed after each analysis are numbered and keyed to the reference list located at the end of this section. The first number indicates the text. The second number indicates the page where information about the questions can be found. For example, (1:219, 384) means that on pages 219 and 384 of reference number 1, information about the question will be found. Frequently, it will be necessary to read beyond the page number indicated to obtain complete information. Therefore, reference to the question will be found either on the page indicated or on subsequent pages.

**IIB2e(3)**

1. D. The BiPAP® unit provides a light-emitting device (LED) readout of the estimated, exhaled tidal volume setting after each transition to IPAP, indicating the last exhaled tidal volume. The estimated, exhaled tidal volume is analyzed via an internal pneumotach to determine which portion of the circuit flow contributes to patient ventilation and which portion leaks out of the circuit. The patient flow portion is converted to volume. Keep in mind that the BiPAP® system is not an air-tight system. You can compensate for small to moderate leaks.

   The flashing estimated, exhaled tidal volume light indicates a possible discrepancy in the tidal volume display. The system has determined that a change in the circuit leak is affecting the accuracy of the display. If the leak is too great, the BiPAP® system might be unable to compensate for it. Therefore, the RRT needs to (1) check for leaks in the tubing system, (2) evaluate the area around the mask for leaks, and (3) observe the patient's breathing to determine whether air is escaping from the mouth. The exhalation ports are not a source for leaks because air flows through this component when the patient exhales.

   (BiPAP® S/T-D Ventilatory Support System product information, Respironics, Inc.), (1:866, 878).

**IIB2n(2)**

2. D. The dome of the strain gauge pressure transducer must be level with the location of the tip of the catheter. In the case of a central venous pressure (CVP) catheter, the dome of the transducer must be level with the patient's mid-chest or phlebostatic axis. The phlebostatic axis is the junction of the patient's mid-axillary line and fourth intercostal space. Figure 4-8 illustrates the proper relationship between the pressure transducer and the tip of the CVP catheter.

   (9:341–342), (14:168–170).

**IA2**

3. D. Glass and metal objects that are ethylene oxide sterilized do not absorb the gas. Therefore, equipment

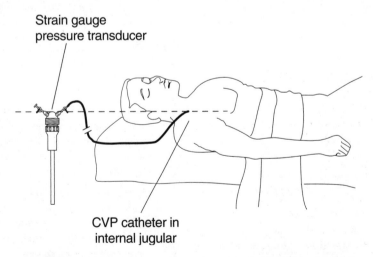

Strain gauge
pressure transducer

CVP catheter in
internal jugular

**Figure 4-8:** Proper pressure transducer–CVP catheter alignment. Note that the strain-gauge pressure-transducer dome is level with the right atrium.

made of these materials that has undergone ethylene oxide sterilization requires no aeration time and can be used immediately upon removal from an ethylene oxide sterilizing chamber.

Porous materials must be adequately aerated for the removal of residual ethylene oxide gas. Equipment that is composed of polyvinyl chloride (PVC) requires the longest aeration time.

(1:47), (13:672–673).

## IIB1r

4. A. The absence of continuous bubbling in the suction-control bottle indicates a malfunction in the pleural drainage system. The RRT needs to check all of the system connections, pressure settings, and water levels. The chest tubes should be checked for the presence of obstructions. The possible causes for system malfunctioning generally include (1) air leaking into the pleural drainage system, (2) air leaking into the intrapleural space around the chest tube, and (3) mechanical failure of the vacuum source. A chest drainage system can be deliberately shut off at the physician's request. The RRT should not assume that the system must always be active.

(9:264–267), (15:1092–1094).

## IIB1d

5. D. Demand-valve, gas-powered resuscitation devices can be operated manually or can be patient triggered. Patient triggering occurs as the negative pressure developed within the patient's thorax is transmitted to the nozzle of the device that houses an exhalation leaf diaphragm, sensing line, and sensing diaphragm. If any of these components malfunction, patient triggering might become compromised.

(13:201).

## IIA1e(1)

6. B. The profile of the ideal home ventilator patient includes the following:

   - having a neuromuscular disease
   - having a neurologic disorder (i.e., sleep apnea)
   - being cardiovascularly stable
   - possessing a good attitude and motivation
   - having a supportive family and nursing care
   - having some degree of ventilatory dependence

Home mechanical ventilation can be a complex matter. A quiet home environment is transformed into a technically oriented, ICU-like situation. Family members are required to perform unfamiliar technical activities. Therefore, the more factors that can be simplified, the less confusing the home setting becomes. The more stable the patient, the less likely complications will

arise. Not all patients fit the ideal home ventilation profile, however. It is not unusual for ventilated patients to require PEEP or to have difficulty creating an adequate seal with their tracheostomy tube cuff.

(1:1122–1125), (13:576).

## IIA1i(3)

7. D. Two types of intermittent mandatory ventilation (IMV) systems are available: continuous-flow IMV and demand flow IMV. One method for adapting an IMV system to a ventilator circuit is the H-valve assembly shown in Figure 4-9.

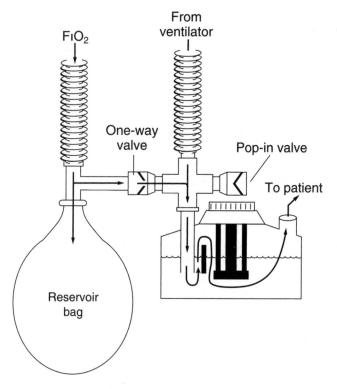

**Figure 4-9:** H-valve assembly for the IMV system attached to the mechanical ventilator.

For this assembly to be used as a continuous-flow system, a one-way valve (not a demand valve) is placed between the continuous-flow system (for spontaneous breathing) and the ventilator circuit (for mandatory breathing) just before the humidifier. The continuous gas flow from this external system (supplied by either a blender or oxygen and air flow meters) should be sufficient enough to keep the one-way valve open so that the patient is not required to increase her work of breathing to open the valve.

This one-way valve also ensures that the patient will receive the benefit of the mandatory breath when the ventilator cycles on to inspiration. During the ventilator's inspiratory cycle, the one-way valve closes as the pressure in the ventilator circuit increases. Closure of the one-way valve at this time also prevents a loss of volume into the H-valve assembly circuitry and reservoir bag.

It is not necessary for the reservoir bag (3 to 5 liters) to have an adjustable screw clamp to vent excessive gas flow. The gas flow from the blender or from the oxygen and air flow meters must be adequate to prevent the reservoir bag from completely collapsing whenever the patient takes a spontaneous breath, however.

A continuous-flow IMV system does not incorporate a demand valve. Such a valve is employed in a demand-flow IMV apparatus and ideally should require about a $-1$ to $-2$ cm $H_2O$ pressure generated by the patient to open. In reality, however, many demand valves fail to meet their functional specifications and often require the patient to generate higher negative inspiratory pressures. The pressure manometer does not always reflect the actual negative pressure developed by the patient to open a demand valve.

(1:861–863), (10:329–330), (15:958, 1053).

## IIB1a(1)

8. D. In the event that a transtracheal catheter dislodges, the patient should be seen by a physician immediately. In the meantime, having the patient use a nasal cannula will minimize the risk of the patient developing hypoxemia.

(Tiep, B., et al. 1990, "Pulsed and Transtracheal Oxygen Delivery," *Chest, 97,* 364–368), (1:744, 1117–1118), (5:70), (13:72–73).

## IIB1e(1)

9. C. The Puritan–Bennett Companion 2801 does not have an $F_IO_2$ control, thus "readjusting the $F_IO_2$ control dial to 0.30" is not a reasonable response. The patient is receiving an $F_IO_2$ of 0.24; therefore, the oxygen bleed-in tube must already be attached. Otherwise, analysis of the ventilator's $F_IO_2$ would have been 0.21. Replacing the ventilator is time-consuming and unnecessary. Increasing the flow rate until the desired $F_IO_2$ is achieved would be the most appropriate course of action.

(13:577, 578, 580), (15:1130).

## IIA1o

10. B. Although the Fleisch pneumotachometer is affected by altitude, gas densities, and temperature alterations, it is the most accurate in terms of measuring volumes and flow rates. It is a pressure differential pneumotach that consists of a capillary mesh to create the pressure

drop as gas flows through the instrument. The pressure gradient is electronically detected, allowing for the continuous monitoring of flow rates, volumes, and ventilatory rates of ventilator patients.

A Wright Respirometer is inaccurate at flow rates of less than 3 L/min. and can be damaged by flow rates greater than 300 L/min. This instrument is relatively delicate. The inertia of the gear mechanism and its rotating vanes affects its accuracy. The Dräger Volumeter experiences the same inertia problem as the Wright Respirometer.

A Tissot spirometer is used to collect large volumes (liters) of exhaled gas. It is sometimes used in conjunction with functional residual capacity (FRC) determinations via helium equilibration tests.

(1:202, 373), (5:294–295), (13:292–293, 295).

## IIA1h(4)

11. B. Transcutaneous electrode placement is critical to obtaining useful data. The electrode must be placed on a non-bony area. It must be situated in a location where it can lie flat and maintain an effective seal around its edges. Hair and folds of skin need to be avoided.

If a transcutaneous electrode is to be used in conjunction with cardiopulmonary resuscitation (CPR), the electrode should be placed on either shoulder. That location affords a lower potential for disturbance or dislodgement. The sternum would be a poor location because the lower two-thirds of the adult sternum is the cardiac compression site. Additionally, placing the transcutaneous electrode on either shoulder avoids interference with ECG leads.

(1:355–356), (5:292–296), (13:267–269), (15:497–498).

## IIB1e(1)

12. C. The Bio-Med MVP-10 transport ventilator is categorized as pneumatically powered and time cycled with continuous flow. The CPAP level on this ventilator can be set as high as 18 cm $H_2O$. Whenever a patient receives continuous-flow CPAP and the pressure during inspiration falls more than 1 to 2 cm $H_2O$, the likelihood is that the flow rate is not meeting the patient's inspiratory demands. When this situation develops, the flow through the system must be increased.

(13:533–534, 564–565).

## IIB2o

13. C. The Wright Respirometer is accurate to $\pm$ 10% of the preset volume. For example, for a volume of 800 cc, the acceptable measured range is 720 to 880 cc.

Because

$$800 \text{ cc}$$
$$\times \ 0.10$$
$$\overline{80 \text{ cc}}$$

then

$$800 \text{ cc} - 80 \text{ cc} = 720 \text{ cc}$$
$$800 \text{ cc} + 80 \text{ cc} = 880 \text{ cc}$$

Therefore, the 740 cc reading is an acceptable value because it represents −7.5% of the set value.

$$\frac{740 \text{ cc}}{800 \text{ cc}} \times 100 = 92.5\%$$

or

$$(800 \text{ cc})(-7.5\%) = -60 \text{ cc}$$
$$800 \text{ cc} - 60 \text{cc} = 740 \text{ cc}$$

(5:276–277), (13:295).

## IIB2a(1)

14. D. Correcting the patient's shortness of breath is the primary goal. A disconnection or obstruction in gas flow to the patient, followed by inadequate flow, are the two most likely equipment causes of this problem.

An empty nebulizer presents several hazards that include drying of secretions, humidity deficits, and pulmonary burns if heat is applied.

Because the patient is ventilating and only complaining of the shortness of breath, there is no need to manually ventilate at this time. Manual ventilation would be indicated if the patient was showing signs of obstruction (i.e., chest movement without airflow or with minimal airflow, restlessness, and cyanosis).

(5:168), (13:78).

## IIB2h(4)

15. D. According to the troubleshooting section of the operator's manual for the IL 182 Co-Oximeter, high hemoglobin readings can be caused by (1) an unmixed sample, (2) a lack of diluent, (3) a blocked diluent feed line, and (4) use of the wrong diluent.

(*Instruction Handbook—IL 182 Co-Oximeter,* Instrumentation Laboratories, Lexington, MA, p. 35).

## IIB2q(2)

16. C. To assure the patency of an arterial line catheter, the system requires a constant and continuous infusion of fluid. The literature recommends 2 to 4 ml/hour, not

12 to 14 ml/hour. All connections must be secured. Flushing the system is essential after blood samples are obtained. In this particular situation, the pressure in the patient's artery is obviously greater than that of the arterial line system. Therefore, the RRT must ensure that the I.V. bag pressure is greater than the patient's arterial pressure. Generally, the I.V. bag pressure is maintained at 300 mm Hg.

(14:205–206), (15:525–529).

## IIA1h(2)

17. D. The following calculations demonstrate how to determine the duration of gaseous oxygen flow from a liquid oxygen system. One must remember that, under ordinary ambient temperature and pressure conditions, one pound of liquid oxygen equals approximately 344 liters of gaseous oxygen.

STEP 1: Determine the weight (lbs) of liquid oxygen remaining in the system.

$$100 \text{ lbs} \times 0.75 = 75 \text{ lbs}$$

STEP 2: Compute the amount (L) of gaseous oxygen equivalent to 75 lbs of liquid oxygen.

$$75 \text{ lbs} \times 344 \text{ L/lb} = 25{,}800 \text{ L}$$

STEP 3: Calculate the duration of flow for the liquid oxygen system.

$$\frac{25{,}800 \text{ L}}{3 \text{ L/min.}} = 8{,}600 \text{ min.}$$

STEP 4: Convert 8,600 minutes to days by using the factor-units method.

$$(8{,}600)\left(\frac{1 \text{ hour}}{60 \text{ min.}}\right)\left(\frac{1 \text{ day}}{24 \text{ hours}}\right) \approx 6.0 \text{ days}$$

(1:1115), (5:28), (17:56–57).

## IIA1p

18. A. There are three groups of electrocardiographic leads: (1) standard bipolar limb leads, (2) augmented unipolar limb leads, and (3) chest or precordial leads. Among the three groups, there are 12 leads. Table 4-2 indicates the specific leads in each group.

The difference among the leads is the positioning of the positive electrode in relation to the negative electrode. Each of the 12 leads offers a different electrical "view" of the conduction of impulses through the heart.

Leads II, III, and aVF are set up in such a manner that the waves of cardiac depolarization travel in the direc-

**Table 4-2** Electrocardiographic Leads

| Standard Bipolar Limb Leads | Augmented Limb Leads | Chest (Precordial) Leads | |
|---|---|---|---|
| Lead I | aVR | V1 | V4 |
| Lead II | aVL | V2 | V5 |
| Lead III | aVF | V3 | V6 |

tion of the positive electrode. Any time a depolarization wave moves toward the positive electrode, an upward deflection will occur.

The augmented limb lead aVR normally displays an inverted ECG because the depolarization wave, which moves from the heart base to the apex, travels away from the positive electrode connected to the right arm. The aVR lead has the positive electrode positioned above and to the right of the heart.

(9:198–201).

## IIA1d

19. A. The only real advantage of gas-powered resuscitators (demand valves) is that they provide 100% oxygen to the patient. Disadvantages include (a) variable delivered volumes, (b) potentially high pressures, and (c) high flow rates. The latter two can contribute to the incidence of barotrauma and massive gastric insufflation.

    (13:201).

## IIB1r

20. A. In this situation, the pressure gauge is indicating line vacuum pressure, which is not the pressure that should be applied to the patient's airways during the suctioning procedure. Most suction regulators have a mode control for switching from line vacuum pressure, which creates a negative pressure as low as −635 mm Hg, to the regulated suction mode, ranging from 0 mm Hg to −200 mm Hg. Therefore, when the patient is about to be suctioned, the mode control must be in the regulated position to enable the appropriate negative pressure to be dialed by using the vacuum-control knob.

    Table 4-3 indicates the generally accepted suction pressure range for neonates, pediatrics, and adults.

For the adult patient referred to here, the vacuum-control knob should not be adjusted to read more negative (subatmospheric) than −120 mm Hg.

(1:616).

## IIA1e(1)

21. D. The Monaghan 225/SIMV ventilator is pneumatically powered and fluidically controlled. Because this ventilator contains no electrical circuits and uses fluidic logic, it is suitable to use in the environment of an MRI device. In fact, the Monaghan Medical Corporation manufacturers a nonmagnetic version of the Monaghan 225/SIMV ventilator for this specific purpose.

    (2:485–486).

## IIB2e(1)

22. C. Based on the RRT's assessment, the patient is ventilating well and is not experiencing respiratory distress. The problem is in the ventilator system. Because either a disconnected inspiratory limb or disconnected tubing to the expiratory diaphragm would be associated with respiratory distress, these possibilities can be eliminated because she is ventilating satisfactorily. Even though replacing the ventilator would probably correct the problem, it is unnecessary to do so at this time because all options have not been explored.

    The Bourns Bear 1 incorporates a vortex-shedding, ultrasonic flow transducer that monitors the exhaled tidal volume by measuring the exhaled gas flow rate and electronically converting it to a volume. The likelihood is that condensation has accumulated on the ultrasonic transducer and/or the sensor.

    (5:406–408), (13:403).

## IIB1e(1)

23. A. A liquid oxygen system is an inappropriate power source for a pneumatically powered device that demands a 50-psig gas source. A liquid oxygen system generally maintains an internal pressure of 20 to 25 psig when not in use. As the cryogenically stored oxygen continues to vaporize, pressure above this level is vented to the atmosphere through a pressure-release valve in the system. Because the internal pressure of a liquid oxygen system does not meet the 50-psig pressure requirements for a pneumatically powered ventilator, the ventilator's low pressure alarm would sound.

**Table 4-3** Recommended Suction Pressures for Patients

| Neonates | Pediatrics | Adults |
|---|---|---|
| −60 to −80 mm Hg | −80 to −100 mm Hg | −100 to −120 mm Hg |

Alternatively, an electrically powered ventilator could be used. If this option is not possible, an electrically driven air compressor can serve as a power source for the pneumatic ventilator, and supplemental oxygen can be provided via an oxygen concentrator connected directly in-line with the ventilator tubing.

(5:548), (13:576).

## IIB3b

24. C. There are two types of quality-control systems: internal and external. Internal quality-control programs are set up to achieve precision of instrumentation within a laboratory. The procedures and protocols set up are intended to detect discrepancies among the instruments used in a laboratory. External quality control is termed *proficiency testing*. It is a mechanism whereby a laboratory can compare the results of its analysis with those derived from other laboratories. The quality-control samples used are received from a central, noncommercial, independent agency. These samples are then analyzed and the data are sent to the central distribution center.

(1:351), (6:295–297).

## IIB3a

25. B. Shifting (i.e., a sudden movement of analyzed data outside the acceptable standard deviation limit) is one type of systematic error. Shifting occurs when there is a sudden shift or movement of the results, followed by a plateauing or clustering of ensuing analyzed data. The diagram in Figure 4-10 demonstrates data shifting.

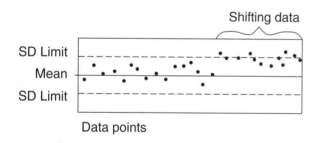

**Figure 4-10:** Analyzed data illustrating the shift outside the acceptable standard deviation (SD) limit (rapid movement of analyzed results away from the mean).

Situations related to blood gas analyzer electrode shifting include (1) contaminated calibration standards, (2) temperature changes in calibration standards, and (3) air bubbles under the membrane.

Another variety of systematic error is trending. Trending describes the continual movement of analyzed results away from the mean. This deviation is not sudden, but gradual. The nature of the deviation from the mean differentiates trending from shifting. The diagram in Figure 4-11 illustrates data trending.

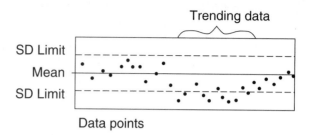

**Figure 4-11:** Analyzed data demonstrating trending (gradual movement of analyzed results away from the mean).

Clinical conditions that can cause trending to occur in conjunction with blood gas analyzer electrodes include (1) mercury battery aging, (2) electrode aging, and (3) protein contamination.

(1:352), (4:47–49).

## IIA1a(1)

26. B. Ventilator circuitry has an inspiratory and an expiratory limb. They converge at a common area called the *patient Y-adaptor*. An exhalation valve is positioned in the expiratory limb and is activated during inspiration with gas from the ventilator. Consequently, gas cannot flow past the exhalation valve and move through the inspiratory limb into the patient's lungs.

At the end of inspiration, the exhalation valve opens, enabling gas from the patient's lungs to flow through the expiratory limb as the gas from the ventilator is trapped or compressed in the inspiratory line. During these events, the only gas that is rebreathed by the patient is about 5 cc located at the patient Y-adaptor.

(5:413).

## IIA1o

27. C. A differential pressure pneumotachometer enables for the direct measurement of a patient's work of breathing. The pneumotachometer is placed between the ventilator and the patient near the proximal airway. The pneumotachometer measures all of the components of the total work of breathing, which include (1) the lung, (2) the thorax, and (3) the imposed work of breathing (ventilator circuitry or ET tube). These components are measured when the work of breathing is performed by the ventilator; therefore, the patient is not spontaneously breathing.

The pneumotachometer directly measures proximal airway pressure. Signals from the pneumotachometer are sent to a computer for volume changes to be calculated (i.e., time × flow = volume). Calculations are also made to compute the area under a pressure-volume curve to render the work of breathing expressed in kg-meter/liter (kg-m/liter) or joules/liter (J/liter).

The normal range of values for the total work of breathing is 0.073 kg-m/liter. Because 1 kg-m is about 10 J, kg-m can be converted to J/liter as follows:

$$0.073 \text{ kg-m/liter} \times 10 \text{ J/kg-m} = 0.73 \text{ J/liter}$$

Table 4-4 illustrates the normal work of breathing ranges for the lungs, thorax, and total system for healthy persons.

**Table 4-4** Normal Work of Breathing Ranges

| Work of Breathing | J/liter | kg-m/liter |
|---|---|---|
| lungs | 0.35–0.50 | 0.035–0.05 |
| thorax | 0.35–0.50 | 0.035–0.05 |
| total | 0.70–1.00 | 0.07–0.10 |

Again, to determine the total work of breathing (WOB) to which the patient is exposed, the lung-thorax system must be inflated with positive pressure when the patient is apneic. This condition enables the following measurement to be obtained:

$$WOB_T = WOB_L + WOB_{CW} + WOB_I$$

where

$WOB_T$ = total work of breathing (J/liter)
$WOB_L$ = lung work of breathing (J/liter)
$WOB_{CW}$ = chest wall work of breathing (J/liter)
$WOB_I$ = imposed (ventilator circuitry) work of breathing (J/liter)

This determination will provide the work of breathing that the patient must perform when he resumes spontaneous breathing in this system.

(1:205–208), (15:19).

## IIA1q(1)

28. D. In addition to measuring hemodynamic pressures and allowing for the calculation of vascular resistances, the pulmonary artery catheter (PAC) is used to determine the cardiac output (C.O.) by the thermodilution method. Usually, 10 cc of injectate (dextrose or normal saline) at either 0°C or room temperature is injected into the proximal injection port or channel, which communicates with an opening about 30 cm from the tip of the catheter. This opening is situated on the catheter such that it will reside in the right atrium when the PAC is properly positioned.

Therefore, the iced (0°C) or room-temperature injectate enters the right atrium and changes temperature in transit through the right ventricle and pulmonary artery. In the pulmonary artery, a thermistor senses the temperature change, which is then displayed on a C.O. computer. (See Figure 4-12 on page 216.)

The diagram depicts (1) the proximal port where the injectate is injected, (2) the opening in the right atrium where the injectate enters the heart, (3) the thermistor located in the pulmonary artery, sensing blood temperature changes, (4) the C.O. computer connected to the thermistor port, and (5) the C.O. curve.

(1:943–949), (9:322–324, 344–345), (15:533–534).

## IIB1o

29. A. The Fleisch pneumotachometer contains a series of parallel capillary tubes through which the gas flows. The resistance across these capillary tubes (resistive elements) can be measured accurately as long as a laminar gas flow pattern exists through the flow resistors. Ordinarily, the Fleisch pneumotach is heated to 37°C to prevent condensation in the capillary tubes, which in turn reduces resistance to flow. If the unit is not adequately heated, condensation will develop in the capillary tubes, causing the resistance through these resistors to increase. Thus, the flow rate measured, based on the pressure gradient and resistance across these resistors, would be inaccurate.

(5:275), (13:294).

## IIA2

30. D. Isopropyl and ethyl alcohol are effective bactericidal and fungicidal agents. They accomplish these activities by denaturation of cellular protein. The most effective concentration of isopropyl alcohol is 70%. This type of solution is common throughout the hospital setting and therefore is easily attainable. Ethyl alcohol is an effective disinfectant at concentrations between 50% and 70%.

(1:44–45), (13:670).

## IIB1n(1)

31. D. Placement of the ET tube is acceptable (i.e., the tip is 2 to 3 cm from the carina), and the patient is stable. Because the ET tube cuff pressure manometer does not indicate zero pressure when it is removed from the pilot balloon line, the manometer is likely malfunctioning. Another cuff pressure manometer needs to be obtained while the previous one is repaired.

The fact that this patient is verbally communicative indicates that air is moving around the cuff and past

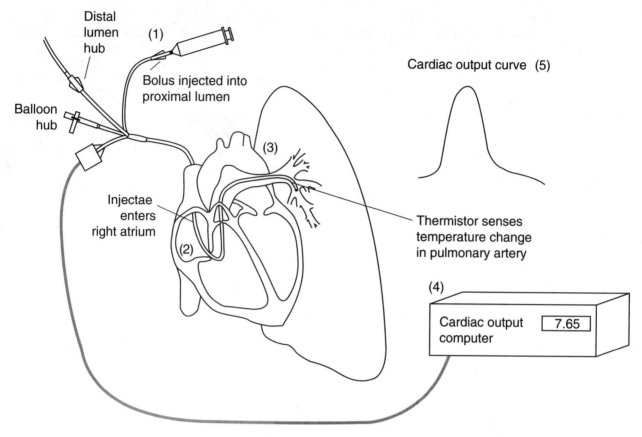

**Figure 4-12:** (1) Proximal port where injectate is injected, (2) opening in right atrium where injectate enters heart, (3) thermistor located in pulmonary artery sensing blood temperature changes, (4) cardiac output computer connected to the thermistor port, and (5) cardiac output curve.

the vocal cords. Therefore, the cuff needs to be inflated. Because the cuff pressure manometer is malfunctioning, however, the instillation of additional air must be withheld until a working pressure manometer is obtained.

(1:609–610), (15:836).

**IIA1i(1)**

32. A. The Bird Mark-series ventilators are unique because they do not require three separate tubings to supply main flow gas to power the nebulizer and to operate the expiratory diaphragm. In fact, one line supplies both the nebulizer and the exhalation valve assembly. Therefore, only two tubes are required for the Bird Mark VII ventilator.

(13:345–349).

**IIB1s**

33. C. The following actions should be taken to troubleshoot the nonfunctioning light source on the bron-

choscope: (1) the tip of the bronchoscope should be wiped with sterile gauze to remove possible residue, (2) the light source should be plugged into the wall outlet, and (3) the bronchoscope should be reseated to the light source connection. Passing a cytology brush has nothing to do with the light source. The brush extends through the accessory port.

(1:623–626), (15:627–634).

**IIA1q(1)**

34. C. Swan–Ganz catheter insertion does not require fluoroscopy because the catheter has flow-directed capabilities (balloon tip) and because each catheter position displays a characteristic waveform, as shown in Figure 4-13.

RA = right atrial pressure
RV = right ventricular pressure
PAP = pulmonary artery pressure
PCWP = pulmonary capillary wedge pressure

(1:943–948), (9:347–352), (15:529–532).

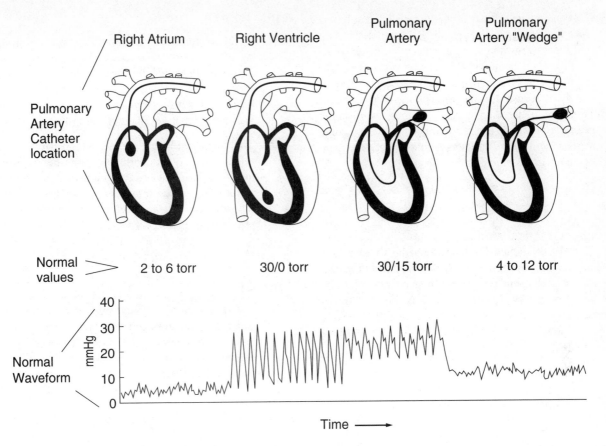

**Figure 4-13:** PAC locations and respective normal pressure ranges and waveforms.

**IIB1h(4)**

35. D. Troubleshooting guides can be obtained from the equipment manufacturer. These guides often facilitate the detection of problems when equipment fails or is not in control. Regarding blood gas and acid-base analyzer electrodes, troubleshooting is indicated when the data have been out of control for at least two daily shifts or when a random error of greater than 3 standard deviations (SD) occurs.

Blood gas analyzer electrodes are considered in control when data are within ±2 SD of known sample values. A random error, an isolated datum outside the control limits, is usually ignored (concerning electrode data) unless it is greater than ±3 SD from the mean.

(1:352), (4:47–49).

**IIB1d**

36. A. Most manual resuscitators have the capability of delivering up to 100% oxygen. A few technical considerations are required to ensure that the highest $FIO_2$ possible is being delivered during a resuscitation procedure. These include (1) ensuring that the reservoir at the oxygen inlet is properly attached, (2) checking the

connection between the flow meter and the resuscitation bag, and (3) determining that the flow meter is delivering 10 to 15 L/min. of oxygen. The pop-off valve on the manual resuscitator has no bearing on the delivered oxygen percentage.

(1:649), (13:195–197).

**IIB1e(1)**

37. D. The condition is normal because the characteristics of a fluidic ventilator include (1) having substantially few mechanical and moving parts (thus the potential for a longer life span), (2) being noisy, and (3) consuming large volumes of compressed gas. Because the patient is not in distress, the last two characteristics are responsible for this situation.

(2:485).

**IIA1h(4)**

38. A. The RRT must ice the sample immediately to maintain sample integrity while troubleshooting the co-oximeter. A common problem that causes a "check cuvette" warning is a blood clot. Generally, the blood

clot can be easily flushed out with cleaning solution. Once the cuvette is cleaned, the RRT will need to install the window and auto-zero the co-oximeter to determine whether the problem has been resolved. The last step is to take apart the tubing and clean it thoroughly. Because this action is time-consuming, it should be undertaken only after other options have been explored. The last result, if none of the preceding actions rectifies the problem, is to telephone the manufacturer for technical assistance.

(1:358–359), (13:239–242).

### IIA1f(2)

39. C. A double-lumen ET tube would be appropriately employed in any case requiring independent lung ventilation. ARDS and pneumonia are generally diffuse bilateral processes. Tracheal malacia is an upper-airway condition. Unilateral interstitial fibrosis is the best representative of a condition requiring independent lung ventilation.

(15:736, 828).

### IIB3

40. C. Dispersion is a form of random error characterized by an increased occurrence of both high and low outliers. An isolated random error generally is not a major problem and is usually ignored. When random errors occur with increased frequency, however, and a pattern is established, the situation is described as *dispersion*.

Trending and shifting are systematic errors. *Trending* refers to a gradual, continuous movement of reported quality-control data away from the mean. *Shifting* describes the sudden movement of analyzed data from the established mean. Each of these types of errors is presented in Figure 4-14 (A–C).

(4:48–49)

### IIB1h(4)

41. C. Co-oximeters are incapable of differentiating between carboxyhemoglobin and fetal hemoglobin. The light absorption characteristics of these two types of hemoglobin are similar at the wavelength used to measure carboxyhemoglobin. Therefore, when blood that

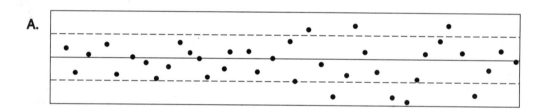

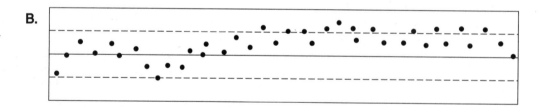

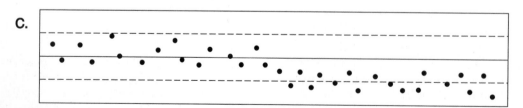

**Figure 4-14:** (A) Dispersion, (B) Trending, (C) Shifting

has a high concentration of fetal hemoglobin is analyzed in a co-oximeter, the carboxyhemoglobin concentration (COHb%) will be erroneously high, whereas the oxyhemoglobin concentration ($O_2$Hb%) will be falsely low. Correction factors are available for normalizing the data.

(1:358–359), (13:239–243), (15:492).

## IIA1k

42. B. A positive expiratory pressure (PEP) mask assists in the mobilization and evacuation of tracheobronchial secretions. The patient places the mask, which has an inspiratory and an expiratory limb, snugly against her face. She inhales room air or oxygen titrated into the unit and exhales against a resistor located in the expiratory limb of the device. The resistance encountered on exhalation prolongs the expiratory phase of the ventilatory cycle, thereby enabling the flowing air to help mobilize the secretions. Similarly, the patient is instructed to inhale slowly and deeply and to initiate an inspiratory pause at end inspiration. This pause enables a more uniform distribution of the inspired air. More air also gets beyond partially obstructed airways by performing this inspiratory maneuver. Therefore, more air can flow past these secretions on exhalation to assist in their removal. More air is also available to improve the efficacy of a cough.

The degree of expiratory resistance against which the patient exhales is in the range of 10 to 15 cm $H_2O$. Patient coughing has also been found to become more effective with this form of therapy.

(1:807–810).

## IIB1i(2)

43. C. The situation illustrated on the pressure-time tracing reflects an increased expiratory pressure. Pressure fluctuations in a CPAP system (continuous flow or demand flow) should not be greater than ±2 cm $H_2O$. The inspiratory phase shown in Figure 4-2 on page 191 depicts an acceptable inspiratory effort (−2 cm $H_2O$). The fact that the inspiratory effort initiated by the patient was only −2 cm $H_2O$ indicates that the demand valve is functioning properly and that the flow rate in the CPAP system is meeting the patient's inspiratory needs.

The pressure shown in Figure 4-2 on exhalation has reached 14 cm $H_2O$. This increase in pressure (6 cm $H_2O$) above the baseline (8 cm $H_2O$) is beyond the acceptable limit of +2 cm $H_2O$. A likely explanation for this increased pressure is that the patient might have coughed. A forced exhalation will elevate the level of positive pressure on exhalation within a CPAP system. Patient accommodation to a CPAP system does not appear to be affected by the type of resistor (threshold or flow) used. Therefore, it is acceptable to incorporate into a CPAP system either a threshold or a flow resistor.

(1:783, 878), (18:292–310).

## IIA1h(2)

44. A. Oxygen concentrators are manufactured in such a manner that as the flow rate is increased, the delivered percent oxygen (*not* the $F_IO_2$) decreases. The converse is also true. Therefore, by virtue of the flow rate being increased from 2 L/min. to 4 L/min., the percent oxygen received by the patient would be lowered, but the patient would actually receive a higher $F_IO_2$ because of the increased oxygen flow rate. In fact, one study revealed little difference in blood oxygen levels in the range of 1 to 4 L/min. regardless of whether the oxygen was delivered by a concentrator or by a 100% source (wall or tank).

(1:1115–1116), (5:17–28), (13:50–51).

## IIB1a(1)

45. B. Transtracheal oxygen administration is a method for delivering oxygen to patients who require home oxygen therapy. This form of oxygen administration affords the patient improved mobility and usually overcomes patient compliance problems. It generally also resolves the issue of cosmetic problems frequently associated with the nasal cannula.

A percutaneous opening into the trachea is performed, and a stenting device is held in place in a needle-wire guide. The stent remains in position for about one week, during which time no oxygen is administered through the trachea. Oxygen is withheld from being delivered through the trachea to minimize the risk of subcutaneous emphysema, bleeding, coughing, and general discomfort. When the stenting device is removed, a 9 Fr catheter is placed into the opening, which has not yet matured, and maintained there for 5 to 7 weeks until the opening matures.

During that time, oxygen is delivered through the catheter, which is periodically cleaned while it is in place. After this period of time, the patient learns to remove, insert, and clean the transtracheal catheter.

A mucous plug located at the tip of a transtracheal catheter will prevent or limit oxygen delivery through the catheter and ultimately into the patient's lungs. Severe oxygen desaturation and hypoxemia may ensue. Irritation by the catheter against the trachea can cause severe airway spasm if uncorrected. A transtracheal catheter creates a port of entry into the trachea, bypassing the normal upper-airway defense mechanisms. Consequently, the potential for the development of infection is constantly present. The patient assumes the responsibility for cleaning and maintaining the device.

(The Clinician's Guide for Scoop™, Transtracheal Systems), (1:1117–1118), (5:70), (13:72–73).

## IIA1e(2)

46. A. Because of the small $V_T$ used to ventilate infants, it is especially important to minimize volume lost to tubing compressibility. A low compressibility factor for the breathing circuit is critical. The normally high infant ventilatory rate requires a machine capable of rapidly responding to patient-initiated breaths for SIMV or assist-control modes. Many infants requiring mechanical ventilatory support have a low pulmonary compliance; therefore, PEEP or CPAP is often used. Thus, these capabilities are desirable characteristics of infant ventilators. For the care of infants with noncompliant lungs, a pressure-limited, time-cycled ventilator is preferred.

(1:1020).

## IIB1e(2)

47. C. In some cases, the preset cartridge temperature setting of 40°C might be too high, resulting in excess condensation near the high–low jet tube. Pressure displayed on the monitor might fluctuate and produce spurious alarms. If the pressures are fluctuating, there is probably too much condensation. The monitor line should be flushed with 10 cc of air in a syringe initially before manipulating the temperature setting. A collection of water in the bacterial filter is a normal occurrence that does not need correction. If the water is inadvertently drained into the jet lumen, most of it will come back out the main lumen without the need to suction the patient.

(Bunnell, Inc., [1991]. *Life Pulse High Frequency Ventilator In-Service Manual*, pp. 9–5).

## IIA2

48. C. Proper treatment of equipment before placement into an ethylene oxide sterilizing chamber is essential for sterilization to occur. All mucus, blood, vomitus, and so on must be removed from the objects before exposure to ethylene oxide (ETO). The equipment must be surgically cleaned before ETO sterilization techniques are used. At the same time, articles must not have beads of water dripping from them when placed in the chamber because water reacts with ETO to form ethylene glycol, which irritates human tissue.

To maintain sterilization after ETO exposure, objects are prewrapped in muslin or wrapping paper. The gas ef-

fectively penetrates these packaging materials to allow sterilization to occur, assuming proper pre-exposure treatment had taken place.

(1:43–46), (13:669–671).

## IIB1h(5)

49. D. Polarographic and galvanic cell oxygen analyzers both contain a cathode and an anode. Oxygen is reduced at the cathode according to the following electrochemical reaction:

$$O_2 + 2H_2O + 4e^- \rightarrow 4OH^-$$

Nitrous oxide, and for that matter, halothane, can participate in this reaction at the cathode, producing more electrons ($e^-$). As more electrons are formed during the cathode reaction, the current flowing through the circuit will be greater, in turn causing a greater deflection of the ammeter. The ammeter indicates the $O_2$ concentration. Therefore, nitrous oxide would cause the polarographic oxygen analyzer to read erroneously high. The diagram in Figure 4-15 illustrates the internal functional components of a polarographic oxygen analyzer.

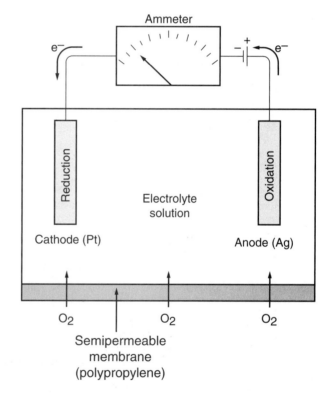

**Figure 4-15:** Internal functional components of a polarographic oxygen analyzer.

(5:281–285), (13:249), (17:209–210, 213).

50.  B. An indwelling arterial catheter or line will enable the measurement of the following hemodynamic data:

- systolic pressure
- diastolic pressure
- pulse pressure
- mean arterial pressure

The pulse pressure is the difference between the systolic and diastolic pressures. For example, if the blood pressure is 120/80 mm Hg, the pulse pressure can be calculated as shown:

pulse pressure = systolic pressure − diastolic pressure

40 mm Hg = 120 mm Hg − 80 mm Hg

The mean arterial pressure (MAP) can be determined from the following relationship:

$$MAP = \frac{\text{systolic pressure} + (2) \text{ diastolic pressure}}{3}$$

A normal arterial waveform and its components are illustrated on the tracing shown in Figure 4-16.

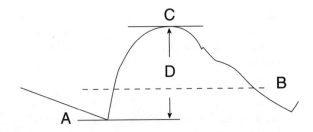

**Figure 4-16:** Components of a normal arterial waveform: (A) diastolic pressure, (B) mean arterial pressure, (C) systolic pressure, and (D) pulse pressure.

A = diastolic pressure
B = mean arterial pressure
C = systolic pressure
D = pulse pressure

For a normal blood pressure of 120/80 mm Hg, the MAP would be:

$$MAP = \frac{120 \text{ mm Hg} + (80 \text{ mm Hg} \times 2)}{3}$$

$$= 93 \text{ mm Hg}$$

(1:942), (9:60–61, 335), (14:110).

51.  B. The efficiency of air entrainment devices are affected by back pressure. As airway resistance through the gas-delivery system increases beyond the point of air entrainment, the velocity of the gas flow rate is reduced and the amount of room air entrained decreases. Therefore, the addition of six feet of large-bore tubing to an oxygen-delivery system already having that length virtually doubles the airway resistance. The impact of extending the length of the tubing to 12 feet would be to increase the $FIO_2$ above 0.40.

Possible ways to circumvent this problem include (1) using an oxygen blender set at 40% with the gas flow passing through a jet nebulizer (set at 100%) for humidification, or (2) employing a T piece inserted along the length of the large-bore tubing for the bleeding in of compressed air with a flow rate titrated with the source flow to provide an analyzed $FIO_2$ of 0.40.

The illustrations shown in Figures 4-17 and 4-18 portray these two alternate approaches.

Consideration must also be given to the accumulation of condensate along the length of the tubing as well as to the possibility of the patient's ventilatory demands changing.

(1:755–758), (13:78–79).

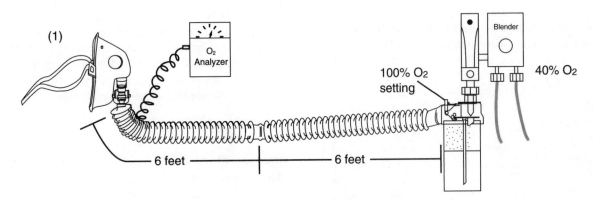

**Figure 4-17:** Oxygen blender at 40% with gas flow through a jet nebulizer at 100% for humidification.

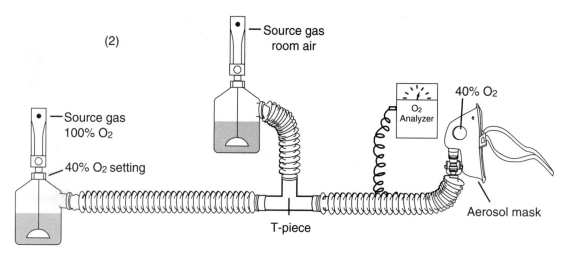

**Figure 4-18:** T piece inserted along the length of large-bore tubing bleeding in compressed air with the flow rate titrated with the source flow to provide analyzed 0.40 $F_{I}O_2$.

### IIB1e(1)

52. A. Fluidic ventilators incorporate basic logic called *fluidic logic,* or fluidic elements. The fluidic logic determines the direction of the gas flow. Three mechanisms are responsible for the direction of flow in fluidic ventilators: (1) back pressure; (2) subatmospheric pressure, or negative inspiratory pressure; and (3) amplification, or cycling pressure.

Therefore, because pressure is responsible for gas flow through a fluidic ventilator, all fluidic circuits and controlling gates require the establishment of pressure gradients from the gas source (air and/or oxygen).

(5:342–346), (13:380).

### IIB1i(1)

53. B. One of the more critical variables in maintaining respiratory stability for patients receiving high-frequency jet ventilation is the position of the jet orifice and its location in the ET tube. Placing the angiocath too proximal or too distal in the tube will have a significant impact on the patient's ventilatory status (and ultimately, his acid-base balance).

(13:616–617).

### IIB1h(5)

54. C. "Zeroing" any analyzer refers to calibrating the instrument to the low-value test signal. The low-value test signal might or might not be zero. Zeroing a gas analyzer is almost equivalent to performing a one-point calibration. During one-point calibration, the analyzer is generally exposed to a certain test value. The

value used varies from device to device. It can be zero or some value greater than zero.

(9:341, 361–362), (14:165–167, 170, 240).

### IIA1q(1)

55. B. When the tip of the pulmonary artery catheter (PAC) is deflated and residing in the pulmonary artery, the diastolic and systolic pulmonary artery pressures will be measured. Pulmonary artery diastolic pressure is usually 5 to 16 mm Hg, and pulmonary artery systolic pressure is ordinarily 15 to 30 mm Hg.

When the balloon tip is inflated, the PAC tip assumes the wedged position and reflects the left ventricular end-diastolic pressure (LVEDP). This measurement should not take longer than 15 seconds to prevent causing a pulmonary infarction.

(1:943–948), (9:344–348).

### IIA1u

56. A. A pulse oximeter and a single-lead ECG monitor are required during bronchoscopy procedures. The pulse oximeter indicates the need to respond to patient desaturation, whereas the ECG monitor affords the ability to assess the presence of cardiac dysrhythmias. In either case, the need for supplemental oxygen is indicated.

(1:623), (*Respiratory Care,* 38:1173–1178, 1993).

### IIB1c

57. A. When water condenses and is allowed to accumulate in the gravity-dependent regions of the large-bore tubing, back pressure is exerted from the point of con-

densate accumulation to the air entrainment port on the nebulizer. The back pressure reduces the amount of air entrainment, thereby causing a greater amount of oxygen to be delivered to the patient. Similarly, less aerosol will be produced because of the reduced entrained airflow. At the same time, the total flow rate delivered to the patient will be reduced.

(1:755–756), (13:78–79).

## IIB2s

58. C. The small-particle aerosol generator (SPAG) is used to administer nebulized ribavirin (Virazole) to infants who have bronchiolitis. The SPAG-2 unit is designed to operate at a pressure of 26 psig. The unit contains two flow meters. One operates the nebulizer, and the other regulates flow to the drying chamber.

When the SPAG-2 unit is being set up for operation, the pressure gauge is adjusted to 26 psig *after* the flow rate (12 to 15 L/min.) to the nebulizer has been established. The pressure gauge is then readjusted to 26 psig *following* the setting of the flow rate going to the

drying chamber. Figure 4-19 illustrates the components of a SPAG-2 unit.

(5:151–153), (13:149–152).

## IIA1h(2)

59. A. Molecular sieve oxygen concentrators deliver lower concentrations of oxygen at higher flow settings. For example, flow settings ranging from 2 to 5 L/min. provide oxygen concentrations somewhere between 80% and 90%. At 10 L/min. approximately 50% oxygen is delivered. The oxygen concentration rises to above 90% when the flow is 1 to 2 L/min.

(5:17–28), (13:50–51).

## IIB1h(4)

60. B. The end-tidal partial pressure of carbon dioxide ($P_{ET}CO_2$) decreases for several reasons. These reasons include (a) circuitry disconnection, (b) ET tube cuff leak, (c) increased alveolar dead space ($V_D/V_T$ ratio increase), (d) decreased C.O., (e) pulmonary embolism,

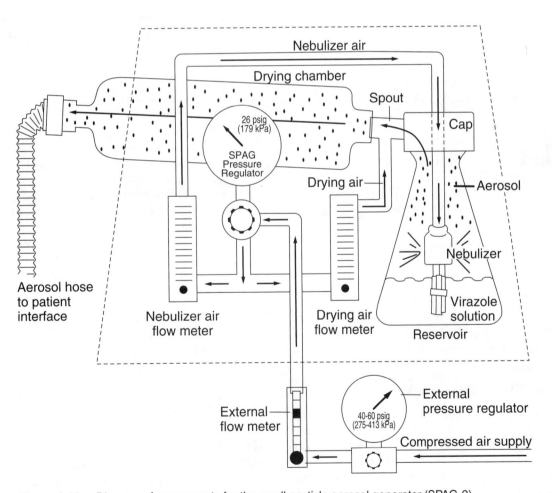

**Figure 4-19:** Diagram of components for the small-particle aerosol generator (SPAG-2).

and (f) chronic hyperventilation. Neither the mainstream nor the sidestream capnometer incorporates a carbon dioxide absorber. It would be fruitless for a device that is designed to measure the carbon dioxide to incorporate a $CO_2$ absorber.

(1:935–936), (10:248, 434).

### IIA1h(5)

61. C. The sensor of a polarographic oxygen analyzer, as well as that of a galvanic cell analyzer, is calibrated with a dry gas. Therefore, humidification of the gas will dilute the sample and render a lower oxygen concentration readout. The sensor of the analyzer must be located in the tubing somewhere before the gas becomes humidified. Placing the analyzer sensor between the ventilator and the humidifier would circumvent this potential problem.

Consider the comparison with dry and saturated oxygen. The general formula used is:

$$\text{analyzed } O_2\% = \left( \frac{P_B - P_{H_2O}}{P_B} \right) F_IO_2 \times 100$$

A. 60% dry oxygen:

$$\text{analyzed } O_2\% = \left( \frac{760 \text{ torr} - 0 \text{ torr}}{760 \text{ torr}} \right) 0.60 \times 100$$

$$= \left( \frac{760 \text{ torr}}{760 \text{ torr}} \right) 0.6 \times 100$$

$$= 60\%$$

B. 60% $O_2$ delivered at 100% saturation at body temperature (47 torr)

$$\text{analyzed } O_2\% = \left( \frac{760 \text{ torr} - 47 \text{ torr}}{760 \text{ torr}} \right) 0.60 \times 100$$

$$= \left( \frac{713 \text{ torr}}{760 \text{ torr}} \right) 0.60 \times 100$$

$$= 56\%$$

Again, humidification will cause the sensor to analyze lower than the actual value because condensation on the polarographic electrode will interfere with the oxygen analysis.

(5:281–285), (13:249), (17:209–210, 213).

### IIA1k

62. C. Positive expiratory pressure (PEP) therapy is applied to mobilize secretions and to decrease and counteract airway closure, which occurs during dynamic compression during a forceful exhalation (coughing). The equipment used with this therapeutic procedure includes (1) a face mask, (2) a one-way valve, (3) ex-

piratory resistors, and (4) a pressure manometer. The diagram in Figure 4-20 illustrates these components and their locations.

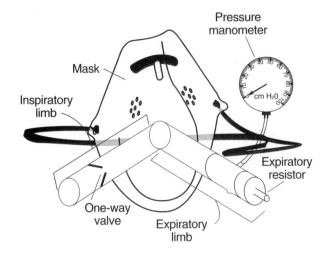

**Figure 4-20:** Positive expiratory pressure (PEP) mask components.

When the patient inhales, the one-way valve along the inspiratory limb opens. Upon exhalation, the inspiratory one-way valve closes, and airflow is directed along the expiratory limb. As the exhaled air encounters the resistor, back pressure develops and opposes exhalation. This back pressure is the PEP and can be sensed by the pressure manometer located anywhere between the resistor and the one-way valve in the inspiratory limb. If the pressure manometer is placed between the one-way valve and the opening of the inspiratory port, the back pressure generated from the resistance to air flow out of the resistor will not be sensed. Also, placing the pressure manometer at the opening of the resistor will not enable the positive expiratory pressure to be measured. If the pressure manometer is placed at the opening of the resistor (opening of the expiratory limb), only the pressure generated from the gas flowing out the expiratory limb opening will be sensed. A number of color-coded resistors with different sized orifices are available for insertion at the distal end of the expiratory limb. The minimum positive pressure that should be exerted during PEP mask therapy is 10 cm $H_2O$. The recommended high limit is 20 cm $H_2O$.

(Astra Meditec A/S [product information], Roskildevej 22, DK-2620 Albertslund, Denmark), (13:353–355).

### IIA1h(4)

63. A. A capnometer is an instrument that measures the carbon dioxide level in the patient's expirate. It takes advantage of the ability of carbon dioxide gas to absorb infrared light.

During cardiopulmonary resuscitation, a capnometer can be used to measure the amount of exhaled $CO_2$ during cardiac compressions. In a cardiac arrest situation, the end-tidal partial pressure of carbon dioxide ($P_{ET}CO_2$) increases with the application of external cardiac compressions. This increase in the $P_{ET}CO_2$ is purported to result from the increased pulmonary circulation. A sudden significant increase in the $P_{ET}CO_2$ might herald the onset of the resumption of spontaneous circulation. Consequently, capnography can be a beneficial tool to quantify the return of spontaneous perfusion.

("Guidelines 2000 for Cardiopulmonary Resuscitation and Emergency Cardiovascular Care," page I–101, (15:500–502).

### IIB3b

64.  B. Balancing an analyzing device refers to making calibration adjustments when the sensor is exposed to the low-value test signal. After an instrument is balanced, the slope can be established. The slope is established by performing calibration adjustments while the device is exposed to the high-value test signal.

(11:386–387).

### IIB1h(4)

65.  D. Clinical experience has revealed that the transcutaneous partial pressure of oxygen ($PtcO_2$) and the arterial partial pressure of oxygen ($PaO_2$) directly correlate. This direct correlation does not mean that the two values are identical, however. Instead, it means that the $PtcO_2$ and $PaO_2$ values increase and decrease to the same degree. This relationship holds true assuming that the $PtcO_2$ electrode has been properly applied and calibrated and that the patient is cardiovascularly stable. The $PtcO_2$ measurement reflects skin perfusion.

Therefore, $PtcO_2$ values should only be relied on as a predictor of oxygen changes.

(1:353–356), (*Respiratory Care*, 39:1176–1179, 1994).

### IIB1n2

66.  C. The phlebostatic axis is at the level of the right atrium. It is located at the juncture of the nipple line and the anterior axillary line. Figure 4-21 shows how the transducer should be aligned with the phlebostatic axis.

Once the transducer has been zeroed (customarily at the phlebostatic axis), it must not be moved. Generally, if the transducer is relocated above the phlebostatic axis after being zeroed, vascular pressures will be erroneously low. Placing the transducer (after it has been zeroed) below the right atrium causes the pressures to read erroneously high.

(9:341, 361–363), (14:165–167, 170, 240).

### IIB1a(1)

67.  C. Most bubble-diffusion humidifiers have a pop-off (pressure-relief) valve designed to activate in the presence of at least 2 psi back pressure. Situations that can cause this pop-off valve to sound include (1) too high a gas source flow rate, (2) too high a water level in the humidifier reservoir, and (3) obstructed oxygen tubing.

(1:663–664), (5:99–98), (13:106).

### IIB1f(2)

68.  B. The brachiocephalic (innominate) artery lies anterior to the trachea. Erosion of the anterior tracheal wall might cause eventual erosion of the brachiocephalic artery, although such an occurrence is uncommon.

(1:605).

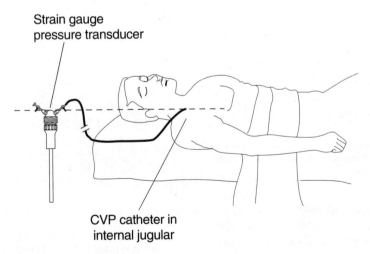

Strain gauge pressure transducer

CVP catheter in internal jugular

**Figure 4-21:** Strain gauge pressure transducer dome aligned with phlebostatic axis (juncture of nipple line and anterior axillary).

69. B. The recommended minimum pressure used in PEP mask therapy is 10 cm $H_2O$. The expiratory resistance can be varied by attaching different sized (color-coded) resistors to the distal end of the expiratory port.

(Astra Meditec A/S [product literature] Roskildevej 22, DK-2620 Albertslund, Denmark), (13:353–355).

70. A. When supplemental oxygen is added to the BiPAP® system, the patient's oxygen saturation should be continuously monitored via pulse oximetry. If the $SpO_2$ is less than 90%, the oxygen flow rate should be increased to deliver more oxygen. The supplemental oxygen should be attached to the mask, rather than to the blower. An oxygen analyzer is not useful because this system is not air tight. Consequently, because of the air leaks in the system, the $F_IO_2$ would fluctuate.

(BiPAP® S/T-D Ventilatory Support System product information, Respironics, Inc.).

71. D. A relatively abrupt change in measurement outcome, followed by clustering or plateauing of analyzed data at any particular time, is known as *shifting*. Shifting might result from (a) air bubbles beneath the electrode membrane, (b) changes in temperature, or (c) contamination of calibration standards.

*Trending* is a systematic error in which progressive controls either increase or decrease (gradually) and might be caused by an aging electrode, an aging mercury battery, or protein contamination of the electrode.

(4:48–49), (6:313).

72. B. Air turbulence, in-flight variables, and pressure fluctuations are not likely to cause function and performance abnormalities for transport ventilators because they are designed to maintain normal function in the face of such adverse factors. The Aequitron LP-10 ventilator serves as a portable, transport ventilator and incorporates an internal battery that can provide an energy source for up to one hour of operation. If the mode of transportation does not have the internal means of providing an energy supply to maintain this function of an electrically operated ventilator, some other external power source must accompany the transport. For example, the Aequitron LP-10 ventilator can be connected to a 12-volt, direct-current battery and remain operational for approximately 10 hours.

(5:550–555).

73. D. The purpose of using the oxygen blender is to deliver a precise and constant $FiO_2$. If the oxygen blender is set at 50%, then 50% oxygen should be reaching the nebulizer (and ultimately, the patient). Because the nebulizer's air entrainment port is open (to the 60% oxygen setting), room air will be entrained at that point, and the $FiO_2$ of the gas operating the nebulizer (gas at 50% $O_2$) will be reduced.

Therefore, with the air entrainment port closed or with the nebulizer set to deliver 100% oxygen, the gas delivered from the blender will not become diluted as it passes through the nebulizer creating aerosol particles.

(5:43–45), (13:81–84).

74. B. The PAC shown in Figure 4-22 contains four lumens. It is called a four-channel PAC.

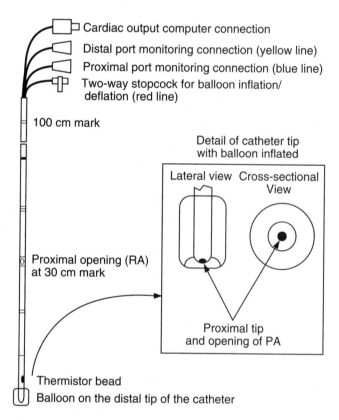

**Figure 4-22:** Four-channel pulmonary artery catheter: (1) distal injection port, (2) proximal injection port, (3) extra injection port, and (4) balloon inflation port.

The distal injection port enables pulmonary artery pressure readings and mixed venous blood sampling. The proximal injection port provides for right atrial or central venous pressure (CVP) measurements as well as fluid infusion or thermal dilution C.O. determinations. The balloon inflation valve provides the means for inflating and deflating the balloon tip. The fourth channel, the extra injection port, is for the continuous infusion of hyperalimentation fluids. The thermistor connector attaches to a bedside cardiac output computer.

The PAC is useful for monitoring the hemodynamic status as well as for rendering data essential for effective patient management (e.g., hypoperfusion conditions, ARDS, permeability pulmonary edema, high-pressure pulmonary edema, and pulmonary vascular disease).

(1:946), (9:346).

## IIA1u

75. D. Fiberoptic bronchoscopy and transtracheal aspiration procedures are two methods that are useful in diagnosing anaerobic lung infections. With either technique, the flora of the upper airway is bypassed, and contamination of the specimen with upper airway flora is avoided. The transtracheal method of obtaining sputum specimens is associated with considerable patient discomfort. Therefore, bronchoscopic retrieval of specimens has made the transtracheal aspiration technique less used. Oral, nasal, and tracheostomy suctioning and expectorated samples are not useful techniques for obtaining such specimens because they often are contaminated with upper airway flora.

(1:434–435), (15:625–626).

## IIB3c

76. C. The Wright Respirometer is a flow-sensing device that measures the tidal volume ($V_T$) and minute ventilation ($\dot{V}_E$). Because this device is not accurate above flow rates of 300 L/min., forced vital capacity maneuvers must not be measured with a Wright Respirometer. Similarly, flow rates of less than 3 L/min. cannot be accurately measured.

Because this flow-sensing device has a range of accuracy between 3 to 300 L/min., the flow rate (120 L/min.) obtained while evaluating the maximum flow provided by the Bennett 7200 is an acceptable value.

(5:276–277).

## IIA1a(1)

77. B. Transtracheal oxygen is often preferred by patients who are greatly concerned about the cosmetic aspects of their oxygen therapy equipment. The diagram in Figure 4-23 shows how the device is situated within the trachea. The catheter is inserted between the sec-

ond and third tracheal rings and is situated just above the carina. The catheter is secured around the patient's neck by a custom-fitted necklace. Oxygen is supplied via standard oxygen tubing connected to a flow meter.

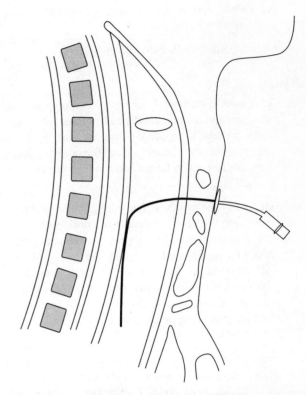

**Figure 4-23:** Position of transtracheal oxygen catheter situated within the trachea above the carina. Note the insertion between the second and third tracheal rings.

In addition to its cosmetic features, transtracheal oxygen delivery conserves oxygen usage by about 50% to 70%. Effective oxygenation can be provided at flow rates as low as 0.25 L/min. for some patients.

(5:70–71), (13:72–73).

## IIA2

78. C. Pasteurization is a physical disinfection technique that employs moist heat to coagulate protein within microorganisms. The microorganism *Clostridium botulinum* is an anaerobic species that cannot survive in an aerobic environment. Therefore, despite the fact that *C. botulinum* is an extremely lethal species and that pasteurization does not kill spores, pasteurization of equipment that has come in contact with a patient so infected is an effective means of disinfection. The equipment is generally immersed for 10 minutes in water that is heated to 75°C.

(1:44), (13:670).

79. A. A low power signal often indicates that the electrode has been placed over a poorly perfused area or that there is poor electrode-to-skin contact. Therefore, the transcutaneous oxygen electrode needs to be removed and repositioned to ensure appropriate location and contact with the skin.

(1:355–356), (5:292–296), (13:265–269).

**IIB1e(1)**

80. A. A double-lumen ET tube is designed to seal off each lung and to enable independent lung ventilation. When the tube is properly positioned, one lumen resides in a mainstem bronchus, and the other is situated in the trachea. Each lumen has a cuff to create a seal for each lung.

Because of the tube's unique configuration and positioning requirements, a number of considerations are critical to its proper deployment. For example, if the entire tube is advanced too deeply, the tip of the lumen that enters the mainstem bronchus might project beyond the lobar bronchus that serves the upper lobe of that lung. Consequently, that lobe might become atelectic, depending on the degree of impaired ventilation that it experiences.

Furthermore, if the double-lumen tube is *not* advanced sufficiently into the airway, both lungs will be subjected to whatever mode of ventilation or therapeutic modality is attached to each of the tube's lumens. This situation is what exists in the question here. Because mainstem bronchus insertion has not occurred, ventilation intended exclusively for the right lung is also flowing to the contralateral side.

The pressure and volume settings on the ventilator have been established for ventilation of the right lung only, not both lungs. Therefore, with ventilation going to both lungs, low PIPs are being generated. Additionally, because a Briggs adaptor is attached to the lumen servicing the left lung and not to a positive pressure ventilation device, that lumen's cuff might not be inflated. The result would be a greater loss of system pressure.

To correct this situation, the location of the double-lumen tube must be verified by either fiberoptic bronchoscopy or chest radiography. Then, the appropriate tube adjustment must be made, followed again by confirmation of the tube position.

(13:166).

**IIB2d**

81. A. Mouth-to-mask resuscitators have emerged upon the clinical scene in the wake of acquired immunodeficiency syndrome (AIDS). In fact, the Centers for Disease Control and Prevention (CDC) recommends that emergency rescuers use a protective barrier between themselves and the victim.

In the situation presented here, the likely problem is the position of the one-way valve associated with the mouth-to-mask device. Only seconds would be taken to reverse the valve. If the problem continued, it would be appropriate for the rescuer to resume mouth-to-mouth resuscitation.

Stopping ventilations until another mouth-to-mask resuscitator was obtained is unacceptable and harmful to the patient. Checking the seal of the mouth-to-mask resuscitator is inappropriate because resistance to ventilation would not be encountered if the problem were an inadequate seal.

(5:191), (13:251).

**IIA1h(2)**

82. D. Because liquid oxygen is cryogenically stored in a liquid oxygen system, room air temperatures cause the liquid oxygen to rapidly evaporate. The evaporation process results in a system pressure increase that causes the pressure-relief valve to vent gaseous oxygen to the atmosphere. This vented oxygen is, of course, not used by the patient but contributes to the depletion of the oxygen supply.

Because this patient is using this liquid oxygen system intermittently, the duration of flow cannot be determined. If the patient were using this system continuously, there would be no evaporative waste, and the patient would be consuming all of the oxygen. Therefore, the duration of flow can be calculated for continuous use situations only.

(5:23–28), (13:47–49).

**IIB1f(2)**

83. A. An endobronchial tube, or double-lumen ET tube, is an artificial airway designed to enable independent lung ventilation. This tube must be positioned accurately. If it is advanced too far down, the portion of the tube extending into the right mainstem bronchus might block the lobar bronchus leading to the right upper lobe and cause right upper lobe atelectasis.

When a double-lumen ET tube is properly positioned, the right mainstem bronchus is intubated for right lung ventilation. The left lung receives its ventilation from a second lumen that resides in the trachea. Two cuffs must be inflated to create a seal for airflow into each lung.

To determine proper tube placement, the RRT can clamp each lumen separately and listen for the movement of air in the contralateral lung via auscultation. To definitively confirm the tube's proper position, fiberoptic bronchoscopy or chest radiography can be employed.

(13:166).

## IIB2e(2)

84. B. Although the SensorMedics 3100 high-frequency oscillatory ventilator can generate an oscillatory pressure amplitude up to 90 cm $H_2O$ measured at the proximal airway, the ET tube greatly attenuates the pressure in the respiratory system. Approximately 90% of the proximal oscillatory pressure amplitude is lost with a 2.5 mm I.D. ET tube. Therefore, the largest tube possible should be used to minimize impedance and subsequent attenuation losses. A 2.8-kg neonate should be able to accommodate a 3.5 mm I.D. ET tube.

(SensorMedics, Corp., 3100 Oscillatory Ventilator Product Information: Clinical Strategies) (5:630).

## IIB3c

85. C. When input signals equal output signals or when observed values equal expected values, an instrument is said to be linear. Linearity checks for gas analyzers can be performed by introducing a series of test gas mixtures into the gas analyzer. First, the analyzer is calibrated and checked for drift. Then, varying percentages (100%, 90%, 80%, etc.) of the test gas are introduced into the analyzer. This method is also called *multiple-point calibration.*

Again, with the expected values plotted on the *y* axis and the observed values on the *x* axis, *x* would equal *y* if the instrument were linear. Most instruments are linear over a limited range. Outside that range (beyond the linear limits), the instrument is said to be alinear. *Drift* refers to the degree of adjustment that must be made to an instrument to bring it within the calibration limits.

(11:396).

## IIB1a(2)

86. D. An air-entrainment mask is a high-flow oxygen-delivery system; therefore, it is not influenced by the patient's (1) ventilatory pattern, (2) ventilatory rate, or (3) tidal volume. An oxygen analyzer that is accurate to ±2% (±0.02) provides reliable readings.

Therefore, something must be partially obstructing the air entrainment ports of the device. Perhaps the patient's gown or the bed sheet is covering or was "sucked" into the air entrainment ports, causing less dilution of the source gas. Note the air entrainment port shown in Figure 4-24.

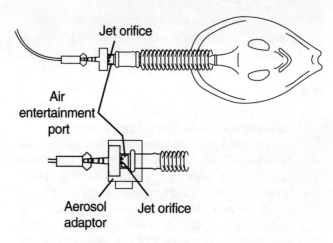

**Figure 4-24:** Note the air entrainment port, where the bedsheet or patient's gown can obstruct.

Some clinicians use the aerosol collar to prevent the patient's gown or bed sheet from obstructing the air entrainment port.

(1:754), (3:50), (13:76).

## IIB1h(4)

87. A. The $PO_2$ obtained from a transcutaneous electrode will be falsely low if the following factors are present:

- reduced capillary perfusion
- hypothermia
- alkalemia
- thickened stratum corneum
- excessive pressure exerted on the electrode, reducing capillary perfusion
- electrode drift

(1:355), (5:268), (13:292).

## IIA1h(3)

88. C. Neither oxygen concentrators nor liquid oxygen systems can generate 50 psig of pressure. In fact, oxygen concentrators develop around 15 psig, whereas liquid oxygen systems produce between 20 psig and 25 psig. An H tank of oxygen can generate source pressures of 50 psig or greater, depending on the type of reducing valve attached to the compressed gas cylinder.

(1:1111), (5:25), (13:22–24).

## IIB1e(1)

89. D. Home care ventilators usually rely on oxygen accumulators, or oxygen lines connected to oxygen concentrators, to enrich the delivered gas with oxygen. Home mechanical ventilators do not utilize continuous gas systems, nor do they enable the attachment of a 50-psig oxygen source. Compressed gas cylinders can be

used in conjunction with home mechanical ventilators. Such an arrangement would be quite costly, however.

(5:547–564), (13:575–589).

## IIB1f(4)

90.  C. A light failure on a laryngoscopy blade is often caused by poor contact between the laryngoscope handle and the blade. Removing and reconnecting the blade might quickly solve the problem. If that effort fails, however, replace the original blade with another blade. This action differentiates a battery failure from a bulb failure. If the bulb on the new blade lights, the problem is most likely in the bulb on the original blade and not the batteries. The RRT will need to replace the bulb on the original laryngoscope blade.

(13:166–167).

## IIA1h(5)

91.  D. A strain gauge pressure transducer, used in the measurement of hemodynamic pressures, incorporates a Wheatstone bridge. Four resistance wires, located below the fluid-filled dome, have their lengths altered as pressure in the dome changes. Varying the lengths of the wires causes a voltage change across the Wheatstone bridge.

Likewise, oxygen analyzers that operate according to the principle of thermoconductivity incorporate a Wheatstone bridge. This type of analyzer consists of a network of four resistances ($R_1$, $R_2$, $R_3$, and $R_4$), as shown in Figure 4-25.

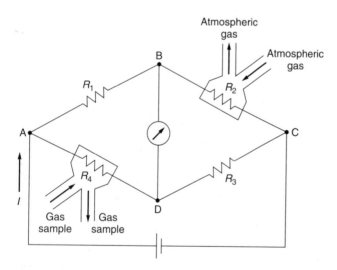

**Figure 4-25:** Internal functional components of a thermoconductive oxygen analyzer incorporating a Wheatstone bridge.

A galvanometer bridges the two parallel electrical circuits (ABC and ADC). The galvanometer is used to sense a voltage difference between these two circuits. A current I is initiated by a battery and travels to point A, where it encounters $R_1$ and $R_4$. When room air enters the gas sample chamber ($R_4$) and the gas cell ($R_2$), current I will be equal through both circuits (i.e., ABC and ADC). An oxygen reading of 20.93% will be indicated on the galvanometer because no potential difference exists between points B and D.

When more oxygen molecules enter the gas sample chamber, however, the temperature of the resistor wire $R_4$ will be reduced, and more current will flow through circuit ADC than through ABC. Consequently, a potential difference (voltage) exists across the galvanometer (between B and D), causing the readout to register an oxygen percentage greater than 20.93% (room air).

(5:335), (13:306), (17:251, 350).

## IIA1e(2)

92.  C. Infants who develop pulmonary interstitial emphysema (PIE) frequently exhibit accumulations of air in the form of unilateral or bilateral cysts. These cysts are frequently aligned linearly and perpendicularly to the lateral pleural edge. Generally, barotrauma is responsible for the rupture of alveoli leading to the movement of this air into the pulmonary interstitium. The air actually accumulates around the airways, blood vessels, and lymphatics. PIE might develop into a pneumomediastinum, pneumopericardium, or pneumothorax. High-frequency jet ventilation is often useful in the treatment of PIE because the mean airway pressure ($\overline{P}_{aw}$) with this mode of mechanical ventilation remains low. Infants with PIE can be ventilated with high-frequency jet ventilation at a reduced risk of aggravating the initial barotrauma.

(18:162–167, 489).

## IIB1q(1)

93.  D. The dome of the strain gauge pressure transducer used in conjunction with a central venous pressure (CVP) catheter must be at the same level as the patient's right atrium. When the patient is supine, the right atrium is approximately midway between the patient's posterior chest and anterior chest. The mid-chest position can be approximated further by measuring 10 cm up from the top of the mattress along the patient's lateral chest. The phlebostatic axis is still another point approximation of the catheter tip or right atrium location. The phlebostatic axis is the junction of the patient's mid-axillary line and fourth intercostal space.

(5:335), (13:306).

## IIB1p

94.  D. The ECG tracing in Figure 4-26 reflects 60-cycle interference possibly caused by improper grounding.

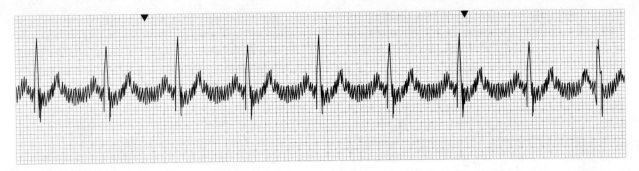

**Figure 4-26:** ECG tracing reflecting 60-cycle interference caused by improper grounding. Note the heavy baseline.

When using electrical equipment, the RRT must consider the problem of current leakage. Most electrically operated equipment leaks a current from the circuitry to the frame. It is recommended that the current leakage for exposed metal surfaces be no greater than 0.01 mA and less than 0.001 mA for patient connections. If ever this characteristic interference appears, the equipment must be checked by the electrical safety engineer.

(1:22–25), (13:16).

**IIB1q(1)**

95. D. The resonant frequency of the components of a monitoring system influences the responsiveness of the fluid-filled tubing system. If the pressure wave produced by the arterial blood has a frequency component equal to or near the fluid-filled tubing system's resonant frequency, the entire system will resonate. The consequences of this condition are (1) an over-shooting of the systolic pressures, (2) an undershooting of the diastolic pressures, and (3) the presence of small oscillations distorting the entire waveform. This situation can be avoided by adhering to the following measures:

- Minimizing catheter and tubing length
- Using noncompliant tubing
- Using large diameter catheters (greater than 7 Fr)
- Removing air bubbles from the system
- Preventing blood clot formation

(14:154–155, 157–158, 174).

**IIB1h(4)**

96. D. Whenever skin perfusion diminishes, the correlation between the transcutaneous partial pressure of oxygen (PtcO$_2$) and the partial pressure of oxygen in the arterial blood (PaO$_2$) likewise diminishes. Specific factors that reduce the PtcO$_2$-PaO$_2$ correlation include (1) hypothermia, (2) severe acidemia, (3) tolazoline, (4) halothane, (5) excessive pressure applied to the electrode, (6) thickened stratum corneum, and (7) electrode shift.

(1:355–356), (13:292–296), (13:268–269).

**IIA1h(4)**

97. C. Capnography is the means by which a patient's exhaled CO$_2$ can be noninvasively measured on a continuous basis. Measurement of the exhaled CO$_2$ is accomplished by a capnometer that contains a capnograph that provides a waveform, called a *capnogram*. A normal capnogram at two speeds (slow and fast) is illustrated in Figure 4-27.

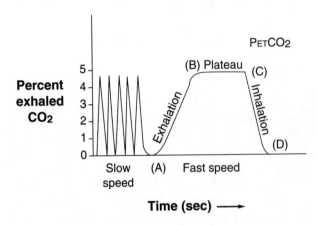

**Figure 4-27:** A normal slow- and fast-speed capnogram.

Different amounts of CO$_2$ are measured at various points throughout exhalation. For example, with the fast-speed capnogram, point A represents the pure, anatomic dead space gas that contains no metabolically produced CO$_2$. Therefore, the exhaled CO$_2$ reading at that point is 0.0%. As exhalation proceeds, traces of alveolar gas begin to mix with remnants of anatomic dead space gas. This event is captured along line A–B. The plateau (line B–C) essentially signifies CO$_2$ from the alveoli. Point C on the plateau represents the end-tidal CO$_2$ (P$_{ET}$CO$_2$). Segment C–D of the capnogram indicates inspiration, characterized by a progressive decrease in the measured CO$_2$, ultimately returning to 0.0% at end inspiration.

Slow capnographic tracings are often used clinically for continuous monitoring of the exhaled CO$_2$ and render information useful in the determination of a variety of pathologic conditions. These conditions include (1) apnea, (2) pulmonary embolism, and (3) cardiac arrest. In each of these clinical conditions, the end-tidal $CO_2$ level would decrease significantly.

(1:363–366, 933), (10:99–101).

## IIB2k

98. A. The purpose of positive expiratory pressure (PEP) mask therapy is to aid in the production of sputum by means of variable expiratory resistance. The correct pressure generally ranges between 10 to 15 cm $H_2O$ at 5 to 15 breaths/min., followed by coughing and expectoration of mucus. The problem here is the patient's inability to develop or maintain 10 to 15 cm $H_2O$ pressure during exhalation. Therefore, all of the connections of the PEP system need to be inspected for leaks. Additionally, the size of the mask being used should be evaluated. It might be too small or too large for the patient's face, thereby resulting in a loss of system pressure. The expiratory limb of the PEP system needs to be inspected to confirm that the appropriate resistor (variable expiratory resistance) has been inserted in the unit.

(1:807–810), (5:190).

## IIA1h(4)

99. C. A capnometer provides a means of continuous, noninvasive exhaled $CO_2$ monitoring. In addition to being beneficial for monitoring a variety of clinical conditions, it is also useful in alerting the RRT to certain equipment malfunctions. For example, a tracheostomy or ET tube cuff leak can be detected by an increase in the end-tidal $CO_2$ ($P_{ET}CO_2$) level as the measured tidal volume decreases. Additionally, a rapid fall in the $P_{ET}CO_2$ of a capnometer sampling a patient's exhaled $CO_2$ in a ventilator circuit might indicate a loose connection or disconnection in the system.

(1:363–366, 598, 933), (10:99–101).

## IIB1h(4)

100. D. If a capnometer is used in-line with a mechanical ventilator, an abrupt fall in the measured exhaled $CO_2$ might indicate a ventilator tubing disconnection. This event would likely be accompanied by a sounding of the ventilator's low-pressure alarm. Certain pathologic states are associated with a decreased $P_{ET}CO_2$ (e.g., apnea, pulmonary embolism and cardiac arrest).

(1:363–366, 598, 933), (10:99–101).

## IIA1e(3)

101. B. The BiPAP® ventilatory support system provides noninvasive pressure-support ventilation. Positive pressure ventilation is applied to spontaneously breathing patients via a mask covering the patient's nose. The sys-

tem is designed to accommodate moderate leaks. The BiPAP® system is not air tight. The patient can receive varying amounts of inspiratory and expiratory positive airway pressure (i.e., IPAP and EPAP, respectively).

This mode of ventilation has proved beneficial for patients who experience postextubation ventilatory distress. The utility of the BiPAP® system in this situation is the avoidance of reintubation. Others who might benefit from BiPAP® are postoperative thoracotomy and laparotomy patients, patients experiencing fluid overload and an increased work of breathing, and patients with hypoxemia as a primary cause of hypoventilation. BiPAP® is not to be used on patients who require full ventilatory support.

(BiPAP® S/T-D Ventilatory Support System product information, Respironics, Inc.), (1:866), (5:366, 571).

## IIB1e(1)

102. D. Substantial evidence exists indicating that the ventilator is not delivering the volume dialed in with the volume-control knob. This condition was ultimately confirmed when the volume was measured along the inspiratory limb before the humidifier, because there are fewer connections between the monitor and ventilator at that point. Therefore, the ventilator must be removed from service and sent to the manufacturer for repair and calibration.

(10:310, 319).

## IIA2i(3)

103. C. The flow rate of gas through the spontaneous breathing system should be at least four times the patient's measured spontaneous minute ventilation (e.g., 60 to 90 L/min). Throughout the patient's ventilatory cycle, mist should be visible leaving the exhalation port. Similarly, the pressure that registers on the pressure manometer of the system must not deflect more than −2 cm $H_2O$ with each inspiratory effort taken by the patient. A deflection more negative than −2 cm $H_2O$ indicates that either (1) the flow rate through the system is insufficient, (2) the one-way valve is malfunctioning, or (3) the one-way valve is positioned incorrectly.

(10:280–283).

## IIB2e(1)

104. B. When the low pressure alarm on a mechanical ventilator sounds, the problem generally is a disconnection in the ventilator circuit. Other situations that can cause the low pressure alarm to sound include a leak in the tubing, a low pressure limit that is set too high, and a large leak around the cuff of the ET tube. If the source of the problem is not readily identifiable, the patient should be disconnected from the ventilator and manually ventilated until help is summoned or until the situation is resolved.

Characteristic features appear on ventilator waveforms or graphics. A normal volume-pressure curve assumes the shape shown in Figure 4-28.

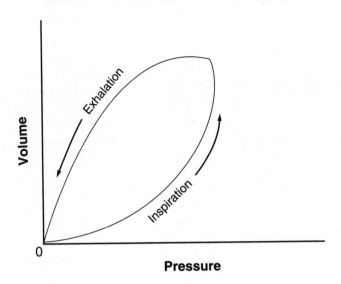

**Figure 4-28:** A normal volume-pressure waveform.

A leak in the system will cause the exhalation limb to fail to return to zero. The volume-pressure loop would appear as shown in Figure 4-29. Observe how the expiratory portion of the loop abruptly terminates. The point where a line drawn horizontally intersects the *y*-axis represents the volume lost from the leak.

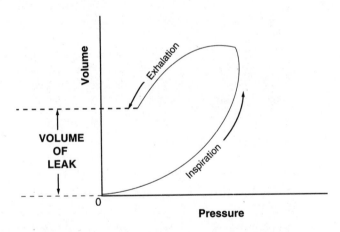

**Figure 4-29:** A volume-pressure loop demonstrating a system leak.

A normal flow-volume loop obtained from a ventilator patient has the appearance of the one shown in Figure 4-30.

If a leak occurs somewhere in the patient-ventilator system, the flow-volume loop will appear as shown in Figure 4-31.

Notice how the expiratory flow loop fails to return to the origin. The distance (volume) from the origin to

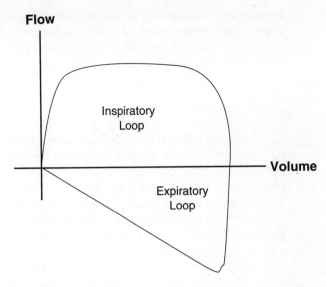

**Figure 4-30:** A normal flow-volume loop obtained from a ventilator patient.

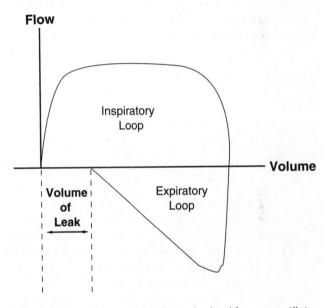

**Figure 4-31:** A flow-volume loop obtained from a ventilator patient demonstrating a leak somewhere in the patient ventilator system.

the point where the expiratory flow contacts the *x*-axis constitutes the volume of the leak.

(1:854), (10:48, 50, 254, 311, 315).

**IIA1d**

105. B. A significant disadvantage of a gas-powered resuscitator is that if the diaphragm were to rupture, the patient would be subjected to 50 psig of pressure. Most of these units are pressure limited, which is not a disadvantage. Some gas-powered resuscitators have demand valves. All units are capable of delivering 100% oxygen and contain a pressure-relief valve. Another disadvantage of these resuscitators is that tidal volume

delivery is compromised in the presence of decreased lung compliance and increased airway resistance.

(5:235–237), (13:201–202).

### IIB1s

106. B. When the patient bit against the ET tube as the fiberoptic bronchoscope was being inserted, she likely broke numerous fiber bundles in the bronchoscope. Any time fiber bundles on the bronchoscope are broken, black dots will appear in the field of vision. A blood clot or dirt on the tip of the bronchoscope will not render this effect. Instead, the vision of the viewer will be blurred. If the light source is unplugged, the entire field will be dark.

(15:627–635).

### IIB3b

107. D. The calibration or measured results in Table 4-5 vary from the predicted value by greater than 10%.

**Table 4-5** Spirometer Calibration Data

| Attempt # | Predicted Volume | Measured Volume | Percent Variation |
|---|---|---|---|
| 1 | 3.00 liters | 2.59 liters | 13.7% |
| 2 | 3.00 liters | 2.56 liters | 14.7% |
| 3 | 3.00 liters | 2.58 liters | 14.0% |

This degree of variation between what has been measured and the predicted value is unacceptable. The measured value must not deviate from the predicted by more than $\pm 3.0\%$. Therefore, the acceptable volume range for calibration of the spirometer with a 3-liter syringe is 2.91 to 3.09 liters. According to the American Thoracic Society-American College of Chest Physicians (ATS-ACCP) standards, at least one of three injected volumes must lie within $\pm 3.0$. These standards also recommend that three different flow rates be used (i.e., 0.5 to 1.0 L/sec., 1.0 to 1.5 L/sec., and 5.0 to 5.5 L/sec.). In the example shown, the spirometer fails to meet these standards and thus must not be used until serviced.

(Zamel, N., et al., 1983, "ACCP Scientific Section Recommendations—Statement on Spirometry; A report of the Section of Respiratory Pathophysiology," *Chest, 83*, 547–550).

### IIB1q(1)

108. A. One of the problems associated with the insertion of a pulmonary artery (Swan–Ganz) catheter (PAC) is coiling of the catheter in either the right atrium or right ventricle. Generally, when the site of insertion is the subclavian vein, the tip of the catheter resides in the

pulmonary artery when about 50 cm of the catheter have been inserted. Suspicions arose when the waveform, characteristic of the right ventricle, did not change despite the insertion of 80 cm of catheter. The normal waveforms experienced during the insertion of a PAC are shown in Figure 4-32.

(1:949–950), (9:348).

### IIA1r

109. C. Ordinarily, when air is present in the intrapleural space, it rises to the apex of the thoracic cavity. Therefore, to evacuate the air from the intrapleural space, a chest tube is usually placed in the third or fourth anterior intercostal space along the mid-axillary line. The chest tubes must always be inserted over the superior aspect of the rib, thereby avoiding injury to the blood vessels and nerves that are located along the inferior aspect of each rib.

(1:489).

### IIB3a

110. C. If it is anticipated that values beyond the usual calibration limits will be measured by an electrode, the RRT should recalibrate the electrode by using standards that exceed the values of the samples to be analyzed.

(1:350), (4:46), (6:304).

### IIA2

111. A. Two percent glutaraldehyde is mixed with sodium bicarbonate, thereby creating an alkaline glutaraldehyde solution. Glutaraldehyde's cidal activity occurs via the denaturation of cell protein. Alkaline glutaraldehyde is tuberculocidal in 10 minutes at room temperature. Additionally, alkaline glutaraldehyde is virucidal, fungicidal, and bactericidal in 10 minutes. Sterilization (sporicidal) occurs after 10 hours of immersion.

(1:44–45), (13:670–671).

### IIA1h(4)

112. A. Co-oximetry might be useful periodically because Isordil (amyl nitrate), an antianginal medication, produces nitrites as the drug is metabolized. Nitrites can cause the dysfunctional hemoglobin methemoglobin to form. Normal hemoglobin contains iron in the ferrous state ($Fe^{+2}$), thereby creating a bond suitable for the carriage of oxygen. Nitrites can oxidize hemoglobin. Specifically, they can oxidize the ferrous ion to the ferric ion ($Fe^{+3}$). When hemoglobin contains iron in the ferric state, hemoglobin can no longer reversibly and chemically combine with oxygen.

Therefore, because co-oximeters are capable of measuring fractional hemoglobin—specifically, carboxyhemoglobin, methemoglobin, oxyhemoglobin, and

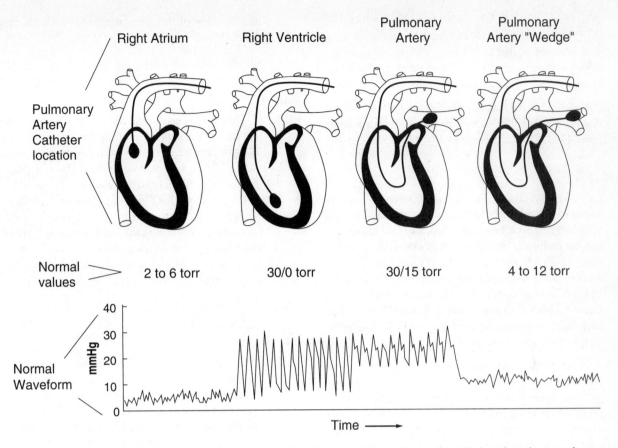

| Pulmonary Artery Catheter location | Right Atrium | Right Ventricle | Pulmonary Artery | Pulmonary Artery "Wedge" |
|---|---|---|---|---|
| Normal values | 2 to 6 torr | 30/0 torr | 30/15 torr | 4 to 12 torr |

**Figure 4-32:** Waveforms observed during PAC insertion. Note the association of the balloon tip location, the waveform, and normal values.

deoxyhemoglobin—patients who receive nitrite medications should have the percentage of methemoglobin in their circulation monitored.

(1:349, 358), (4:199), (5:297–298).

### IIB1h(4)

113. C. The transcutaneous $PCO_2$, or $PtcCO_2$, generally overestimates the arterial $PO_2$ because heating the $PtcCO_2$ electrode causes more carbon dioxide to diffuse through the skin. Despite the disparity between the actual values of these two measurements, however, the $PtcCO_2$ and the $PaCO_2$ generally correlate well. Their correlation will be lost when skin perfusion decreases and when the patient experiences an acidosis.

(1:354–355), (10:104).

### IIB2e(1)

114. C. Sidestream capnometers incorporate a water trap immediately before the sample gas enters the analyzer. The purpose of the water is to prevent condensation from entering the analyzer. The volume of the water is apparently critical, however, especially when the patient is mechanically ventilated with high PIPs. Therefore, the combination of a sidestream capnometer with

a large-volume (30-ml) water trap and high PIPs causes the capnograph tracing to deflect upward (expiratory deflection) during inspiration.

(1:363–365), (5:314–317), (13:257).

### IIB2e(1)

115. D. When the patient Y on the ventilator circuit disconnects from the ET tube, the PIP will suddenly drop to 0 cm $H_2O$. The patient's lung compliance and airway resistance affect the PIP also. An increased lung compliance and/or a decrease in the patient's airway resistance will result in a lower PIP. Neither of these two physiologic changes will cause the PIP to fall to 0 cm $H_2O$, however. If the exhalation valve is stuck in the inspiratory position, the PIP will increase because exhalation will not be complete. The next breath would be delivered while a portion of the preceding breath remains in the lungs.

(10:33, 109, 210–211, 254, 356).

### IIB2k

116. A. Positive expiratory pressure (PEP) mask therapy does not require the use of a positive pressure source. The patient exhales against a fixed orifice resistor placed

in the device's expiratory limb. Depending on their caliber, these resistors establish a positive expiratory pressure between 10 and 20 cm $H_2O$. The patient generally initiates therapy at a lower level, then gradually increases the positive expiratory pressure to a higher level.

("AARC Clinical Practice Guideline: Use of Positive Airway Pressure Adjuncts to Bronchial Hygiene Therapy," 1993, *Respiratory Care, 38,*(5), pp. 516–519).

## IIA1f(2)

117.  C. A double-lumen ET, or endobronchial, tube is sometimes used in conjunction with independent lung ventilation. This tube has two lumens. One lumen enters the mainstem bronchus (usually the right), and the other resides in the trachea. Each lumen has its own cuffs to allow sealing the airway for mechanical ventilation of one or both lungs. The diameter of each lumen is smaller than that of conventional ET tubes. The cuffs of these tubes vary from high-volume, low-pressure to low-volume, high-pressure types.

A number of considerations regarding positioning of this tube are critical to proper ventilation. For example, the lumen that is intended to enter the mainstem bronchus must not be inserted too deeply because ventilation to the upper lobe of that lung might be compromised, leading to atelectasis of that lobe. Similarly, if the tube is not advanced far enough into the airway, both lungs will receive the same ventilation.

(13:166).

## IIA1e(2)

118.  B. The high-frequency oscillator, which can ventilate at a frequency of 60 to 3,600 breaths/min. or 1 to 60 Hertz, offers a rather simple means of humidification compared with the high-frequency positive pressure ventilator (HFPPV) and high-frequency jet ventilator (HFJV). The bias gas flow is humidified, therefore conventional humidification systems are compatible with high-frequency oscillation (HFO).

(5:620–621), (13:614–618).

## IIA1o

119.  B. A vortex-shedding, flow-sensing device incorporates a strut to create turbulent flow between an ultrasonic transducer and an ultrasonic receiver. Each vortex of air interferes with the sound sensed by the receiver. This interference creates a change in current that is proportional to the gas flow. Also, as the ultrasound wave interference takes place, the pulses sensed by the ultrasonic receiver are proportional to a volume. The electronic sum of these pulses produces a volume readout. Ventilatory rate is also available on this device. Therefore, because the vital capacity is a volume,

the accuracy of this measurement is accurate despite the high flow rate limit of 250 L/min.

(5:276, 335), (13:296).

## IIB1d

120.  C. This brief scenario did not indicate that the rescuer was having difficulty depositing air through the device. The problem here focused on not seeing the patient's chest wall rise with each inspiration. Therefore, because the question did not refer to any problem or difficulty on the part of the RRT exhaling through the device, one can infer that the one-way valve is properly aligned and functioning. Vomitus in the mask would also create resistance to airflow, making the rescuer's exhalation difficult. At this point, it is reasonable to assume that the mask is not sealed well against the patient's face.

(1:649–650), (13:191).

## IIA1e(1)

121.  C. The Omni-Vent D/MRI is a pneumatically powered and pneumatically controlled transport ventilator that is designed intentionally for ventilation during magnetic resonance imaging (MRI). The Monaghan 225 can also be accommodated within an MRI unit. It is not a transport ventilator, however. Both the Newport E100i and the Bio-Med MVP 10 are transport ventilators, but neither one can function in an MRI unit.

(5:602), (13:561).

## IIB2e(2)

122.  B. The Life Pulse high-frequency jet ventilator comes equipped with a patient box. This satellite component to the jet ventilator contains (1) a pinch valve, (2) an inhalation valve release button, (3) a purge (solenoid) valve, (4) a pressure transducer, and (5) a patient box connector.

The pinch valve breaks the flow of pressurized gas delivered by the jet ventilator into small bursts. This operation is accomplished by a rapid pinching action (compression and decompression) on the portion of the patient breathing circuit situated in the patient box. The inhalation valve release button (PUSH-TO-LOAD button) enables the attachment of the patient breathing circuit to the patient box.

The purge (solenoid) valve maintains the pressure monitoring lumen of the Hi-Low Jet tracheal tube free of moisture or secretions. The pressure transducer enables measuring the pressure in the patient's trachea via the monitoring lumen. The patient box connector connects the patient box to the jet ventilator.

The CANNOT-MEET-PIP alarm lights under the following circumstances:

1. when a leak develops in the humidifier cartridge/patient breathing circuit
2. when the humidifier/cartridge patient breathing circuit is not properly connected to the Hi-Lo Jet tracheal tube
3. when the Hi-Lo Jet tracheal tube is damaged or defective (e.g., too much restriction to the high-frequency pulses in the jet tubing)
4. when the patient is too large for the Life Pulse ventilator
5. when the pinch valve is not opening enough, causing high servo pressures to meet the settings

(Life Pulse High-Frequency Jet Ventilator, Operator's Manual, p. VI-14, September 1990).

## IIB1e(2)

123. C. The SensorMedics 3100 ventilator is a high-frequency oscillatory ventilator only. It cannot function in a conventional mechanical ventilation mode. Therefore, the 3100 does not interface with a conventional ventilator as high-frequency jet ventilators do. The presence of a conventional ventilator along with the 3100 high-frequency oscillatory ventilator indicates that the patient might be about to be weaned from high-frequency mechanical ventilation.

(SensorMedics Corporation, product information), (5:630).

## IIA1a(1)

124. D. An ECG exhibiting ST-segment deviation and T-wave flattening often indicates the presence of an acute myocardial infarction. Because supplemental oxygen is believed to improve myocardial oxygenation and decrease the incidence of cardiac dysrhythmias, providing oxygen to the patient via a nasal cannula at 2 to 4 L/min. is generally the appliance of choice.

Neither a Brigg's adaptor nor a trach collar is appropriate here because the patient's condition does not warrant a tracheostomy. Both of these appliances are used in conjunction with a tracheostomy. An aerosol mask is not indicated here because high humidity is not warranted, nor is 60% oxygen. The high oxygen concentration (greater than 50%) provided by a non-rebreathing mask is unnecessary.

Because the patient here is showing no signs of respiratory distress, it is presumed that (1) his ventilatory pattern is normal and regular, (2) his tidal volume is normal, and (3) his ventilatory rate is normal. Therefore, he meets the criteria for a low-flow oxygen-delivery system. A cannula at 2 to 4 L/min. will provide an $F_IO_2$ between 0.28 to 0.36. This amount of oxygen might be sufficient to reduce the work of the heart.

(1:651), (3:54–58), (9:201–202), (13:66).

## IIA1a(1)

125. B. This patient is experiencing high-pressure (cardiogenic) pulmonary edema as indicated by the frothy, pink sputum being produced. The patient is hyperventilating ($PaCO_2$ 29 torr) and is moderately hypoxemic ($PaO_2$ 55 torr). The attempt here is to correct the hypoxemia causing the hyperventilation. Although a non-rebreathing mask is a low-flow device, it meets the low-flow criteria exhibited by this patient (i.e., a regular ventilatory pattern, a tidal volume between 300 cc to 700 cc, and a ventilatory rate of less than 25 breaths/min.).

The non-rebreathing mask at 10 L/min. can deliver up to 90% oxygen, depending on the patient's ventilatory pattern. If this device is unable to correct the patient's hypoxemia, intubation and CPAP might be required.

(1:749–750), (3:71–73), (13:75).

## IIA1f

126. C. Whenever a volume of gas is delivered by a mechanical ventilator, some of the volume remains in the ventilator tubing at end inspiration. Therefore, to determine the actual tidal volume or actual minute ventilation received by the patient, the volume "lost" or compressed in the ventilator circuit must be obtained. To perform this calculation, however, the compliance or compressibility factor of the ventilator tubing must be known.

To derive the tubing compressibility factor, a low tidal volume must be set and the patient Y connector must be occluded. When the ventilator cycles to inspiration, the PIP (opened maximally) must then be noted. The procedure for calculating the tubing compliance factor is outlined below.

STEP 1: Determine the tidal volume delivered by the Siemens Servo 900C.

$$V_T = \frac{\dot{V}_E}{f}$$

where

$V_T$ = tidal volume (cc)
$\dot{V}_E$ = minute ventilation (L/min.)
$f$ = ventilatory rate (breaths/min.)

$$V_T = \frac{2 \text{ L/min.}}{10 \text{ breaths/min.}}$$

$$= 0.2 \text{ L/breath or}$$
$$200 \text{ cc/breath}$$

STEP 2: Calculate the tubing compliance factor by using the following formula.

$$C_T = \frac{V_T}{PIP - PEEP}$$

where

$C_T$ = tubing compliance (cc/cm $H_2O$)
$V_T$ = tidal volume (cc)
PIP = peak inspiratory pressure (cm $H_2O$)
PEEP = positive end-expiratory pressure (cm $H_2O$)

$$C_T = \frac{200\ cc}{55\ cm\ H_2O - 5\ cm\ H_2O}$$
$$= 4\ cc/cm\ H_2O$$

This value indicates that for each cm $H_2O$ pressure generated during inspiration, 4 cc of volume is compressed ("lost") in the ventilator tubing.

(1:937), (10:208, 257).

## IA1f(3)

127.  C.

STEP 1:   Determine the delivered tidal volume.

$$V_T = \frac{\dot{V}_E}{f}$$

$$= \frac{8\ L/min.}{10\ breaths/min.}$$

$$= 0.8\ L/breath\ or\ 800\ cc/breath$$

STEP 2:   Determine the volume compressed ("lost") in the tubing by solving for $V_{lost}$.

$$C_T = \frac{V_{lost}}{PIP - PEEP}$$

therefore,

$$V_{lost} = C_T(PIP - PEEP)$$
$$= (4\ cc/cm\ H_2O)(40\ cm\ H_2O - 5\ cm\ H_2O)$$
$$= (4\ cc/cm\ H_2O)(35\ cm\ H_2O)$$
$$= 140\ cc$$

STEP 3:   Calculate this patient's actual tidal volume.

$$V_T = ventilator\ volume - compressed\ volume$$
$$= 800\ cc - 140\ cc$$
$$= 660\ cc$$

(1:937), (10:208, 257).

## IIIB2c

128.  D. The patient's IBW is given in pounds; therefore, it must be converted to kg.

$$kg = \frac{145\ lbs}{2.2\ lbs/kg}$$
$$= 65.9\ kg$$

Now, knowing the patient's IBW in kilograms, the tidal volume recommended by the physician (10 cc/kg) can be determined.

$$V_T = (10\ cc/kg)(65.9\ kg)$$
$$= 659\ cc$$

Because the tidal volume set on the ventilator is 800 cc and the volume "lost" in the ventilator tubing is 140 cc, the patient's actual tidal volume is already 660 cc. Therefore, no change in the ventilator setting is necessary. If it were necessary to alter the tidal volume, however, the change could be accomplished by either (1) adjusting the ventilatory rate or (2) manipulating the minute ventilation. The following formula can be rearranged to solve for either $\dot{V}_E$ or f:

$$V_T = \frac{\dot{V}_E}{f}$$

Keep in mind that the SIMV rate setting will have no influence on the tidal volume but must always be set equal to, or less than, the breaths per minute (rate) control located on the panel immediately above the SIMV rate control.

(1:937), (10:208, 257).

## IA1a

129.  A. These grossly obese patients actually exhibit the signs and symptoms of sleep apnea. During sleep, they experience a loss of pharyngeal muscle tone. Similarly, the genioglossus muscle of the tongue becomes flaccid and rests against the posterior pharyngeal wall. The combination of these events creates an upper airway obstruction during sleep, or *obstructive sleep apnea*. These patients often present with a variety of clinical manifestations also known as obesity-hypoventilation syndrome. This condition was formerly called Pickwickian Syndrome, named after the obese messenger, Joe, in Charles Dickens' first novel, *The Pickwick Papers*. These clinical manifestations include lethargy, hypersomnolence, pulmonary hypertension, and congestive heart failure.

The excessive weight carried by these persons creates a restrictive breathing condition. Diaphragmatic and thoracic excursions are limited. Arterial blood gases (ABGs) reveal alveolar hypoventilation, either partially compensated or noncompensated respiratory acidosis (depending on the severity of the restrictive condition) and the resultant effects of the increased work of breathing. It is a condition producing a low $\dot{V}_A/\dot{Q}_C$ ratio caused almost entirely by a decreased alveolar ventilation. These patients can improve their alveolar ventilation on command and ordinarily respond well when they lose weight.

(1:554–557), (9:358–359), (15:250, 304, 306, 751–752).

## IIA1a

130. A. The ordinarily high $CO_2$ of the obesity-hypoventilation syndrome patient has, in essence, produced the same effects as a chronic $CO_2$ retainer who is breathing in response to his hypoxic drive. Unlike COPD patients, however, these patients generally respond well to ventilatory stimulants. The starting baseline for oxygen administration is a low $F_IO_2$. Of course, oxygen administration should be correlated to ABG analysis and the oxygen percentage adjusted according to the patient's expected normals. The first therapeutic intervention should be directed toward relieving the hypoxemia and the work of breathing. In the absence of further complications (i.e., pulmonary infection), the implementation of IPPB, aerosol therapy, or CPT is not indicated at the onset. Assessment should be performed to determine whether the immediate oxygen therapy has relieved the patient's ventilatory distress and improved alveolar ventilation. If it has not, consideration should be given to mechanical ventilatory support (intermittent or continuous). In terms of long-term therapy, these patients often respond favorably to nocturnal CPAP or BIPAP®. Tracheostomy is sometimes performed to circumvent the obstructive apnea problem.

(1:554–557), (9:358–359), (15:250, 304, 306, 751–752).

# References

1. Scanlan, C., Spearman, C., and Sheldon, R., *Egan's Fundamentals of Respiratory Care*, 7th ed., Mosby-Year Book, Inc., St. Louis, MO, 1999.

2. Kacmarek, R., Mack, C., and Dimas, S., *The Essentials of Respiratory Care*, 3rd ed., Mosby-Year Book, Inc., St. Louis, MO, 1990.

3. Shapiro B., Peruzzi, W., and Kozlowska-Templin, R., *Clinical Applications of Blood Gases*, 5th ed., Mosby-Year Book, Inc., St. Louis, MO, 1994.

4. Malley, W., *Clinical Blood Gases: Application and Noninvasive Alternatives*, W.B. Saunders Co., Philadelphia, PA, 1990.

5. White, G., *Equipment Theory for Respiratory Care*, 3rd ed., Delmar, Albany, NY, 1999.

6. Ruppel, G., *Manual of Pulmonary Function Testing*, 7th ed., Mosby-Year Book, Inc., St. Louis, MO, 1998.

7. Barnes, T., *Core Textbook of Respiratory Care Practice*, 2nd ed., Mosby-Year Book, Inc., St. Louis, MO, 1994.

8. Rau, J., *Respiratory Care Pharmacology*, 5th ed., Mosby-Year Book, Inc., St. Louis, MO, 1998.

9. Wilkins, R., Sheldon, R., and Krider, S., *Clinical Assessment in Respiratory Care*, 4th ed., Mosby-Year Book, Inc., St. Louis, MO, 2000.

10. Pilbeam, S., *Mechanical Ventilation: Physiological and Clinical Applications*, 3rd ed., Mosby-Year Book, Inc., St. Louis, MO, 1998.

11. Madama, V., *Pulmonary Function Testing and Cardiopulmonary Stress Testing*, 2nd ed., Delmar, Albany, NY, 1998.

12. Koff, P., Eitzman, D., and New, J., *Neonatal and Pediatric Respiratory Care*, 2nd ed., Mosby-Year Book, Inc., St. Louis, MO, 1993.

13. Branson, R., Hess, D., and Chatburn, R., *Respiratory Care Equipment*, J.B. Lippincott, Co., Philadelphia, PA, 1995.

14. Darovic, G., *Hemodynamic Monitoring: Invasive and Noninvasive Clinical Application*, 2nd ed., W.B. Saunders Company, Philadelphia, PA, 1995.

15. Pierson, D, and Kacmarek, R., *Foundations of Respiratory Care*, Churchill Livingston, Inc., New York, NY, 1992.

16. Burton, et al., *Respiratory Care: A Guide to Clinical Practice*, 4th ed., Lippincott-Raven Publishers, Philadelphia, PA, 1997.

17. Wojciechowski, W., *Respiratory Care Sciences: An Integrated Approach*, 3rd ed., Delmar, Albany, NY, 2000.

18. Aloan, C., *Respiratory Care of the Newborn and Child*, 2nd ed., Lippincott-Raven Publishers, Philadelphia, PA, 1997.

19. Dantzker, D., MacIntyre, N., and Bakow, E., *Comprehensive Respiratory Care*, W.B. Saunders Company, Philadelphia, PA, 1998.

20. Farzan, S., and Farzan, D., *A Concise Handbook of Respiratory Diseases*, 4th ed., Appleton & Lange, Stamford, CT, 1997.

# CHAPTER 5 ———— THERAPEUTIC PROCEDURES

**PURPOSE:** This chapter consists of 222 items intended to assess your understanding and comprehension of subject matter contained in the therapeutic procedures portion of the Written Registry Examination for Advanced Respiratory Therapy Practitioners. In this chapter, you are required to answer questions regarding the following activities:

A. Evaluating, monitoring, and recording the patient's response to respiratory care
B. Conducting therapeutic procedures in order to maintain a patent airway, achieving adequate ventilation and oxygenation, and removing bronchopulmonary secretions
C. Making necessary modifications to therapeutic procedures based on patient response
D. Initiating, conducting, and modifying respiratory care
E. Assisting the physician, initiating and conducting pulmonary rehabilitation

> **NOTE:** Please refer to the examination matrix key located at the end of this chapter. This examination matrix key will enable you to identify the specific areas on the Written Registry Examination Matrix that require remediation, based on your performance on the test items in this chapter. Use the answer sheet located at the front of this chapter to record your answers as you work through questions relating to therapeutic procedures. Remember to study the analyses that follow the questions in this chapter. The purpose of each analysis is to present you with the rationale for the correct answer (and, in many instances, reasons are given for why the distractors are incorrect). The references at the end of each analysis provide you with resources to seek more information regarding each question and its associated Written Registry Examination Matrix item. Please keep in mind that this chapter is too lengthy to complete in one sitting. Be realistic about your approach here. Consider completing this chapter in four sessions according to the following breakdown:

SESSION 1: 1 to 52 questions, analyses, and matrix items
SESSION 2: 53 to 104 questions, analyses, and matrix items
SESSION 3: 105 to 156 questions, analyses, and matrix items
SESSION 4: 157 to 208 questions, analyses, and matrix items

# Therapeutic Procedures Answer Sheet

**DIRECTIONS:** Darken the space under the selected answer.

|  | A | B | C | D |  |  | A | B | C | D |
|---|---|---|---|---|---|---|---|---|---|---|
| 1. | ❏ | ❏ | ❏ | ❏ |  | 25. | ❏ | ❏ | ❏ | ❏ |
| 2. | ❏ | ❏ | ❏ | ❏ |  | 26. | ❏ | ❏ | ❏ | ❏ |
| 3. | ❏ | ❏ | ❏ | ❏ |  | 27. | ❏ | ❏ | ❏ | ❏ |
| 4. | ❏ | ❏ | ❏ | ❏ |  | 28. | ❏ | ❏ | ❏ | ❏ |
| 5. | ❏ | ❏ | ❏ | ❏ |  | 29. | ❏ | ❏ | ❏ | ❏ |
| 6. | ❏ | ❏ | ❏ | ❏ |  | 30. | ❏ | ❏ | ❏ | ❏ |
| 7. | ❏ | ❏ | ❏ | ❏ |  | 31. | ❏ | ❏ | ❏ | ❏ |
| 8. | ❏ | ❏ | ❏ | ❏ |  | 32. | ❏ | ❏ | ❏ | ❏ |
| 9. | ❏ | ❏ | ❏ | ❏ |  | 33. | ❏ | ❏ | ❏ | ❏ |
| 10. | ❏ | ❏ | ❏ | ❏ |  | 34. | ❏ | ❏ | ❏ | ❏ |
| 11. | ❏ | ❏ | ❏ | ❏ |  | 35. | ❏ | ❏ | ❏ | ❏ |
| 12. | ❏ | ❏ | ❏ | ❏ |  | 36. | ❏ | ❏ | ❏ | ❏ |
| 13. | ❏ | ❏ | ❏ | ❏ |  | 37. | ❏ | ❏ | ❏ | ❏ |
| 14. | ❏ | ❏ | ❏ | ❏ |  | 38. | ❏ | ❏ | ❏ | ❏ |
| 15. | ❏ | ❏ | ❏ | ❏ |  | 39. | ❏ | ❏ | ❏ | ❏ |
| 16. | ❏ | ❏ | ❏ | ❏ |  | 40. | ❏ | ❏ | ❏ | ❏ |
| 17. | ❏ | ❏ | ❏ | ❏ |  | 41. | ❏ | ❏ | ❏ | ❏ |
| 18. | ❏ | ❏ | ❏ | ❏ |  | 42. | ❏ | ❏ | ❏ | ❏ |
| 19. | ❏ | ❏ | ❏ | ❏ |  | 43. | ❏ | ❏ | ❏ | ❏ |
| 20. | ❏ | ❏ | ❏ | ❏ |  | 44. | ❏ | ❏ | ❏ | ❏ |
| 21. | ❏ | ❏ | ❏ | ❏ |  | 45. | ❏ | ❏ | ❏ | ❏ |
| 22. | ❏ | ❏ | ❏ | ❏ |  | 46. | ❏ | ❏ | ❏ | ❏ |
| 23. | ❏ | ❏ | ❏ | ❏ |  | 47. | ❏ | ❏ | ❏ | ❏ |
| 24. | ❏ | ❏ | ❏ | ❏ |  | 48. | ❏ | ❏ | ❏ | ❏ |

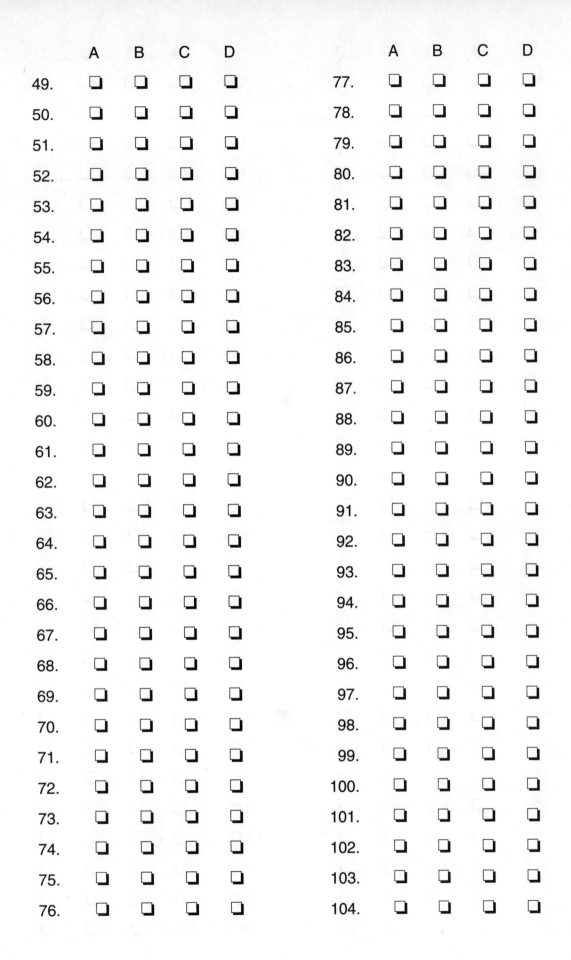

|  | A | B | C | D |  | A | B | C | D |
|---|---|---|---|---|---|---|---|---|---|
| 49. | ❏ | ❏ | ❏ | ❏ | 77. | ❏ | ❏ | ❏ | ❏ |
| 50. | ❏ | ❏ | ❏ | ❏ | 78. | ❏ | ❏ | ❏ | ❏ |
| 51. | ❏ | ❏ | ❏ | ❏ | 79. | ❏ | ❏ | ❏ | ❏ |
| 52. | ❏ | ❏ | ❏ | ❏ | 80. | ❏ | ❏ | ❏ | ❏ |
| 53. | ❏ | ❏ | ❏ | ❏ | 81. | ❏ | ❏ | ❏ | ❏ |
| 54. | ❏ | ❏ | ❏ | ❏ | 82. | ❏ | ❏ | ❏ | ❏ |
| 55. | ❏ | ❏ | ❏ | ❏ | 83. | ❏ | ❏ | ❏ | ❏ |
| 56. | ❏ | ❏ | ❏ | ❏ | 84. | ❏ | ❏ | ❏ | ❏ |
| 57. | ❏ | ❏ | ❏ | ❏ | 85. | ❏ | ❏ | ❏ | ❏ |
| 58. | ❏ | ❏ | ❏ | ❏ | 86. | ❏ | ❏ | ❏ | ❏ |
| 59. | ❏ | ❏ | ❏ | ❏ | 87. | ❏ | ❏ | ❏ | ❏ |
| 60. | ❏ | ❏ | ❏ | ❏ | 88. | ❏ | ❏ | ❏ | ❏ |
| 61. | ❏ | ❏ | ❏ | ❏ | 89. | ❏ | ❏ | ❏ | ❏ |
| 62. | ❏ | ❏ | ❏ | ❏ | 90. | ❏ | ❏ | ❏ | ❏ |
| 63. | ❏ | ❏ | ❏ | ❏ | 91. | ❏ | ❏ | ❏ | ❏ |
| 64. | ❏ | ❏ | ❏ | ❏ | 92. | ❏ | ❏ | ❏ | ❏ |
| 65. | ❏ | ❏ | ❏ | ❏ | 93. | ❏ | ❏ | ❏ | ❏ |
| 66. | ❏ | ❏ | ❏ | ❏ | 94. | ❏ | ❏ | ❏ | ❏ |
| 67. | ❏ | ❏ | ❏ | ❏ | 95. | ❏ | ❏ | ❏ | ❏ |
| 68. | ❏ | ❏ | ❏ | ❏ | 96. | ❏ | ❏ | ❏ | ❏ |
| 69. | ❏ | ❏ | ❏ | ❏ | 97. | ❏ | ❏ | ❏ | ❏ |
| 70. | ❏ | ❏ | ❏ | ❏ | 98. | ❏ | ❏ | ❏ | ❏ |
| 71. | ❏ | ❏ | ❏ | ❏ | 99. | ❏ | ❏ | ❏ | ❏ |
| 72. | ❏ | ❏ | ❏ | ❏ | 100. | ❏ | ❏ | ❏ | ❏ |
| 73. | ❏ | ❏ | ❏ | ❏ | 101. | ❏ | ❏ | ❏ | ❏ |
| 74. | ❏ | ❏ | ❏ | ❏ | 102. | ❏ | ❏ | ❏ | ❏ |
| 75. | ❏ | ❏ | ❏ | ❏ | 103. | ❏ | ❏ | ❏ | ❏ |
| 76. | ❏ | ❏ | ❏ | ❏ | 104. | ❏ | ❏ | ❏ | ❏ |

|      | A | B | C | D |      | A | B | C | D |
|------|---|---|---|---|------|---|---|---|---|
| 105. | ❏ | ❏ | ❏ | ❏ | 134. | ❏ | ❏ | ❏ | ❏ |
| 106. | ❏ | ❏ | ❏ | ❏ | 135. | ❏ | ❏ | ❏ | ❏ |
| 107. | ❏ | ❏ | ❏ | ❏ | 136. | ❏ | ❏ | ❏ | ❏ |
| 108. | ❏ | ❏ | ❏ | ❏ | 137. | ❏ | ❏ | ❏ | ❏ |
| 109. | ❏ | ❏ | ❏ | ❏ | 138. | ❏ | ❏ | ❏ | ❏ |
| 110. | ❏ | ❏ | ❏ | ❏ | 139. | ❏ | ❏ | ❏ | ❏ |
| 111. | ❏ | ❏ | ❏ | ❏ | 140. | ❏ | ❏ | ❏ | ❏ |
| 112. | ❏ | ❏ | ❏ | ❏ | 141. | ❏ | ❏ | ❏ | ❏ |
| 113. | ❏ | ❏ | ❏ | ❏ | 142. | ❏ | ❏ | ❏ | ❏ |
| 114. | ❏ | ❏ | ❏ | ❏ | 143. | ❏ | ❏ | ❏ | ❏ |
| 115. | ❏ | ❏ | ❏ | ❏ | 144. | ❏ | ❏ | ❏ | ❏ |
| 116. | ❏ | ❏ | ❏ | ❏ | 145. | ❏ | ❏ | ❏ | ❏ |
| 117. | ❏ | ❏ | ❏ | ❏ | 146. | ❏ | ❏ | ❏ | ❏ |
| 118. | ❏ | ❏ | ❏ | ❏ | 147. | ❏ | ❏ | ❏ | ❏ |
| 119. | ❏ | ❏ | ❏ | ❏ | 148. | ❏ | ❏ | ❏ | ❏ |
| 120. | ❏ | ❏ | ❏ | ❏ | 149. | ❏ | ❏ | ❏ | ❏ |
| 121. | ❏ | ❏ | ❏ | ❏ | 150. | ❏ | ❏ | ❏ | ❏ |
| 122. | ❏ | ❏ | ❏ | ❏ | 151. | ❏ | ❏ | ❏ | ❏ |
| 123. | ❏ | ❏ | ❏ | ❏ | 152. | ❏ | ❏ | ❏ | ❏ |
| 124. | ❏ | ❏ | ❏ | ❏ | 153. | ❏ | ❏ | ❏ | ❏ |
| 125. | ❏ | ❏ | ❏ | ❏ | 154. | ❏ | ❏ | ❏ | ❏ |
| 126. | ❏ | ❏ | ❏ | ❏ | 155. | ❏ | ❏ | ❏ | ❏ |
| 127. | ❏ | ❏ | ❏ | ❏ | 156. | ❏ | ❏ | ❏ | ❏ |
| 128. | ❏ | ❏ | ❏ | ❏ | 157. | ❏ | ❏ | ❏ | ❏ |
| 129. | ❏ | ❏ | ❏ | ❏ | 158. | ❏ | ❏ | ❏ | ❏ |
| 130. | ❏ | ❏ | ❏ | ❏ | 159. | ❏ | ❏ | ❏ | ❏ |
| 131. | ❏ | ❏ | ❏ | ❏ | 160. | ❏ | ❏ | ❏ | ❏ |
| 132. | ❏ | ❏ | ❏ | ❏ | 161. | ❏ | ❏ | ❏ | ❏ |
| 133. | ❏ | ❏ | ❏ | ❏ | 162. | ❏ | ❏ | ❏ | ❏ |

|      | A | B | C | D |      | A | B | C | D |
|------|---|---|---|---|------|---|---|---|---|
| 163. | ❏ | ❏ | ❏ | ❏ | 186. | ❏ | ❏ | ❏ | ❏ |
| 164. | ❏ | ❏ | ❏ | ❏ | 187. | ❏ | ❏ | ❏ | ❏ |
| 165. | ❏ | ❏ | ❏ | ❏ | 188. | ❏ | ❏ | ❏ | ❏ |
| 166. | ❏ | ❏ | ❏ | ❏ | 189. | ❏ | ❏ | ❏ | ❏ |
| 167. | ❏ | ❏ | ❏ | ❏ | 190. | ❏ | ❏ | ❏ | ❏ |
| 168. | ❏ | ❏ | ❏ | ❏ | 191. | ❏ | ❏ | ❏ | ❏ |
| 169. | ❏ | ❏ | ❏ | ❏ | 192. | ❏ | ❏ | ❏ | ❏ |
| 170. | ❏ | ❏ | ❏ | ❏ | 193. | ❏ | ❏ | ❏ | ❏ |
| 171. | ❏ | ❏ | ❏ | ❏ | 194. | ❏ | ❏ | ❏ | ❏ |
| 172. | ❏ | ❏ | ❏ | ❏ | 195. | ❏ | ❏ | ❏ | ❏ |
| 173. | ❏ | ❏ | ❏ | ❏ | 196. | ❏ | ❏ | ❏ | ❏ |
| 174. | ❏ | ❏ | ❏ | ❏ | 197. | ❏ | ❏ | ❏ | ❏ |
| 175. | ❏ | ❏ | ❏ | ❏ | 198. | ❏ | ❏ | ❏ | ❏ |
| 176. | ❏ | ❏ | ❏ | ❏ | 190. | ❏ | ❏ | ❏ | ❏ |
| 177. | ❏ | ❏ | ❏ | ❏ | 200. | ❏ | ❏ | ❏ | ❏ |
| 178. | ❏ | ❏ | ❏ | ❏ | 201. | ❏ | ❏ | ❏ | ❏ |
| 179. | ❏ | ❏ | ❏ | ❏ | 202. | ❏ | ❏ | ❏ | ❏ |
| 180. | ❏ | ❏ | ❏ | ❏ | 203. | ❏ | ❏ | ❏ | ❏ |
| 181. | ❏ | ❏ | ❏ | ❏ | 204. | ❏ | ❏ | ❏ | ❏ |
| 182. | ❏ | ❏ | ❏ | ❏ | 205. | ❏ | ❏ | ❏ | ❏ |
| 183. | ❏ | ❏ | ❏ | ❏ | 206. | ❏ | ❏ | ❏ | ❏ |
| 184. | ❏ | ❏ | ❏ | ❏ | 207. | ❏ | ❏ | ❏ | ❏ |
| 185. | ❏ | ❏ | ❏ | ❏ | 208. | ❏ | ❏ | ❏ | ❏ |

# Therapeutic Procedures Assessment

**DIRECTIONS:** Each of the questions or incomplete statements below is followed by four suggested answers or completions. Select the one that is best in each case, and then blacken the corresponding space on the answer sheet found in the front of this chapter. Good luck.

1. The RRT has just administered a bronchodilator to a mechanically ventilated patient. The before and after flow-volume loop is displayed in Figure 5-1. How should the RRT record this patient's response to therapy?

    A. The patient did *not* exhale forcefully enough.
    B. The after bronchodilator study was performed too soon following bronchodilator administration.
    C. The bronchodilator had a beneficial effect on the patient's expiratory flow rates.
    D. A more potent β-2 agonist needs to be administered.

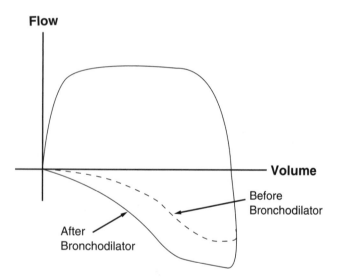

**Figure 5-1:** Flow-volume obtained from a mechanically ventilated patient. Dotted line below baseline indicates exhalation before brochodilator. Heavy line below baseline represents exhalation after brochodilator.

2. A 6-year-old child has experienced an accidental drug overdose. A 4 mm I.D. endotracheal tube has been inserted, and mechanical ventilation has been initiated. The low pressure alarm sounds with each mechanical breath. What action would correct this problem?

    A. re-intubating the child with a 6 mm I.D. endotracheal tube
    B. performing endotracheal suctioning
    C. increasing the delivered tidal volume
    D. inflating the cuff of the endotracheal tube with more air

3. A patient treated for a tension pneumothorax with chest tubes in the ICU needs to be transported by air to another hospital. A portable suction device is being considered for the transport. Which of the following considerations must be taken into account?

    A. A battery-powered, portable suction system must be used.
    B. A Heimlich valve can be used during transport.
    C. The chest tubes can be clamped during transport.
    D. A trial for the anticipated transport time must be conducted in the ICU by using the portable system chosen.

4. Which of the following mechanical ventilators would be most likely chosen to ventilate a patient with adult respiratory distress syndrome (ARDS) complicated with a bronchopulmonary fistula?

    A. high-frequency jet ventilator
    B. negative pressure ventilator
    C. a ventilator providing SIMV with pressure support
    D. pressure control with inverse ratio ventilation

5. A patient who has left ventricular failure, causing an increased preload, has been admitted to the coronary care unit (CCU). He has received pharmacologic intervention to increase myocardial contractility. Which of the following therapeutic interventions would be most beneficial at this time?

    A. nasal cannula at 5 L/min.
    B. 5 to 10 cm $H_2O$ of mask continuous positive airway pressure (CPAP) with 30% oxygen
    C. continuous ultrasonic nebulization with supplemental oxygen
    D. ET intubation and 40% oxygen via a Briggs adaptor

6. Calculate the arterial–venous oxygen content difference when given a cardiac output (C.O.) of 5 L/min. and an oxygen consumption of 250 ml/min.

    A. 3.5 volumes %
    B. 4.0 volumes %
    C. 4.5 volumes %
    D. 5.0 volumes %

7. Which of the following hazards are associated with changing a tracheostomy tube?

I. injury to the recurrent laryngeal nerve
II. right mainstem intubation
III. placement of the tube in pretracheal space
IV. cuff laceration

   A. I, II, III, IV
   B. II, III only
   C. I, III, IV only
   D. II, IV only

8. Determine an appropriate flow rate needed to deliver a 40-ml $V_T$ to an infant breathing 45 breaths/min. while receiving mechanical ventilation. The desired inspiratory:expiratory (I:E) ratio is 1:2.

   A. 90 ml/sec.
   B. 120 ml/sec.
   C. 126 ml/sec.
   D. 150 ml/sec.

9. Which ventilation variable(s) is(are) set by the RRT when ventilating a patient in the pressure-support mode?

   I. tidal volume
   II. pressure plateau level
   III. peak inspiratory flow rate
   IV. ventilatory rate

   A. II only
   B. I, III, IV only
   C. II, III only
   D. I only

10. A 32-week-old neonate is receiving CPAP of 2 cm $H_2O$ at an $FiO_2$ of 0.35. Arterial blood gas (ABG) and acid-base data reveal the following:

PO$_2$ 85 torr
PCO$_2$ 35 torr
pH 7.44
HCO$_3^-$ 23 mEq/liter
B.E. 0 mEq/liter

What should the neonatal RRT do at this time?

   A. Extubate the infant and provide 35% $O_2$.
   B. Terminate the CPAP and institute a T-piece at 40%.
   C. Increase the $FiO_2$ to 0.40.
   D. Increase the CPAP to 4 cm $H_2O$.

11. Which of the following statements are true concerning pressure-control inverse-ratio ventilation (PC-IRV)?

   I. The patient must be sedated and paralyzed with this mode of ventilation.
   II. Peak airway pressures are reduced with this ventilation mode.
   III. The delivered tidal volume decreases as the ventilatory rate or the I:E ratio increases.
   IV. This mode is useful for patients who have dynamic flow limitation.

   A. I, II, III, IV
   B. I, II, III only
   C. II, III only
   D. I, II only

12. Which of the following statements are true regarding mean airway pressure ($\overline{P}_{aw}$)?

   I. The $\overline{P}_{aw}$ is greater with sine waveflow patterns than with square waveflow patterns.
   II. High $\overline{P}_{aw}$ can cause venous obstruction in patients who have improving lung compliance.
   III. Increasing the $\overline{P}_{aw}$ in neonates who have respiratory distress syndrome usually increases the arterial PO$_2$.
   IV. The $\overline{P}_{aw}$ is ordinarily affected by changes in the I:E ratio, positive end-respiratory pressure (PEEP), and peak inspiratory pressure (PIP).

   A. I, IV only
   B. II, III, IV only
   C. II, IV only
   D. I, III only

13. Which of the following medications can be given in combination to sedate a patient for ET intubation?

   I. midazolam and morphine
   II. fentanyl and morphine
   III. diazepam and fentanyl
   IV. chlordiazepoxide and benzocaine

   A. II, IV only
   B. I, II only
   C. I, III only
   D. II, III, IV only

14. Which inspiratory time percent setting on the Siemens Servo 900C ventilator enables the establishment of inverse-ratio ventilation?

   A. 25%
   B. 33%
   C. 50%
   D. 67%

15. The most effective method for the administration of artificial surfactant is by:

   A. intramuscular injection.
   B. aerosolization.
   C. intravenous injection.
   D. instillation into the ET tube.

16. Which of the following therapeutic interventions would be appropriate to recommend for a patient who has a neuromuscular disease requiring nocturnal ventilatory support at home?

   I. tracheostomy
   II. mechanical ventilation via a portable positive pressure ventilator

III. negative pressure ventilation via a chest cuirass

IV. bilevel, noncontinuous pressure-support ventilation (PSV)

A. I, II, III, IV
B. II only
C. I, IV only
D. III, IV only

17. Calculate the percent shunt for a mechanically ventilated patient who is receiving 100% oxygen and who has a pulmonary artery catheter (PAC) in place. This patient's arterial and mixed venous blood gas data are as follows:

| Arterial | Venous |
| --- | --- |
| $PaO_2$ 325 torr | $P\bar{v}O_2$ 55 torr |
| $PaCO_2$ 35 torr | $P\bar{v}CO_2$ 48 torr |
| $SaO_2$ 100% | $S\bar{v}O_2$ 80% |

This patient has a normal respiratory quotient and a hemoglobin concentration of 13 g/dl.

A. 10%
B. 20%
C. 30%
D. 40%

18. The RRT is confronted with the problem of stabilizing the particle size of an aerosol from a small-volume nebulizer. How can this goal be accomplished?

A. Fill the nebulizer with 15 ml of solution.
B. Have the patient hold the nebulizer firmly in his hand with his fingers enveloping the nebulizer.
C. Use a compressed air cylinder to supply the gas to the nebulizer.
D. Reduce the humidity of the gas supplying the nebulizer.

19. A mechanically ventilated patient develops subcutaneous emphysema. The patient appears dyspneic, cyanotic, and is achieving high peak inspiratory pressures with each mechanical ventilatory breath. Which of the following actions should the RRT recommend?

A. application of inverse ratio ventilation
B. insertion of chest tubes
C. thoracentesis
D. pleurodesis

20. While performing cardiopulmonary resuscitation on a patient, the RRT is questioned by the physician as to when endotracheal intubation is appropriate. The RRT should respond by saying:

A. "Intubation should be attempted as soon as possible during the resuscitative effort."
B. "Intubation should be delayed until the victim has received bag-mask ventilation for at least 15 minutes."
C. "Intubation should be performed when serial ABG data demonstrate the patient's $PaCO_2$ is rising."
D. "Intubation should be performed after the initial ventilation of the victim has been accomplished and when the procedure can be performed without jeopardizing effective resuscitative efforts."

21. A neuromuscular disease patient is experiencing ventilatory muscle fatigue. Room air ABGs at this time reveal the following:

$PO_2$ 65 torr
$PCO_2$ 55 torr
pH 7.32
$HCO_3^-$ 26 mEq/liter
B.E. 1 mEQ/liter

Over the past hour, his maximum inspiratory pressure (MIP) has changed from $-65$ cm $H_2O$ to $-40$ cm $H_2O$. The patient has a spontaneous ventilatory rate of 8 breaths/min. and is currently receiving BiPAP® in the spontaneous mode. Which intervention would be most appropriate at this time?

A. intubating and mechanically ventilating the patient
B. changing the BiPAP® to the spontaneous-timed mode and adding oxygen
C. switching the BiPAP® to the timed mode and providing oxygen
D. adjusting the BiPAP® to the CPAP/EPAP mode and supplying oxygen

22. A neonate is being mechanically ventilated via a ventilator displaying a square pressure waveform. Given the following data, calculate the mean airway pressure:

ventilatory rate: 45 breaths/min.
peak inspiratory flow: 9 L/min.
peak inspiratory pressure (PIP): 22 cm $H_2O$
$FiO_2$: 0.50
PEEP: 5 cm $H_2O$
I:E ratio: 1:1.6

A. 8.3 cm $H_2O$
B. 11.5 cm $H_2O$
C. 13.4 cm $H_2O$
D. 15.5 cm $H_2O$

23. An RRT is discussing discharge orders with an emphysematous patient. The most important aspect of the discharge orders concerning this patient's pulmonary status is:

A. avoiding air pollution.

B. avoiding individuals with respiratory tract infections.

C. quitting smoking.

D. avoiding traveling by air.

24. To establish an I:E ratio of 2:1 on a patient who is receiving controlled mechanical ventilation from the Siemens Servo 900C, which of the following inspiratory time % and pause time % settings need to be set?

A. 25% inspiratory time %;
   30% pause time %

B. 25% inspiratory time %;
   5% pause time %

C. 67% inspiratory time %;
   5% pause time %

D. 67% inspiratory time %;
   0% pause time %

25. Which of the following adjustments need to be made to initiate airway pressure-release ventilation (APRV)?

   I. Set two levels of CPAP.
   II. Set the high CPAP level at 10 to 30 cm $H_2O$.
   III. Set the low or baseline CPAP level at 2 to 10 cm $H_2O$.
   IV. Maintain an inverse I:E ratio.

A. I only

B. II only

C. III only

D. I, II, III, IV

26. A patient is receiving mechanical ventilation from a ventilator that is delivering a square wave flow pattern. The ventilatory settings are as follows:

$FiO_2$: 0.40
PIP: 55 cm $H_2O$
PEEP: 10 cm $H_2O$
peak inspiratory flow rate: 60 L/min.
high-pressure limit: 65 cm $H_2O$
tidal volume: 800 cc
plateau pressure: 35 cm $H_2O$

Calculate the airway resistance of this patient–ventilator system.

A. 10 cm $H_2O$/L/sec.

B. 20 cm $H_2O$/L/sec.

C. 30 cm $H_2O$/L/sec.

D. 40 cm $H_2O$/L/sec.

27. If subglottic edema develops after ET extubation, what procedures could be implemented to reduce the airway narrowing?

   I. Nebulized racemic epinephrine could be administered.
   II. The patient might need to be reintubated.
   III. Instituting mist tent therapy would be helpful.
   IV. A tracheotomy might be required.

A. I, IV only

B. II, IV only

C. I, II, IV only

D. I, III only

28. Which of the following ventilator setting changes should the RRT recommend to correct an uncompensated respiratory acidosis in an infant receiving high-frequency ventilation?

   I. instituting PEEP
   II. increasing the driving pressure
   III. increasing the inspiratory time
   IV. increasing the ventilatory rate

A. II, III, IV only

B. II, IV only

C. III, IV only

D. I, II only

29. The RRT has obtained a mixed venous blood sample from a patient who has a PAC inserted. The patient is also receiving mechanical ventilatory support for adult respiratory distress syndrome (ARDS) caused by gram-negative sepsis.

Analysis of the blood sample reveals the following:

$P\bar{v}O_2$ 50 torr
$P\bar{v}CO_2$ 46 torr
pH 7.32
$HCO_3^-$ 23 mEq/liter
B.E. 0 mEq/liter
$S\bar{v}O_2$ 80%
blood lactate 3.6 moles/liter

What is the likely cause of these data?

A. These are normal mixed venous blood values.

B. The patient has recently had a left ventricular myocardial infarction.

C. The patient is experiencing peripheral microcirculation shunting.

D. The patient might have just received a dose of corticosteroids.

30. A patient in the ICU has just had a pulmonary artery catheter inserted. The RRT is about to recommend a chest radiograph to verify the position of the catheter tip within the pulmonary artery. Which of the following types of chest radiographs should the RRT recommend?

A. an overpenetrated, portable AP chest radiograph

B. a lateral chest X-ray

C. a standard PA chest film

D. an overpenetrated, lateral decubitus chest radiograph

31. To effectively hemodynamically monitor a patient who has left ventricular dysfunction, which of the following hemodynamic measurements should the RRT record?

   I. central venous pressure
   II. pulmonary capillary wedge pressure
   III. mean pulmonary artery pressure
   IV. cardiac output

   A. II, III only
   B. I, IV only
   C. II, III, IV only
   D. I, II, III, IV

32. The RRT is about to institute PSV on a patient and is accumulating data to determine the appropriate level of pressure support. The following data have been obtained:

   PIP: 55 cm $H_2O$
   static pressure: 35 cm $H_2O$
   mechanical inspiratory flow rate: 60 L/min.
   patient inspiratory flow rate: 30 L/min.

   What level of pressure support should the RRT establish for this patient?

   A. 5 cm $H_2O$
   B. 10 cm $H_2O$
   C. 15 cm $H_2O$
   D. 20 cm $H_2O$

33. A patient who has chronic bronchitis is about to leave the hospital. His room air ABGs are:

   $PO_2$ 52 torr
   $PCO_2$ 64 torr
   pH 7.37
   $HCO_3^-$ 36 mEq/liter
   B.E. 12 mEq/liter

   Which of the following considerations are important components of a discharge plan for this patient?

   I. dietary guidelines
   II. plans for smoking cessation
   III. recreational and vocational counseling
   IV. detailed information concerning the physiological effects of medications
   V. education on various relaxation techniques

   A. I, II, III, IV, V
   B. II, III, IV only
   C. I, II, III, V only
   D. III, IV only

34. A 155-pound COPD patient has been receiving synchronized intermittent mandatory ventilation (SIMV) for 5 hours and has been having difficulty adjusting to mechanical ventilation. The SIMV settings include the following:

   mechanical ventilatory rate: 12 breaths/min.
   $FIO_2$: 0.30
   mechanical tidal volume: 800 cc

   The patient's spontaneous ventilatory rate is 16 breaths/min. ABGs and acid-base data reveal the following:

   $PO_2$ 70 torr
   $PCO_2$ 30 torr
   pH 7.59
   $HCO_3^-$ 28 mEq/liter
   B.E. 4 mEq/liter

   What should the RRT recommend in this situation?

   A. to decrease the tidal volume to 650 cc
   B. to institute PSV
   C. to institute a PEEP of 5 cm $H_2O$
   D. to sedate the patient and institute controlled mechanical ventilation

35. During polysomnography, the RRT frequently observes the absence of snoring concurrent with the cessation of ventilatory efforts and airflow from the patient's nose and mouth. During this period, pulse oximetry indicates mild desaturation. Which of the following clinical conditions is this patient likely to display?

   A. mixed sleep apnea
   B. central sleep apnea
   C. obstructive sleep apnea
   D. paroxysmal nocturnal dyspnea

36. A patient is 6'1", weighs 195 lbs, and has a cardiac output of 6.0 liters/min. Determine this patient's cardiac index. Use the nomogram shown in Figure 5-2 on page 251.

   A. 3.08 liters/min./m²
   B. 2.80 liters/min./m²
   C. 2.25 liters/min./m²
   D. 1.56 liters/min./m²

37. The volume-pressure curve shown in Figure 5-3 was obtained from a patient who was receiving positive pressure mechanical ventilation.

   What interpretation can the RRT make about the patient based on the graphic?

   A. The patient's airway resistance has increased.
   B. The patient's lung compliance has decreased.

## Dubois Body Surface Chart

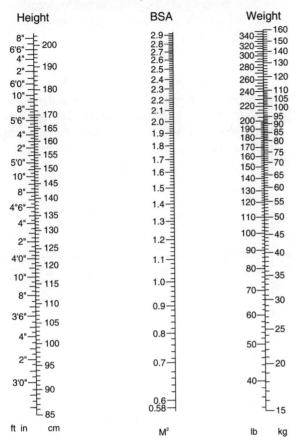

Figure 5-2

**Volume**

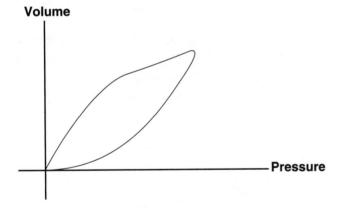

Figure 5-3: Volume-pressure loop.

C. The patient has recently been endotracheally suctioned.

D. The patient's endotracheal tube cuff is leaking.

38. A physician asks an RRT to recommend an aerosol-delivery device for continuous use to a recently tracheotomized COPD patient who has previously been receiving oxygen via a nasal cannula. Which of the following aerosol generators would be most appropriate to recommend?

A. hydrodynamic nebulizer
B. ultrasonic nebulizer
C. large-volume jet nebulizer
D. small-particle aerosol generator

39. Calculate the pulmonary vascular resistance when given the following hemodynamic profile:

central venous pressure: 10.9 cm $H_2O$
right atrial pressure: 8 mm Hg
mean pulmonary artery pressure: 17 mm Hg
mean pulmonary artery wedge pressure: 7 mm Hg
stroke volume: 70 ml/beat
heart rate: 65 beats/min.

A. 1.32 mm Hg/L/min.
B. 1.97 mm Hg/L/min.
C. 2.20 mm Hg/L/min.
D. 2.28 mm Hg/L/min.

40. Chest physiotherapy (CPT) has been administered to both lower lobes for seven days to a patient who had streptococcal pneumonia. Chest radiography and auscultation indicate both lower lobes are clear, but involvement appears in the right middle lobe. What is the appropriate action to take at this time?

A. Switch to incentive spirometry.
B. Continue CPT to the lower lobes and include the right middle lobe.
C. Administer CPT only to the involved area.
D. Place the patient on aerosol therapy only.

41. Which of the following physiologic measurements needs to be measured before a cardiopulmonary stress test?

I. end-tidal $PCO_2$
II. carbon dioxide production
III. minute ventilation
IV. ventilatory rate

A. II, III, IV only
B. I, II only
C. III, IV only
D. I, II, III, IV

42. A patient produces a moderate amount of sputum following a sputum induction for culture and sensitivity and cytology. The sputum is mucoid in character. The specimen is sent to the lab. Twenty-four hours later, the following results are obtained: "Small amounts of gram-negative cocci are present; many eosinophils are seen." Based on this report, the most likely diagnosis would be:

A. bronchiectasis.
B. lung cancer.
C. tuberculosis.
D. bronchial asthma.

43. A patient who has atelectasis is receiving an intermittent positive pressure breathing (IPPB) treatment. The patient's exhaled volume is less than his inspiratory capacity. To increase this patient's exhaled volume, the RRT should:

I. increase the inspiratory flow rate.
II. increase the preset pressure.
III. decrease the inspiratory time.
IV. use a shorter length of tubing.

A. I only
B. II, IV only
C. I, III, IV only
D. II, III, IV, only

44. While performing cardiopulmonary resuscitation (CPR), the RRT notices on the monitor the ECG pattern shown in Figure 5-4.

What should he recommend at this time?

A. that the patient be defibrillated
B. that more bicarbonate be administered
C. that the depth of cardiac compression be increased
D. that the patient be intubated

45. A patient who has chronic bronchitis enters the emergency department complaining of shortness of breath. His admitting ABGs while receiving oxygen at 1 L/min. via a nasal cannula are as follows:

$PO_2$ 38 mm Hg
$PCO_2$ 64 mm Hg
pH 7.39
$HCO_3^-$ 36 mEq/liter
B.E. + 12 mEq/liter

The cannula's liter flow is increased to 3 L/min. The RRT observes that the patient is increasingly lethargic, appears confused, and complains of a headache. Based on this information, what would be the most reasonable evaluation of this patient?

A. The patient is receiving too much oxygen.
B. He is tired and should be allowed to sleep.
C. The cannula's liter flow should be increased to 5 L/min.
D. A non-rebreather mask set at 10 L/min. should be instituted.

46. A patient is being mechanically ventilated in a volume-controlled, time-cycled mode. The flow waveform shown in Figure 5-5 is displayed on the ventilator's monitor.

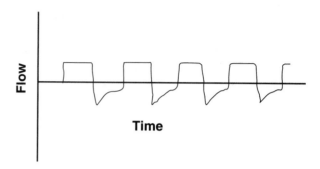

**Figure 5-5:** Flow-time waveform.

Which of the following ventilator setting adjustments would be appropriate at this time?

A. Decrease the tidal volume.
B. Decrease the peak inspiratory flow.
C. Decrease the ventilatory rate.
D. Decrease the expiratory time.

47. Given the following cardiovascular data, calculate the patient's stroke volume:

blood pressure: 125/80 mm Hg
C.O.: 6.0 L/min.
heart rate: 75 beats/min.
C.I.: 2.65 L/min./m²

A. 45 ml
B. 65 ml
C. 70 ml
D. 80 ml

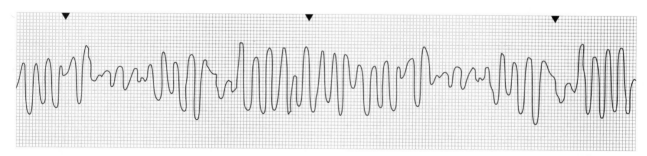

**Figure 5-4:** Lead II ECG tracing.

48. A patient with a stable cardiopulmonary status receiving mechanical ventilation has an arterial $PO_2$ of 153 torr on 70% oxygen. The physician wants the arterial $PO_2$ between 90 torr and 100 torr. What $FIO_2$ would likely achieve the desired arterial $PO_2$?

A. 0.60
B. 0.55
C. 0.45
D. 0.35

49. A mechanically ventilated, chronic bronchitic has just been admitted to the surgical ICU following a cholecystectomy. Humidification is being provided via a heat–moisture exchanger. The RRT notices that the patient's secretions are becoming thicker. At the same time, it is also observed that the PIP is gradually increasing while the plateau pressure remains constant. What should the RRT do at this time?

A. Administer ultrasonic treatments in-line Q1h.
B. Replace the heat–moisture exchanger.
C. Remove the heat–moisture exchanger, and insert a wick humidifier.
D. Irrigate the tracheobronchial tree with normal saline and perform ET suctioning.

50. A 24-year-old, 70-kg motor vehicle accident victim receiving mechanical ventilation in the SIMV mode displays the following data:

tidal volume: 800 ml
SIMV rate: 12 breaths/min.
peak flow rate: 60 L/min.
$FIO_2$: 0.50
PEEP/CPAP: 8 cm $H_2O$

ABG data and vital signs indicate the following:

$PO_2$ 62 torr
$PCO_2$ 44 torr
pH 7.35
$HCO_3^-$ 23 mEg/liter
B.E. 0 mEq/liter
pulse rate 118 beats/min.
blood pressure 92/63 mm Hg

The patient also has a spontaneous ventilatory rate during mechanical ventilation of 40 breaths/min. He is diaphoretic, anxious, and thrashing about in the bed. The patient is fighting the ventilator and is generating a PIP of 70 cm $H_2O$. The patient has been given morphine for pain and sedation. Which of the following actions should the RRT recommend?

A. Increase the tidal volume to 1,200 ml.
B. Increase the $FIO_2$ to 0.80.
C. Administer Norcuron and benzodiazepine.
D. Administer Doxapram and Pavulon.

51. The RRT is assisting a physician during the insertion of a pulmonary artery catheter (PAC). As the catheter is being floated into position, the ECG in Figure 5-6 suddenly appears on the monitor.

The ventricular rate is greater than 150 beats/min. The RRT should:

A. recommend cardioversion.
B. recommend defibrillation.
C. recommend the injection of isoproterenol hydrochloride.
D. recommend continuing floating the catheter.

52. The RRT is performing ventilator rounds in the pediatric ICU and hears the high pressure alarm sounding from the ventilator set up on a 5-year-old boy. The RRT observes that the PIP has increased but the $P_{plateau}$ has remained constant. Gurgling sounds are also heard coming from the child's 5.5 mm I.D. endotracheal tube. Which of the following actions are appropriate?

A. Use a 12 Fr suction catheter to perform endotracheal suctioning.
B. Reintubate the patient with a 6.5 mm I.D. endotracheal tube.
C. Set the vacuum pressure to −100 mm Hg.
D. Increase the level of the high pressure alarm.

53. A 62-year-old COPD patient has been prescribed to begin a pulmonary rehabilitation program. The patient has a 138 pack-year smoking history, is 5'10" tall, and

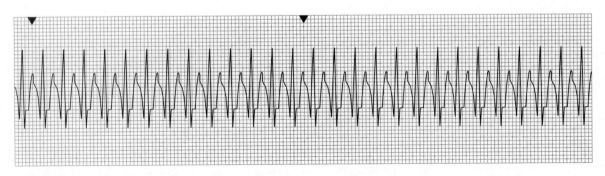

**Figure 5-6:** Lead II ECG tracing.

weighs 230 lbs. The patient complains of dyspnea at rest and receives oxygen 24 hours a day via a reservoir nasal cannula at $\frac{1}{2}$ liter/min. Which of the following goals should the RRT consider reasonable for the initial two weeks of the pulmonary rehabilitation program?

I. improve the activities of daily living
II. understand the importance of diet and nutrition
III. increase the duration and intensity of exercise
IV. acquire knowledge of the pathophysiology of COPD

A. I, II only
B. II, III only
C. II, IV only
D. I, III, IV only

54. The volume-pressure curve displayed in Figure 5-7 was generated by a spontaneously breathing patient.

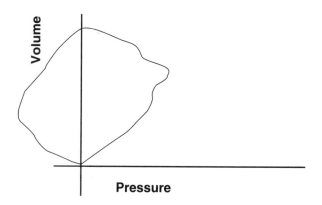

**Figure 5-7:** Volume-pressure loop.

How should the RRT interpret this graphic?

A. a normal spontaneous breath curve
B. an increased work of breathing
C. a decreased pulmonary compliance
D. an increased airway pressure

55. A patient who has chronic ventilatory failure is able to adequately ventilate while awake but requires nocturnal ventilation. Spontaneous mode BiPAP is instituted with an inspiratory positive airway pressure (IPAP) of 8 cm $H_2O$ and an EPAP of 5 cm $H_2O$. The patient complains of shortness of breath. At the same time, a low exhaled tidal volume is measured. Which of the following changes would the RRT recommend to alleviate this problem?

A. Increase the EPAP to 8 cm $H_2O$.
B. Increase the IPAP to 10 cm $H_2O$.
C. Change the mode to timed ventilation.
D. Increase the IPAP time % to 40%.

56. Which range represents the normal, room-air $P(A-a)O_2$ for a 25-year-old person?

A. 20 to 25 torr
B. 15 to 20 torr
C. 10 to 15 torr
D. 5 to 10 torr

57. A newborn in the ICU is receiving 30% oxygen via an oxyhood. Which of the following setups would be most appropriate if the oxyhood needs 8 L/min. of humidified gas?

A. a heated, all-purpose nebulizer set on 30%, operating at an oxygen flow rate of 8 L/min.
B. a blender set on 30% with a flow rate set at 8 L/min. to a heated humidifier.
C. an entrainment adaptor set on 30% and an oxygen flow rate of 8 L/min. to a heated humidifier.
D. an oxygen flow rate of 1 L/min. and an air flow rate of 7 L/min., both delivered to a heated humidifier.

58. The RRT is performing chest physiotherapy on a patient who had a coronary artery bypass graft 3 days previously. The RRT looks at the ECG monitor and observes the cardiac pattern shown in Figure 5-8.

What would be the most appropriate *initial* action for the RRT to take?

A. Stop the treatment and allow the patient to recover.
B. Obtain the patient's pulse.
C. Start cardiopulmonary resuscitation.
D. Check the patient's pupil status.

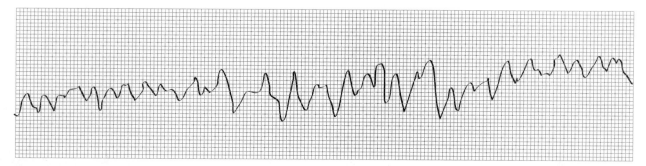

**Figure 5-8:** ECG tracing.

59. Carbon dioxide monitoring has been determined necessary for a nonintubated COPD patient who has a bleeding disorder (platelets: 40,000/mm³). Which of the following monitoring modalities would provide the most accurate *estimate* of the carbon dioxide in his arterial blood?

   A. $V_D/V_T$ calculations
   B. $PtcCO_2$ monitoring
   C. capnometry
   D. alveolar air equation

60. A COPD patient in a pulmonary rehabilitation program has been working with a resistive training device for the past week. During one of the rehabilitation sessions, she tells the RRT that she has been able to tolerate breathing through the resistive training device for 15 minutes. What should the RRT do?

   A. Inform the patient to try breathing with larger volumes through the device.
   B. Insert a smaller restrictive orifice in the device.
   C. Instruct the patient to increase her breathing time through the device to 30 minutes.
   D. Congratulate the patient for successfully completing the inspiratory muscle-training program.

61. Which conditions would indicate the performance of a cricothyroidotomy on a nonhospitalized cardiac arrest victim?

   I. obstructive laryngeal edema
   II. a noticeable inability to provide adequate ventilation via mouth-to-mouth or mouth-to-nose ventilation
   III. deviated nasal septum
   IV. diffuse bronchospasm

   A. I, III only
   B. I, II only
   C. II, III only
   D. III, IV only

62. Which of the following modes of communication can be used by patients to express their subjective response to therapy during a treatment?

   I. verbal
   II. facial expressions
   III. tone of voice
   IV. body language

   A. I, IV only
   B. I, II, IV only
   C. II, IV only
   D. I, II, III, IV

63. A patient who is receiving mechanical ventilation is about to undergo bronchoscopy. The ventilator settings are as follows:

tidal volume: 800 ml
$FiO_2$: 0.40
ventilatory rate: 12 breaths/min.
PEEP: 10 cm $H_2O$

Which of the following ventilator adjustments should the RRT consider during the bronchoscopy procedure?

   I. increasing to the $FiO_2$ to 1.0
   II. increasing the high-pressure limit
   III. increasing the PEEP to 15 cm $H_2O$
   IV. increasing the tidal volume

   A. I, II only
   B. II, IV only
   C. I, II, III only
   D. I, IV only

64. An 18-year-old female sustained a blunt chest injury in an automobile accident. She has been orally intubated and is now receiving mechanical ventilation. Inspection shows diminished chest wall expansion on the left side. Palpation indicates a midline trachea. Auscultation of the thorax reveals diminished breath sounds on the left side. Percussion of the chest demonstrates hyperresonance on the left side. Based on these physical findings, the RRT should suspect:

   A. The patient has a flail chest on the right side.
   B. The endotracheal tube is situated in the right mainstem bronchus.
   C. The patient has developed a right-sided pneumothorax.
   D. The patient has severe atelectasis on the left side.

65. An 80-kg patient is receiving mechanical ventilatory support with the following settings:

mode: SIMV
$FiO_2$: 0.60
mechanical rate: 8 breaths/min.
mechanical $V_T$: 800 cc
PEEP: 15 cm $H_2O$

How can the RRT determine whether the amount of PEEP administered is inappropriate?

   I. by measuring the cardiac output
   II. by measuring the urinary output
   III. by measuring the dead space-tidal volume ratio
   IV. by measuring the transcutaneous $PCO_2$

   A. I only
   B. I, II only
   C. I, II, III only
   D. II, III, IV only

66. A 35-week-old neonate is receiving continuous flow, nasotracheal CPAP. She is receiving an $FiO_2$ of 0.50 and a CPAP of 3 cm $H_2O$. ABG data reveal the following:

PO$_2$ 80 torr
PCO$_2$ 43 torr
pH 7.35
HCO$_3^-$ 23 mEq/liter
B.E. −1 mEq/liter

What should the neonatal RRT do at this time?

A. Increase the CPAP to 5 cm H$_2$O.
B. Decrease the CPAP to 1 cm H$_2$O.
C. Decrease the F$_1$O$_2$ by 0.05.
D. Increase the F$_1$O$_2$ by 0.10.

67. The RRT has been asked to prepare a patient for a transtracheal aspiration procedure. What patient preparations must she make?

I. Position the patient supine with his neck hypoflexed.
II. Inform the patient that the procedure will cause coughing.
III. Encourage the patient to swallow while the cricothyroid membrane is being punctured.
IV. Explain that after the procedure the puncture site will be compressed for 5 minutes.

A. II, III only
B. II, IV only
C. I, III only
D. I, II, III, IV

68. Which ventilatory patterns or breathing maneuvers provide for a more effective delivery of a nebulized medication to the lungs?

I. inspiratory hold
II. mouth breathing
III. deep inspirations
IV. pursed-lip breathing

A. I, II only
B. II, IV only
C. III, IV only
D. I, II, III, IV

69. The following data are from a post-op, coronary bypass patient who is receiving 40% oxygen via an all-purpose nebulizer operating at 10 L/min.

| Ventilatory | Cardiovascular |
| --- | --- |
| ventilatory rate: 26 breaths/min. | heart rate: 115 beats/min. |
| minute ventilation: 7.8 L/min. | blood pressure: 110/85 torr |

When the patient's SpO$_2$ fell to 90% 2 hours postextubation, the physician ordered the F$_1$O$_2$ to be increased to 0.60. The following data were obtained after the patient had been breathing an F$_1$O$_2$ of 0.60 for 30 minutes.

| Ventilatory | Cardiovascular |
| --- | --- |
| ventilatory rate: 28 breaths/min. | heart rate: 117 beats/min. |
| minute ventilation: 9.8 L/min. | blood pressure: 105/90 torr |

How should the RRT evaluate this patient's response to oxygen therapy?

A. The second set of data indicates a need for oxygen greater than 60%.
B. The second set of data reflects an improvement in the patient's oxygenation status.
C. The second set of data indicates a need for oxygen less than 60%.
D. The total flow rate delivered to the patient is inadequate, indicating that the F$_1$O$_2$ is less than 0.60.

70. A patient with interstitial pulmonary fibrosis is receiving oxygen at 6 L/min. via a nasal cannula and is ready for discharge. What home oxygen system is appropriate for this patient?

A. an oxygen enricher
B. an oxygen concentrator
C. gas oxygen cylinders
D. a liquid oxygen system

71. Which procedure appropriately refers to the process of weaning a neonate from a high level of CPAP and high F$_1$O$_2$?

A. The CPAP level should be reduced before F$_1$O$_2$ reductions are made.
B. F$_1$O$_2$ and CPAP pressure reductions should be alternately made, beginning with the pressure.
C. The F$_1$O$_2$ should be lowered before the pressure reductions are made.
D. CPAP pressure and F$_1$O$_2$ reductions should be performed simultaneously.

72. A patient is receiving airway pressure-release ventilation with a baseline pressure of 5 cm H$_2$O and a high-level pressure of 10 cm H$_2$O. What should the RRT recommend to improve alveolar ventilation?

A. Increase the baseline pressure to 10 cm H$_2$O.
B. Increase the high-pressure level to 15 cm H$_2$O.
C. Decrease the baseline pressure to 2 cm H$_2$O.
D. Decrease the high-pressure level to 8 cm H$_2$O

73. The RRT is preparing to administer an 80/20 helium-oxygen mixture to a patient who has an upper airway lesion causing acute distress. An oxygen flowmeter is the only flowmeter available to the RRT for use. If the liter flow on the oxygen flowmeter is set at 10 liters/min., what will be the actual helium-oxygen flow rate received by the patient?

A. 25 liters/min.
B. 18 liters/min.
C. 10 liters/min.
D. 7 liters/min.

74. A 21-year-old male was the driver of a vehicle involved in an automobile accident. He was not wearing a seat belt and was hurtled against the steering wheel. Upon entering the emergency department, he is conscious, exhibits intense chest pain, and presents with severe respiratory distress. Paradoxical chest-wall movement of the left chest is apparent on observation. His trachea is midline with breath sounds apparent in both lungs but greatly diminished on the left side. ABG data reveal the following:

$PO_2$ 65 mm Hg
$PCO_2$ 29 mm Hg
pH 7.49
$HCO_3^-$ 22 mEq/liter
B.E. −3 mEq/liter

What should the RRT recommend for this patient at this time?

A. IMV at a mechanical rate of 4 breaths/min. with an $FIO_2$ of 0.60
B. controlled mechanical ventilation with a ventilatory rate of 20 breaths/min. and an $FIO_2$ of 1.0
C. CPAP with an $FIO_2$ of 0.50
D. nasal cannula at 3 L/min. with incentive spirometry QID

75. If the preset pressure is being prematurely achieved when an IPPB treatment is being administered to a patient, what action(s) should be taken?

I. Increase the machine sensitivity.
II. Reduce the flow rate.
III. Increase the pressure limit.
IV. Institute negative pressure during exhalation.

A. II, IV only
B. II only
C. III only
D. II, III only

76. When a COPD patient is about to be discharged from the hospital to the home and still requires medical attention, a discharge plan must be established. Which of the following components comprise a discharge plan?

I. patient transportation needs after arriving back home
II. the physician's plan of treatment
III. how the family will pay for the care
IV. the capability of the patient to participate in a pulmonary rehabilitation program

A. I, IV only
B. II, III only
C. II, III, IV only
D. I, II, III, IV

77. The RRT is asked by the physician to help position a patient who is about to have a thoracentesis. How should the patient be positioned?

A. lying flat on the affected side
B. lying flat on the unaffected side
C. lying on the affected side with the head and thorax 45° to the horizontal
D. sitting up with the feet over the bedside with the arms and hands supported at the shoulder level

78. An ARDS patient is receiving mechanical ventilation via a volume ventilator. The following ventilator data are obtained:

PIP: 68 cm $H_2O$
PEEP: 20 cm $H_2O$
minute ventilation: 20 L/min.

The following values represent the patient's 24-hour intake and output:

| Intake | Output |
| --- | --- |
| $D_5W$ I.V.: 1,500 ml | Urine: 900 ml |
| Hyperalimentation: 1,000 ml | Chest tube: 200 ml |
| Lipids: 200 ml | Cholostomy: 500 ml |

This patient is diaphoretic, and his urine has a specific gravity of 1.025. What are possible reasons for this negative fluid balance?

I. Atrial natriuretic peptide levels are elevated.
II. C.O. is decreased.
III. Plasma level of antidiuretic hormone is increased.
IV. Insensible water loss is increased.

A. I, III only
B. II, III only
C. II, III, IV only
D. I, II, III, IV

79. A patient is being mechanically ventilated at the following settings.

mode: control
tidal volume: 950 cc
ventilatory rate: 30 breaths/min.
$FIO_2$: 1.0

The ventilator indicates a PIP of 35 cm $H_2O$ and an I:E ratio of 1:1. ABG data indicate severe hypoxemia. What recommendation(s) should be made to improve this patient's oxygenation status?

I. Institute PEEP.
II. Increase the inspiratory time.
III. Increase the expiratory time.
IV. Initiate PCV with inverse-ratio ventilation.

A. IV only
B. I, II only
C. I, II, IV only
D. I, III only

80. A patient is receiving BiPAP® in the timed mode. The IPAP rate is set at 12 breaths/min. What %IPAP should be set by the RRT to establish an I:E ratio of 1:1.5?

A. 20%
B. 30%
C. 40%
D. 50%

81. A patient has an extremely peripheral lung mass inaccessible to a bronchoscope. The physician asks the RRT to recommend a procedure enabling the evaluation of the lung mass. Which of the following procedures would the RRT recommend?

A. fine needle biopsy
B. cutting needle biopsy
C. thoracentesis
D. pleuroscopy

82. Which statements relate to the administration of sodium bicarbonate during CPR?

I. Excessive administration of this drug can lead to iatrogenic metabolic alkalosis.
II. It decreases cardiac contractility and corrects acidemia by supplying more sodium ions to the sodium pump in the mycocardium.
III. The use of this drug in correcting the metabolic acidosis is associated with increased arterial carbon dioxide tension.
IV. It inhibits the occurrence of cardiac dysrhythmias.

A. I, III only
B. I, IV only
C. II, III only
D. II, IV only

83. A patient who is suffering from nocturnal apnea is receiving negative-pressure ventilation. The RRT observes that over the course of one evening, the delivered tidal volume has decreased. What conditions might have caused this change to occur?

I. increased lung compliance
II. decreased negative pressure
III. increased airway resistance
IV. decreased ventilatory rate

A. I, III only
B. II, III only

C. III, IV only
D. I, II, III only

84. A post-MI patient with a pulmonary artery catheter inserted has been breathing 100% oxygen for 20 minutes. Calculate this patient's shunt fraction based on the following data. Assume a normal respiratory quotient and normal ambient conditions.

| Arterial | Venous |
| --- | --- |
| $PaO_2$ 500 torr | $P\bar{v}O_2$ 70 torr |
| $PaCO_2$ 60 torr | $P\bar{v}CO_2$ 65 torr |
| $SaO_2$ 100% | $S\bar{v}O_2$ 85% |

This patient's [Hb] is 16 g%.

A. 0.093
B. 0.139
C. 0.156
D. 0.223

85. The RRT is performing CPT on the lateral basal segment of the right lower lobe of an 80-year-old female patient. Suddenly, the patient complains of a sharp pain that intensifies during inspiration. The patient indicates that the pain is localized along the right mid-axillary line at about the level of the seventh rib. After terminating the treatment and returning the patient to a semirecumbent position, what should the RRT do?

A. Contact the physician and suggest an increase in $FiO_2$.
B. Contact the physician and suggest a STAT ECG.
C. Contact the physician and request pain medication.
D. Contact the physician and request a STAT chest X-ray.

86. A patient is receiving high-density aerosol therapy by using an ultrasonic nebulizer with 0.45% NaCl. The therapy is ordered QID for 30 minutes. Following 5 minutes of therapy, the RRT assesses the patient and compares the information with the pretreatment values shown in Table 5-1.

**Table 5-1** Evaluation of High-Density Aerosol Therapy

| Assessments | Pretreatment Values | Values After 5 Minutes of Ultrasonic Nebulization |
| --- | --- | --- |
| pulse | 84 beats/min. | 102 beats/min. |
| ventilatory rate | 15 breaths/min. | 28 breaths/min. |
| breath sounds | clear | expiratory wheezing |

What should the RRT do at this time?

A. Administer two puffs of albuterol and continue the therapy.
B. Terminate the therapy and notify the physician.
C. Continue the therapy as ordered and monitor the patient carefully.
D. Decrease the amplitude on the ultrasonic nebulizer.

87. A spontaneously breathing patient displays a calibrated tracing recorded from the distal port of a PAC during a pulmonary capillary wedge-pressure (PCWP) reading (Figure 5-9).

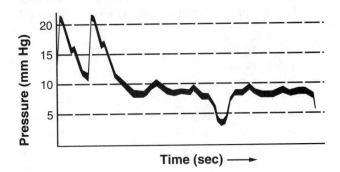

**Figure 5-9:** PAC tracing from distal port during pulmonary capillary wedge-pressure (PCWP) determination.

From the tracing, determine this patient's approximate PCWP.

A. 20 to 22 mm Hg
B. 12 to 13 mm Hg
C. 8 to 9 mm Hg
D. 3 to 4 mm Hg

88. The RRT is asked by a physician to evaluate a patient's progress after involvement in a pulmonary rehabilitation program. Which of the following outcomes would be expected to realistically improve?

I. pulmonary function
II. exercise tolerance and endurance
III. ABG
IV. quality of life

A. II, IV only
B. I only
C. I, II, III only
D. I, II, III, IV

89. While performing ET suctioning on a patient, the RRT notes that the patient's heart rate decreased from 85 beats/min. to 45 beats/min. What is the possible cause of this response?

A. increased intracranial pressure
B. vagal reflex
C. Hering–Breuer reflex
D. transient hypoxemia

90. A severe COPD patient is about to be discharged from the hospital. The physician has prescribed nocturnal oxygen at 1 L/min. with a nasal cannula. Which of the following home oxygen delivery systems is most appropriate for this patient?

A. oxygen concentrator
B. oxygen gas cylinders
C. liquid oxygen systems
D. oxygen blender

91. The RRT extubates a patient who has been nasotracheally intubated for the last three weeks. Following the extubation procedure, the RRT hears inspiratory stridor via auscultation of the patient's lateral neck and notices that the patient is speaking with a hoarse voice. What should the RRT do as this time?

A. *No* action is necessary because these postextubation findings are normal.
B. The patient should be reintubated immediately.
C. Fiberoptic bronchoscopy should be performed.
D. Administer nebulized racemic epinephrine.

92. When interpreting the values obtained from a capillary blood sample, which of the following measurements is the *least* accurate when correlated with an arterial blood sample?

A. pH
B. $PO_2$
C. $PCO_2$
D. base excess

93. The physician has asked the RRT to determine whether an anion gap is present in a patient who is displaying a metabolic acidosis. The RRT should refer to which of the following laboratory profiles to gather the necessary information?

A. complete blood count (CBC)
B. serum electrolytes
C. differential diagnosis of white blood cells
D. urinalysis

94. While an RRT performs a ventilator check, he observes that the PIP is progressively increasing as the preset tidal volume is being delivered. Auscultation of the patient's thorax reveals diminished breath sounds over the left upper lobe; percussion renders a hyperresonant note also on the left side. What should the RRT recommend at this time?

A. Increase the high-pressure limit.
B. Increase the tidal volume.
C. Insert a chest tube in the left thorax.
D. Change mechanical ventilators.

95. Persistent pulmonary hypertension of the newborn is suspected in an infant who has underlying meconium

aspiration syndrome. The physician requests two transcutaneous oxygen monitors to reflect preductal and postductal oxygen tension. Which of the following sites are most appropriate for obtaining these measurements?

A. the left upper chest quadrant and right inner thigh
B. the right upper chest quadrant and left inner thigh
C. the right and left side of the anterior abdomen
D. the right lower back and left upper shoulder

96. The following ABG data were obtained from a chronic $CO_2$ retaining patient who was breathing room air:

PO₂ 40 torr
PCO₂ 65 torr
pH 7.30

Which type of oxygen therapy would be appropriate?

A. nasal cannula at 2 L/min.
B. partial rebreathing mask at 10 L/min.
C. simple $O_2$ mask at 10 L/min.
D. air entrainment mask at 24% $O_2$

97. A 60-kg, 24-year-old patient with neuromuscular disease is about to be ventilated via a chest cuirass. An appropriate *initial* negative-pressure setting would be:

A. $-5$ cm $H_2O$.
B. $-10$ cm $H_2O$.
C. $-20$ cm $H_2O$.
D. $-40$ cm $H_2O$.

98. Which medications would be useful for reducing respiratory mucosal edema?

I. albuterol
II. metaproternerrol
III. racemic epinephrine

A. I only
B. III only
C. I, III only
D. II, III only

99. Which of the of the following exercise protocols would provide for the determination of the workload at which the subject achieves maximum oxygen uptake?

A. a cycle ergometer at 50 watts for 10 minutes
B. a treadmill at a speed of 5 miles/hour with a 10% grade increased by 2% every 3 minutes
C. a constant grade treadmill with increasing speed every 8 minutes
D. a cycle ergometer at 50 watts for 8 minutes

100. A patient who is 2 days postop for a transurethral resection of the prostate develops a fever and chills. Which of the following laboratory studies should the RRT recommend to rule out the presence of an infectious process?

A. prothrombin time
B. partial thromboplastin time
C. CBC
D. platelet count

101. Which of the following statements are true concerning positive expiratory pressure (PEP) therapy?

I. It is applied to intubated and mechanically ventilated patients.
II. Between 10 to 20 breaths should be performed before the patient attempts to evacuate secretions.
III. Each therapy session should last at least one hour.
IV. The patient should achieve an I:E ratio of about 1:3.

A. I, II, III only
B. II, III only
C. II, IV only
D. I, II, IV only

102. An infant receiving positive pressure ventilation through tubing with a heated wire circuit has been reintubated twice because of mucous plugging. The house staff suggests that the humidifier is malfunctioning. The inspired gas temperature of the wick humidification system has been maintained at 36°C. The wick humidifier is *not* malfunctioning. How will the RRT determine that the inspired humidity is optimal?

A. by changing the humidifier temperature to 37°C
B. by checking the patient Y for signs of mild condensation
C. by increasing the temperature of the heated wire circuit
D. by adjusting the heated wire temperature to the "rain cloud" setting

103. A patient is being treated with intrapulmonary percussive ventilation for atelectasis caused by retained secretions. Which of the following physical findings support an improved pulmonary status?

A. decreased early inspiratory crackles
B. decreased late inspiratory crackles
C. increased vocal fremitus
D. decreased bronchial breath sounds

104. A post-myocardial infarction (MI) patient is being hemodynamically monitored and is receiving mechanical ventilation with the following settings:

peak inspiratory flow rate: 50 L/min.
tidal volume: 800 cc
ventilatory rate: 12 breaths/min.
F₁O₂: 0.40
PEEP: 5 cm $H_2O$
C.O.: 5.1 L/min.

ABG data reveal the following:

PO$_2$ 75 torr
PCO$_2$ 48 torr
pH 7.34
HCO$_3^-$ 25 mEq/liter
B.E. 1 mEq/liter

After a PEEP of 10 cm H$_2$O was instituted, the following ABG and hemodynamic data were obtained:

PO$_2$ 68 torr
PCO$_2$ 56 torr
pH 7.31
HCO$_3^-$ 27 mEq/liter
B.E. 3 mEq/liter
C.O. 2.4 L/min.

What should the RRT do at this time?

A. Increase the PEEP to 15 cm H$_2$O and increase the FIO$_2$ to 0.50.
B. Increase the FIO$_2$ to 0.50 and administer a volume expander.
C. Increase the tidal volume to 900 cc, maintain the FIO$_2$ at 0.40, and decrease the PEEP to 5 cm H$_2$O.
D. Decrease the PEEP to 5 cm H$_2$O and increase the FIO$_2$ to 0.50.

105. PCV should be considered in which of the following situations?

   I. PIPs greater than 60 cm H$_2$O
   II. refractory hypoxemia on moderate to high levels of PEEP
   III. to improve the arterial PCO$_2$

   A. I only
   B. II only
   C. I, II only
   D. I, III only

106. The following ABG data were obtained from a patient who was receiving mechanical ventilation:

PaO$_2$ 95 torr
PaCO$_2$ 44 torr
pH 7.32
HCO$_3^-$ 24 mEq/liter
B.E. 0 mEq/liter
SaO$_2$ 96.5%

Which of the following interpretations of the acid-base status is appropriate?

A. uncompensated respiratory acidosis
B. compensated metabolic acidosis
C. mixed acidosis
D. The data are erroneous.

107. A postoperative right thoracotomy patient has been prescribed incentive spirometry (IS) Q2h following extubation. Breath sounds during therapy are bronchial in the posterior segment of the right lower lobe, with wheezes in the posterior segment of the left lower lobe. ABG data are marginal on 40% oxygen via an all-purpose nebulizer. The incentive spirometry volume is set at 10 ml/kg. Which of the following recommendations is appropriate for this patient?

A. Have the patient perform diaphragmatic or lateral chest-expansion breathing exercises during IS to increase inspiratory volumes.
B. Administer volume-oriented IPPB therapy with volumes of 20 ml/kg.
C. Apply intermittent mask CPAP therapy for 20 minutes Q4h at 5 cm H$_2$O.
D. Perform postural drainage and percussion specifically over the right lower lobe.

108. A 65-year-old COPD patient is admitted to the emergency department complaining of shortness of breath. His family informs the physician that the patient recently caught the flu and that his condition has worsened during the past few days. He appears dyspneic and has an irregular ventilatory pattern with a ventilatory rate of 30 breaths/min. His V$_T$ is 400 cc, and his radial pulse is 122 beats/min. The patient is lucid and responds to questioning. Room air ABGs reveal the following:

PO$_2$ 50 torr
PCO$_2$ 68 torr
pH 7.29
HCO$_3^-$ 32 mEq/liter
SO$_2$ 75%
[Hb] 18 g%.

A nasal cannula with a flow rate of 6 L/min. is installed for this patient per physician's orders. When the RRT returned to this patient's room after being away for about 20 minutes, she observes the patient to be asleep. His ventilatory rate is now 10 breaths/min., and his tidal volume has fallen to 300 cc. He responds lethargically as his name is called. He is confused, does not respond well to questioning, and slumbers off to sleep again. Which statement(s) correctly describe(s) this situation?

   I. The fact that this patient is *no* longer tachypneic is a sign of improvement.
   II. His somnolence and reduced sensorium indicate the possibility of CO$_2$ narcosis.
   III. The oxygen administered to this patient is being provided by the appropriate device for this situation.
   IV. The patient should be left alone (i.e., *not* awakened) because this is the first time in a few days that he has been able to rest.

   A. I, IV only
   B. III, IV only

C. II only

D. I only

109. While receiving full ventilatory support, a COPD patient is experiencing difficulty exhaling to resting levels despite prolonged expiratory times. What should the RRT suggest to assure complete exhalation?

A. Adding expiratory resistance.

B. Adding 5 cm $H_2O$ PEEP.

C. Initiating BiPAP®.

D. Initiating inverse-ratio ventilation.

110. A patient is receiving BiPAP® via a nasal mask at the following settings:

mode: timed

inspiratory positive airway pressure (IPAP): 6 cm $H_2O$

expiratory positive airway pressure (EPAP): 3 cm $H_2O$

ventilatory rate: 14 breaths/min.

The patient's $PaCO_2$ is 48 mm Hg. What change should the RRT recommend to lower the $PaCO_2$?

A. Increase EPAP to 5 cm $H_2O$.

B. Increase IPAP to 11 cm $H_2O$.

C. Change the device to the spontaneous mode.

D. Increase the ventilatory rate to 20 breaths/min.

111. Which of the following statements represent acceptable, optional therapeutic goals for a patient to achieve in a pulmonary rehabilitation program?

I. increased activities of daily living

II. improvement in cardiopulmonary status

III. reduction in hospitalizations

IV. control of respiratory infections

A. I, IV only

B. II, III only

C. I, III, IV only

D. I, II, III, IV

112. How should the family or caregivers of a home respiratory care patient be instructed by the RRT to clean reusable respiratory therapy equipment?

A. Rinse the equipment in hot water from a faucet weekly.

B. Wash the equipment in warm tap water and immerse it in a commercial disinfectant as needed.

C. Wash the equipment in soap and water, then immerse it in a vinegar solution as needed.

D. Package equipment for transport to the hospital for disinfection periodically.

113. A 165-pound patient has been receiving mechanical ventilatory support with the following settings:

mode: assist/control

tidal volume: 600 ml

$FiO_2$: 0.50

ventilatory rate: 6 breaths/min.

sigh volume: 900 ml

sigh rate: 10 breaths/hour

The physician now orders this patient to receive control-mode ventilation with a tidal volume of 12 ml/kg at a rate of 12 breaths/min. at an $FiO_2$ of 0.50. What other change should the RRT make?

A. Eliminate the sigh mode.

B. Increase the sensitivity setting.

C. Decrease the high-pressure limit.

D. Decrease the inspiratory flow rate.

114. An emphysema patient to whom the RRT is administering an IPPB treatment experiences air trapping from generating a forceful cough that terminates at mid-expiration. This patient *cannot* create an adequate intrathoracic pressure to overcome this air trapping and produce an inspiration, nor can he complete his previous exhalation. What action should the RRT take?

A. Obtain a mask and deliver positive pressure to the patient's airways.

B. Attempt to coach the patient into relaxing and spontaneously breathing slowly and deeply.

C. Have the patient breathe a bronchodilator administered via a hand-held nebulizer.

D. Perform the Heimlich maneuver on this patient.

115. It is becoming increasingly difficult to oxygenate a mechanically ventilated patient despite increasing PEEP and $FiO_2$ levels. Which of the following maneuvers might improve the patient's distribution of ventilation and oxygenation?

A. expiratory resistance

B. BiPAP® ventilation

C. inspiratory hold

D. APRV

116. A patient who is receiving mechanical ventilation has the following data recorded on his bedside flowsheet:

| Day 1: | Day 2: |
| --- | --- |
| Total intake: 2,500 cc | Total intake:2,200 cc |
| Total output: 1,500 cc | Total output: 1,400 cc |
| PCWP: 12 mm Hg | PCWP: 18 mm Hg |
| PIP: 28 cm $H_2O$ | PIP: 35 cm $H_2O$ |

Based on this information, which of the following conditions is most likely occurring?

A. The patient is developing ARDS.
B. The patient is developing cor pulmonale.
C. The patient is overhydrated.
D. The patient is developing airway obstruction.

117. A patient who has pneumonia in the lower and middle lobes of the right lung is receiving mechanical ventilation with SIMV and pressure support. The patient is displaying severe hypoxemia despite an $FIO_2$ of 1.0 and a PEEP of 12 cm $H_2O$. Which of the following recommendations made by the RRT is appropriate?

A. Sedate the patient and use control mode ventilation.
B. Institute airway pressure release ventilation.
C. Apply any form of high frequency ventilation.
D. Administer independent lung ventilation.

118. An ECG-monitored, 3-year-old child weighing 35 pounds is experiencing ventricular fibrillation. The decision has been made to defibrillate the patient for the first time. What energy level on the defibrillator should the RRT recommend?

A. 15 joules
B. 32 joules
C. 54 joules
D. 70 joules

119. A COPD patient enters the emergency department with labored breathing and shortness of breath. He is administered oxygen via a non-rebreather mask after ABG data reveal severe hypoxemia. The RRT is called to evaluate the patient, who is now lethargic and hypoventilating. ABG and acid-base data now reveal the following:

$PO_2$ 90 torr
$PCO_2$ 70 torr
pH 7.32
$HCO_3^-$ 32 mEq/liter
B.E. 8 mEq/liter

What should the RRT recommend at this time?

A. intubating and mechanically ventilating the patient
B. administering 30% oxygen via an air entrainment mask
C. instituting CPAP at 10 cm $H_2O$
D. administering oxygen via a nasal cannula at 3 L/min.

120. For which of the following conditions might independent lung ventilation be useful?

I. adult respiratory distress syndrome (ARDS)
II. bronchopleural fistula
III. massive hemoptysis
IV. acute exacerbation of COPD

A. I, III only
B. II, IV only
C. II, III only
D. I, II, III only

121. Which of the following evaluations are necessary before a bronchoscopic biopsy is performed?

I. activated partial thromboplastin time
II. history of hemoptysis
III. history of malabsorption
IV. prothrombin time

A. I, II, III, IV
B. I, IV only
C. II, III only
D. I, II, IV only

122. Over the past three hours, the RRT has recorded the data in Table 5-2 on the ventilator flowsheet of a 70-kg patient who is receiving mechanical ventilation in the control mode.

**Table 5-2** Ventilator Flowsheet Data

| TIME | VT$_{EXHALED}$ | P$_{plateau}$ | PIP |
| --- | --- | --- | --- |
| 1900 | 700 cc | 20 cm $H_2O$ | 30 cm $H_2O$ |
| 2000 | 700 cc | 21 cm $H_2O$ | 35 cm $H_2O$ |
| 2100 | 700 cc | 22 cm $H_2O$ | 50 cm $H_2O$ |

What should the RRT do in response to this data?

I. Reposition the endotracheal tube.
II. Increase the pressure limit.
III. Perform endotracheal suctioning.
IV. Administer a bronchodilator.

A. I only
B. II only
C. III, IV only
D. I, III only

123. A 70-kg asthmatic is receiving mechanical ventilation for an acute episode that has *not* favorably responded to routine therapy. The ventilator settings as follows:

mode: control
ventilatory rate: 12 breaths/min
$V_T$: 850 cc
$V_I$: 60 liters/min
$FIO_2$: 0.30

The ventilator is displaying the volume-pressure loop presented in Figure 5-10 on page 264.

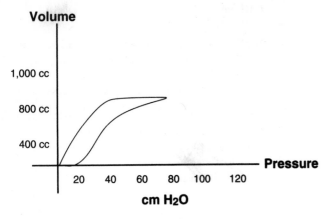

**Volume**

1,000 cc

800 cc

400 cc

**Pressure**

20    40    60    80    100    120

**cm H₂O**

**Figure 5-10:** Volume-pressure loop.

What should the RRT do at this time to correct the situation?

A. Decrease the peak inspiratory flow.
B. Add PEEP.
C. Decrease the patient's tidal volume.
D. Do *nothing*, because this condition is acceptable for this patient.

124. Given the hemodynamic data shown here, calculate the cardiac output (C.O.).

$SaO_2$ 90%
$CaO_2 - C\bar{v}O_2$ 6.0 vol%
$\dot{V}O_2$ 245 ml/min.
PCWP 12 mm Hg

A. 4.08 L/min.
B. 3.83 L/min.
C. 2.05 L/min.
D. 1.50 L/min.

125. A patient has been intubated with an 8.0 mm I.D. oral ET tube. The patient develops coarse breath sounds and there are visible secretions in the ET tube. The RRT, using a 16 Fr suction catheter, begins to clear the tube after appropriately preoxygenating the patient. The patient now develops tachycardia and desaturation as determined by a pulse oximeter. What can the RRT do to try to prevent these developments?

A. Wait to suction the patient until the procedure is indicated.
B. Increase the amount of negative pressure applied to 150 mm Hg.
C. Turn off the pulse oximeter to prevent an alarm from sounding.
D. Use a 12 Fr suction catheter.

126. A 20-year-old male experienced massive blood loss in an automobile accident. Following surgery, he re-

ceived mechanical ventilatory support for 24 hours, after which he was placed on a T-piece at 40% oxygen. Shortly thereafter, he developed ARDS. His spontaneous breathing and hemodynamic status evaluated at that time are as follows:

ventilatory rate: 40 breaths/min.
tidal volume: 325 cc
heart rate: 135 beats/min.
blood pressure: 155/105 torr
C.O.: 13 L/min.
C.I.: 7.5 L/min./m²
$FiO_2$: 0.90

ABG data reveal the following:

$PO_2$ 45 torr
$PCO_2$ 25 torr
pH 7.53
$HCO_3^-$ 20 mEq/liter
B.E. −4 mEq/liter

Immediately, a CPAP of 10 cm $H_2O$ was instituted, and the following ventilatory and hemodynamic data were obtained:

ventilatory rate: 22 breaths/min.
tidal volume: 325 cc
heart rate: 80 beats/min.
blood pressure: 125/75 torr
C.O.: 6 L/min.
C.I.: 3.3 L/min./m²
$FiO_2$: 0.90

ABG data at this time are as follows:

$PO_2$ 80 torr
$PCO_2$ 35 torr
pH 7.42
$HCO_3^-$ 22 mEq/liter
B.E. 0 mEq/liter

What should the RRT do at this time?

A. Reduce the CPAP level to restore the C.O.
B. Recommend that the patient receive a volume expander to return the C.I. to normal.
C. Sedate the patient somewhat to normalize the ventilatory rate.
D. Monitor the patient and evaluate his response to this therapeutic modality.

127. While performing ventilator rounds in the ICU, the RRT observes a patient being weaned from mechanical ventilation via a T-piece. The RRT notices asymmetrical chest wall movement as the patient breathes. Auscultation of the patient's thorax revealed breath sounds on the right side but *none* on the left. What action should the RRT take at this time?

A. Reconnect the patient to the mechanical ventilator.
B. Extubate and reintubate the patient.
C. Recommend the insertion of chest tubes.
D. Check the position of the endotracheal tube.

128. While performing endotracheal suctioning on a post-MI patient in the coronary ICU, the RRT notices on the ECG monitor that the patient's heart rate decreases from 80 beats/min. to 60 beats/min. What should the RRT do at this time?

A. Terminate the suctioning procedure.
B. Instill 3 cc of normal saline into the lungs and continue suctioning.
C. Use a smaller size suction catheter.
D. Change the vacuum pressure to $-80$ mm Hg and continue suctioning.

129. A 13-year-old, cystic fibrosis, home care patient has been producing large amounts of sputum daily. The patient has been non-compliant with chest physiotherapy. What type of therapy could the RRT recommend to the patient to increase secretion mobilization?

A. deep breathing with cough
B. BiPAP® therapy
C. PEP mask therapy
D. sustained maximal inspiration

130. Under normal and stable cardiovascular conditions, the end-tidal carbon dioxide tension values are normally approximate to which of the following measurements?

I. venous carbon dioxide tension
II. mean exhaled carbon dioxide tension
III. alveolar carbon dioxide tension
IV. arterial carbon dioxide tension

A. I only
B. III only
C. I, II only
D. III, IV only

131. A 32-year-old, 150-pound (IBW) male Guillain–Barré patient is receiving controlled mechanical ventilation with a volume-cycled ventilator with the following settings:

ventilatory rate: 10 breaths/min.
peak inspiratory flow: 50 L/min.
tidal volume: 800 cc
F$I$O$_2$: 0.40

ABG data reveal the following:

PO$_2$ 90 torr
PCO$_2$ 60 torr
pH 7.29

HCO$_3^-$ 28 mEq/liter
B.E. 3 mEq/liter

Which of the following ventilatory rate and tidal volume setting combinations would most likely result in an arterial PCO$_2$ of 50 torr?

A. ventilatory rate 14 breaths/min.; 750 cc tidal volume
B. ventilatory rate 14 breaths/min.; 800 cc tidal volume
C. ventilatory rate 12 breaths/min.; 800 cc tidal volume
D. ventilatory rate 10 breaths/min.; 850 cc tidal volume

132. A patient is receiving controlled mechanical ventilation to support a severe lung injury. She is requiring high inspiratory pressures, an oxygen concentration of 100%, and a PEEP level of 15 cm H$_2$O. Her ABG data indicate the following:

PO$_2$ 70 torr
PCO$_2$ 55 torr
pH 7.32
HCO$_3^-$ 28 mEq/liter
B.E. 4 mEq/liter

Her C.I. is falling despite pharmacological support. What mode of ventilation might be helpful in improving her oxygenation and ventilation without further cardiovascular embarrassment?

A. PC-IRV
B. PSV
C. mandatory minute ventilation
D. APRV

133. A 22-year-old, female auto accident victim is admitted to the emergency department for evaluation and treatment of a closed head injury. She is breathing spontaneously and is agitated and combative. She is also receiving oxygen at 40% via an air entrainment mask and is in *no* apparent respiratory distress. She has *no* history of pulmonary disease and is a nonsmoker. After obtaining an ABG sample with some difficulty, the presence of air bubbles in the syringe is noted. What are the probable effects of the bubbles on the results of the blood gas analysis?

I. The PaO$_2$ will be decreased.
II. The PaO$_2$ will be increased.
III. The PaCO$_2$ will be increased.
IV. The PaCO$_2$ will be decreased.
V. The pH will be more acidotic.

A. I, III only
B. II, IV only
C. I, III, V only
D. I, IV only

134. While performing ventilator rounds in the ICU, the RRT approaches the bed of a patient who is receiving

mechanical ventilation in the control mode. The patient is also being monitored with capnography. The capnogram in Figure 5-11 appears on the monitor.

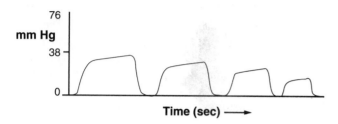

**Figure 5-11:** Capnogram.

Which of the following interpretations should the RRT make concerning the capnogram?

A. The patient has become disconnected from the ventilator.
B. The patient has suffered a cardiac arrest and continues to be ventilated.
C. The patient is hyperventilating.
D. The patient has retained secretions causing partial airway obstruction.

135. An intubated patient is being endotracheally suctioned by an RRT, who notices the ECG pattern in Figure 5-12 just as he is about to apply suction to the suction catheter.

What should he do at this time?

A. Immediately withdraw the suction catheter.
B. Momentarily refrain from applying suction pressure.
C. Continue with the procedure.
D. Use a less mucosal-irritating suction catheter.

136. After assisting a physician with an ET intubation, the RRT is asked to evaluate the placement of the ET tube.

Which of the following procedures should the RRT perform?

I. Listen for bilateral breath sounds.
II. Auscultate the epigastrium.
III. Obtain an ABG.
IV. Measure the patient's negative inspiratory force.

A. I, II only
B. II, III only
C. I, IV only
D. I, II, IV only

137. A patient who is undergoing a bronchoscopic procedure is extremely anxious regarding the procedure. Which of the following medications would help sedate this patient?

A. naloxone
B. meperidine
C. lidocaine
D. succinylcholine

138. Which of the following physiologic effects are associated with PEEP?

I. decreased intracranial pressure
II. decreased urinary output
III. decreased C.O.
IV. increased pulmonary vascular resistance

A. I, III, IV only
B. II, III, IV only
C. I, II only
D. II, III only

139. When a patient is nasally or orally intubated, generally how much time should elapse before a tracheotomy is considered?

A. If the patient is comatose, a tracheotomy should be done 24 hours after the patient is intubated.
B. A tracheotomy should be done immediately if tracheobronchial secretions are thick.

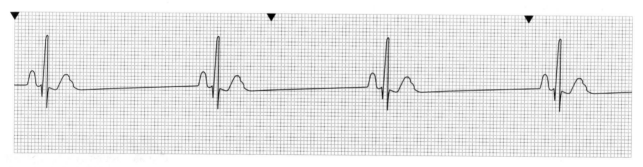

**Figure 5-12:** ECG tracing.

C. If the patient appears to be in further need of the artificial airway, a tracheotomy should be done 72 hours after intubation.

D. Because each clinical condition and situation is different, the decision to perform a tracheotomy is an individualized medical determination.

140. A patient is receiving mechanical ventilation with the following settings:

mode: assist-control
tidal volume: 1,000 cc
ventilatory rate: 14 breaths/min.
PEEP: 15 cm $H_2O$
$FiO_2$: 1.0

The PIP generated is 65 cm $H_2O$, and the I:E ratio is 1:1. ABGs at this time reveal the following:

$PO_2$ 45 torr
$PCO_2$ 44 torr
pH 7.35
$HCO_3^-$ 24 mEq/liter
B.E. 0 mEq/liter

Chest X-rays reveal diffuse, bilateral infiltrates. The patient's lung compliance has been steadily decreasing. What ventilator recommendation would be most appropriate for this patient?

A. Switch to SIMV at a ventilatory rate of 14 breaths/min.

B. Institute PCV at 30 cm $H_2O$.

C. Increase the PEEP level to 25 cm $H_2O$.

D. Maintain the current settings and continue monitoring the patient.

141. While performing endotracheal suctioning on a patient who is attached to a cardiac monitor, the RRT observes the ECG pattern shown in Figure 5-13.

What should the RRT recommend at this time?
A. Administer lidocaine.
B. Perform cardioversion.

C. Begin cardiopulmonary resuscitation.
D. Administer a precordial thump.

142. When noting a patient's fluid status, which of the following pressures is the best clinical indicator of left ventricular preload?

A. central venous pressure
B. pulmonary artery systolic pressure
C. pulmonary artery diastolic pressure
D. pulmonary capillary wedge pressure

143. A 25-year-old football player incurred a flail chest injury in an automobile accident while en route to his home after practice. While receiving volume ventilation with an $FiO_2$ of 0.30, he displayed the following ABGs:

$PO_2$ 120 torr
$PCO_2$ 44 torr
pH 7.38
$HCO_3^-$ 25 mEq/liter
B.E. 0 mEq/liter

A PEEP of 5 cm $H_2O$ has been ordered by the physician. What is the probable rationale for this decision? This person has never had a pleural effusion or pneumothorax.

A. to increase the patient's $PaO_2$ without having to increase the $FiO_2$

B. to overcome the patient's severe shunting problem

C. to assist in stabilizing the chest wall

D. to overcome the patient's lung parenchymal problem

144. A patient has been switched from assist-control ventilation to SIMV in preparation for weaning from the mechanical ventilator. Which of the following modes of ventilation could be included in the orders to supplement the weaning process?

A. inverse-ratio ventilation
B. APRV
C. PSV
D. PCV

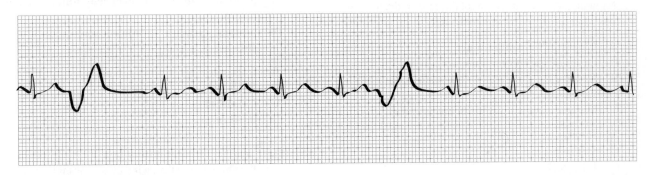

**Figure 5-13:** Lead II ECG tracing.

145. The RRT is assisting the physician in the emergency department with performing oral endotracheal intubation on a patient who has a depressed level of consciousness and has reportedly consumed lunch 20 minutes ago. Which of the following actions would be appropriate for the RRT to take at this time?

    A. have the physician use a Miller laryngoscope blade
    B. apply gentle pressure with a finger against the patient's cricoid cartilage
    C. suggest using a laryngeal mask airway
    D. recommend to the physician to administer 0.5 of midazolam I.V.

146. An RRT working in the emergency department sees an 18-year-old smoke-inhalation victim arrive. En route to the hospital, the EMTs administered oxygen to this patient with a simple mask at 8 L/min. ABGs drawn upon arrival indicate the following:

$PO_2$ 130 mm Hg
$PCO_2$ 25 mm Hg
pH 7.43
$HCO_3^-$ 16 mEq/liter
[Hb] 15 g%
COHb% 45%

Vital signs taken at this time reveal the following:

blood pressure: 130/85 torr
heart rate: 80 beats/min.
ventilatory rate: 20 breaths/min.

What should the RRT do at this time?

    A. Intubate and mechanically ventilate the patient.
    B. Administer mask CPAP with 100% oxygen.
    C. Administer an $FIO_2$ of 0.50 via a partial rebreathing mask.
    D. Intubate and administer an $FIO_2$ of 0.40 via a T-piece with 50 cc of reservoir tubing.

147. A patient is receiving oxygen therapy via a simple mask operated at a flow rate of 15 L/min. The RRT observes the patient having a nonproductive cough. Additionally, the patient is complaining of a dry mouth, nose, and throat. What should the RRT do at this time?

    I. Check the humidifier water level.
    II. Decrease the oxygen flow rate.
    III. Replace the apparatus with a small-volume nebulizer.
    IV. Suggest a Mucomyst treatment.

    A. II only
    B. I, II only
    C. I, IV only
    D. III, IV only

148. A patient is receiving continuous-flow intermittent mandatory ventilation (IMV). The ventilator settings and spontaneous measurements are as follows:

mechanical ventilatory rate: 6 breaths/min.
spontaneous ventilatory rate: 8 breaths/min.
mechanical tidal volume: 900 cc
spontaneous tidal volume: 300 cc
$FIO_2$: 0.35
PEEP: 12 cm $H_2O$

As the RRT conducts ventilator rounds, she notices that while the patient breathes spontaneously, the pressure gauge registers 3 cm $H_2O$ on inspiration and 12 cm $H_2O$ during expiration. What should she do at this time?

    A. Increase the mechanical ventilatory rate.
    B. Increase the gas flow rate through the continuous-flow system.
    C. Decrease the mechanical tidal volume.
    D. Reduce the PEEP level.

149. The physician requests the RRT to perform percutaneous catheter insertion into a patient's trachea in preparation for performing a transtracheal aspiration procedure. Where should the RRT perform the percutaneous insertion of the catheter?

    A. 1 centimeter above the manubrium
    B. between the first and second tracheal rings
    C. at the level of the cricothyroid membrane
    D. immediately below the cricoid cartilage

150. A 58-year-old, male COPD patient has the following respiratory care orders:

atrovent (ipratropium bromide) MDI: two puffs QID
albuterol MDI: two puffs QID
postural drainage with chest percussion QID

The physician requests the RRT "space out the therapy to maximize the benefits." Which of the following sequence of therapies would be most appropriate?

    I. albuterol at 7 A.M., 11 A.M., 3 P.M., and 7 P.M.
    II. atrovent at 9 A.M., 1 P.M., 5 P.M., and 9 P.M.
    III. postural drainage to immediately follow each albuterol treatment
    IV. postural drainage to immediately precede each atrovent treatment

    A. I, III only
    B. II, IV only
    C. I, II, III only
    D. II, III only

151. A patient has a recent history of a dry, nonproductive cough. Which of the following conditions might be the cause of this problem?

I. pulmonary fibrosis
II. asthma
III. bronchitis
IV. congestive heart failure

A. I only
B. II, III only
C. I, IV only
D. II, IV only

152. Which mode of mechanical ventilation along with the settings listed will result in the *least* elevation in the patient's mean intrathoracic pressure?

   A. mode: SIMV
      ventilatory rate: 10 breaths/min.
      tidal volume: 15 cc/kg
      PEEP: 5 cm $H_2O$
   B. mode: controlled mechanical ventilation
      ventilatory rate: 12 breaths/min.
      tidal volume: 12 cc/kg
      PEEP: 5 cm $H_2O$
   C. mode: IMV
      ventilatory rate: 6 breaths/min.
      tidal volume: 15 cc/kg
      PEEP: 5 cm $H_2O$
   D. mode: assisted mechanical ventilation
      ventilatory rate: 14 breaths/min.
      tidal volume: 10 cc/kg

153. A patient is receiving mechanical ventilation via a microprocessor ventilator with the following settings established:

   mode: assist-control
   flow wave pattern: square
   tidal volume: 800 cc
   ventilatory rate: 12 breaths/min.
   peak flow rate: 60 L/min.

   The RRT has noticed a change in the PIP from 40 cm $H_2O$ to 50 cm $H_2O$ while the plateau pressure remained at 25 cm $H_2O$. Calculate this patient's airway resistance.

   A. 25 cm $H_2O$/L/sec.
   B. 40 cm $H_2O$/L/sec.
   C. 50 cm $H_2O$/L/sec.
   D. 90 cm $H_2O$/L/sec.

154. Calculate a patient's C.O. when given the following data:

   heart rate: 100 beats/min.
   blood pressure: 135/90 mm Hg
   stroke volume: 60 ml/beat

   A. 6.5 L/min.
   B. 6.0 L/min.

C. 5.5 L/min.
D. 5.0 L/min.

155. Calculate the mean exhaled carbon dioxide tension for a 75-kg (IBW) patient who has a tidal volume of 520 cc. This patient's ABG data reveal the following:

   $PO_2$ 95 torr
   $PCO_2$ 44 torr
   pH 7.35
   $HCO_3^-$ 24 mEq/liter
   B.E. 0 mEq/liter

   Assume *no* dead space disease is present.

   A. 70 torr
   B. 68 torr
   C. 51 torr
   D. 30 torr

156. When implementing a graded exercise program, which of the following components first need to be established?

   I. duration
   II. frequency
   III. intensity
   IV. mode of exercise

   A. I, II, III, IV
   B. II, IV only
   C. I, II, IV only
   D. I, III only

157. Which of the following hemodynamic values are needed to determine the effects of an increased mean airway pressure on the C.O.?

   I. stroke volume index
   II. heart rate
   III. PCWP
   IV. central venous pressure (CVP)
   V. stroke volume

   A. II, V only
   B. III, IV only
   C. I, II, IV only
   D. III, IV, V only

158. While assisting a physician performing oral endotracheal intubation, the RRT is asked how the patient's head and neck should be positioned during this procedure. The RRT should respond by saying that the head and neck need to be:

   A. in the sniffing position
   B. maximally flexed
   C. in a neutral position
   D. moderately flexed

159. A post-MI patient has a pulmonary artery catheter in place. A blood sample has been obtained from the distal port of the catheter. An arterial blood sample has also been obtained from the radial artery. Calculate this patient's $C(a-\bar{v})O_2$. This patient has a [Hb] of 15 g%.

Arterial and Mixed Venous Blood Gas and
Acid-Base Data

| Arterial | Mixed Venous |
| --- | --- |
| $PaO_2$ 100 torr | $P\bar{v}O_2$ 40 torr |
| $PaCO_2$ 40 torr | $P\bar{v}CO_2$ 46 torr |
| $HCO_3^-$ 24 mEq/L | $HCO_3^-$ 24 mEq/L |
| pH 7.40 | pH 7.36 |
| $SaO_2$ 97% | $S\bar{v}O_2$ 70% |

A. 5.6 vol%
B. 6.4 vol%
C. 7.0 vol%
D. 7.8 vol%

160. Which of the following procedures should be performed by the RRT immediately after ET intubation?

I. Auscultate the patient's chest.
II. Note the position of the tube at the teeth or gum line.
III. Auscultate the patient's epigastrum.
IV. Recommend that a chest X-ray be ordered.

A. I, II, III only
B. II, III only
C. I, II, IV only
D. I, II, III, IV

161. Calculate the C.I. when given the following data. Use the Dubois Body Surface Chart (Figure 5-14).

systolic pressure: 190 mm Hg
diastolic pressure: 100 mm Hg
heart rate: 82 beats/min.
stroke volume: 65 ml
height: 78 inches
weight: 210 pounds

A. 2.05 L/min./m²
B. 2.31 L/min./m²
C. 4.69 L/min./m²
D. 5.33 L/min./m²

162. Calculate the percent shunt by using the following data:

end-pulmonary capillary $O_2$ content: 24.78 vol%
total arterial $O_2$ content: 24.36 vol%
total mixed-venous $O_2$ content: 20.86 vol%

A. 8.9%
B. 10.7%
C. 12.0%
D. 13.8%

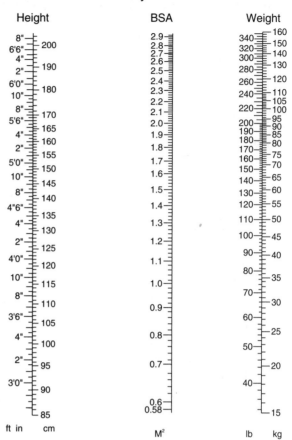

Dubois Body Surface Chart

Figure 5-14: Find the patient's height in either feet or centimeters in the left column and the patient's weight in pounds or kilograms in the right column. Connect these two points with a ruler. The body surface area (BSA) is indicated at the point where the ruler crosses the middle column.

163. A 25-year-old female complaining of dyspnea has an arterial $PO_2$ of 35 torr and a $P(A-a)O_2$ of 95 torr while breathing room air. After receiving 100% $O_2$, her arterial $PO_2$ was 55 torr and her $P(A-a)O_2$ became 625 torr. What is the cause of this patient's hypoxemia?

A. diffusion defect
B. venous admixture
C. capillary shunting
D. shunt effect

164. A patient who has been receiving CPT for 5 days has been noted as coughing more frequently and producing more sputum. The sputum has changed from mucoid to purulent during this time frame. Which of the following therapeutic modalities would be beneficial to this patient?

I. increasing the duration of vibration during CPT
II. having the patient receive a heated aerosol before CPT

III. administering a bronchodilator before CPT
IV. having the patient perform incentive spirometry Q1h

A. II, III only
B. III only
C. II, IV only
D. I, II, III only

165. A post-laparotomy patient has been receiving incentive spirometry and daily therapeutic assessments for 4 days since her surgery. Her presurgical pulmonary function data are as follows:

vital capacity: 4.2 liters
inspiratory capacity: 3.0 liters

On the fourth postsurgical day, her inspiratory capacity has been determined to be 2.0 liters. What should the RRT recommend at this time?

A. instituting IPPB therapy
B. discontinuing incentive spirometry
C. continuing with the current therapy and daily evaluations
D. instituting PEP mask therapy

166. A physician seeking a therapeutic modality to reduce air trapping and to mobilize secretions in a COPD patient asks the RRT for his recommendation. Which of the following modalities would be appropriate?

A. IS
B. IPPB
C. PEP
D. CPT

167. While performing ventilator rounds, the RRT observes that the patient's PIP increased from 40 cm $H_2O$ to 50 cm $H_2O$ while the plateau pressure remained at 25 cm $H_2O$. Which of the following conditions might have accounted for these pressure changes?

I. bronchospasm
II. pneumothorax
III. right mainstem bronchus intubation
IV. accumulation of secretions

A. I, IV only
B. I, II only
C. III only
D. I, III, IV only

168. An adult female who has micrognathia is orally intubated with a 6.5 mm I.D. ET tube. She is a recovering ARDS patient with a reliable ventilatory drive. She has been on assist-control ventilation previously. The physician asks the RRT to recommend a mode of ventilation that would reduce the patient's work of breath-

ing and prepare the patient for weaning. Which of the following recommendations would be appropriate?

A. PCV
B. controlled mechanical ventilation
C. PSV
D. inverse ratio ventilation

169. A postoperative thoracotomy patient has been receiving incentive spirometry for 7 days. His preoperative pulmonary function values are listed as follows:

vital capacity: 4.8 liters
inspiratory capacity: 3.6 liters

As of the patient's seventh day of incentive spirometry and therapeutic evaluation, his inspiratory capacity is measured to be 3.0 liters. What should the RRT recommend at this time?

A. discontinuing incentive spirometry
B. discontinuing daily therapeutic evaluations
C. adding CPT to the regimen
D. changing to IPPB

170. The RRT receives an order to administer a 70–30, helium–oxygen mixture to a patient who is having an acute asthmatic episode. The only flow meter available to deliver this helium–oxygen gas mixture is an oxygen flow meter. What flow rate needs to be set on the oxygen flow meter for 12 L/min. of this mixture to be delivered?

A. 6.5 L/min.
B. 7.5 L/min.
C. 9.0 L/min.
D. 10.0 L/min.

171. Which of the following tracheostomy tubes can be used to train a tracheotomized patient to become an upper-airway breather and still allow for positive-pressure ventilation?

A. Kamen–Wilkinson tube
B. Lanz tube
C. fenestrated tube
D. tracheal button

172. A 25-year-old, post-op thoracotomy patient is receiving mechanical ventilation in the SIMV mode with a mechanical ventilatory rate of 8 breaths/min. The patient also has a closed tracheal suction system attached to the patient Y. The patient is receiving an $FIO_2$ of 0.50 and PEEP of 5 cm $H_2O$. To what level should the $FIO_2$ be raised before suctioning?

A. The $FIO_2$ should be increased to 1.00.
B. The $FIO_2$ should be raised to 0.60.

C. The presence of the PEEP of 5 cm H$_2$O obviates the need for elevating the F$_I$O$_2$.

D. Closed suction catheter systems do *not* require increasing the F$_I$O$_2$.

173. The RRT is preparing to perform ET suctioning on a mechanically ventilated patient and observes on the cardiac monitor the ECG tracing in Figure 5-15.

During the suctioning procedure, she notices the ECG pattern on the cardiac monitor as shown in Figure 5-16.

What should she do at this time?

A. Continue suctioning and monitor the patient.

B. Remove the suction catheter immediately.

C. Adjust the suction pressure to be less subatmospheric.

D. Instill 3 to 5 ml of normal saline into the trachea.

174. The RRT is monitoring the intracuff pressure of a tracheostomy tube inserted in a patient who is receiving mechanical ventilation. She observes the pressure manometer indicating a pressure of 42 cm H$_2$O. What should she do at this time?

A. Inject more air through the pilot balloon.

B. Release some of the air from the cuff.

C. Insert a new tracheostomy tube.

D. Do *nothing*, because the cuff pressure reading is acceptable.

175. Which of the following considerations must be taken into account when providing 80–20 helium–oxygen therapy using an oxygen flow meter?

I. An uncompensated flow meter needs to be used.

II. A high-flow flow meter must be used.

III. 1.8 L/min. of helium–oxygen is delivered for each L/min. indicated on the flow meter.

A. I, II, III

B. II, III only

C. I, II only

D. III only

176. During CPR (basic life support), the RTT checks the victim's pupillary size and reactivity. She observes that the pupils are dilated but react to light. What is the significance of this finding?

A. The victim has irreversible brain damage.

B. The victim is experiencing adequate cerebral circulation.

C. Cerebral oxygenation is inadequate.

D. Cerebral circulation is inadequate.

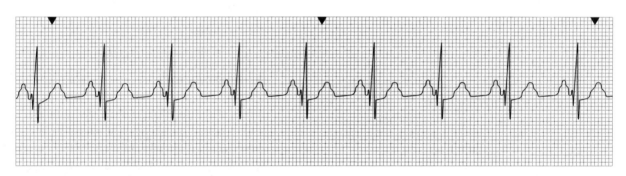

**Figure 5-15:** Lead II ECG tracing.

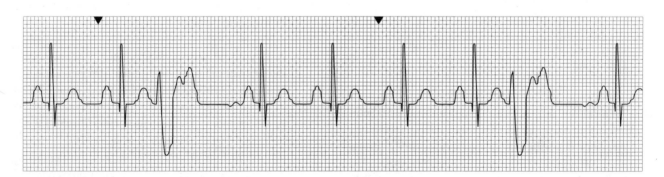

**Figure 5-16:** Lead II ECG tracing.

177. A patient is being mechanically ventilated with a ventilator classified as a flow controller. How will the peak inspiratory pressure be affected when the patient's airway resistance increases?

  A. unaffected
  B. increased
  C. decreased
  D. will fluctuate

178. During advanced cardiac life support, the decision has been made to endotracheally administer epinephrine to the victim. Which of the following concerns should be considered?

  I. Ten milliliters of distilled water will enhance ET absorption.
  II. The arterial $PO_2$ might decrease.
  III. External cardiac compressions should *not* be withheld to instill the medication.
  IV. The medication should be rapidly sprayed down the ET tube.

  A. I, II, IV only
  B. II, III, IV only
  C. I, III only
  D. I, II, III, IV

179. While administering an IPPB treatment to a patient, the RRT notices that the machine pressure gauge deflects to −2 cm $H_2O$ before the machine is cycled on by the patient. What should the RRT do in this situation?

  A. Do *nothing* and continue with the treatment.
  B. Adjust the sensitivity control to allow the machine to cycle on more easily.
  C. Reduce the preset pressure because it is probably too high for the patient to tolerate.
  D. Terminate the treatment because the patient's inspiratory effort is adequate; therefore, IPPB probably is *not* indicated.

**Situational Sets**

**Questions 180 and 181 refer to the same patient.**

A 65-kg patient is receiving mechanical ventilation via a microprocessor ventilator with the following settings.

tidal volume: 850 cc
ventilator rate: 15 breaths/min.
peak inspiratory flow rate: 60 L/min.
$FIO_2$: 0.80

The patient's pulmonary compliance and airway resistance have been determined to be 0.07 L/cm $H_2O$ and 12 cm $H_2O$/L/sec., respectively. The ventilator has been programmed to deliver a square waveflow pattern.

180. Calculate this patient's static pressure.

  A. 4 cm $H_2O$
  B. 12 cm $H_2O$
  C. 14 cm $H_2O$
  D. 17 cm $H_2O$

181. Calculate the PIP.

  A. 12 cm $H_2O$
  B. 16 cm $H_2O$
  C. 24 cm $H_2O$
  D. 29 cm $H_2O$

**Questions 182 and 183 refer to the same patient.**

182. The flow-time waveform in Figure 5-17 was obtained from a patient who was receiving mechanical ventilation.

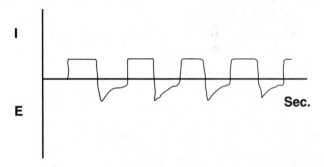

**Figure 5-17:** Flow-time waveform (I equals inspiration; E equals expiration.)

How should the RRT interpret this waveform?

  A. It is normal.
  B. The patient has to exert a large negative pressure to initiate inspiration.
  C. Auto-PEEP is present.
  D. The patient-ventilator system has a leak somewhere in it.

183. What action should the RRT take to correct this situation?

  I. *No* action is necessary because the flow time waveform is normal.
  II. Increase the tidal volume and decrease the ventilatory rate.
  III. Increase the peak inspiratory flow rate.
  IV. Add more volume to the cuff on the endotracheal tube.
  V. Adjust the sensitivity to facilitate patient triggering.

  A. I only
  B. IV only

C. II, III only

D. IV, V only

**Questions 184, 185, and 186 refer to the same patient.**

The RRT is monitoring the cardiopulmonary status of a patient who has a PAC and a radial arterial pressure line inserted. She is also receiving continuous positive pressure ventilation (CPPV). Hemodynamic, ventilatory, and blood gas data are as follows:

### Hemodynamic Data

pulmonary artery systolic pressure: 40 mm Hg
pulmonary artery diastolic pressure: 20 mm Hg
central venous pressure: 17 cm $H_2O$
pulmonary artery wedge pressure: 12 mm Hg
oxygen consumption: 285 ml/min.
cardiac output: 3.5 L/min.

### Ventilatory Data

mode of ventilation: control
$FiO_2$: 0.80
ventilatory rate: 12 breaths/min.
tidal volume: 750 cc

### Arterial and Mixed Venous Blood Gas and Acid-Base Data

| Arterial | Mixed Venous |
|----------|--------------|
| $PO_2$ 80 torr | $PO_2$ 29 torr |
| $PCO_2$ 65 torr | $PCO_2$ 75 torr |
| pH 7.30 | pH 7.24 |
| $HCO_3^-$ 31 mEq/liter | $HCO_3^-$ 31 mEq/liter |

184. Calculate the mean pulmonary artery pressure ($\overline{PAP}$).

    A. 26.7 mm Hg

    B. 24.0 mm Hg

    C. 21.3 mm Hg

    D. 20.0 mm Hg

185. Calculate this patient's pulmonary vascular resistance.

    A. 2.8 mm Hg/L/min.

    B. 3.5 mm Hg/L/min.

    C. 4.2 mm Hg/L/min.

    D. 5.1 mm Hg/L/min.

186. What is the possible cause of this particular pulmonary vascular resistance value?

    A. decreased venous return

    B. pulmonary vasoconstriction

    C. hypervolemia

    D. high-pressure pulmonary edema

**Questions 187, 188, and 189, refer to the same patient.**

A 34-year-old, 130-pound, 5ft. 6-in. female is brought into the emergency department by her family. The chief complaints are general muscle weakness, paresthesia, and difficulty breathing. The medical staff is informed that this patient had a cytomegalovirus infection 2 weeks ago and experienced numbness and weakness of the hands and feet for the last few days. Data from a number of diagnostic tests indicated an increased protein concentration in the cerebrospinal fluid and a normal leukocyte count. ABG analysis on room air revealed the following:

$PO_2$ 80 torr
$PCO_2$ 48 torr
pH 7.33
$HCO_3^-$ 24 mEq/liter
B.E. 0 mEq/liter

Two hours later, the patient became progressively weaker. At this time, her vital capacity was 15 cc/kg and her maximum inspiratory pressure was $-20$ cm $H_2O$. Her room air ABGs now indicated the following:

$PO_2$ 70 torr
$PCO_2$ 55 torr
pH 7.29
$HCO_3^-$ 26 mEq/liter
B.E. 1 mEq/liter

187. What action should now be taken by the RRT?

    A. Administer 40% $O_2$ via an air entrainment mask.

    B. Institute nasal CPAP at 10 cm $H_2O$.

    C. Intubate the patient and administer an $FiO_2$ of 0.40 via a T-piece.

    D. Intubate and mechanically ventilate the patient.

188. What type of mechanical ventilatory support would be appropriate for this patient?

    A. Sedation and controlled mechanical ventilation at a rate of 12 breaths/min.

    B. IMV at a rate of 4 breaths/min.

    C. Assist-control ventilation with a controlled rate of 8 to 10 breaths/min.

    D. PSV with a pressure plateau level of 5 cm $H_2O$.

189. Which of the following ventilator settings are appropriate for this patient? Use the Dubois BSA chart in Figure 5-18.

    A. $\dot{V}_E$ 6.0 L/min.; $V_T$ 700 cc; f 8 breaths/min.

    B. $\dot{V}_E$ 5.0 L/min.; $V_T$ 800 cc; f 6 breaths/min.

    C. $\dot{V}_E$ 8.0 L/min.; $V_T$ 650 cc; f 12 breaths/min.

    D. $\dot{V}_E$ 8.0 L/min.; $V_T$ 800 cc; f 10 breaths/min.

## Dubois Body Surface Chart

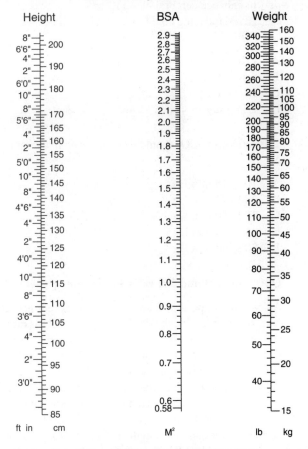

**Figure 5-18:** Find the patient's height in either feet or centimeters in the left column and the patient's weight in pounds or kilograms in the right column. Connect these two points with a ruler. The BSA is indicated at the point where the ruler crosses the middle column.

**Questions 190 and 191 refer to the same patient.**

An 90-kg (IBW) patient is receiving controlled volume-cycled ventilation with the following settings:

$V_T$: 800 cc
ventilatory rate: 15 breaths/min.
peak inspiratory flow rate: 50 L/min.
$FiO_2$: 0.60

190. Calculate this patient's approximate $\dot{V}_A$.

   A. 120 cc/min.
   B. 2.97 L/min.
   C. 7.56 L/min.
   D. 9.03 L/min.

191. If this patient had the following ABG values,

   $PO_2$ 50 torr
   $PCO_2$ 45 torr
   pH 7.37

$HCO_3^-$ 25 mEq/liter
B.E. 0 mEq/liter

what therapeutic intervention would be most appropriate for this situation?

   A. Decrease the ventilatory rate.
   B. Increase the $FiO_2$.
   C. Add PEEP.
   D. Decrease the tidal volume.

**Questions 192, 193, and 194 refer to the following data.**

A patient is being mechanically ventilated on the Siemens Servo 900C. The ventilator settings include the following:

ventilatory rate: 10 breaths/min.
minute ventilation ($\dot{V}_E$): 6 L/min.
inspiratory time percent ($T_{I\%}$): 30%

192. Calculate this patient's tidal volume.

   A. 60 cc
   B. 200 cc
   C. 333 cc
   D. 600 cc

193. Calculate this patient's inspiratory time.

   A. 1.00 sec.
   B. 1.98 sec.
   C. 2.18 sec.
   D. 3.02 sec.

194. Calculate this patient's expiratory time ($T_E$).

   A. 6.00 sec.
   B. 5.08 sec.
   C. 4.02 sec.
   D. 3.18 sec.

**Questions 195, 196, and 197 refer to the same patient.**

The RRT has been asked to establish mechanical ventilation with a Siemens Servo 900C on a 10-year-old girl who has an IBW of 87 pounds. Before connecting the patient to the ventilator, the RRT sets the machine in the volume-control mode with a minute ventilation of 2 L/min. and a ventilatory rate of 12 breaths/min. When the ventilator cycles to inspiration, he occludes the Y connector and notes that the PIP achieves 50 cm $H_2O$ in the presence of a PEEP of 5 cm $H_2O$.

195. Calculate the tubing compliance factor for this ventilator.

   A. 4.00 cc/cm $H_2O$
   B. 3.71 cc/cm $H_2O$

C. 3.03 cc/cm $H_2O$

D. 2.67 cc/cm $H_2O$

196. The RRT establishes the following settings.

   minute ventilation: 8 L/min.
   ventilatory rate: 12 breaths/min.
   $FIO_2$: 0.60
   inspiratory time %: 25%
   PEEP: 5 cm $H_2O$
   mode: SIMV
   SIMV rate: 6 breaths/min.

   When the ventilator cycles to inspiration, the PIP achieved is 35 cm $H_2O$. Calculate this patient's actual tidal volume.

   A. 277 cc

   B. 556 cc

   C. 667 cc

   D. 890 cc

197. The physician has requested that the patient's tidal volume be equal to 12 cc/kg of IBW. What ventilator setting adjustment must be made?

   A. *No* adjustment is necessary.

   B. Increase the ventilatory rate to 15 breaths/min.

   C. Decrease the minute ventilation to 6 L/min.

   D. Decrease the minute ventilation to 7 L/min.

### Questions 198, 199, and 200 refer to the same patient.

An automobile accident victim is admitted to the emergency department. Clinical examination of the victim reveals massive head injury with cerebral hemorrhage. The victim presents as comatose with an irregular ventilatory pattern, a spontaneous ventilatory rate of 7 breaths/min., and a $V_T$ of 270 cc. The victim weighs approximately 72 kg and is 52 years of age.

198. What therapeutic intervention is immediately recommended for this patient?

   A. CPAP

   B. controlled mechanical ventilation, maintaining a low $PaCO_2$

   C. assist-control mechanical ventilation

   D. mechanical ventilation with an IMV rate of 10 breaths/min.

199. How should intracranial pressure be managed for this patient?

   I. Maintain an adequate $PaO_2$ to reduce cerebral vasodilatation.

   II. Maintain a low $PaCO_2$.

III. Reduce the resistance of the cerebral vasculature to enhance cerebral blood flow.

IV. Avoid inducing coughing, gagging, and excessive PIPs.

   A. I, II, IV only

   B. I, II only

   C. III, IV only

   D. I, IV only

200. The patient's $PaCO_2$ should be maintained in the range of ___.

   A. 10 to 15 mm Hg

   B. 20 to 25 mm Hg

   C. 30 to 50 mm Hg

   D. 35 to 45 mm Hg

   E. 50 to 60 mm Hg

### Questions 201 and 202 refer to the same patient.

A 45-year-old, postop laparotomy patient is returned to his room after leaving the PACU room. The RRT is evaluating this patient for postoperative respiratory care. Upon inspection of the chest wall, the RRT observes less chest-wall movement on the left side than on the right. Palpation findings include increased tactile fremitus over the lower left lobe and reduced left chest excursion. Percussion reveals dullness over the left lower lobe and normal percussion notes on the right side. Auscultation reveals diminished breath sounds on the left side and normal sounds on the right. The anteroposterior chest roentgenogram shows left hemidiaphragm elevation and an increased opacity in the region of the left lower lobe.

201. What is the basis for these findings?

   A. a pleural effusion in the lower left intrapleural space

   B. a left lower lobe atelectasis

   C. a left-sided pneumothorax

   D. consolidation of the left lower lobe

202. Based on these assessment findings, which of the following modalities should the RRT recommend for this patient?

   A. CPT

   B. aerosol therapy

   C. bronchodilator therapy

   D. IPPB

### Questions 203 and 204 refer to the same patient.

A term neonate having Apgar scores of 4 and 6 at 1 and 5 minutes, respectively, is placed in an oxyhood at an $FIO_2$ of 0.40. ABGs obtained from both the right radial artery and the umbilical artery catheter are as follows:

ABG and Uac Values

| Right Radial Artery | Umbilical Artery Catheter |
|---|---|
| $PO_2$ 45 torr | $PO_2$ 28 torr |
| $PCO_2$ 55 torr | $PCO_2$ 58 torr |
| pH 7.26 | pH 7.23 |
| $HCO_3^-$ 24 mEq/liter | $HCO_3^-$ 24 mEq/liter |

Physical examination of the neonate reveals cyanosis, respiratory distress, and clear breath sounds. A chest radiograph indicates clear lung fields and cardiomegaly.

203.    What is the neonate's likely diagnosis?

A.   respiratory distress syndrome
B.   apnea of prematurity
C.   meconium aspiration syndrome
D.   persistent pulmonary hypertension of the newborn

The neonate is now receiving mechanical ventilation via a time-cycled, pressure-limited ventilator with the following settings:

$FIO_2$: 1.0
PIP: 55 cm $H_2O$
ventilatory rate: 50 breaths/min.

ABGs at this time reveal the following:

$PO_2$ 22 torr
$PCO_2$ 30 torr
pH 7.50
$HCO_3^-$ 23 mEq/liter
B.E. 0 mEq/liter

204.    What action should the RRT recommend at this time?

A.   Decrease the $FIO_2$.
B.   Suggest giving tolazoline I.V.
C.   Increase the ventilatory rate.
D.   Decrease the PIP.

**Questions 205 and 206 refer to the same patient.**

A 4-year-old boy presents in the emergency department with a 104°F fever. The boy appears anxious and frightened and is sitting leaning forward with his head held in the sniffing position. In a muted, muffled voice, the boy complains of dyspnea and dysphagia, and he drools as he speaks. Both inspiratory and expiratory stridor are clearly audible. A lateral neck radiograph indicates an obliterated vallecula, a ballooning hypopharynx, and the thumb sign.

205.    Which diagnosis can be made based on the foregoing clinical data?

A.   subglottic stenosis
B.   laryngotracheobronchitis

C.   epiglottitis
D.   tracheal malacia

206.    Which therapeutic or diagnostic procedure is most appropriate at this time?

A.   ET intubation
B.   laryngoscopy
C.   fiberoptic bronchoscopy
D.   tracheostomy

**Questions 207 and 208 refer to the same patient.**

A patient is being mechanically ventilated via a mechanical ventilator with the following settings, and programmed to deliver a square waveflow pattern:

tidal volume: 1,000 cc
ventilatory rate: 12 breaths/min.
peak inspiratory flow rate: 50 L/min.
$FIO_2$: 0.30
PEEP: 5 cm $H_2O$

The RRT has charted the pressure readings over a 4-hour period as shown in Table 5-3

**Table 5-3** Peak and Static Pressure Readings

| Time of Ventilator Check | Peak | Static |
|---|---|---|
| 4:10 P.M. | 36 cm $H_2O$ | 24 cm $H_2O$ |
| 5:15 P.M. | 38 cm $H_2O$ | 26 cm $H_2O$ |
| 6:05 P.M. | 41 cm $H_2O$ | 29 cm $H_2O$ |
| 7:15 P.M. | 42 cm $H_2O$ | 30 cm $H_2O$ |
| 8:10 P.M. | 45 cm $H_2O$ | 33 cm $H_2O$ |

207.    How has this patient's airway resistance changed over the 4-hour period?

A.   It has *not* changed at all.
B.   It has initially increased then decreased.
C.   It has continuously decreased.
D.   It has initially decreased then increased.

208.    Which of the following conditions might have accounted for the change in the PIP?

I.    tracheobronchial secretions
II.   pneumothorax
III.  atelectasis
IV.   slippage of the ET tube into the right mainstem bronchus

A.   I, II, III, IV
B.   II, III, IV only
C.   I, III, IV only
D.   I, II, III only

209. A patient who has severe COPD *cannot* perform the normal directed cough technique because high intrapleural pressures tend to compress the patient's small airways, limiting the effectiveness of the technique. What modification to this procedure should the RRT recommend?

I. forced expiratory technique
II. splinting
III. autogenic drainage
IV. postural drainage with percussion and vibration

A. I, II only
B. I, III only
C. II, IV only
D. I, III, IV only

210. A 10-year-old cystic fibrosis patient who lives with her elderly grandmother receives postural drainage along with percussion and vibration. The child's grandmother has expressed, "My arthritis makes it hard keeping up with my granddaughter's therapy." Which of the following forms of bronchial hygiene therapy would be suitable for the RRT to recommend?

I. PEP therapy
II. forced expiratory technique
III. mechanical percussor
IV. intrapulmonary percussive ventilation

A. I, II only
B. I, IV only
C. II, III only
D. I, III, IV only

211. While delivering a β-2 agonist via a small-volume nebulizer, the RRT notices the patient breathing slowly through her mouth and using a normal tidal volume. What should the RRT recommend to optimize the technique for using a small-volume nebulizer?

A. Do *nothing,* because the patient is breathing appropriately.
B. Instruct the patient to take deep breaths.
C. Have the patient hold her breath at end-inspiration.
D. Coach the patient to breathe through her nose.

212. The RRT has been summoned by a physician to evaluate a patient's inability to clear pulmonary secretions. The RRT finds a non-smoking, 35-year-old female, 5'4" tall, weighing 225 lbs, recovering from lower abdominal surgery performed under general anesthesia two hours ago. The patient is alert and intubated with an oral endotracheal tube attached to a Briggs adaptor delivering an $FiO_2$ of 0.40. The patient is receiving morphine I.V. for pain. Which of the following factors are preventing this patient from evacuating her pulmonary secretions?

I. obesity
II. narcotic analgesic
III. oral endotracheal tube
IV. post-surgical pain

A. I, III only
B. II, IV only
C. I, III, IV only
D. I, II, III, IV

213. While assessing a patient's use of an metered-dose inhaler (MDI), the RRT observes the patient slowly inhale a normal tidal volume and breathhold for 10 seconds following the actuation of the MDI. Based on this observation, what should the RRT do to improve the patient's use of this device?

A. Do *nothing*, because the patient is breathing appropriately.
B. Instruct the patient to inspire to total lung capacity.
C. Coach the patient to inspire forcefully (greater than 40 L/min) to total lung capacity.
D. Have the patient refrain from breathholding.

214. The RRT is asked to evaluate for bronchial hygiene therapy a patient who has a neuromuscular disease and is experiencing retained secretions. Which of the following techniques would be most effective for this type of patient?

A. PEP therapy
B. flutter therapy
C. manually assisted coughing
D. intrapulmonary percussive ventilation

215. The RRT is evaluating a patient's use of a dry powder inhaler (DPI). The RRT observes the patient holding the opening of the DPI about 4 cm from her open mouth, inhaling deeply and forcefully, and breathholding for 10 seconds. What should the RRT recommend at this time?

I. Do *nothing*, because the patient is using the DPI correctly.
II. The patient must *not* inhale forcefully.
III. The patient's lips must be sealed around the DPI mouthpiece.
IV. The patient must be instructed to avoid breathholding.

A. I only
B. II, III only
C. III, IV only
D. II, III, IV only

216. A patient is receiving mechanical ventilation from a volume ventilator. When the RRT approaches the patient's bed, he notices the build-up of condensate along the inspiratory limb of the recyclable breathing circuit.

Which of the following modifications should the RRT make at this time?

A. Drain the condensate from the ventilator breathing circuit.
B. Replace the recyclable tubing with a heated-wire circuit.
C. Replace the volume ventilator with a pressure ventilator.
D. Raise the temperature of the humidifier to increase the relative humidity of the gas.

217. A patient receiving assisted volume ventilation develops a respiratory alkalosis. The RRT reduces the mandatory rate on the ventilator, but the respiratory alkalosis persists because all the breaths are initiated by the patient. The RRT then decreases the tidal volume in response, but the patient has increased her spontaneous ventilatory rate. What action should the RRT take at this time?

A. Use a ventilator breathing circuit of shorter length.
B. Institute 5 cm $H_2O$ of PEEP.
C. Assess the patient for the presence of auto-PEEP.
D. Add mechanical dead space.

**Questions 218 and 219 refer to the same patient.**

218. An RRT is summoned to the emergency department to treat a patient having an acute asthmatic attack. A 70-30 heliox gas mixture has been ordered for this patient. Which of the following delivery devices is appropriate to use to administer this gas mixture?

A. nasal cannula
B. nonrebreathing mask
C. partial rebreathing mask
D. large oxyhood

219. The heliox is being supplied by a brown and green compressed gas cylinder labeled 70% helium and 30% oxygen. During the treatment, the patient becomes cyanotic and complains of shortness of breath and is demonstrating an increased work of breathing. What action should be taken by the RRT at this time?

A. Administer 100% oxygen to the patient.
B. Administer a bronchodilator via a small-volume nebulizer.
C. Intubate the patient and administer the heliox via a intermittent positive pressure device.
D. Continue with the prescribed mode of therapy until the $PaCO_2$ rises above 50 torr.

220. The RRT is paged to see a 45-year-old, one-day post-op laparotomy patient. The RRT performs a physical examination on the patient, who appears *not* to be in respiratory distress. The patient is breathing spontaneously at a rate of 12 breaths/min. Auscultation reveals inspiratory and expiratory crackles that clear whenever the patient manages to cough. Which of the following therapeutic interventions should the RRT recommend at this time?

I. incentive spirometry
II. aerosol therapy
III. postural drainage
IV. cough training

A. I, II only
B. III, IV only
C. I, III, IV only
D. I, II, III, IV

221. A patient has a fenestrated tracheostomy tube inserted. Before applying the decannulation cannula and weaning the patient from the tracheostomy tube, which of the following actions should the RRT perform?

I. Deflate the cuff on the tracheostomy tube.
II. Remove the inner cannula.
III. Perform endotracheal and oropharyngeal suctioning.
IV. Cap the opening of the tracheostomy tube.

A. I, III only
B. II, IV only
C. I, II, IV only
D. I, II, III, IV

222. A 65-year-old woman weighing 45 kg (IBW) is receiving mechanical ventilation for an acute exacerbation of her COPD. She is receiving a $V_T$ of 450 ml from the ventilator. Her measured exhaled $V_T$ is 400 ml because her endotracheal tube cuff has been inflated via the minimal leak technique.

While receiving mechanical ventilation, she developed a pneumothorax and had chest tubes inserted. The same $V_T$ is set on the ventilator, but she is now exhaling 250 ml. How much volume is she losing through the chest tubes?

A. 250 ml
B. 200 ml
C. 150 ml
D. 100 ml

# Therapeutic Procedures Matrix Categories

1. IIIA1e
2. IIIC6a
3. IIIC8b
4. IIIC8a
5. IIIB4a
6. IIIA1m(1)
7. IIIB1a
8. IIIA1h
9. IIIB2c
10. IIIB4c
11. IIIB2c
12. IIIA1h
13. IIIE1l
14. IIIB4b
15. IIIC7d
16. IIIE2a
17. IIIA1m(1)
18. IIIB1b
19. IIIE1j
20. IIID1b
21. IIIB2c
22. IIIA1h
23. IIIE2b
24. IIIB2c
25. IIIB2c
26. IIIA1h
27. IIIB1c
28. IIIB2b
29. IIIA1b
30. IIIA1a
31. IIIA1f
32. IIIB2c
33. IIIE2f
34. IIIB2c
35. IIIE1g
36. IIIA1l
37. IIIA1e
38. IIIC3a
39. IIIA1l
40. IIIC5
41. IIIE1e
42. IIIA1c
43. IIIC1a
44. IIID1b
45. IIIC3a
46. IIIB2c

47. IIIA1l
48. IIIC3a
49. IIIB1b
50. IIIE1l
51. IIIE1h
52. IIIC7c
53. IIIE2b
54. IIIA1e
55. IIIB4a
56. IIIA1m(1)
57. IIIC3a
58. IIIC5
59. IIIA1b
60. IIIE2e
61. IIID1b
62. IIIA1c
63. IIIE1a
64. IIIB1e
65. IIIA1f
66. IIIC3a
67. IIIE1c
68. IIIC2
69. IIIC3a
70. IIIC3b
71. IIIB4a
72. IIIB2c
73. IIIC4
74. IIIB4a
75. IIIC1a
76. IIIE2b
77. IIIE1b
78. IIIA1d
79. IIIB4b
80. IIIB4a
81. IIIE1f
82. IIID1b
83. IIIE1g
84. IIIA1l
85. IIIC5
86. IIIA2d
87. IIIA1f
88. IIIE2b
89. IIIC7a
90. IIIE2d
91. IIIB1c
92. IIIA1b

93. IIIA1g
94. IIIE1j
95. IIIA1b
96. IIIB4c
97. IIIB2c
98. IIIB1c
99. IIIE1e
100. IIIA1g
101. IIIB3
102. IIIB1b
103. IIIA2a(2)
104. IIIB4a
105. IIIB2c
106. IIIA2b
107. IIIC5
108. IIIA2a(1)
109. IIIA1h
110. IIIB4a
111. IIIE2b
112. IIIE2a
113. IIIA1h
114. IIIC1c
115. IIIB4b
116. IIIA1d
117. IIIE2a
118. IIID1c
119. IIIC3a
120. IIIB2d
121. IIIE1a
122. IIIC6b
123. IIIA2c
124. IIIA1l
125. IIIC7b
126. IIIA1m(3)
127. IIIC6a
128. IIIC7a
129. IIIC5
130. IIIA1m(2)
131. IIIA1h
132. IIIB2c
133. IIIA1b
134. IIIA2a(4)
135. IIIC7a
136. IIIE1i
137. IIIE1l
138. IIIA2a(1)

139. IIIB1a
140. IIIB2c
141. IIID1b
142. IIIA1f
143. IIIB4a
144. IIIB4b
145. IIIE1i
146. IIIB4a
147. IIIC3a
148. IIIA1i
149. IIIE1c
150. IIIC5
151. IIIA2a(2)
152. IIIA1h
153. IIIA1e
154. IIIA1d
155. IIIA1m(2)
156. IIIE2e
157. IIIA1l
158. IIIE1i
159. IIIA1m(1)
160. IIIB1e
161. IIIA1l
162. IIIA1m(1)
163. IIIA1l
164. IIIC5
165. IIIC5
166. IIIB3
167. IIIA1h
168. IIIB2c
169. IIIA1e
170. IIIC4
171. IIIB1a
172. IIIC3a
173. IIIC7a
174. IIIB1a
175. IIIC4
176. IIID1a
177. IIIA1a
178. IIID1b
179. IIIC1a
180. IIIA1h
181. IIIA1h
182. IIIA1e
183. IIIA1e
184. IIIA1f

185. IIIA1l
186. IIIA1m(3)
187. IIIB1a
188. IIIB2c
189. IIIB2c
190. IB9c
191. IIIB4a
192. IB9b
193. IIIA1h
194. IIIA1h

195. IIIA1e
196. IIIA1h
197. IIIA1e
198. IIIB2c
199. IIIB2c
200. IIIB2c
201. IB2b
202. IIIC1a
203. IA1h
204. IIIA1b

205. IA1b
206. IIIB1a
207. IA1f(4)
208. IIIC6a
209. IIIC5
210. IIIC5
211. IIIC2
212. IIIB3
213. IIIC2
214. IIIB3

215. IIIC2
216. IIIC8a
217. IIIC8c
218. IIIC4
219. IIIC4
220. IIIB3
221. IIIC6b
222. IIIC8b

# Chapter 5 Therapeutic Procedures: Written Registry Examination Matrix Scoring Form

| Content Area | Therapeutic Procedures Item Number | Therapeutic Procedures Content Area Score | |
|---|---|---|---|
| IIIA1. Evaluate and monitor patient's response to respiratory care. | 1,6,8,12,17,22,26, 29,30,31,36,37,39,42, 47,54,56,59,62,65,78, 84,87,92,93,95,100, 109,113,116,124,126, 130,131,133,142,148,152, 153,154,155,157,159, 161,162,163,167,169, 177,180,181,182,183, 184,185,186,193,194, 195,196,197,204 | $\frac{}{62} \times 100 = \_\_\_\_\%$ | $\frac{}{70} \times 100 = \_\_\_\_\%$ |
| IIIA2. Maintain records and communication | 86,103,106,108,123, 134,138,151 | $\frac{}{8} \times 100 = \_\_\_\_\%$ | |
| IIIB1. Maintain a patent airway including the care of artificial airways. | 7,18,27,49,64,91, 98,102,139,160,171, 174,187,206 | $\frac{}{14} \times 100 = \_\_\_\_\%$ | $\frac{}{56} \times 100 = \_\_\_\_\%$ |
| IIIB2. Achieve adequate spontaneous and artificial ventilation. | 9,11,21,24,25,28,32, 34,46,72,97,105,120, 132,140,168,188,189, 198,199,200 | $\frac{}{21} \times 100 = \_\_\_\_\%$ | |
| IIIB3. Remove bronchial pulmonary secretions by using bronchial pulmonary hygiene techniques. | 101,166,212, 214,220 | $\frac{}{5} \times 100 = \_\_\_\_\%$ | |
| IIIB4. Achieve adequate arterial and tissue oxygenation. | 5,10,14,55,71,74,79, 80,96,104,110,115, 143,144,146,191 | $\frac{}{16} \times 100 = \_\_\_\_\%$ | |
| IIIC1. Modify IPPB. | 43,75,114,179,202 | $\frac{}{5} \times 100 = \_\_\_\_\%$ | |
| IIIC2. Modify patient breathing pattern during aerosol therapy. | 68,211,213,215 | $\frac{}{4} \times 100 = \_\_\_\_\%$ | |
| IIIC3. Modify oxygen therapy. | 38,45,48,57,66,69, 70,119,147,172 | $\frac{}{10} \times 100 = \_\_\_\_\%$ | |

| Content Area | Therapeutic Procedures Item Number | Therapeutic Procedures Content Area Score | |
|---|---|---|---|
| IIIC4. Modify specialty gas therapy. | 73, 170, 175, 218, 219 | $\frac{}{5} \times 100 = $ _____ % | |
| IIIC5. Modify bronchial hygiene therapy. | 40,58,85,107,129, 150,164,165,209,210 | $\frac{}{10} \times 100 = $ _____ % | |
| IIIC6. Modify artificial airway management. | 2,122,127,208,221 | $\frac{}{5} \times 100 = $ _____ % | $\frac{}{51} \times 100 = $ _____ % |
| IIIC7. Modifying suctioning | 15,52,89,125, 128,135,173 | $\frac{}{7} \times 100 = $ _____ % | |
| IIIC8. Modify mechanical ventilation | 3,4,216,217,222 | $\frac{}{5} \times 100 = $ _____ % | |
| IIID. Initiate, conduct, and modify respiratory care techniques in an emergency setting. | 20,44,61,82, 118,141,176,178 | $\frac{}{8} \times 100 = $ _____ % | $\frac{}{8} \times 100 = $ _____ % |
| IIIE1. Assist physician performing special procedures. | 13,19,35,41,50,51,63, 67,77,81,83,94,99,121, 136,137,145,149,158 | $\frac{}{19} \times 100 = $ _____ % | $\frac{}{31} \times 100 = $ _____ % |
| IIIE2. Initiate and conduct pulmonary rehabilitation and home care. | 16,23,33,53,60, 76,88,90,111, 112,117,156 | $\frac{}{12} \times 100 = $ _____ % | |

The following questions were part of situational sets and are not located on this scoring form because they do not pertain to section III, Therapeutic Procedures:

- 190 IB9c
- 192 IB9b
- 201 IB2b
- 203 IA1h
- 205 IA1b
- 207 IA1f(4)

# NBRC Written Registry Examination for Advanced Respiratory Therapists (RRTs) Content Outline

## III. Initiate, Conduct, and Modify Prescribed Therapeutic Procedures

**SETTING:** In any patient care setting, the RRT evaluates, monitors, and records the patient's response to care. The therapist maintains patient records and communicates with other healthcare team members. The therapist initiates, conducts, and modifies prescribed therapeutic procedures to achieve the desired objectives. The therapist provides care in emergency settings, assists the physician, and conducts pulmonary rehabilitation and homecare.

| | RECALL | APPLICATION | ANALYSIS |
|---|---|---|---|
| III. Initiate, Conduct, and Modify Prescribed Therapeutic Procedures | 6 | 8 | 49 |
| **A. Evaluate, monitor, and record patient's response to respiratory care.** | 2 | 3 | 13 |
| 1. Evaluate and monitor patient's response to respiratory care: | | | |
| a. recommend and review chest X-ray | X | X | |
| b. perform arterial puncture, capillary blood gas sampling, and venipuncture; obtoain blood from arterial or pulmonary artery lines; perform transcutaneous $O_2/CO_2$, pulse oximetry, co-oximetry, and capnography monitoring | X | X | |
| c. observe changes in sputum production and consistency, note patient's subjective response to therapy and mechanical ventilation | X | X | |
| d. measure and record vital signs, monitor cardiac rhythm, evaluate fluid balance (intake and output) | X | X | |
| e. perform spirometry/determine vital capacity, measure lung compliance and airway resistance, interpret ventilator flow, volume, and pressure waveforms, measure peak flow | X | X | |
| f. determine and record central venous pressure, pulmonary artery pressures, pulmonary capillary wedge pressure and/or cardiac output | | | |

| | RECALL | APPLICATION | ANALYSIS |
|---|---|---|---|
| g. recommend measurement of electrolytes, hemoglobin, CBC and/or chemistries | | | |
| h. monitor mean airway pressure, adjust and check alarm systems, measure tidal volume, respiratory rate, airway pressures, I:E, and maximum inspiratory pressure (MIP) | X | X | |
| i. measure $FIO_2$ and/or liter flow | X | X | |
| j. monitor endotracheal or tracheostomy tube cuff pressure | X | X | |
| k. auscultate chest and interpret changes in breath sounds | X | X | |
| l. perform hemodynamic calculations [e.g., shunt studies ($\dot{Q}s/\dot{Q}t$), cardiac output, cardiac index, pulmonary vascular resistance and systemic vascular resistance, stroke volume] | | | |
| m. interpret hemodynamic calculations: | | | |
| (1) calculate and interpret $P(A-a)O_2$, $C(a-\bar{v})\,O_2$, $\dot{Q}s/\dot{Q}t$ | | | |
| (2) exhaled $CO_2$ monitoring, $V_D/V_T$ | | | |
| (3) cardiac output, cardiac index, pulmonary vascular resistance and systemic vascular resistance, stroke volume | | | |
| 2. Maintain records and communication: | | | |
| a. record therapy and results using conventional terminology as required in the healthcare setting and/or by regulatory agencies by noting and interpreting: | | | |
| (1) patient's response to therapy including the effects of therapy, adverse reactions, patient's subjective and attitudinal response to therapy | X | X | |
| (2) auscultatory findings, cough and sputum production and characteristics | X | X | |
| (3) vital signs [e.g., heart rate, respiratory rate, blood pressure, body temperature] | X | X | |
| (4) pulse oximetry, heart rhythm, capnography | X | X | |
| b. verify computations and note erroneous data | X | X | |

| | RECALL | APPLICATION | ANALYSIS |
|---|---|---|---|
| c. apply computer technology to patient management [e.g., ventilator waveform analysis, electronic charting, patient care algorithms] | | X | X |
| d. communicate results of therapy and alter therapy per protocol(s) | | X | X |
| **B. Conduct therapeutic procedures to maintain a patent airway, achieve adequate ventilation and oxygenation, and remove bronchopulmonary secretions.** | **1** | **1** | **10** |
| 1. Maintain a patent airway including the care of artificial airways: | | | |
| a. insert oro- and nasopharyngeal airway, select endotracheal or tracheostomy tube, perform endotracheal intubation, change tracheostomy tube, maintain proper cuff inflation, position of endotracheal or tracheostomy tube | | X | X |
| b. maintain adequate humidification | | X | X |
| c. extubate the patient | | X | X |
| d. properly position patient | | X | X |
| e. identify endotracheal tube placement by available means | | X | X |
| 2. Achieve adequate spontaneous and artificial ventilation: | | | |
| a. initiate and adjust IPPB therapy | | X | X |
| b. initiate and select appropriate settings for high frequency ventilation | | | |
| c. initiate and adjust ventilator modes [e.g., A/C, SIMV, pressure support ventilation (PSV), pressure control ventilation (PCV)] | | X | X |
| d. initiate and adjust independent (differential) lung ventilation | | | |
| 3. Remove bronchopulmonary secretions by instructing and encouraging bronchopulmonary hygiene techniques [e.g., coughing techniques, autogenic drainage, positive expiratory pressure device (PEP), intrapulmonary percussive ventilation (IPV), Flutter®, High Frequency Chest Wall Oscillation (HFCWO)] | | X | X |
| 4. Achieve adequate arterial and tissue oxygenation: | | | |
| a. initiate and adjust CPAP, PEEP, and noninvasive positive pressure | | X | X |
| b. initiate and adjust combinations of ventilatory techniques [e.g., SIMV, PEEP, PS, PCV] | | X | X |

| | RECALL | APPLICATION | ANALYSIS |
|---|---|---|---|
| c. position patient to minimize hypoxemia, administer oxygen (on or off ventilator), prevent procedure-associated hypoxemia [e.g., oxygenate before and after suctioning and equipment changes] | | X | X |
| **C. Make necessary modifications in therapeutic procedures based on patient response.** | **0** | **1** | **10** |
| 1. Modify IPPB: | | | |
| a. adjust sensitivity, flow, volume, pressure, $FIO_2$ | | X | X |
| b. adjust expiratory retard | | X | X |
| c. change patient—machine interface [e.g., mouthpiece, mask] | | X | X |
| 2. Modify patient breathing pattern during aerosol therapy | | X | X |
| 3. Modify oxygen therapy: | | | |
| a. change mode of administration, adjust flow, and $FIO_2$ | | X | X |
| b. set up an $O_2$ concentrator or liquid $O_2$ system | | X | X |
| 4. Modify specialty gas [e.g., $He/O_2$, $O_2/CO_2$] therapy [e.g., change mode of administration, adjust flow, adjust gas concentration] | | X | |
| 5. Modify bronchial hygiene therapy [e.g., alter position of patient, alter duration of treatment and techniques, coordinate sequence of therapies, alter equipment used and PEP therapy] | | X | X |
| 6. Modify artificial airway management: | | | |
| a. alter endotracheal or tracheostomy tube position, change endotracheal or tracheostomy tube | | X | X |
| b. initiate suctioning | | X | X |
| c. inflate and deflate the cuff | | X | X |
| 7. Modify suctioning: | | | |
| a. alter frequency and duration of suctioning | | X | X |
| b. change size and type of catheter | | X | X |
| c. alter negative pressure | | X | X |
| d. instill irrigating solutions | | X | X |
| 8. Modify mechanical ventilation: | | | |
| a. change patient breathing circuitry, change type of ventilator | | X | X |
| b. measure volume loss through chest tube(s) | | X | |
| c. change mechanical dead space | | X | X |

| | RECALL | APPLICATION | ANALYSIS |
|---|:---:|:---:|:---:|
| **D. Initiate, conduct, or modify respiratory care techniques in an emergency setting.** | **1** | **1** | **10** |
| 1. Treat cardiopulmonary collapse according to: | | | |
|    a. BCLS | X | X | |
|    b. ACLS | X | X | |
|    c. PALS | X | X | |
|    d. NRP | X | X | |
| 2. Treat tension pneumothorax | | | |
| 3. Participate in land/air patient transport | | | |
| **E. Assist physician, initiate, and conduct pulmonary rehabilitation.** | **2** | **2** | **6** |
| 1. Act as an assistant to the physician performing special procedures including: | | | |
|    a. bronchoscopy | X | X | |
|    b. thoracentesis | X | X | |
|    c. transtracheal aspiration | | | |
|    d. tracheostomy | X | X | |
|    e. cardiopulmonary stress testing | | | |
|    f. percutaneous needle biopsies of the lung | | | |
|    g. sleep studies | | | |
|    h. cardioversion | X | X | |
|    i. intubation | X | X | |
|    j. insertion of chest tubes | | | |
|    k. insertion of lines for invasive monitoring [e.g., central venous pressure, pulmonary artery catheters, Swan-Ganz, arterial lines] | | | |
|    l. conscious sedation | | | |
| 2. Initiate and conuct pulmonary rehabilitation and home care within the prescription: | | | |
|    a. monitor and maintain home respiratory care equipment, maintain apnea monitors | | | |
|    b. explain planned therapy and goals to patient in understandable terms to achieve optimal therapeutic outcome, counsel patient and family concerning smoking cessation, disease management | X | X | |
|    c. assure safety and infection control | X | X | |
|    d. modify respiratory care procedures for use in the home | X | X | |
|    e. implement and monitor graded exercise program | | | |
|    f. conduct patient education and disease management programs | X | X | |
| **TOTALS** | **12** | **15** | **73** |

# Therapeutic Procedures Answers and Analyses

**NOTE:** The references listed after each analysis are numbered and keyed to the reference list located at the end of this section. The first number indicates the text. The second number indicates the page where information about the question can be found. For example, (1:219, 384) means that on pages 219 and 384 of reference number 1, information about the question will be found. Frequently, it will be necessary to read beyond the page number indicated to obtain complete information. Therefore, reference to the question will be found either on the page indicated or on subsequent pages.

## IIIA1e

1. C. The graphics obtained from a mechanically ventilated patient display the inspiratory loop above the baseline and the expiratory limb below the baseline. The patient's before bronchodilator tracing (dotted line) demonstrated air flow obstruction, as characterized by a scooped out appearance of the expiratory tracing. The after bronchodilator (continuous line) tracing shows definite air flow improvement because it extends significantly more to the left of the pre-bronchodilator, expiratory tracing.

   (1:958), (10:321).

## IIIC6a

2. C. Children under the age of 8 are able to use an uncuffed ET tube because the cricoid cartilage ring is the narrowest point in the upper airway. This area enables a properly sized, cuffless endotracheal tube to provide a seal for positive pressure ventilation. However, the mucosa in this area is fragile and prone to trauma. To determine the size of uncuffed tube, the following formula is used:

   $$\text{I.D. of uncuffed ET tube} = \frac{18 + \text{Age in years}}{4}$$

   Therefore,

   $$\text{I.D. of uncuffed ET tube} = \frac{18 + 6}{4} = 6 \text{ mm}$$

   The appropriate action in this situation would be for the RRT to reintubate the child with a 6 mm I.D. endotracheal tube.

   (18:402, 410, 432).

## IIIC8b

3. D. A water seal chest drainage system cannot be assured of being maintained below the patient's chest throughout the entire transport. Therefore, to ensure a portable suction device will evacuate a sufficient volume of gas to avoid an inadvertent pneumothorax, a test trial should be conducted for the expected duration of transport while the patient is still in the ICU.

   A water seal suction system cannot be used during air transport because of the risk that the water seal will rise above the patient's chest. Regardless of the portable suction system used, a trial run must be conducted in the ICU before the transport occurs to determine that the transport system chosen will remove a sufficient volume of gas to prevent an inadvertent pneumothorax.

   (1:487–489), (15:1131).

## IIIB2b

4. A. A bronchopulmonary fistula (BPF) is the persistence of an air leak from the lungs into the intrapleural space after the placement of chest tubes for the treatment of a pneumothorax.

   High-frequency jet ventilation (HFJV) is sometimes used in cases of BPF, or air leak syndromes. HFJV is associated with low tidal volumes (smaller than the patient's anatomic dead space) and lower peak inspiratory pressures. Both of these favor reduced lung expansion and pulmonary healing.

   (1:488, 821), (10:368–369), (15:1090).

## IIIB4a

5. B. Patients who experience left ventricular failure, accompanied by an increased left ventricular preload, generally require pharmacologic intervention directed toward increasing the strength of the myocardial contractility. In addition, they usually need supplemental oxygen and a reduction of the left ventricular preload.

   The application of 5 to 10 cm $H_2O$ via mask CPAP might prove beneficial from the standpoint that it might reduce venous return, thereby reducing the left ventricular preload. The decreased venous return also decreases the transudation of fluid from the pulmonary vasculature into the pulmonary interstitium. The effect results from the lower pulmonary hydrostatic pressures associated with a decreased venous return. Less fluid in the pulmonary interstitium should enhance oxygenation.

Other possible benefits from the application of this low CPAP level include (1) increased left-ventricular ejection fraction, (2) decreased left-ventricular end-diastolic pressure (LVEDP), and (3) an increased C.O.

This low level of positive airway pressure might help stabilize these types of patients and, perhaps, eliminate the need to intubate. At the same time, this approach during the outset of management affords the medication time to act.

(1:186–187, 783), (9:315–316), (15:901).

## IIIA1m(1)

6. D. The arterial–venous oxygen content difference $(CaO_2 - C\bar{v}O_2)$ can be calculated by using the Fick equation when the oxygen consumption $(\dot{V}O_2)$ and the C.O. $(\dot{Q}_T)$ are known. The Fick equation is as follows:

$$\dot{Q}_T = \frac{\dot{V}O_2}{CaO_2 - C\bar{v}O_2}$$

Because $\dot{Q}_T$ and $\dot{V}O_2$ have been given, the equation can be rearranged to solve for the $CaO_2 - C\bar{v}O_2$. The equation then becomes:

$$CaO_2 - C\bar{v}O_2 = \frac{\dot{V}O_2}{\dot{Q}_T}$$

Calculate the $CaO_2 - C\bar{v}O_2$.

$$CaO_2 - C\bar{v}O_2 = \frac{\dot{V}O_2}{\dot{Q}_T}$$
$$= \frac{250 \text{ ml } O_2/\text{min.}}{(5 \text{ L/min.})(10 \text{ dl/liter})}$$
$$= 5 \text{ ml } O_2/\text{dl}$$
$$= 5.0 \text{ vol\%}$$

Alternatively,

$$\left(\frac{250 \text{ ml } O_2}{\text{min.}}\right)\left(\frac{1 \text{ min.}}{5 \text{ L/min.}}\right)\left(\frac{1/\text{L}}{10 \text{ dl/L}}\right) = \frac{5 \text{ ml } O_2}{\text{dl}}$$
$$= 5.0 \text{ vol\%}$$

STEP 1: Convert the $\dot{Q}_T$ from L/min. to ml/min.

(5 L/min.)(1,000 ml/liter) = 5,000 ml/min.

STEP 2: Calculate the $CaO_2 - C\bar{v}O_2$.

$$CaO_2 - C\bar{v}O_2 = \frac{\dot{V}O_2}{\dot{Q}_T}$$
$$= \frac{250 \text{ ml } O_2/\text{min.}}{5 \text{ L/min.} (10 \text{ dl/L})}$$

$$= 5 \text{ ml } O_2/\text{dl, or}$$
$$= 5.0 \text{ vol\%}$$

(1:225–226, 930), (9:323–324).

## IIIB1a

7. C. The performance of a tracheostomy is associated with many complications, many of which also might occur during the insertion of a new tracheostomy tube.

- bleeding
- thyroid injury
- inappropriate incision position
- injury to the recurrent laryngeal nerve
- pneumothorax
- tracheoesophageal fistula
- subcutaneous emphysema
- pneumomediastinum
- placement of the tube into the pretracheal space
- cuff laceration during insertion
- cardiac arrest
- hypoxia

During the routine care of the tracheostomy tube of a patient requiring mechanical ventilation, the RRT should remove the inner cannula and insert a second, sterile inner cannula so that the patient can continue to receive positive pressure ventilation. The RRT can then clean the first inner cannula without interrupting the mechanical ventilation of the patient. When inserting a new tracheostomy tube, she should use the removable obturator to facilitate entry of the tracheostomy tube into the patient's stoma.

(1:605), (16:599).

## IIIA1h

8. A.

STEP 1: Determine the length of the ventilatory cycle by using the following relationship:

$$\frac{\text{sec./min.}}{\text{ventilatory rate}} = \text{length of ventilatory cycle}$$

$$\frac{60 \text{ sec./min.}}{45 \text{ breaths/min.}} = 1.33 \text{ sec./breath}$$

STEP 2: Determine the number of time segments comprising the desired I:E ratio. The desired I:E ratio of 1:2 has three time segments (i.e, 1 + 2 = 3).

STEP 3: Compute the inspiratory time by dividing the length of the ventilatory cycle by the number of time segments comprising the I:E ratio.

$$\frac{1.33 \text{ sec.}}{3} = 0.443 \text{ sec. } (T_I)$$

STEP 4:    Calculate the inspiratory flow rate by dividing the tidal volume by the inspiratory time.

$$\frac{V_T}{T_I} = \dot{V}$$

$$\frac{40 \text{ ml}}{0.443 \text{ sec.}} = 90 \text{ ml/sec.}$$

(1:860), (10:205–206).

## IIIB2c

9.  A. Pressure support ventilation (PSV) is a mode of ventilatory support that augments a patient's spontaneous breathing. Based on the patient's needs, the RRT selects a pressure plateau level to reduce the work of breathing imposed by the ET tube, the ventilator circuitry, demand values, as well as that resulting from the patient's pulmonary pathophysiology. The pressure-time waveforms illustrated in Figure 5-19 contrast PSV (tracing A) and continuous positive pressure breathing (CPPB) in the control mode.

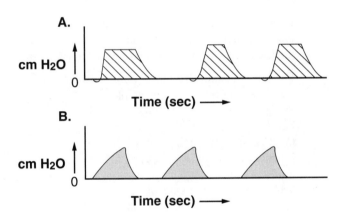

**Figure 5-19:**   (A) Pressure support ventilation (PSV) pressure-time waveform. Note the unequal intervals between the pressure-support breaths and variable tidal volumes (hatched areas). (B) Continuous positive pressure breathing (CPPB) pressure-time waveform. Note the equal intervals between the CPPB breaths and equal tidal volumes (shaded areas).

While the patient breathes in the PSV mode, she determines her own tidal volume, peak inspiratory flow rate, ventilatory rate, and inspiratory:expiratory (I:E) ratio. The interval between each of the three pressure support breaths is unequal (i.e., the patient determines her own ventilatory rate). Note that in Tracing A, the patient generates a negative pressure (deflection below baseline), which results in a flow rate. The inspiratory

flow rate reaches its peak rapidly and decays gradually as the airway pressure and ventilator pressure gradient decreases. The preset pressure-support plateau is maintained throughout inspiration, however. The inspiratory flow rate terminates when the inspiratory flow rate falls to 25% of its initial level. With CPPB in the control mode (Tracing B), the spacing between each breath is exact, as is the tidal volume, inspiratory flow rate, and I:E ratio.

(1:864, 877), (10:84, 199, 331), (15:960).

## IIIB4c

10.  A. If an infant can maintain an arterial $PO_2$ between 50 mm Hg and 70 mm Hg at a CPAP level of 2 cm $H_2O$ on an $FiO_2$ equal to or less than 0.40, the neonate should be extubated and placed in an oxyhood at an $FiO_2$ of 0.40 or less. The neonatal RRT should not wait until the CPAP level is reduced to 0 cm $H_2O$ before extubation. Also, when the CPAP is removed, the patient should also be extubated to prevent a decrease in the functional residual capacity (FRC), and to reduce airway resistance. It is difficult to maintain a normal ventilatory status while intubated.

(1:1015–1019), (18:292).

## IIIB2c

11.  D. The pressure-control inverse-ratio ventilation (PC-IRV) utilizes a rapid lung insufflation with a decelerating flow pattern, maintaining a preset pressure throughout the inspiratory phase. During PC-IRV, the inspiratory time ($T_I$) is prolonged beyond the expiratory time ($T_E$). As a result of the prolonged inspiratory phase, a pressure-limited plateau develops during inspiration. A patient who is receiving PC-IRV must be sedated and paralyzed to eliminate spontaneous ventilatory efforts that would disrupt this ventilatory pattern. The pressure and flow curves for PC-IRV are illustrated in Figure 5-20 on page 290.

Again, the flow pattern is decelerating following a rapid insufflation of the lungs. The ventilatory rate is set based on each inspiration set to begin as the terminal expiratory flow approaches zero. This point is labeled and indicated by the arrows on the flow pattern shown previously.

Initiating a new inspiration before the preceding expiration is completed establishes auto-PEEP (previous pressure pattern). Because the peak inspiratory pressure (PIP) set in the PC-IRV mode is dialed to be about 50% of the PIP in the volume-cycled mode, airway pressures with PC-IRV are quite moderate.

Patients who have lung disease characterized by dynamic flow limitation (e.g., COPD and asthma) are not

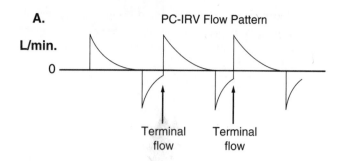

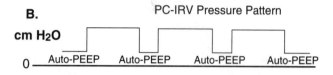

**Figure 5-20:** Pressure-control inverse-ratio ventilation (PC-IRV) flow: (A) flow-time waveform highlighting terminal flow and (B) pressure-time waveform illustrating auto-PEEP.

considered likely candidates for PC-IRV because this ventilation mode does not enable complete exhalation. These types of patients generally require longer expiratory time than those used with PC-IRV. The tidal volume received by the patient will decrease as either the ventilatory rate or I:E ratio increases because more auto-PEEP will develop as a consequence.

(1:876), (10:156, 215, 285–287), (15:968, 993).

**IIIA1h**

12. B. The mean airway pressure ($\overline{P}_{aw}$) represents the average airway pressure developed or maintained from the beginning of one inspiration to the onset of the next (the entire ventilatory cycle). The hatched area under the curve in the illustration in Figure 5-21 indicates the $\overline{P}_{aw}$.

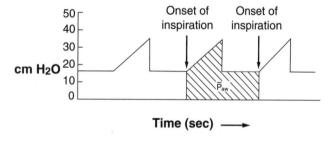

**Figure 5-21:** Pressure-time waveform highlighting mean airway pressure ($\overline{P}_{aw}$). Note that $\overline{P}_{aw}$ extends from inspiration to inspiration.

The area under the curve ($\overline{P}_{aw}$) can be calculated according to the following expression:

$$\overline{P}_{aw} = K(PIP - PEEP)\left(\frac{T_I}{TCT}\right) + PEEP$$

If the PIP and the inspiratory time ($T_I$) are equal, the $\overline{P}_{aw}$ will be lower with a sine waveflow pattern than with a square waveflow pattern. The PIP, I:E ratio, and PEEP greatly influence the $\overline{P}_{aw}$. Increasing the $\overline{P}_{aw}$ in hypoxemic neonates with respiratory distress syndrome generally improves oxygenation by reducing right-to-left shunting. High levels of $\overline{P}_{aw}$ can reduce venous return and decrease the C.O., especially in patients who have cardiovascular disease and those whose lung compliance is improving.

(1:888, 912), (10:143–144, 265).

**IIIE1l**

13. C. Many ET intubations are performed while the patient is awake. In fact, sedation of a patient to perform ET intubation is generally limited to a few special situations (e.g., head injury, spinal cord injury, and patient combativeness). Intubation under sedation implies that the establishment of an ET tube is not an emergency because it does take time to titrate the proper amount of medication. The usual route by which sedatives are administered is the intravenous (I.V.) route.

The two commonly used classes of drugs are opioid analgesics and benzodiazapines. Opioid analgesics tend to cause analgesia, respiratory depression, mood change, and sedation. Opioid analgesics include morphine, fentanyl (Sublimaze), meperidine (Demerol), methadone (Dolophine), and propoxyphene (Darvon).

For ET intubation, fentanyl (Sublimaze) has advantages over morphine. For example, fentanyl is about 80 times more potent, has almost immediate onset, and has a short half-life (duration). An advantage of fentanyl is an early, slight depression of left-ventricular function, resulting in a reduced risk of hypotension. Furthermore, fentanyl does not cause histamine release, which, in the case of morphine, produces vasodilatation and increases venous capacitance.

Benzodiazapines clinically used include diazepam (Valium), midazolam (Versed), chlordiazepoxide (Librium), and lorazepam (Ativan). Midazolam is often favored for sedative intubation because of its rapid-onset and short-duration characteristics. The effects brought about by benzodiazapines include relief of anxiety, skeletal muscle relaxation, and sedation. The combination of a benzodiazapine and an opioid analgesic will provide the necessary effects to enable ET intubation to take place.

(16:591–592).

**IIIB4(b)**

14. D. Setting the inspiratory time percent control on the Siemens Servo 900C ventilator to 67% will provide an I:E ratio of approximately 2:1. Any time the inspira-

tory time exceeds the expiratory time, the I:E ratio becomes inversed.

Normal spontaneous breathing has an I:E ratio of about 1:2. Simimlarly, a 1:2 I:E ratio is customary for adult positive pressure ventilation to minimize the adverse cardiovascular effects that are sometimes associated with mechanical ventilation.

(1:899–900), (10:205–206).

## IIIC7d

15. D. For artificial surfactant to be effective, it needs to reach the distal airways. The most effective way to accomplish this end is to instill the medication directly into the ET tube before a manual ventilation is given (or, if the patient is receiving mechanical ventilation, before an inspiratory cycle).

(1:520–521), (*Resp. Care* 39(8) 824–829, 1994).

## IIIE2a

16. D. A chest cuirass or BiPAP® ventilator offer a noninvasive approach to providing nocturnal ventilation. These devices are portable and relatively easy to use. Both have been used effectively by neuromuscular disease patients who are able to maintain adequate ventilation during their waking hours.

(1:895, 982, 1122), (10:190, 399), (15:1200–1201).

## IIIA1m(1)

17. B. The shunt equation that can be used to solve this problem is represented as follows:

$$\frac{\dot{Q}_S}{\dot{Q}_T} = \frac{Cc'O_2 - CaO_2}{Cc'O_2 - C\bar{v}O_2}$$

where

$\dot{Q}_S$ = shunted C.O. (L/min.)
$\dot{Q}_T$ = total C.O. (L/min.)
$Cc'O_2$ = end-pulmonary capillary oxygen content (vol%)
$CaO_2$ = total arterial oxygen content (vol%)
$C\bar{v}O_2$ = total mixed venous oxygen content (vol%)

This equation is a ratio of the shunted C.O. ($\dot{Q}_S$) compared with the total C.O. ($\dot{Q}_T$). As $\dot{Q}_S$ nears zero, the $CaO_2$ approaches the $Cc'O_2$. The $Cc'O_2$ will always be greater than the $CaO_2$ as long as a shunt exists. The diagram in Figure 5-22 illustrates the relationship among the factors present in the shunt equation.

The following steps demonstrate the calculation of the percent shunt.

STEP 1: Calculate the $PaO_2$ by using the alveolar air equation.

$$P_AO_2 = F_IO_2(P_B - P_{H_2O}) - PaCO_2\left(F_IO_2 + \frac{1 - F_IO_2}{R}\right)$$

$$= 1.0(760 \text{ torr} - 47 \text{ torr}) - 35 \text{ torr}\left(1.0 + \frac{1 - 1.0}{0.8}\right)^*$$

$$= 1.0(713 \text{ torr}) - 35 \text{ torr}$$

$$= 678 \text{ torr}$$

Assuming complete equilibration of oxygen across the alveocapillary membrane, the $PaO_2$ will equal the end-pulmonary capillary oxygen tension.

*When the $F_IO_2$ is 1.0, the expression $\left(F_IO_2 + \frac{1 - F_IO_2}{R}\right)$ in the alveolar air equation is equal to one.

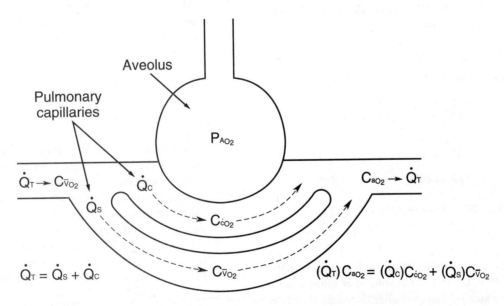

**Figure 5-22:** Relationship among pulmonary capillary blood flow ($\dot{Q}_C$), shunted C.O. ($\dot{Q}_S$), and total C.O. ($\dot{Q}_T$).

STEP 2: Calculate the end-pulmonary capillary oxygen content ($C\acute{c}O_2$).

$$C\acute{c}O_2 = \left(\begin{array}{c}\text{combined}\\\text{end-pulmonary}\\\text{capillary oxygen}\end{array}\right) + \left(\begin{array}{c}\text{dissolved}\\\text{end-pulmonary}\\\text{capillary oxygen}\end{array}\right)$$

$$= (13 \text{ g/dl} \times 1.0 \times 1.34)$$
$$+ (678 \text{ torr} \times 0.003 \text{ vol\%/torr})$$
$$= 17.42 \text{ vol\%} + 2.03 \text{ vol\%}$$
$$= 19.45 \text{ vol\%}$$

STEP 3: Calculate the total arterial oxygen content ($CaO_2$).

$$CaO_2 = \left(\begin{array}{c}\text{combined}\\\text{arterial oxygen}\end{array}\right) + \left(\begin{array}{c}\text{dissolved}\\\text{arterial oxygen}\end{array}\right)$$

$$= (13 \text{ g/dl} \times 1.0 \times 1.34)$$
$$+ (325 \text{ torr} \times 0.003 \text{ vol\%/torr})$$
$$= 17.42 \text{ vol\%} + 0.98 \text{ vol\%}$$
$$= 18.40 \text{ vol\%}$$

STEP 4: Calculate the total mixed venous oxygen content ($C\bar{v}O_2$).

$$C\bar{v}O_2 = \left(\begin{array}{c}\text{combined mixed}\\\text{venous oxygen}\end{array}\right) + \left(\begin{array}{c}\text{dissolved mixed}\\\text{venous oxygen}\end{array}\right)$$

$$= (13 \text{ g/dl} \times 0.8 \times 1.34)$$
$$+ (55 \text{ torr} \times 0.003 \text{ vol\%/torr})$$
$$= 13.94 \text{ vol\%} + 0.17 \text{ vol\%}$$
$$= 14.11 \text{ vol\%}$$

STEP 5: Calculate the percent shunt by using the shunt equation.

$$\frac{\dot{Q}_S}{\dot{Q}_T} = \frac{C\acute{c}O_2 - CaO_2}{C\acute{c}O_2 - C\bar{v}O_2}$$

$$= \frac{19.45 \text{ vol\%} - 18.40 \text{ vol\%}}{19.45 \text{ vol\%} - 14.11 \text{ vol\%}}$$

$$= \frac{1.05 \text{ vol\%}}{5.34 \text{ vol\%}}$$

$$= 0.20, \text{ or } 20\%$$

(1:930), (15:487–488), (16:329), (17:46–51).

## IIIB1b

18. B. Small-volume nebulizers generally have a capacity between 10 ml to 15 ml. The volume of solution nebulized in a small-volume nebulizer is ordinarily 2 to 6 ml, however.

Four factors affect the particle size delivered by a small-volume nebulizer: (1) the temperature of the nebulized solution, (2) the humidity of the source or driving gas, (3) the temperature of the entrained gas, and (4) the humidity of the entrained gas.

The temperature within the nebulizer is approximately 8°F to 12°F below that of room temperature because of evaporation and adiabatic expansion. As gas temperature decreases, less evaporation takes place. Therefore, particle size is larger.

The evaporative loss can be minimized by having the patient hold the nebulizer cup firmly in his hand with his fingers extending around the nebulizer cup. The warmth from the patient's fingers and hand tends to lessen the extent of the temperature drop within the nebulizer, thereby stabilizing aerosol particle size. Alternatively, using an air compressor instead of a compressed air cylinder will tend to stabilize the particle size because of the higher water vapor content of the room air from the air compressor.

(1:693–694), (13:137–142), (15:806).

## IIIE1j

19. B. Subcutaneous emphysema is the presence or accumulation of air in the soft or subcutaneous tissues of the body. Frequently described as crepitus, the affected tissues when palpated make a sound resembling crumpled cellophane.

When a patient develops subcutaneous emphysema, a pneumothorax should be suspected—especially a patient who is receiving mechanical ventilation. In such cases, the subcutaneous air often accumulates in the soft tissues in the face, neck, and chest areas. The patient often looks grotesque; however, the condition itself seldom creates physiologic problems. The underlying cause, nonetheless, must be ascertained. The placement of chest tubes is generally the approach when subcutaneous emphysema develops in patients who are receiving mechanical ventilation.

(1:483), (15:1078, 1082–1083).

## IIID1b

20. D. The first concern when ventilating during CPR is to provide oxygenated air to the victim as quickly as possible. Mouth-to-mouth or bag-mask ventilation can accomplish this end more quickly than ET intubation in most circumstances. Consuming time to intubate upon finding a victim is contrary to basic principles of ventilating during CPR. Once the early stages of CPR have passed and intubation can be accomplished in a controlled manner, maintenance of a patent airway is best accomplished with the insertion of an ET tube.

(1:630–634), (16:820–821).

21. B. The BiPAP® provides a spontaneous-timed mode that is appropriate for patients who have an inadequate ventilatory rate and who can benefit from a backup frequency. During this ventilatory mode, the patient's ventilatory effort triggers inspiratory positive airway pressure (IPAP) to expiratory positive airway pressure (EPAP). A ventilatory frequency is also set to supplement the patient's ventilatory rate. In BiPAP® spontaneous mode, the patient establishes his tidal volume and inspiratory flow rate for each IPAP cycle. Both the IPAP and EPAP levels are the only settings operating in the spontaneous mode.

The patient in this situation might benefit from a backup rate and supplemental oxygen. This attempt to avoid intubation and mechanical ventilation is worth the effort. Following the change to the spontaneous–timed mode, the patient must be monitored. Arterial blood gases (ABGs), pulse oximetry, vital capacity, maximum inspiratory pressure, spontaneous minute ventilation, and tidal volume need to be evaluated. If this patient deteriorates further, then intubation and full ventilatory support will be required.

(BiPAP® S/T-D Ventilation Support System product information, Respironics, Inc.), (1:866, 878), (16:673–674, 902).

22. B. The following four steps outline the calculation of the mean airway pressure ($\overline{P}_{aw}$).

STEP 1:   Determining the inspiratory time ($T_I$).

$T_I$ = inspiratory time (sec.)
f = ventilatory rate (breaths/min.)
$T_I$% = inspiratory time percent

$$T_I = \left( \frac{60 \text{ sec./min.}}{45 \text{ breaths/min.}} \right)\left( \frac{1}{1 + 1.6} \right)$$

$$= (1.3 \text{ sec./breath})(0.4)$$

$$= 0.5 \text{ sec.}$$

STEP 2:   Calculate the expiratory time ($T_E$).

$$T_E = \left( \frac{60 \text{ sec./min.}}{f} - T_I \right)$$

$$= \frac{60 \text{ sec./min.}}{45 \text{ breaths/min.}} - 0.5 \text{ sec.}$$

$$= 1.3 \text{ sec./breath} - 0.5 \text{ sec.}$$

$$= 0.8 \text{ sec.}$$

STEP 3:   Determine the total cycle time (TCT).

$$T_I + T_E = TCT$$

$$0.5 \text{ sec.} + 0.8 \text{ sec.} = 1.3 \text{ sec.}$$

STEP 4:   Calculate the mean airway pressure ($\overline{P}_{aw}$).

$$\overline{P}_{aw} = K*(PIP - PEEP)\left( \frac{T_I}{TCT} \right) + PEEP$$

$$= 1.0(22 \text{ cm H}_2\text{O} - 5 \text{ cm H}_2\text{O})\left( \frac{0.5 \text{ sec.}}{1.3 \text{ sec}} \right) + 5 \text{ cm H}_2\text{O}$$

$$= (17 \text{ cm H}_2\text{O})(0.38) + 5 \text{ cm H}_2\text{O}$$

$$= 6.50 \text{ cm H}_2\text{O} + 5 \text{ cm H}_2\text{O}$$

$$= 11.5 \text{ cm H}_2\text{O}$$

*K equals 0.5 for triangular pressure waveforms (ascending or descending ramp). For square or rectangular pressure waveforms, K equals 1.0.

(10:143–144, 256–266), (16:319, 323).

23. C. Avoidance of smoking is the single-most important factor in the management of a COPD patient. Evidence indicates that smoking cessation early in the progression of airway disease might alter the course of COPD. Nicotine chewing gum and nicotine patches are two techniques that help ease the process of quitting smoking.

Avoiding areas with high air-pollution levels, preventing exposure to people with respiratory tract infections, and not traveling by air (low $PIO_2$s during flight) are important considerations for a COPD patient. Smoking cessation is critical if the patient hopes to alter the progression of respiratory deterioration, however.

Health-education classes might help the COPD patient understand the tremendous cost associated with cigarette smoking. Unfortunately, education concerning the risks of cigarette smoking should begin while an individual is young for maximum effectiveness and it might have little impact on older people.

(1:448), (16:883–886, 1093–1094).

24. D. When the Siemens Servo 900C ventilator operates in the control mode, the inspiratory:expiratory (I:E) ratio is a function of the inspiratory time % control and the pause time % control. Once these two settings are set, the total time devoted to inspiration is established. The balance of the duration of the ventilatory cycle will be the expiratory time.

Therefore, to establish an inverse I:E ratio of 2:1, the RRT needs to set the inspiratory time % to 67% and the pause time % to 0%. Two-thirds or 67% of the total cycle time is spent in inspiration. Because the pause time % is 0%, the remainder of the cycle time (33%) will be in expiration. These settings create an I:E ratio where two parts are devoted to inspiration and one to exhalation, hence a 2:1 (inverse) I:E ratio.

On the 900C, the inspiratory time % can be set at either 20%, 25%, 33%, 50%, 67%, or 80%. The pause time % settings available are 0%, 5%, 10%, 20%, and 30%. When the patient assists the 900C, the expiratory time is variable.

(13:516–521).

## IIIB2c

25. D. Airway pressure-release ventilation (APRV) is a mode of mechanical ventilation that is commercially available on the Irisa ventilator. Two levels of CPAP are set with APRV. The high CPAP level is set at 10 to 30 cm H$_2$O, and the low or baseline CPAP is set at about 2 to 10 cm H$_2$O. Generally, an inverse I:E ratio (high CPAP to low CPAP) is set, and the frequency or ventilatory rate is adjusted to maintain ventilation. The patient can breathe spontaneously throughout the APRV cycle. The waveform produced by APRV is similar to that associated with PC-IRV.

(1:830, 876), (10:200, 216–217), (15:961–962).

## IIIA1h

26. B. The peak inspiratory pressure (PIP) is composed of two components (i.e., the elastic and nonelastic components of the work of breathing). The elastic component represents the work of breathing performed to overcome the compliance of the respiratory system. The nonelastic component is reflected by the pressure generated to overcome airway resistance.

When an inspiratory hold is initiated, the static or plateau pressure is obtained. This pressure provides the means of partitioning the two components of the PIP. The pressure generated to overcome the compliance component is calculated by subtracting the PEEP from the static pressure. The difference between the static pressure and the PEEP represents the pressure maintaining the lungs in their distended state during the time of no gas flow.

The difference between the PIP and the static pressure is the pressure generated to overcome airway resistance (nonelastic component). The airway resistance (R$_{aw}$) can be calculated according to the following formula:

$$R_{aw} = \frac{(PIP - \text{static pressure})}{\text{peak inspiratory flow rate}}$$

$$= \frac{55 \text{ cm H}_2\text{O} - 35 \text{ cm H}_2\text{O}}{60 \text{ L/min.}}$$

$$= 0.333 \text{ cm H}_2\text{O/L/min.}$$

Customarily, airway resistance is expressed as cm H$_2$O/L/sec. Therefore, 0.333 cm H$_2$O/L/min. can be converted to cm H$_2$O/L/sec. as follows:

(0.333 cm H$_2$O/L/min.)(60 sec./min.) ≃ 20 cm H$_2$O/L/sec.

This calculation for airway resistance applies only to those ventilators that exhibit a square wave, peak flow rate pattern because the flow rate is held reasonably constant. This calculation will render drastically lower values if the ventilator used displays either a sine wave or a decelerating waveform.

(1:937–938), (10:257–258, 436), (15:976–977).

## IIIB1c

27. C. Glottic edema is commonly treated by applying a topical alpha-adrenergic medication (nebulized racemic epinephrine) or steroid therapy. Subglottic edema poses a much more serious problem, however. It generally requires reintubation, and might sometimes require a tracheostomy.

(15:564–565).

## IIIB2b

28. B. An uncompensated respiratory acidosis is caused by hypoventilation, producing carbon dioxide retention. The following ventilator adjustments for high-frequency ventilation can help eliminate retained carbon dioxide: (1) increasing the ventilatory rate, (2) decreasing the inspiratory time, or (3) increasing the driving pressure. The CO$_2$ retention would be corrected by increasing the ventilatory rate, because more gas exchange would occur each minute. Decreasing the inspiratory time would devote more time to exhalation, thereby enhancing CO$_2$ removal. By increasing the driving pressure, more uniform ventilation would be promoted (also improving CO$_2$ elimination).

(18:108).

## IIIA1b

29. C. Sepsis is known to cause peripheral vascular shunting. This condition results in tissue oxygen deprivation and the buildup of lactic acid (lactate ions) caused by anaerobic metabolism. Additionally, because the arterial blood is not allowed to deliver an adequate supply of oxygen (caused by the altered peripheral microcirculation), mixed venous blood exhibits an inordinately higher P$\bar{\text{v}}$O$_2$ and S$\bar{\text{v}}$O$_2$. On room air, the normal P$\bar{\text{v}}$O$_2$ is 46 torr, and the S$\bar{\text{v}}$O$_2$ ranges between 70% to 75%. Other indices, such as, SaO$_2$, C.O., and blood lactate levels, need to be evaluated because mixed venous blood analysis alone is inadequate.

(1:207, 511), (15:534).

## IIIA1a

30. A. An overpenetrated chest radiograph will allow for observing the location of the pulmonary artery catheter. A standard portable AP chest film will not reveal the catheter's location as clearly as an overpenetrated film. The overpenetration of the X-ray reveals

the catheter's normal location in the pulmonary artery (usually the right). Overpenetration enables the entire length of the catheter to be visualized within the cardiovascular structures.

(9:151), (14:278–279).

## IIIA1f

31. C. One of the indications for inserting a pulmonary artery catheter is left ventricular dysfunction, or congestive heart failure. Because the pulmonary artery catheter measures pressures reflecting the left heart status, certain hemodynamic measurements indicate left ventricular failure.

As the left ventricle becomes a less efficient pump, blood flow backs up in the pulmonary vasculature. Consequently, pulmonary vascular pressures rise. Data useful for monitoring left ventricular dysfunction include (1) pulmonary artery pressures, such as pulmonary artery systolic and pulmonary artery diastolic, (2) mean pulmonary artery pressure, (3) pulmonary capillary wedge pressure, and (4) cardiac output.

In left ventricular dysfunction, all the pulmonary artery pressures and the pulmonary capillary wedge pressure will be elevated because of the pulmonary vascular engorgement. The cardiac output will be decreased because the left ventricle is a less efficient pump. These hemodynamic measurements are useful when evaluating and treating a patient who has left ventricular dysfunction.

The central venous pressure value is not an essential hemodynamic value when monitoring left ventricular failure.

Knowing that the cardiac output is low in light of an elevation of all the other hemodynamic values given in the question differentiates left ventricular dysfunction from hypervolemia. In left ventricular dysfunction, the pulmonary vascular pressures and the pulmonary capillary wedge pressure will be increased, but the cardiac output will be decreased. In hypervolemia, all the pulmonary vascular pressures and the pulmonary capillary wedge pressure will be high along with the cardiac output.

(1:511–512, 942–949), (9:314–315).

## IIIB2c

32. B. The formula for calculating the level of pressure-support ventilation (PSV) is as follows:

$$P_{PS} = \frac{(PIP) - (\text{static pressure})}{\left(\begin{array}{c}\text{mechanical inspiratory} \\ \text{flow rate}\end{array}\right)} \times \left(\begin{array}{c}\text{spontaneous} \\ \text{inspiratory} \\ \text{flow rate}\end{array}\right)$$

STEP 1: Convert the mechanical and spontaneous inspiratory flow rates from L/min. to L/sec.

A) mechanical inspiratory flow rate:

$$\frac{60 \text{ L/min.}}{60 \text{ sec./min.}} = 1 \text{ L/sec.}$$

B) spontaneous inspiratory flow rate:

$$\frac{30 \text{ L/min.}}{60 \text{ sec./min.}} = 0.5 \text{ L/sec.}$$

STEP 2: Use the formula for calculating the level of pressure support ($P_{PS}$).

$$P_{PS} = \frac{55 \text{ cm H}_2\text{O} - 35 \text{ cm H}_2\text{O}}{1 \text{ L/sec.}} (0.5 \text{ L/sec.})$$

$$= 20 \text{ cm H}_2\text{O/L/sec.} \times 0.5 \text{ L/sec.}$$

$$= 10 \text{ cm H}_2\text{O}$$

(1:980), (10:214).

## IIIE2f

33. C. Although fully compensated, the ABGs indicate that this patient has a significant history of hypercapnia. A cardiopulmonary rehabilitation program would benefit this patient, barring any malignant neoplasms of the respiratory system and so on. A complete cardiopulmonary rehabilitation program should include the following components:

- A basic review of the anatomy, physiology, and pathophysiology of the respiratory system
- Diaphragmatic and pursed-lip breathing techniques
- Methods of relaxation and stress management
- Personalized exercise techniques
- Instruction on postural drainage, chest physiotherapy, vibration, and so on
- Home care administration and cleaning of respiratory care equipment
- Medications
- Dietary guidelines
- Recreation and vocational couseling

The depth of this program should be dictated by the educational level of the participants. Too detailed of an explanation would frustrate many of the participants and could increase attrition.

(1:1084, 1089–1090), (15:1139–1151).

## IIIB2c

34. B. This patient is experiencing an increased work of breathing, as evidenced by his high spontaneous ventilatory rate (16 breaths/min.) despite the relatively high SIMV rate (12 breaths/min.). As a result, he is being overventilated. His oxygenation status is fine, especially for a COPD patient. His arterial $PCO_2$ level is quite low for his pulmonary pathophysiology, however.

A COPD patient is expected to have carbon dioxide retention, and his pH should be less than 7.40.

Pressure-support ventilation (PSV) would provide a reasonable alternative to the SIMV along with its demand valve system, which contributes to the patient's increased work of breathing. PSV is a mode of ventilation that augments the patient's spontaneous ventilation. The RRT presets a pressure plateau level that is maintained throughout the patient's inspiratory cycle. During PSV, the patient is able to establish his own tidal volume, ventilatory rate, inspiratory flow rate, and I:E ratio. This pressure-limited, flow-cycled, assisted ventilation should decrease the patient's work of breathing and allow his acid-base status to normalize (i.e., the arterial $PCO_2$ should rise above 50 torr, his pH should drop to below 7.40, and the $HCO_3^-$ level should rise with renal compensation for the increased arterial $PCO_2$).

(1:910), (10:198, 199), (15:960).

### IIIE1g

35. B. The diagnosis of sleep apnea syndrome requires polysomnography. Suspicion of this disorder can arise from patient complaints, such as daytime hypersomnolence, snoring, persistent headaches, and reduced mental acuity. Frequently, the complaint of snoring as well as flailing of the limbs during sleep is made by a discontented spouse whose own sleep is disturbed.

During polysomnography, airflow-detection devices sense the degree of movements of air from the nose and mouth. Similarly, thoracic and abdominal movements are sensed by an inductance plethysmograph. Oxygen saturation via pulse oximetry is continuously monitored. Sleep staging by way of EEG is also studied. The cessation of airflow from the nose and mouth for at least 10 seconds defines an apneic episode. Patients who have 30 or more apneic episodes during 7 hours of nocturnal sleep are diagnosed as having sleep apnea.

Three forms of sleep apnea exist (i.e., central sleep apnea, obstructive sleep apnea, and mixed sleep apnea). Table 5-4 outlines the major diagnostic differences among these three forms.

(1:557–558), (9:410–413), (15:261–276, 579–584).

### IIIA1l

36. B. The DuBois body surface chart in Figure 5-23 enables the determination of the patient's body surface area (BSA). A straight edge is placed across the chart connecting the patient's height (6'1") and body weight (195 lbs). The point where the straight edge intersects the BSA line is the body surface area.

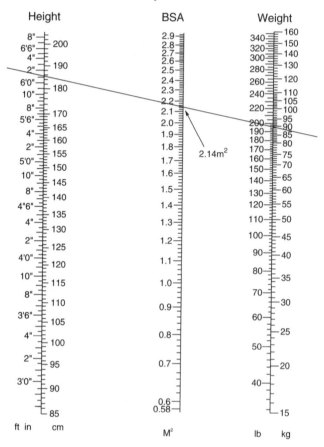

Dubois body surface chart

**Figure 5-23:** Connect the patient's height and the patient's weight with a straightedge. The BSA is the point where the line drawn crosses the middle column. From DuBois, E.F., Basal Metabolism in Health and Disease, 3rd ed., Lea & Febiger, Philadelphia, 1936.

The cardiac index (C.I.) is calculated according to the following formula:

**Table 5-4** Characteristic Findings of the Forms of Sleep Apnea Syndrome

| Central Sleep Apnea | Obstructive Sleep Apnea | Mixed Sleep Apnea |
| --- | --- | --- |
| • snoring absent<br>• airflow absent<br>• ventilatory efforts absent<br>• mild to moderate desaturation | • loud, intermittent snoring<br>• airflow absent<br>• paradoxical thoracic and abdominal movements<br>• moderate to severe desaturation | • central sleep apnea findings preceding those of obstructive sleep apnea<br>• moderate to severe desaturation |

$$C.I. = \frac{C.O.}{BSA} = \frac{6.0 \text{ liters/min.}}{2.14 \text{ m}^2} = 2.8 \text{ liters/min./m}^2$$

The C.I. enables the cardiac output of different size people to be compared. The C.I. eliminates the differences in body build. The normal value ranges between 2.5 to 4.2 liters/min./m². Essentially, the C.I. represents the blood flow relative to the body surface area in square meters.

(14:324–325).

## IIIA1e

37. B. A normal volume-pressure curve generated from a positive mechanical ventilation breath is shown in Figure 5-24.

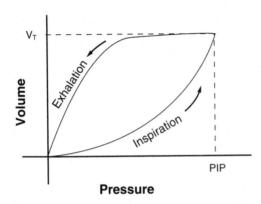

**Figure 5-24:** Normal volume-pressure loop displaying hysteresis. Different inspiratory and expiratory curves during the same ventilatory cycle demonstrates hysteresis. PIP on the *x*-axis and V$_T$ on the *y*-axis.

Notice how the inspiratory limb differs from the expiratory limb. This phenomenon is termed hysteresis. The hysteresis in the volume-pressure curve of the lung results from the surface tension forces in the lungs. During inspiration, the volume-pressure relationships (surface tension forces increase) differ from the volume-pressure relationships experienced during exhalation, as the surface tension forces decrease.

On such a volume-pressure curve, the maximum point achieved on the *y*-axis is the tidal volume (V$_T$) and the maximum point reached on the *x*-axis is the peak inspiratory pressure (PIP).

Changes in lung compliance alter the characteristics of the volume-pressure curve. For example, when the lungs become stiff (decreased compliance), more pressure is required to deliver any volume of air into the lungs. The volume-pressure loop changes shape. It tends to flatten and move down toward the *x*-axis and to the right.

Conversely, when lung compliance increases (pulmonary emphysema), less pressure is needed to deposit any volume of air into the lungs. Under this circumstance, the curve bends towards the *y*-axis and to the left.

(1:199–200, 958), (10:48–49), (17:317–319).

## IIIC3a

38. C. Neither the hydrodynamic (Babbington or hydrosphere) nebulizer nor the ultrasonic nebulizer is appropriate for continuous use, because both produce outputs as high as 6 ml/min. and are a potential hazard for fluid overload. These two types of aerosol generators are usually used for sputum induction or for short-term application for reducing the viscosity of tenacious secretions.

The small-volume nebulizer is not suitable for humidifying the airway. Rather, it is primarily used for medication delivery. The small-particle aerosol generator (SPAG) is used exclusively for the delivery of ribavirin in children who have bronchiolitis.

The aerosol generator of choice here is the large-volume jet nebulizer because its output is only about 1 ml/min. Ordinarily, it sufficiently humidifies the airway as well as provides an effective vehicle for oxygen delivery. This device should also be heated.

(1:673, 675, 693, 755), (13:115, 120, 130), (15:805–806).

## IIIA1l

39. C. The general formula for calculating the resistance of any fluid (air or liquid) is as follows:

$$R = \Delta P / \dot{V}$$

where

R = resistance (cm H$_2$O/L/sec.)
$\Delta$P = pressure change or driving pressure (cm H$_2$O)
$\dot{V}$ = flow rate (L/min.)

This formula is used for calculating airway resistance as well as vascular resistance. To calculate the pulmonary vascular resistance, one needs to know the driving pressure across the pulmonary vasculature (i.e., from the pump [right ventricle] to the reservoir [left atrium]).

The mean pulmonary artery pressure ($\overline{PAP}$) represents the pump pressure. The left ventricular end-diastolic pressure (LVEDP) is approximated by the pulmonary capillary wedge pressure (PCWP). The C.O. is the flow rate.

The formula for calculating pulmonary vascular resistance (PVR) is:

$$PVR = \frac{\overline{PAP} - PCWP}{C.O.}$$

STEP 1: Calculate the C.O.

$$C.O. = SV \times HR$$
$$= 70 \text{ ml/beat} \times 65 \text{ beats/min.}$$
$$= 4,550 \text{ ml/min.}$$

STEP 2: Convert the C.O. to L/min.

$$C.O. = \frac{4,550 \text{ ml/min.}}{1,000 \text{ ml/liter}}$$
$$= 4.55 \text{ L/min.}$$

STEP 3: Calculate the PVR.

$$PVR = \frac{\overline{PAP} - PCWP}{C.O.}$$
$$= \frac{17 \text{ mm Hg} - 7 \text{ mm Hg}}{4.55 \text{ L/min.}}$$
$$= 2.20 \text{ mm Hg/L/min.}$$

The normal PVR range is 1.5 to 3.0 mm Hg/L/min. Multiplying the PVR value expressed in mm Hg/L/min. by 79.9 converts to the units of dynes-sec./cm$^5$, the normal range of which is 150 to 250 dynes-sec./cm$^5$. Alternatively, the units for PVR can also be expressed as dynes-sec-cm$^{-5}$, or dynes • sec/cm$^5$.

(1:949), (9:317–318), (10:136), (15:530).

### IIIC5

40. C. Chest physiotherapy (CPT) has been effective in clearing both lower lobes, as evidenced by chest radiography and auscultation. CPT to the lower lobes should be abandoned at this time because they are clear, but it should be applied exclusively to the right middle lobe, which has been identified as a recent area of involvement.

Incentive spirometry is not effective in mobilizing secretions. Its utility includes overcoming and preventing atelectasis. Aerosol therapy only would be inappropriate because a mechanical means of mobilizing the secretions would also be needed. Aerosol therapy could perhaps be used in conjunction with CPT.

(1:774–775, 792), (16:504, 529–532, 1153).

### IIIE1e

41. D. Essentially, the cardiopulmonary measurements that are made during an exercise test must also be made before the test is conducted. Table 5-5 outlines the physiologic measurements that must be made before and during a cardiopulmonary stress test.

(1:1092), (16:879–880).

### IIIA1c

42. D. When analyzing a sputum sample, the RRT should ask the patient questions concerning the duration of sputum production, the character of the sputum, and whether blood is present. Mucoid sputum is frequently produced by patients who have diseases that inflame or irritate the airway, such as asthma and chronic bronchitis. The sputum is thin, elastic (consistency), and clear. Purulent sputum is yellow-green, more viscous (sticky), has numerous pus cells, and usually indicates a bacterial infection. Fetid sputum often occurs in large quantities, is foul smelling, and usually represents an airway infection, such as bronchiectasis, lung abscess, or aspiration pneumonia. Expectoration of bloody or blood-tinged sputum is termed *hemoptysis* and can occur in conditions ranging from bronchiectasis to pulmonary emboli.

Because the Gram stain was taken from a sputum sample coughed by the patient and the sample was mucoid, the gram-negative cocci probably represent a contaminant from the mouth (Neisseriae). The fact that the sputum contained a large number of eosinophils indicates that the condition is an *allergic* one, such as asthma. If a large number of polymorphonuclear leukocytes (neutrophils) were present, a *bacterial* infection, rather than an allergic condition, would be suspected.

(1:299, 795), (9:112–113), (15:622).

### IIIC1a

43. B. The goal of a volume-oriented IPPB treatment should be to increase a patient's inspiratory capacity by at least 20%. To achieve this goal, the RRT would increase the preset pressure, which should increase the exhaled volume. Other goals of volume-oriented IPPB can include

**Table 5-5** Physiologic Measurements Associated with Cardiopulmonary Stress Testing

| Pulmonary Measurements/Monitoring | Cardiovascular Measurements/Monitoring |
| --- | --- |
| • ventilatory rate (f) | • heart rate (HR) |
| • minute ventilation ($\dot{V}_E$) | • blood pressure (BP) |
| • end-tidal oxygen tension ($P_{ET}O_2$) | • electrocardiography (ECG) |
| • end-tidal carbon dioxide tension ($P_{ET}CO_2$) | |
| • data to obtain mixed exhaled $O_2$ and $CO_2$ values | |

(1) improved breath sounds, (2) an improved chest radiograph, and (3) a forced vital capacity 70% of predicted.

(1:777–778, 780), (15:845–846).

## IIID1b

44. A. The ECG indicates that the patient has gone into ventricular fibrillation. The ECG pattern is characterized by irregular, widened, and poorly defined QRS complexes. Once this cardiac pattern develops, the patient must be defibrillated immediately.

(1:331, 652), (9:206, 207), (15:1119–1120).

## IIIC3a

45. A. The liter flow, and consequently the $FIO_2$, are too high for the patient. This patient has a chronically elevated $PaCO_2$ and likely ventilates via stimulation of his hypoxic drive, as opposed to increases in his arterial carbon dioxide levels. The hypoxic drive, controlled by the peripheral chemoreceptors, is triggered when the $PaO_2$ drops below 50 mm Hg, as shown in Figure 5-25.

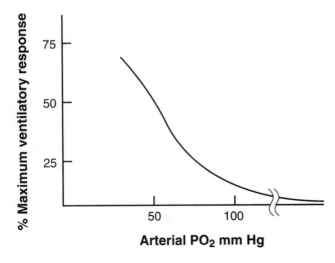

**Figure 5-25:** Ventilatory response to decreased arterial $PO_2$. Note the ventilatory response to the $PaO_2$ below 50 mm Hg. This ventilatory response is carried out by the peripheral chemoreceptors.

The increased $FIO_2$ provided by the nasal cannula at 3 L/min. has caused this patient's $PaO_2$ to rise above the level stimulating his peripheral chemoreceptors, and as a result has caused him to decrease his minute ventilation, causing his $PaCO_2$ to increase to dangerously high levels. As a result of this hypercapnia, the patient is increasingly somnolent and confused. The signs and symptoms associated with hypercapnia include the following:

- lethargy
- coma
- peripheral vasoconstriction
- hypertension
- CNS vasodilatation
- headache
- papilledema
- shock

At this time, the RRT should administer 24% $O_2$ via an air entrainment mask, remain with the patient, and obtain an ABG. An air entrainment mask is appropriate in this situation because it is a high-flow oxygen-delivery device, which means that the $FIO_2$ is not influenced by changes in either the patient's ventilatory pattern, ventilatory rate, or tidal volume.

On the contrary, a nasal cannula is a low-flow oxygen-delivery device (i.e., its $FIO_2$ is inversely proportional to the patient's minute ventilation). Therefore, if a COPD patient who breathes via his hypoxic drive experiences shortness of breath, he must not be administered oxygen via a low-flow delivery device.

If adequate oxygenation cannot be maintained without eliminating the hypoxic drive, the patient might require ET intubation and mechanical ventilation until his condition improves.

(1:742), (15:877–878), (16:375, 1124).

## IIIB2c

46. C. The problem encountered in this mechanical ventilation situation is auto-PEEP. The patient is receiving an inspiration before the expiratory phase is complete. The expiratory flow is displayed below the baseline. Failure of the expiratory flow to return to the baseline before the next inspiration produces auto-PEEP. Auto-PEEP develops in such a situation because air is "trapped" in the lungs.

Patients who are receiving mechanical ventilation at high ventilatory rates and with a high minute ventilation are prone to developing auto-PEEP.

Auto-PEEP can be minimized via the techniques listed in Table 5-6 on page 300.

(1:917, 951–952), (10:153–156).

## IIIA1l

47. D. The stroke volume (SV) is the volume of blood ejected from the heart per beat. The normal range is 50 ml/beat to 80 ml/beat. The stroke volume can be calculated as follows.

$$SV = \frac{C.O.}{HR}$$

**Table 5-6** Techniques Used to Reduce Auto-Peep

- Decrease the ventilatory rate and increase the tidal volume
- Increase the peak inspiratory flow
- Decrease the tidal volume and allow the $PaCO_2$ to increase (permissive hypercapnia)
- Alter the ventilatory pattern
- Decrease the inspiratory time in relation to the total cycle time
- Apply bronchial hygiene techniques to eliminate tracheobronchial secretions
- Administer bronchodilators
- Apply low rate SIMV
- Evaluate the size of the ETT; use a larger I.D. tube if appropriate
- Administer PEEP or CPAP

STEP 1: Convert the C.O. to ml/min.

$$C.O. = 6.0 \text{ ł/minute} \times 1,000 \text{ ml/ł}$$
$$= 6,000 \text{ ml/min.}$$

STEP 2: Calculate the SV.

$$SV = \frac{C.O.}{HR}$$
$$= \frac{6,000 \text{ ml/min.}}{75 \text{ beats/min.}}$$
$$= 80 \text{ ml/beat}$$

(1:949), (10:136), (15:76, 530).

## IIIC3a

48. C. An $FIO_2$ of 0.45 would likely bring the arterial $PO_2$ within the range of 90 to 100 torr. When the patient's cardiopulmonary status (C.O., $\dot{V}_A/\dot{Q}_C$, $\dot{V}_A$) is stable, the following method can be used to approximate the $FIO_2$ that would yield a desired arterial $PO_2$.

STEP 1: Use the following equation to calculate the approximate $FIO_2$ that would render a desired arterial $PO_2$:

$$\frac{\text{actual } PaO_2}{\text{actual } F_IO_2} = \frac{\text{desired } PaO_2}{\text{desired } F_IO_2}$$

STEP 2: Insert the known values into the equation.

$$\frac{153 \text{ torr}}{0.70} = \frac{95 \text{ torr}}{X}$$

$$153 \text{ torr } X = 66.5 \text{ torr}$$

$$X = \frac{66.5 \text{ torr}}{153 \text{ torr}}$$

$$X = 0.43 \text{ (Set } FIO_2 \text{ at } 0.45.)$$

Therefore, an $FIO_2$ of approximately 0.45 in this situation should produce an arterial $PO_2$ between 90 torr and 100 torr.

Alternatively, the $PaO_2/PaO_2$ ratio can be used to establish a new $FIO_2$. This ratio also provides an indication of oxygenation and lung function (i.e., the available alveolar oxygen that is diffusing into the pulmonary capillary blood). A $PaO_2/PaO_2$ ratio, or a/A ratio, of less than 0.60 reflects the need for oxygen therapy, whereas an a/A ratio below 0.15 signifies refractory hypoxemia caused by intrapulmonary shunting (capillary shunt and shunt effect).

To use the a/A ratio to calculate an estimated $FIO_2$ for achieving a desired $PaO_2$, one would need to employ the alveolar air equation. Therefore, the $FIO_2$, $PaO_2$, and $PaCO_2$ need to be known. Also, a respiratory quotient (R) of 0.8 would be presumed. Using the a/A ratio to predict the $FIO_2$ needed to achieve a certain $PaO_2$ is rather lengthy, as outlined below.

STEP 1: Use the shortened form of the alveolar air equation to calculate the actual $PaO_2$.

$$\text{actual } P_AO_2 = (P_B - P_{H_2O})F_IO_2 - PaCO_2(1.25)$$

STEP 2: Determine the $PaO_2$ needed to achieve the desired $PaO_2$.

$$\text{needed } (P_AO_2) = \frac{\text{desired } PaO_2}{\text{actual } PaO_2/\text{actual } P_AO_2}$$

STEP 3: Use the alveolar air equation again, but rearrange it to solve for the desired $FIO_2$.

$$\text{desired } F_IO_2 = \frac{\text{needed } P_AO_2 + (PaCO_2 \times 1.25)}{(P_B - P_{H_2O})}$$

Again, all these calculations require a constant cardiopulmonary status (C.O., $\dot{V}_A/\dot{Q}_C$, $\dot{V}_A$).

(1:911), (10:263–264).

## IIIB1b

49. C. Although heat–moisture exchangers (HMEs) or hygroscopic condensing humidifiers (HCHs) are useful during anesthesia and short-term mechanical ventilation, especially in the postoperative period, they are contraindicated in patients who have copious amounts of secretions. The secretions often compromise the humidification function of the HME as well as increase resistance to gas flow through the unit. Similarly, thick, tenacious secretions pose the threat of obstructing the patient's airway. Therefore, if a patient who is using an HME or HCH is discovered to have thick and/or copious secretions, the humidification device needs to be removed immediately and replaced by an

alternate form of humidification (e.g., a heated cascade humidifier or a wick humidifier).

(1:679, 903), (15:799).

**IIIE1l**

50. C. The patient should be sedated and paralyzed to facilitate mechanical ventilation. Pavulon and Norcuron are nondepolarizing neuromuscular blocking agents that would enable complete control of ventilation by paralyzing the patient. Neither Pavulon nor Norcuron should be given without a sedative or tranquilizer, such as an I.V. benzodiazepine (Valium or Librium), because neither one has any effect on the level of consciousness. Also, if a neuromuscular blocking agent is used and a ventilator malfunction or disconnection occurred, the patient would be unable to breathe spontaneously. This situation could result in a ventilator catastrophe. Many clinicians prefer to try other methods of sedation, such as the use of narcotic analgesics (morphine, etc.) or benzodiazepine-related tranquilizers (Ativan, Valium, etc.) before resorting to neuromuscular blocking agents.

(10:298–299), (15:715).

**IIIE1h**

51. A. Cardioversion is the application of electrical energy through the chest wall to the heart. This energy is discharged from a defibrillation device that is mechanically set or manually triggered to generate an electric current during ventricular depolarization (i.e., in synchrony with the R-wave).

The ECG tracing indicates supraventricular tachycardia (SVT), which in this situation is associated with a ventricular rate of greater than 150 beats/min. This condition warrants immediate cardioversion. When the ventricular rate is less than 150 beats/min., immediate cardioversion is generally not necessary. In such cases, vagal maneuvers can be performed to increase parasympathetic tone and to slow AV node conduction time. Vagal maneuvers include carotid sinus pressure or massage, breath holding, and squatting.

If any of these techniques fails, the patient should be given adenosine and/or verapamil I.V. If these medications do not help, other pharmacologic considerations include digoxin, b-blockers, diltiazem, lidocaine, and procainamide. Unsuccessful pharmacologic intervention with this dysrhythmia is usually then followed by cardioversion. (Nonsynchronized cardioversion, i.e., the application of electrical energy to the heart any time during the cardiac cycle, is called *defibrillation.*)

("Guidelines 2000 for Cardiopulmonary Resuscitation and Emergency Cardiovascular Care," 2000, American Heart Association, Inc., pages I–91 and I–92), (1:657).

**IIIC7c**

52. C. The clinical situation described strongly indicates the need for endotracheal suctioning. Despite conflicting information among texts (e.g., reference #1 states −80 to −100 mm Hg, while reference #18 advocates −100 to −120 mm Hg) for the appropriate vacuum pressure level for endotracheal suctioning of children, a vacuum pressure of −100 mm Hg is reasonable. A 10 Fr suction catheter would be appropriate for an endotracheal tube ranging in size from 5 to 7 mm I.D. A 12 Fr catheter is suggested for ET tubes 7.5 to 8.0 mm I.D.

(1:616), (18:402,432).

**IIIE2b**

53. C. The initial, or short-term, goals for a pulmonary rehabilitation program differ from the long-term goals. The ultimate goals of a pulmonary rehabilitation program include (1) improving activities of daily living, (2) reducing the number of hospitalizations, and (3) increasing the intensity and duration of exercise. Early on in a pulmonary rehabilitation program the goals differ. They often include (1) teaching the patient about medications, (2) instructing the patient on the pathophysiology of the disease, and (3) providing the patient with information regarding proper nutrition.

(1:1088–1094).

**IIIA2c**

54. A. Figure 5-26 illustrates a normal volume-pressure loop for a spontaneous breath.

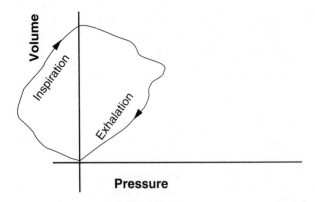

**Figure 5-26:** A normal volume-pressure loop from a spontaneously breathing patient.

The area to the left of the *y*-axis signifies inspiration while the region to the right of the *y*-axis represents exhalation. The origin is the point of end-exhalation, or the beginning of inspiration.

(10:48).

55. B. In PSV, as used with the BiPAP® system, the tidal volume is controlled by the patient's effort, lung compliance, airway resistance, and inspiratory positive airway pressure (IPAP) level. This patient has efforts greater than that which have been set by the IPAP level. With the BiPAP® system, the tidal volume is determined by the IPAP settings and the patient's inspiratory effort; therefore, increasing the IPAP enables a larger tidal volume. The additional flow in the circuit will enhance the patient's own inspiratory efforts. IPAP augments the patient's ventilatory efforts, whereas expiratory positive airway pressure (EPAP) augments the patient's oxygenation requirement.

(1:563, 866, 878, 910), (10:89–90, 201, 217).

## IIIA1m(1)

56. D. The passive diffusion of oxygen across the alveolar-capillary membrane occurs because a partial pressure gradient exists between the alveoli and the pulmonary capillary blood. The magnitude of this gradient on room air is normally within the range of 5 to 10 torr. Venous blood entering the pulmonary capillaries ordinarily has a $PO_2$ of 40 torr and is arterialized ($PO_2$ 100 torr) within about 0.25 sec. That is the amount of time that the blood resides in the pulmonary capillary at a normal, resting C.O.

Atmospheric (environmental) changes or pathophysiologic conditions can adversely influence the diffusion of oxygen across the alveolar-capillary membrane. For example, ascending to a higher altitude reduces the alveolar oxygen tension, whereas pulmonary fibrosis impedes the diffusion of oxygen by thickening the alveolar-capillary membrane. Such situations cause hypoxemia and an increased alveolar arterial oxygen tension gradient [$P(A\text{-}a)O_2$].

The cause of hypoxemia can often be determined when the room air $P(A\text{-}a)O_2$ is evaluated in conjunction with the arterial $PCO_2$. For example, when the $P(A\text{-}a)O_2$ is widened in the presence of either normocapnia or hypocapnia, the hypoxemia generally results from ventilation–perfusion ($\dot{V}_A/\dot{Q}_C$) abnormalities. $\dot{V}_A/\dot{Q}_C$ abnormalities include conditions such as diffusion defects, shunting, perfusion in excess of ventilation (venous admixture or shunt effect), and capillary shunting. Furthermore, when the room air $P(A\text{-}a)O_2$ increases or remains normal and the arterial $PCO_2$ increases, the hypoxemia ordinarily stems from hypoventilation.

Similarly, capillary shunting and diffusion defects, both of which cause a widened $P(A\text{-}a)O_2$, can be differentiated as the cause of hypoxemia when supplemental oxygen is administered. In the case of capillary shunting, the hypoxemia will not be relieved by the additional oxygen deposited in the lungs because the oxygen-enriched gas cannot enter the unventilated alveoli. Therefore, the $P(A\text{-}a)O_2$ actually worsens (increases), and the hypoxemia is not ameliorated. In essence, hypoxemia caused by capillary shunting is not amenable to oxygen therapy.

On the other hand, when the $F_IO_2$ is increased in the presence of a diffusion defect or $\dot{V}_A/\dot{Q}_C$ abnormalities, the $P(A\text{-}a)O_2$ decreases. The decreased $P(A\text{-}a)O_2$ results from the diffusion of more oxygen across the alveolar-capillary membrane, or more oxygen available in low $\dot{V}_A/\dot{Q}_C$ units. The calculation of the room-air $P(A\text{-}a)O_2$ is as follows.

*GIVEN:*

$P_B$: 760 torr
Body temperature: 37°C
$PaCO_2$: 40 torr
$PaO_2$: 95 torr
R: 0.8

STEP 1:  Use the alveolar air equation to calculate the alveolar $PO_2$.

$$P_AO_2 = F_IO_2(P_B - P_{H_2O}) - PaCO_2\left( F_IO_2 + \frac{1 - F_IO_2}{R}\right)$$

$$= 0.21(760 \text{ torr} - 47 \text{ torr})$$

$$- 40 \text{ torr} \left( 0.21 + \frac{1.0 - 0.21}{0.8}\right)$$

$$= 0.21(713 \text{ torr}) - 40 \text{ torr}(1.19)$$

$$= 149.7 \text{ torr} - 47.6 \text{ torr}$$

$$= 102 \text{ torr}$$

STEP 2:  Calculate the $P(A\text{-}a)O_2$.

$$P(A\text{-}a)O_2 = P_AO_2 - PaO_2$$

$$= 102 \text{ torr} - 95 \text{ torr}$$

$$= 7 \text{ torr}$$

Alternatively, a shortened formula is available to obtain a rapid approximation of the $P(A\text{-}a)O_2$:

$$\text{predicted } P(A\text{-}a)O_2 = (\text{Age} \times F_IO_2) + 2.5$$

$$= (25 \times 0.21) + 2.5$$

$$= 7.75 \text{ torr}$$

(1:217, 234–235, 821, 929), (10:21, 181, 274).

## IIIC3a

57. B. Air entrainment devices produce excessively high noise levels inside an oxyhood. Therefore, they are not acceptable. Besides, the total flow as described would be 64 L/min., which is entirely too much for such a small patient. Although 1 L/min. of oxygen mixed

with 7 L/min. air will result in the delivery of 30% oxygen and a total flow rate of 8 L/min., this setup is cumbersome and should be used only when a blender is not available. Therefore, a blender on 30% with a flow rate of 8 L/min. to a heated humidifier is the appropriate modality.

(5:75), (13:79–81), (18:282–284).

## IIID1b

58. C. The ECG monitor is showing ventricular fibrillation. According to the American Heart Association (AHA) standards for cardiopulmonary resuscitation, basic life support (BLS) must be administered immediately when ventricular fibrillation occurs. CPR must be maintained until a defibrillator is attached to the patient. The only effective treatment for ventricular fibrillation is electrical defibrillation.

(16:813–814).

## IIIA1b

59. B. Unlike an arterial puncture procedure for obtaining ABG values, noninvasive monitoring methods can provide a continuous report of a patient's oxygenation and ventilatory status. Many factors affect the accuracy of each of these forms of noninvasive monitoring. The $PtcCO_2$ is more accurate than the $PtcO_2$ values because carbon dioxide is more diffusible across the epidermis than oxygen. Factors affecting the $PtcO_2$ and $PtcCO_2$ measurements are shown in Table 5-7.

**Table 5-7** Factors Affecting $PtcD_2$ and $PtcCO_2$ Values

| Factors | $PtcO_2$ | $PtcCO_2$ |
|---|---|---|
| *Patient Factors* | Skin thickness | Acidosis |
| | Perfusion | Perfusion |
| | Blood pressure | |
| | Vasodilators | |
| | Age | |
| *Electrode Factors* | Calibration | |
| | Membrane condition | |
| | Contact | |
| | Probe placement | |

End-tidal $CO_2$ monitoring is difficult in a nonintubated patient. The difference between $PaCO_2$ and $PetCO_2$ will increase in a number of conditions, including pulmonary hypoperfusion, high ventilatory rate, low tidal volume, positive pressure ventilation, cardiac arrest, and pulmonary embolism. Increases in $PetCO_2$ include an increased $CO_2$ production, decreased alveolar ventilation, and equipment malfunctions. The $PetCO_2$ will decrease in conditions causing a fall in $CO_2$ pro-

duction, increased alveolar ventilation, and equipment malfunctions.

(1:355, 364), (9:290, 227, 232, 301).

## IIIE2e

60. B. Three types of ventilatory muscle-training techniques are available: (1) resistive training, (2) hypercapnic training, and (3) threshold load training. Restrictive training requires the patient to breathe through smaller orifices in consecutive training sessions as the load is placed on the muscles during inspiration. Expiration is passive (unrestricted). Patients using resistive breathing devices begin with the largest size orifice. They are instructed to continue using a particular orifice size until they are able to tolerate (breathe relatively comfortably) 15 minutes of breathing through a given orifice. The patients are then informed to insert a smaller size orifice until they can tolerate the smaller orifice. They continue this pattern until they have used all the possible resistors. They are expected to breathe normally through the device. The program generally extends from 4 to 8 weeks. These devices will increase the strength and endurance of the muscles of ventilation.

(1:1096), (15:1146–1147).

## IIID1b

61. B. Any situation that does not enable ventilation to occur (e.g., laryngeal edema or extensive facial trauma) is an indication for the use of the cricothyroidotomy procedure on cardiac arrest victims. Similarly, conditions preventing the passage and/or insertion of ancillary airway equipment warrant consideration of this emergency airway procedure.

The cricothyroid membrane is horizontally cut to create a relatively large opening through which an ET tube can be inserted. Transtracheal catheterization is another procedure that enables the establishment of an emergency airway. A 12- to 16-gauge needle encased by a plastic catheter is inserted through the cricothyroid membrane at a 45° angle. When the catheter is in place, ventilation is supplied by a high-pressure oxygen source with automatic airflow direction.

(1:163), (1:39).

## IIIA1c

62. D. Subjective responses and attitudes are not measurable. These responses include feelings, pain, discomfort, uneasiness, and other psychoemotional perceptions. As such, they are difficult to directly assess. They are often presented in the way people speak, rather than what they say. The patient's posture (body language), eye contact, choice of phrases, tone of voice, and facial expressions can all provide clues to the alert and sensitive observer.

Dyspnea is an important and common subjective finding in a patient who has pulmonary disease.

(1:26), (10:16, 18).

## IIIE1a

63. A. When a mechanically ventilated patient is about to undergo bronchoscopy, a number of ventilator considerations need to be taken into account. First, because oxygen desaturation is commonplace during the procedure, the $FIO_2$ must be increased to 1.0. At the same time, pulse oximetry should be performed during the bronchoscopy to monitor the patient's saturation. A swivel adaptor must be used to maintain the PEEP level throughout the procedure. Loss of PEEP during the bronchoscopy can lead to desaturation. The fact that the bronchoscope acts as a partial obstruction increases the likelihood for auto-PEEP to develop because the time required for exhalation will become inadequate. If the time needed to empty the lungs increases to the point where the ensuing inspiration begins, auto-PEEP will develop. Similarly, as the bronchoscope partially obstructs the airway, airway resistance increases—resulting in the possibility that the high pressure limit will be reached. Therefore, to prevent premature termination of inspiration, the high pressure limit needs to be increased.

(15:633–634).

## IIIB1e

64. B. The physical findings presented in this situation reflect an increase in air flow to the right lung (percussion findings) and a decrease to the left (auscultation and observation findings). These findings are consistent with the migration or placement of the endotracheal tube in the right mainstem bronchus.

A flail chest would include paradoxical chest wall movement. A pneumothorax would be characterized by a deviated trachea from the midline and considerable patient distress. The atelectasis is occurring on the left side in this situation because all the ventilation is flowing into the right lung.

(1:164–174), (9:74–80), (10:161–162).

## IIIA1f

65. C. Administering PEEP raises the mean intrathoracic pressure. As the mean intrathoracic pressure increases, venous return to the right side of the heart is reduced. Consequently, the amount of blood entering and leaving the right ventricle decreases. Furthermore, the volume of blood flowing through the pulmonary vasculature diminishes, thereby compromising blood oxygenation. Ultimately, less blood fills the left ventricle and the cardiac output decreases.

A reduction in the cardiac output also affects the renal output of urine. A lower urinary output accompanies a decreased cardiac output.

Because inappropriate PEEP increases dead space, the dead space-tidal volume ratio ($V_D/V_T$) would increase.

The foregoing scenario highlights the importance of conducting a PEEP study to ascertain the best, or optimum, PEEP.

Other detrimental effects of inappropriate PEEP include the following:

- increased risk of barotrauma
- increased work of breathing
- increased pulmonary vascular resistance
- increased intracranial pressure
- increased dead space
- increased mean airway pressure

(1:880), (10:268–269).

## IIIC3a

66. C. Generally, CPAP levels are changed by increments of 2 cm $H_2O$ to 3 cm $H_2O$ until a minimum CPAP level of 2 cm $H_2O$ is achieved. The reduction of CPAP requires the neonate to maintain spontaneous breathing without fatiguing, while having an adequate $PaO_2$ on an $FIO_2$ of about 0.40.

$FIO_2$ levels are progressively reduced to 0.40 as long as the arterial $PO_2$ remains between 50 torr and 70 torr. In this situation, the $FIO_2$ is 0.50 with a CPAP of 3 cm $H_2O$. Therefore, the likely action to take is to reduce the $FIO_2$ by about 0.05 to 0.45, and not change the CPAP until the $FIO_2$ gets below 0.40.

Extubation, or removal from CPAP, often occurs when the newborn can maintain an adequate alveolar ventilation and oxygenation at a CPAP level of around 2 cm $H_2O$ on an $FIO_2$ of 0.40.

(1:783, 865), (10:285).

## IIIE1c

67. B. Transtracheal aspiration involves percutaneously aspirating tracheal secretions through a punctured cricothyroid membrane. The purpose of this procedure is to obtain lower respiratory tract specimens that are uncontaminated by secretions or microorganisms in the oro- and nasopharynx. This technique of obtaining specimens is especially useful in diagnosing anaerobic lung infections, because specimens that pass through the pharynx become contaminated with a variety of anaerobic organisms from that region.

Additionally, the transtracheal aspiration technique is sometimes used to encourage coughing by patients who are unable to generate an effective cough. Once the catheter is in place, 2 to 5cc of normal saline are instilled into the trachea, causing paroxysms of coughing.

In preparation for the procedure, the RRT must inform the patient that coughing will occur and that the puncture site will be locally anesthetized. The patient should be placed supine with a pillow situated under the shoulders and the neck hyperextended. This position optimally exposes the cricothyroid membrane. The patient must be cautioned not to swallow or talk while the cricothyroid membrane is being punctured by the needle. The patient also needs to be informed that the puncture site will be gently pressurized (compressed) for approximately 5 minutes after the catheter is removed. The purpose of this precaution is to reduce the risk of subcutaneous or mediastinal emphysema.

(15:625).

## IIIC2

68. D. Performing an inspiratory hold provides for a more even distribution of the medication as well as an increase in the time available for the drug's penetration and deposition. Nasal breathing is accompanied by turbulent air movement and increased contact between the nasal mucosa and the medication, in addition to the nasal filtering apparatus. Therefore, mouth breathing is preferred. Slow, deep inspirations favor increased aerosol penetration. Pursed-lip breathing extends the time of exhalation, providing the opportunity for more particle deposition.

(1:696), (15:802).

## IIIC3a

69. D. Oxygen-delivery systems that are set to deliver greater than 40% oxygen often fail to do so because of the decreased air:oxygen entrainment ratios. For example, an $FIO_2$ of 0.60 has an air:oxygen entrainment ratio of 1:1.

The total gas flow rate delivered to this patient is inadequate because a source flow rate of 10 L/min., delivering 60% oxygen, provides a total flow rate of only 20 L/min. The following calculation illustrates how the total flow rate for these settings (60% $O_2$ at 10 L/min.) is determined.

STEP 1: Use the following relationship to determine the total delivered flow rate.

$$\dot{V}_{DEL} = \dot{V}_S + \dot{V}_{ENT}$$

where

$\dot{V}_{DEL}$ = total delivered flow rate (L/min.)

$\dot{V}_S$ = source or oxygen flow rate (L/min.)

$\dot{V}_{ENT}$ = entrained or air flow rate (L/min.)

STEP 2: Determine the entrained flow rate ($\dot{V}_{ENT}$) knowing that an $FIO_2$ of 0.60 has an air:$O_2$ ratio of 1:1.

$$\frac{\text{air flow rate}}{\text{oxygen flow rate}} = \frac{X}{10 \text{ L/min.}} = 1$$

$$X = 10 \text{ L/min.} \times 1.0$$

$$= 10 \text{ L/min. of air flow rate}$$

STEP 3: Insert the known values into the expression presented in STEP 1.

$$\dot{V}_{DEL} = \dot{V}_S + \dot{V}_{ENT}$$

$$= 10 \text{ L/min.} + 10 \text{ L/min.}$$

$$= 20 \text{ L/min.}$$

The estimated spontaneous peak flow for a patient is approximately three times the patient's minute ventilation ($\dot{V}_E$) (i.e., $3 \times 9.8$ L/min. $= 29.4$ L/min. from the second data set). The prescribed oxygen concentration (60%) is not being delivered because the total delivered flow rate from the system is only 20 L/min., whereas the patient's estimated spontaneous peak flow is 29.4 L/min.

For this patient to actually receive an $FIO_2$ of 0.60, the delivered (total) flow rate ($\dot{V}_{DEL}$) should be at least three times the patient's minute ventilation ($3 \times \dot{V}_E$) to accommodate further increases in the patient's inspiratory demands. To accomplish this requirement, a double flow meter setup would be necessary.

If each all-purpose nebulizer were set at 60%, operating at a source flow rate of 15 L/min., the patient would experience a delivered (total) flow rate of 60 L/min. (i.e., 30 L/min. from each system). This total flow rate would greatly exceed the patient's estimated spontaneous peak flow of 29.4 L/min. (i.e., $3 \times 9.8$ L/min.).

Setting up a dual flow meter system with each flow meter set at 10 L/min. would also exceed this patient's present ventilatory demands because 20 L/min. would be delivered by each flow meter. A total flow rate of 40 L/min. would be delivered.

The RRT must be mindful of the patient's minute ventilation when setting up an oxygen-delivery system. Focusing only on setting a prescribed oxygen percentage is sometimes inadequate. Anticipating changes in the patient's ventilatory demands is equally important.

(15:883), (17:134, 281–284).

## IIIC3b

70. D. The high-flow rate (6 L/min.) requirements of this patient make a liquid oxygen system the most cost-effective.

An oxygen concentrator would not meet this patient's oxygen needs because the oxygen concentration decreases at higher flow rates. Gas cylinders would be too costly at this rate of use.

(1:1111–1114).

### IIIB4a

71. C. Ordinarily, weaning from CPAP commences with incremental reductions in the $FIO_2$. The degree of $FIO_2$ reduction will be dictated by the clinical response of the infant, ABG data, transcutaneous $O_2$ and $CO_2$ monitoring, and pulse oximetry. As a guideline, the $FIO_2$ should not be reduced by more than 0.15 each time.

Once the $FIO_2$ is reduced to 0.40 while the arterial $PO_2$ is maintained at 70 torr or better, the CPAP should then be reduced in decrements of 2 to 3 cm $H_2O$ until a minimum CPAP level of 2 to 3 cm $H_2O$ is attained.

(1:783, 865), (10:285).

### IIIB2c

72. B. APRV is a mode of ventilation that is currently available only on the Irisa ventilator. When using APRV, two levels of CPAP are established. The low CPAP level is generally set at 2 to 10 cm $H_2O$, and the high level CPAP is set at 10 to 30 cm $H_2O$. An inverse ratio (high pressure to low pressure) can be used. The patient can breathe spontaneously throughout the high and low pressure cycles. An increase in the high-level CPAP will tend to increase tidal volume and in turn improve ventilation and lower the $PaCO_2$.

(1:830, 876, 910), (10:200, 216–217).

### IIIC4

73. B. An 80/20 helium-oxygen mixture is less dense than oxygen. Therefore, the helium-oxygen flow rate through an oxygen flowmeter will actually be greater than the flow rate set on the oxygen flowmeter.

Regarding the situation stated in this question, the flow rate of 80/20 heliox will be as follows:

$$\begin{aligned}
\text{actual} \atop \text{80/20 heliox} \atop \text{flow rate} &= \frac{\sqrt{\text{density of } O_2}}{\sqrt{\text{density of 80/20 heliox}}} \left( \begin{array}{c} \text{flow rate} \\ \text{set on} \\ \text{flowmeter} \end{array} \right) \\
&= \frac{\sqrt{1.43 \text{ g/L}}}{\sqrt{0.43 \text{ g/L}}} \times 10 \text{ L/min.} \\
&= \frac{1.20 \text{ g/L}}{0.66 \text{ g/L}} \times 10 \text{ L/min.} \\
&= 1.82 \times 10 \text{ L/min.} \\
&= \sim 18 \text{ L/min.}
\end{aligned}$$

(1:717, 768), (16:349, 396).

### IIIB4a

74. C. This patient has a flail chest condition resulting from the blunt chest-wall trauma. A flail chest is commonly accompanied by a pneumothorax and a hemothorax, neither of which is apparent in this situation. Chest X-rays would help to further assess the degree of injury. However, because of the proximity of the lungs to the chest wall, the patient must be monitored closely for the possibility of a lung contusion. It may take 2 to 3 days for lung contusions to become manifest. Lung contusions can produce refractory hypoxemia or ventilatory failure, in which case mechanical ventilation is generally needed.

The patient in this problem displays respiratory distress and hypoxemia. His ABGs reveal no hypercapnia; in fact, his ventilatory status appears quite reasonable. At this point, he could be placed on CPAP to help splint the chest wall and receive oxygen to treat his hypoxemia. Once the flail segment heals, CPT might be indicated.

(1:550), (9:76, 260, 262), (1:1077–1079).

### IIIC1a

75. D. If a pressure-limited, volume-variable device cycles off prematurely, either the flow rate can be reduced to promote laminar flow or the pressure limit can be increased. Decreasing the flow rate will increase inspiratory time and decrease ventilatory frequency. Increasing the pressure while maintaining a constant flow increases inspiratory time and decreases frequency.

(1:843–844), (10:79–80).

### IIIE2b

76. B. A discharge plan should contain the following components:

- physician's plan of treatment
- professional services required to administer the plan
- equipment needed to treat the patient
- financial status/reimbursement issues
- determination of caregivers
- advanced directives

Considerations of patient transportation once he is at home becomes the responsibility of the family and caregivers. The capability of the patient to participate in a pulmonary rehabilitation program is not an issue at the time of discharge. This aspect becomes a component of pulmonary rehabilitation if and when the physician decides to prescribe a pulmonary rehabilitation program.

(*Respiratory Care* 40:1308–1312, 1995), (16:891).

### IIIE1b

77. D. Thoracentesis is performed to aspirate fluid that has accumulated in the intrapleural space. The procedure

is usually performed with the patient sitting upright with his feet over the side of the bed while both hands and arms are supported at the shoulder level. Support is often provided by using a bedside tray and elevating it to the appropriate level.

The procedure, performed for either diagnostic or therapeutic purposes, is ordinarily painless because a local anesthetic is generously applied to the skin and to the periosteum of the rib at the puncture site. A 22-gauge needle, used for intrapleural fluid aspiration, is advanced just above the superior aspect of the anesthetized rib to avoid the possibility of injuring vessels and/or nerves that run along the inferior surface of each rib.

(1:479–482), (9:264–265), (15:636).

### IIIA1d

78. C. During mechanical ventilation, the intrathoracic pressures become elevated—which in turn can cause a negative fluid balance. The increased intrathoracic pressures adversely affect venous return. The body perceives this reduced venous return as fluid depletion. To compensate, the plasma levels of antidiuretic hormone (ADH), or vasopressin, increase. ADH is secreted by the posterior pituitary gland. Normally, ADH release is triggered by an increase in the tonicity of the extracellular fluid and the dehydration of the osmoreceptor cells in the supraoptic nuclei of the hypothalamus. If venous return is diminished, however, the autonomic nervous system will trigger the release of vasopressin independently of the osmoreceptors. As a result, maximum concentration of urine occurs because of the increased water permeability of the collecting duct within the kidney.

Additionally, the elevated intrathoracic pressure causes a decrease in the degree of left-atrial stretch. The baroreceptors responding to the decreased stretch within the left atrium cause a *decrease* in plasma levels of atrial natriuretic peptide (ANP). This decreased level of ANP results in an increased retention of sodium by the body and a decreased urine output.

Blood flow to the kidneys might be reduced during mechanical ventilation because the C.O. is adversely affected. This drop in C.O. will decrease the glomerular filtration rate and the urine output. Finally, the patient's high minute ventilation will increase the insensible water loss from the patient's respiratory tract. Insensible water loss cannot be measured and occurs through the skin (excluding sweating) and through the lungs. Table 5-8 summarizes the daily water exchange in the body.

The patient in this question had a total fluid intake of 2,700 ml and a total fluid output of 1,600 ml. This

**Table 5-8** Daily Water Exchange in the Body

|  | Average Daily Volume | Maximum Daily Volume |
|---|---|---|
| Water losses |  |  |
| • Insensible |  |  |
| Skin | 700 ml | 1,500 ml |
| Lung | 200 ml |  |
| • Sensible |  |  |
| Urine | 1,000 to 1,200 ml | > 2,000 ml/hour |
| Intestinal | 200 ml | 8,000 ml |
| Sweat | 0 ml | > 2,000 ml/hour |
| Water gain |  |  |
| • Ingestion |  |  |
| Fluids | 1,500 to 2,000 ml | 1,500 ml/hour |
| Solids | 500 to 600 ml | 1,500 ml/hour |
| • Body metabolism | 250 ml | 1,000 ml |

negative fluid balance resulted from the elevated intrathoracic pressures and the high minute ventilation (irreversible water loss).

(1:885–890), (10:141–143), (15:121–123).

### IIIB4b

79. C. Instituting PEEP, lengthening the inspiratory time, and initiating PCV with an inverse ratio are measures that might help improve oxygenation when the patient appears to have refractory hypoxemia. Prolonging inspiratory time can help prevent alveolar and airway collapse. Keeping the alveoli open longer can reduce alveolar dead space and improve gas exchange.

Some of these measures should be considered independently and not concurrently. For example, it is counterproductive to institute PEEP and PC-IRV at the same time. Similarly, it would be fruitless to simultaneously increase both the inspiratory and expiratory times. Prolonging the inspiratory time and shortening expiratory time establishes an inverse I:E ratio, however.

(1:912), (10:215, 263), (15:968).

### IIIB4a

80. C. To provide an I:E ratio of 1:1.5 with an IPAP rate of 12 breaths/min., the RRT needs to set the %IPAP to 40%. The following calculation shows how the %IPAP needed to be set was determined.

STEP 1: Determine the total parts in the I:E ratio by adding the inspiratory component to the expiratory components.

$$I:E = 1:1.5$$

Therefore,

$$1.0 + 1.5 = 2.5$$

Calculate the inspiratory time percent by dividing the inspiratory component by the total parts in the I:E ratio.

$$\frac{\text{inspiratory component}}{\text{total I:E parts}} = \frac{1.0}{2.5}$$

$$= 0.4, \text{ or } 0.4 \times 100$$

$$= 40\%$$

The general formula for determining the inspiratory time percent is as follows:

$$\% \, T_I = \frac{T_I}{T_I + T_E} \times 100$$

(1:860, 910), (10:205–206, 216).

## IIIE1f

81. A. Fine-needle aspiration is performed by using a long, narrow-bore needle. This procedure is conducted to puncture and aspirate cellular material from chest masses for diagnostic purposes. Fine needle aspiration is generally used with chest masses inaccessible via bronchoscopy or for those having been sampled by bronchoscopy and yielding no diagnosis.

A cutting needle biopsy provides for the sampling of large fragments of tissue. A thoracentesis is a procedure whereby fluid from the intrapleural space can be aspirated via a needle inserted into that space. Pleuroscopy, or thoracoscopy, provides for direct visualization of the parietal and visceral pleurae. A thoracotomy is unnecessary with a pleuroscopy.

(15:636–638).

## IIID1b

82. A. When the salt of a weak acid and the weak acid itself are dissolved in the same solution, the solution is capable of reacting with both bases and acids. Small additions of either acids or bases produce little change in the pH of a buffer solution.

Physiologically, the body has such a buffer system. Sodium bicarbonate ($NaHCO_3$) is a salt of a weak acid, and carbonic acid ($H_2CO_3$) is a weak acid. When a cardiac arrest occurs, biologic death does not immediately occur. The cells of the body continue to metabolize. They do so via the anaerobic route, however, producing lactic acid as one of their metabolites. The $CO_2$ levels increase because ventilation and gas exchange have become impaired. The accumulation of $CO_2$ ($H_2CO_3 \rightarrow CO_2 + H_2O$) and lactic acid depletes the body's store of $NaHCO_3$ which is essential for effective physiologic buffering. In this clinical condition, exogenous $NaHCO_3$ must be administered to alleviate the acidosis by replenishing the body's buffer stores.

Excessive administration of $NaHCO_3$ can result in medically induced (iatrogenic) metabolic alkalosis. During CPR, ventilation must be adequate, of course, to eliminate the increased $CO_2$ from $NaHCO_3$ administration.

$$HCO_3^- + H^+ \rightarrow H_2CO_3 \rightarrow H_2O + CO_2$$

The law of mass action favors this reaction to the right in this situation. The amount of bicarbonate required to treat a metabolic acidosis is calculated as follows:

$$[HCO_3^-] = \text{body weight (kg)} \times \text{base excess} \times 0.3$$

One-half of the calculated amount is given. ABG data must be obtained in about 15 minutes. If necessary, the calculation is performed again. One-half of the calculated $HCO_3^-$ value is always administered.

(3:178–179), (15:291–292).

## IIIE1g

83. B. Tidal volume delivery via negative-pressure ventilators is dependent on the patient's lung characteristics (lung compliance and airway resistance) as well as on the amount of negative pressure delivered. Changes in the lung characteristics, such as a decreased pulmonary compliance and an increased airway resistance, will cause the pressure difference to be met more quickly. Therefore, a smaller tidal volume will be delivered. Less negative pressure applied will also decrease the delivered tidal volume.

(1:1123–1129), (10:31, 190), (15:1200–1201).

## IIIA1l

84. A.

Step 1: Calculate the $P_{A}O_2$ using the alveolar air equation.

$$P_AO_2 = F_IO_2(P_B - P_{H_2O}) - PaCO_2\left(F_IO_2 + \frac{1 - F_IO_2}{R}\right)$$

$$= 1(760 \text{ torr} - 47 \text{ torr}) - 60 \text{ torr} (1)$$

$$= (1) \, 713 \text{ torr} - 60 \text{ torr}$$

$$= 653 \text{ torr}$$

Because the $P_AO_2$ equals 653 torr, the end-pulmonary capillary oxygen tension, or $P\dot{c}O_2$, is also assumed to be 653 torr.

Step 2: Calculate the end pulmonary capillary $O_2$ content ($C\dot{c}O_2$).

$$C\dot{c}O_2 = \text{combined } O_2 \text{ (vol\%)} + \text{dissolved } O_2 \text{ (vol\%)}$$

$$= ([Hb] \times 1.34 \times 100\%) +$$

$$(P_AO_2 \times 0.003 \text{ vol\%/torr})$$

$$= (16\ g\% \times 1.34 \times 100\%) +$$

$$(653\ torr \times 0.003\ vol\%/torr)$$

$$= 21.44\ vol\% + 1.96\ vol\%$$

$$= 23.4\ vol\%$$

STEP 3: Calculate the total arterial $O_2$ content ($CaO_2$).

$$CaO_2 = combined\ O_2\ (vol\%) + dissolved\ O_2\ (vol\%)$$

$$= ([Hb] \times 1.34 \times SaO_2) +$$

$$(P\textsc{a}O_2 \times 0.003\ vol\%/torr)$$

$$= (16\ g\% \times 1.34 \times 100\%) +$$

$$(500\ torr \times 0.003\ vol\%/torr)$$

$$= 21.44\ vol\% + 1.5\ vol\%$$

$$= 22.94\ vol\%$$

STEP 4: Calculate the total mixed venous $O_2$ content ($C\bar{v}O_2$).

$$C\bar{v}O_2 = combined\ O_2\ (vol\%) + dissolved\ O_2\ (vol\%)$$

$$= ([Hb] \times 1.34 \times S\bar{v}O_2) +$$

$$(P\bar{v}O_2 \times 0.003\ vol\%/torr)$$

$$= (16\ g\% \times 1.34 \times 85\%) +$$

$$(70\ torr \times 0.003\ vol\%/torr)$$

$$= 18.22\ vol\% + 0.21\ vol\%$$

$$= 18.43\ vol\%$$

STEP 5: Set up the shunt equation.

$$\frac{\dot{Q}_S}{\dot{Q}_T} = \frac{Cc'O_2 - CaO_2}{Cc'O_2 - C\bar{v}O_2}$$

$$= \frac{23.4\ vol\% - 22.94\ vol\%}{23.4\ vol\% - 18.43\ vol\%}$$

$$= \frac{0.46\ vol\%}{4.97\ vol\%}$$

$$= 0.093,\ or\ 9.3\%$$

(1:930), (10:272), (17:46–50).

### IIIC5

85. D. The patient is elderly and has brittle, demineralized bones. CPT, which includes postural drainage, percussion (clapping), vibration, and coughing might result in iatrogenic fractures (i.e., "cough fractures"). This complication generally occurs with ribs 6 to 9 (usually the seventh rib) along the posterior, mid-axillary line. Sudden onset of a sharp, localized pain in this area while coughing during CPT warrants a STAT chest X-ray to rule out or confirm fracture(s) as the most likely cause of such an elderly patient's pain.

(16:507).

### IIIA2d

86. B. A hazard of aerosol therapy is bronchospasm, especially when using ultrasonic nebulizers. The therapy should be terminated (based on the breath sounds, pulse, and respirations), and the physician should be notified. A bronchodilator would be appropriate. A physician's order or preapproved protocol is required, however.

(*Respiratory Care* 40:1300–1307, 1995).

### IIIA1f

87. C. The following graphic illustrates the various components of a pulmonary artery catheter (PAC) waveform as the balloon tip of the catheter is being inflated to obtain a recording of the pulmonary capillary wedge pressure (PCWP) (Figure 5-27).

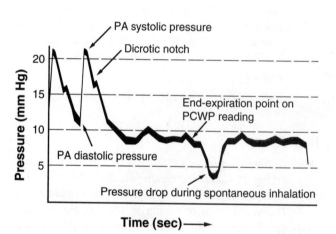

**Figure 5-27:** Components of a pulmonary artery catheter (PAC) waveform with the catheter in the wedge position. Note the pressure drop during spontaneous inspiration (arrow).

The first two pressure waves represent the pressure changes occurring within the pulmonary artery. The highest reading is the PA systolic (PAs) pressure. The dicrotic notch represents the closing of the pulmonic valve, and the lowest pressure is the PA diastolic (PAd) pressure. The RRT then inflates the balloon on the distal tip of the PA catheter to obtain the PCWP tracing. The PCWP's a, c, and v waves (representing atrial contraction, closure of the mitral valve, and filling of the left atrium, respectively) are difficult to see on most PCWP tracings. During a spontaneous inhalation, the drop in intrathoracic pressure is transmitted to the thoracic blood vessels and heart. This pressure drop causes the fall in pressure seen during the PCWP tracing.

Normal values for the PAs, PAd, and PCWP are listed as follows.

| Pressure | Normal Range |
|----------|--------------|
| PA systolic | 15 to 30 mm Hg |
| PA diastolic | 10 to 15 mm Hg |
| PCWP a/v | less than 12 to 15 mm Hg |
| PCWP (mean) | 4 to 12 mm Hg |

*All* PAC pressure readings should be obtained at end-exhalation, because this point in the ventilatory cycle is where intrathoracic pressure closely approaches atmospheric pressure and ventilatory artifacts are minimal.

(1:946–948), (9:349–354), (10:125–127).

### IIIE2b

88. A. Studies have shown an increase in exercise tolerance and endurance following a 10-week pulmonary rehabilitation program. Positive changes in pulse, ventilation, and anaerobic threshold have been noted. Also, after rehabilitation, a number of patients reported a reduction in respiratory symptoms and an increased level of physical activity. These outcomes have led to improved self-esteem and psychological function.

(1:1094–1095), (15:1148–1149), (16:882–883).

### IIIC7a

89. B. Impingement of the suction catheter on the carina during ET suctioning can initiate the vagal reflex. The vagal reflex results in bradycardia and hypotension. Tachycardia can occur during the suctioning procedure if hypoxemia develops. Inadequate preoxygenation or prolonged suction catheter insertion and the application of suction can reduce the arterial $PO_2$, thereby increasing the rate of myocardial contraction. Similarly, patient anxiety can result in tachycardia.

(1:154, 286).

### IIIE2d

90. A. Because the patient will be using oxygen on a limited basis, it will be cost-effective to use an oxygen concentrator. A liquid oxygen system would be too costly because the oxygen will be used for only a short time. Although the liquid oxygen remained unused during the day, substantial volumes of it would vaporize, vent, and be wasted. A compressed oxygen gas cylinder would be useful as a backup system to the concentrator in the event of a concentrator malfunction or power outage.

(1:1115–1116), (16:896–897).

### IIIB1c

91. D. Hearing inspiratory stridor via auscultation of the lateral neck and noting that the patient has a hoarse voice following ET extubation are common occurrences. The inspiratory stridor might be a harbinger of severe subglottic edema. Therefore, administering nebulized racemic epinephrine is often useful in reducing the inflammation in the glottic and subglottic regions. Dexamethasone is sometimes given in these circumstances, although its utility is doubtful because corticosteroids generally require longer than 12 hours to take effect.

Most patients who have been endotracheally intubated will experience some degree of laryngeal edema, which can usually be ascertained by (1) complaints of a sore throat, (2) inspiratory stridor heard via auscultation of the neck, and (3) hoarseness or loss of voice.

(1:312, 988), (15:564–565), (16:443–444).

### IIIA1b

92. B. An adequately "arterialized" capillary sample should correlate well with arterial pH, $PCO_2$, and base excess. The $PO_2$ of a capillary sample correlates minimally with the $PO_2$ in arterial blood, however. Additionally, the difference between the two values becomes greater as the arterial $PO_2$ increases.

(*Respiratory Care* 39:1180–1183, 1994), (9:226–227), (16:271).

### IIIA1g

93. B. To calculate the anion gap, one needs to know the patient's serum sodium, chloride, and bicarbonate values (the additional use of serum potassium is optional). These measurements are found only in the serum electrolyte profile in the patient's chart.

The anion gap provides a basis for determining the cause of metabolic acidosis. Quantitatively, the anion gap is the difference between the sodium ion concentration and the sum of the bicarbonate and chloride ion concentrations. The bicarbonate ion concentration is estimated from the total blood carbon dioxide, or $[(PaCO_2 \times 0.03) + HCO_3^-] = TCO_2$. The anion gap $(A^-)$ equation reads as follows:

$$A^- = [Na^+] - ([TCO_2] + [Cl^-])$$

Inserting the normal values for these factors, we can calculate the $A^-$ (anion gap).

$$A^- = 142 \text{ mEq/liter} - (27 \text{ mEq/liter} + 103 \text{ mEq/liter})$$

$$= 12 \text{ mEq/liter}$$

The normal range is 12 to 14 mEq/liter. An anion gap greater than 14 mEq/liter signifies an increase in blood fixed acids. An $A^-$ less than 12 mEq/liter is rare.

Based on the anion gap concept, two types of metabolic acidoses can develop. One results from a loss of bicarbonate (base) and is associated with a normal anion gap (12 to 14 mEq/liter). The other is caused by the presence of increased fixed acids in the blood, which leads to a high anion gap (greater than 14 mEq/liter).

(1:274), (4:249), (1:125–126).

### IIIE1j

94. C. This patient has developed a pneumothorax. The progressively increasing PIPs causes suspicion. The PIP continuously rises as portions of the delivered tidal volume leak into the intrapleural space, resulting in ensuing breaths being deposited into a compressed left lung. Physical assessment of the thorax reveals diminished left upper-lobe air movement and hyperresonant percussion notes. These findings are characteristic of a pneumothorax. Treatment involves having chest tubes inserted into the upper region on the affected side—specifically, along either the mid-axillary or posterior axillary lines between the sixth and seventh intercostal space on the left side.

(1:485–486), (9:92–93), (15:1090).

### IIIA1b

95. B. The right brachiocephalic (innominate) artery leaves the aortic arch just before the ductus arteriosus attaches to the aorta. This artery perfuses the head and right arm. Hence, a transcutaneous oxygen ($PtcO_2$) electrode placed on the right upper chest quadrant is the most appropriate site to measure preductal oxygen tension. A $PtcO_2$ electrode placed on the left side of the neonate's body would reflect postductal oxygen tension. A preductal oxygen tension greater than postductal oxygen tension is indicative of right-to-left intracardiac shunting of blood through a patent ductus arteriosus.

(15:496), (18:225).

### IIIC3a

96. D. Patients who are chronic $CO_2$ retainers should judiciously receive $O_2$ therapy because they potentially can have their hypoxic drive obliterated. Some $CO_2$ retainers maintain their spontaneous ventilation via the hypoxic drive, elicited through the stimulation of the carotid and aortic bodies. If the arterial $PO_2$ is elevated in these patients to the extent of eliminating the peripheral chemoreceptor stimulation, these patients will hypoventilate or stop breathing. Increased levels

of $CO_2$ in the blood and cerebrospinal fluid no longer serve as a sufficient stimulus to the central chemoreceptors.

Therefore, it is extremely important to use a high-flow oxygen-delivery device (e.g., an air-entrainment mask) to administer a precise, constant, and low oxygen concentration. Low-flow oxygen-delivery systems, such as the nasal cannula, simple mask, and partial rebreathing mask, do not deliver precise and constant $O_2$ concentrations when the patient's ventilatory pattern, ventilatory rate, and tidal volume change.

For example, a patient who has a regular and constant ventilatory pattern, a ventilatory rate of fewer than 25 breaths/min., and a tidal volume between 300 and 700 ml receiving $O_2$ via a nasal cannula operating at 2 L/min. would be expected to receive an $FIO_2$ of 0.28. If the patient's minute ventilation decreased, however (↓ ventilatory rate and/or ↓$V_T$), the $FIO_2$ delivered by the nasal cannula at 2 L/min. would increase. The converse is likewise true.

(1:742), (16:375, 1124).

### IIIB2c

97. C. An appropriate initial negative-pressure setting for a patient who is to be ventilated via a chest cuirass would be $-20$ cm $H_2O$. The negative pressure would then be adjusted, following clinical assessment of the patient, to ensure adequate ventilation.

(10:7, 190), (13:570, 571).

### IIIB1c

98. B. There are two general categories of adrenergic receptors: alpha and beta. In turn, two subtypes of these exist. For example, alpha-one adrenergic receptors are generally located on the postsynaptic membrane and produce vasoconstriction. The alpha-two receptors are considered to be located on the presynaptic membrane of peripheral sympathetic nerves and act as a negative feedback mechanism, turning off the release of the neurotransmitter norepinephrine. In the central nervous system, the alpha-two receptors are thought to reside on the postsynaptic membrane.

The beta-one and beta-two adrenergic receptors cause positive inotropism and positive chronotropism and bronchodilatation, respectively. Racemic epinephrine stimulates the alpha-one adrenergic receptors, thereby causing vasoconstriction. Metaproterenol and albuterol cause bronchodilatation by primarily stimulating $\beta$-2 receptors and are therefore not useful for the condition described here.

(1:442, 480), (15:178).

99. B. Steady-state exercise tests and progressive multi-stage, steady-state exercise tests constitute the two types of exercise protocols that are used. Steady-state protocols are intended to evaluate cardiopulmonary physiologic activity during a constant metabolic demand. Steady state is achieved after the subject has performed an exercise at a constant workload for 5 to 8 minutes. The physiologic functions that ordinarily define the steady state are the (1) oxygen consumption, (2) ventilation, and (3) heart rate.

Progressive, multi-stage exercise tests involve the use of plateau-like increases in the workload throughout the test. The incremental changes in the workload are generally instituted every 1 to 3 minutes without necessarily permitting a steady state to be achieved. The purpose of this protocol is to obtain values for the maximum oxygen consumption ($\dot{V}O_2max$), the maximum heart rate, and the maximum ventilation.

Exercise workload is varied by using either a cycle ergometer or a treadmill. The cycle ergometer provides for the adjustment of the workload by changing the resistance and frequency of pedaling. On the other hand, the treadmill enables the alteration of the workload by manipulating the speed and percent grade of the walking platform. Therefore, a treadmill at a speed of 5 miles per hour with a 10% grade initially established, followed by a 2% incremental grade increase every three minutes, constitutes a progressive, multi-stage exercise protocol. This type protocol permits the $\dot{V}O_2max$, the maximum heart rate, and the maximum ventilation to be measured. A steady state would likely be achieved with (1) a cycle ergometer at 50 watts for 10 minutes, (2) a constant-grade treadmill with increasing speeds every eight minutes, and (3) a cycle ergometer at 50 watts for eight minutes.

(1:1092), (16:242–245).

100. C. The complete blood count (CBC) supplies the RRT with a number of important values relating to the patient's blood. These values and the clinical significance of their alterations are summarized in Table 5-9.

Frequently, physicians and other health-care providers use a form of shorthand to record the patient's current values. Using this shorthand convention and Table 5-9, decide the clinical significance of the following entry in a patient's chart. This patient has an elevated RBC, Hb, and Hct. This finding is common in patients who have chronic hypoxia or in patients who have hemoconcentration caused by an inadequate parenteral administration of I.V. fluids. The elevation in the WBC could indicate the presence of an infection. Correlation with other signs and symptoms is indicated.

(1:332–333), (9:99–102), (16:178).

101. C. Positive expiratory pressure (PEP) mask therapy is a bronchial hygiene technique that requires the patient to breathe against some level of positive pressure during exhalation. Following a slow, deep inspiration with a one to three second inspiratory pause, the patient exhales slowly against a resistance, attempting to achieve an I:E ratio of approximately 1:3.

The physiologic theory is that the slow, deep inspirations and momentary breath-hold enables a more uniform distribution of inspired air. Furthermore, this breathing pattern is intended to have air move behind airway obstructions. The prolonged exhalations against a fixed resistance is expected to help move tracheobronchial secretions from the smaller and/or midsized airways to the larger airways, facilitating expectoration.

**Table 5-9** Complete Blood Count Values and Significance

| Test | Normals | Clinical Significance |
| --- | --- | --- |
| Red Blood Cells (RBC) | Male: 4.6–6.2 3 $10^6$/mm³ Female: 4.2–5.4 3 $10^6$/mm³ | Oxygen transport is decreased in the presence of a reduced RBC count. Chronic hypoxia (altitude or COPD) will result in an increase in the RBC count. |
| Hemoglobin (Hb) | 14.5–16.5 g/dl | Oxygen transport is decreased in the presence of a decreased Hb. Chronic hypoxia (altitude or COPD) will result in an increase in the Hb concentration. |
| Hematocrit (Hct) | Male: 40%–50% Female: 38%–47% | If there is inadequate fluid intake, hemoconcentration might occur (Hct will be high). If too much fluid is administered, hemodilution will occur, and the Hct will be low. The Hct will increase if the Hb is increased (by a 3:1 ratio). |
| White blood cells (WBC) | 4.5–10 K/mm³ | If the WBC is high, it is indicative of an infection. If the WBC is low, the patient will have a reduced immunity. |

The patient is instructed to take 10 to 20 PEP breaths in the manner just described and then perform huffing. In the course of one PEP therapy session, 10 to 20 PEP breaths are repeated about 4 to 6 times. The PEP therapy session should not be longer than 20 minutes.

(NBRC Horizons, March/April, Vol. 19, No. 2, 1993), (1:807–810), (16:516, 534).

## IIIB1b

102. B. The percent relative humidity (%RH) is as important as the actual humidity in heated-wire circuits. When the heated-wire temperature is excessively greater than the humidifier temperature, the %RH will drop. Inadequate %RH will increase evaporation from the trachea and larger airways, leading to inspissated secretions and mucous plugging.

(13:114–115), (15:794).

## IIIA2a(2)

103. B. Atelectasis is characterized from a physical assessment standpoint by (1) rapid and shallow breathing, (2) decreased to absent breath sounds, (3) decreased to absent vocal fremitus, (4) dullness to percussion, (5) cyanosis, and (6) mediastinal shift to the affected side.

Crackles are discontinuous sounds heard during inspiration and exhalation as air flows through airways partially filled with secretions, for example. Inspiratory crackles are often categorized as either early inspiratory crackles or late inspiratory crackles. Early inspiratory crackles are heard early during inspiration or originate from proximal bronchi that close during exhalation when an increase in bronchial compliance is experienced or when retractive pressures around the bronchi are low. Early inspiratory crackles are not related to atelectasis.

Late inspiratory crackles tend to arise from peripheral alveoli and airways that close during exhalation when intrathoracic pressure increases. These crackles are heard when these collapsed structures pop open late in the inspiratory phase. Late inspiratory crackles are associated with atelectasis. Therefore, if the amount of late inspiratory crackles decreases, the likelihood is atelectasis is decreasing.

Vocal fremitus is perceived during palpation and decreases when atelectasis is present. Bronchial breath sounds are heard over the trachea.

(1:308–309, 311–314), (9:85–86).

## IIIB4a

104. D. After the initiation of the PEEP of 10 cm $H_2O$, the patient displayed hypoxemia (as reflected by the arterial $PO_2$ of 68 torr). In fact, the rationale for administering the PEEP of 10 cm $H_2O$ was to relieve the hypoxemia.

The additional PEEP exceeded the optimum level, however, because the C.O. dropped from 5.1 L/min. to 2.4 L/min. while the arterial $PO_2$ decreased further and the $PaCO_2$ increased. Evidently, the additional PEEP decreased the lung compliance significantly enough to adversely affect the arterial $PCO_2$, rendering the patient more hypoxemic and creating cardiovascular embarrassment.

The RRT should reduce the PEEP back to 5 cm $H_2O$ in an attempt to lower the mean intrathoracic pressure and to improve the C.O. At the same time, reducing the PEEP is intended to increase lung compliance and return the arterial $CO_2$ to normal. The $FIO_2$ should then be elevated to try to relieve the hypoxemia.

(1:880, 879, 901–902), (15:725–727).

## IIIB2c

105. C. Pressure-control ventilation (PCV) is a time-cycled, pressure-limited, volume-variable mode of mechanical ventilation. The clinician establishes a preset pressure that is attained rapidly and early during the inspiratory phase. This preset pressure is sustained throughout inspiration by adjusting the inspiratory flow rate. After a predetermined time, inspiration ends.

PCV might be useful in lowering the PIP in patients who are receiving a high $FIO_2$ and a moderate to high level of PEEP. PCV and PC-IRV might also improve the $PaO_2$ in these patients.

(1:837, 878, 900–901), (10:198–199, 214–215).

## IIIA2b

106. D. Neither the $PaCO_2$ nor the $HCO_3^-$ value is consistent with the pH. Both the $PaCO_2$ (44 torr) and the $HCO_3^-$ (24 mEq/liter) are normal. Therefore, an acidemic pH is impossible. The blood gas analyzer should be calibrated, or perhaps the pH electrode should be checked.

(1:268–270), (9:127–128).

## IIIC5

107. A. The inspiratory volume must increase to facilitate bronchial hygiene. Because no mention is made of the efficiency of IS administration in this example, one can assume that minimal attention was given to the patient's breathing pattern. Diaphragmatic breathing exercises, in conjunction with IS, should be attempted before more costly and hazardous modalities are used.

(1:775, 777), (16:529, 1034, 1153).

## IIIA2a(1)

108. C. The patient was administered an inappropriate oxygen device. He did not meet the low-flow oxygen-delivery system criteria: (1) a regular ventilatory pattern, (2) a ventilatory rate not greater than 25 breaths/min., and (3) a tidal volume of 300 to 700 cc. The patient's ventilatory pattern was irregular, and his ventilatory rate was 40 breaths/min. Therefore, he should have been given an air entrainment mask at a low $F_IO_2$, perhaps 0.24 to 0.28.

Under the conditions stipulated for a low-flow oxygen device, a cannula at 6 L/min. can be expected to deliver approximately 44% oxygen. With the clinical conditions presented here, the $FiO_2$ would be even greater because low-flow oxygen-delivery systems will provide a higher than predicted $FiO_2$ as the tidal volume ($V_T$) or ventilatory rate (i.e., minute ventilation or a $\dot{V}_E$), decreases.

The high oxygen concentration received by this COPD patient likely obliterated his hypoxic stimulus, causing hypercarbia and possibly $CO_2$ narcosis. It should be kept in mind that hypercapnia resulting from hyperoxia is usually *not* associated with a decreased minute ventilation. The belief is that ventilation–perfusion ratio changes have taken place. In particular, perfusion in excess of ventilation (shunt effect or venous admixture) develops.

(1:743–745, 754–756), (15:711–714, 876–877).

## IIIA1h

109. A. COPD patients, especially those who have pulmonary emphysema, use pursed-lip breathing to prevent air trapping. Expiratory resistance, or expiratory retard, is a mechanical means that mimics this breathing action. Adding expiratory resistance is thought to facilitate lung emptying and to minimize premature airway collapse.

In conjunction with mechanical ventilation, expiratory resistance enables a more complete emptying of the lungs by prolonging exhalation. Contrasted with PEEP, airway pressure returns to atmospheric levels when expiratory resistance is used. When expiratory resistance is instituted, the patient's FRC is not increased as it is with PEEP.

(10:88, 225), (16:649, 657–658).

## IIIB4a

110. B. The $PaCO_2$ will decrease with an increase in the tidal volume or the ventilatory rate. An increase in the IPAP will increase the tidal volume. Therefore, increasing the IPAP is the appropriate change for this patient. If the ventilatory rate is increased to 20 breaths/

min., the $PaCO_2$ will be lowered too much. It would decrease to approximately 34 mm Hg.

(1:866, 1127), (10:217), (16:673–674, 1121).

## IIIE2b

111. D. Exercising ventilatory muscles increases muscle strength and endurance. This improvement certainly would promote increased activities of daily living and would likely improve the patient's cardiopulmonary status. A number of studies have reported a decrease in hospitalizations and better control of infections by patients after completion of a pulmonary rehabilitation program.

(1:1092), (15:1139–1151), (16:879).

## IIIE2a

112. C. Home respiratory therapy equipment must be clean and disinfected to be eliminated as a source of patient infection. The recommended procedure is as follows:

1. Completely disassemble the equipment.
2. Wash in cool water to loosen attached debris if applicable.
3. Soak the equipment in warm soapy water for a few minutes.
4. Scrub the equipment of adhering material if applicable.
5. Rinse the equipment of residual soap.
6. Immerse the equipment in the disinfectant solution, usually a vinegar solution, for at least 15 minutes.
7. Rinse the disinfectant from the equipment and allow equipment to dry.

(1:1136–1137).

## IIIA1h

113. A. The sigh mode on a mechanical ventilator is designed to mimic the normal sigh mechanism of a normal, spontaneously breathing person. Physiologically, a sigh represents a hyperinflation of the lungs to periodically expand the lungs beyond the normal, resting tidal volume to prevent the development of microatelectasis. A normal, spontaneously breathing person usually sighs a few times each hour.

Some patients who are mechanically ventilated at low lung volumes receive sigh breaths that range between 1.5 to 2.0 times the delivered tidal volume. Patients who receive large mechanical tidal volumes (10 to 15 ml/kg) do not require sighs because the larger than tidal volume breaths sufficiently distend the lungs, thus avoiding the problem of atelectasis.

The patient in this problem was receiving a low tidal volume (600 ml or 8 ml/kg). Therefore, it was clinically acceptable to provide him with a sigh breath 1.5 times his tidal volume (i.e., 900 ml). When the order was received to increase the tidal volume to 12 ml/kg (165 lbs ÷ 2.2 lbs/kg = 75 kg), or 900 ml (12 ml/kg × 75 kg = 900 ml) at a rate of 12 breaths/min., however, periodic hyperinflations or sighs became unnecessary.

(1:847–848, 903), (10:225, 248), (15:969).

## IIIC1c

114. D. The RRT should approach the patient from the back side, place her fist on the patient's epigastrium, place her other hand on top of the hand held in a fist, and apply successive compressions to the epigastrium until the patient is relieved. Essentially, the practitioner should perform the Heimlich maneuver in this situation.

It is also imperative to instruct pulmonary emphysema patients not to generate a cough from the maximum end-inspiratory (total lung capacity) position. Rather, coughing from the mid-inspiratory position might prevent the buildup of too great an intrathoracic pressure, thus preventing airway collapse.

Pulmonary emphysema patients ordinarily need to avoid generating deep coughs to prevent dynamic compression of the airways. The rapid ascent of the diaphragm elevates the intrapleural pressure to supra-atmospheric levels, resulting in air trapping. The air trapping can occur beyond the equal pressure point in the airways. During a forced exhalation (i.e., deep coughing), an equal pressure point develops in the tracheobronchial tree. At this point, the extraluminal pressure (intrapleural pressure) equals the intraluminal pressure. Airway collapse can occur beyond this equal pressure point where the extraluminal pressure exceeds the intraluminal pressure.

(15:664).

## IIIB4b

115. C. An inspiratory hold maneuver is a mechanical means of sustaining lung inflation at end inspiration. The duration of the sustained inflation varies from one to two seconds. During this time, the delivered volume is allowed to become distributed throughout the lungs, especially to those regions that have large time constants (compliance times resistance = time constant). Affording this additional time for air distribution enhances gas exchange in otherwise poorly ventilated areas, thereby potentially improving oxygenation.

(10:85, 146, 213), (15:243–244).

## IIIA1d

116. C. The intake–output record clearly demonstrates a fluid imbalance indicative of overhydration. In addi-

tion, patients who are overhydrated will demonstrate an elevation in the pulmonary capillary wedge pressure (PCWP) and a fall in pulmonary compliance, illustrated in this example by the increasing PCWP and PIP.

(1:926), (9:314).

## IIIB2d

117. D. The application of independent lung ventilation is without clinical guidelines. Clinical practice has demonstrated a few pathophysiologic conditions that have responded favorably to this mode of ventilation, however. These conditions include (1) massive hemoptysis, (2) bronchopleural fistula, (3) severe unilateral lung disease, and (4) single lung transplant patients.

(1:829).

## IIID1c

118. B. According to the American Heart Association Guidelines 2000 for Cardiopulmonary Resuscitation and Emergency Cardiovascular Care, the recommendation for pediatric defibrillation is 2 joules/kg for the initial defibrillation and 4 joules/kg for each ensuing defibrillation. Therefore, a child weighing 35 pounds should receive 32 joules of energy for an initial defibrillation effort. The following calculations outline how this energy level is determined.

STEP 1: Convert the body weight expressed in lbs to kg.

$$\frac{35 \text{ lbs}}{2.2 \text{ lbs/kg}} = 15.9 \text{ kg}$$

STEP 2: Calculate the energy level in joules that is recommended for an initial pediatric defibrillation.

$$(15.9 \text{ kg})(2 \text{ joules/kg}) = 31.9 \text{ joules}$$

For adults, the recommended guidelines for defibrillation of a cardiac arrest caused by ventricular fibrillation are (1) 200 joules for the first attempt, (2) 200 to 300 joules for the second, and (3) 360 joules thereafter.

("Guidelines 2000 for Cardiopulmonary Resuscitation and Emergency Cardiovascular Care," 2000, American Heart Association, page I–91 and I–291 to I–292).

## IIIC3a

119. B. This patient's ABGs reveal a chronic $CO_2$ elevation. From inspection of the pH, it is evident that the $CO_2$ change was not acute. For example, had the arterial $PCO_2$ risen rapidly to 70 torr, the pH would have been 7.22 ± 0.03. Because the measured pH is 7.32 and the

bicarbonate level has increased, a chronic elevation of the arterial $PCO_2$ has taken place (i.e., the patient exhibits a chronic [compensated] respiratory acidosis).

Administering a high $FIO_2$ via a non-rebreather mask has caused oxygen-induced hypoventilation, signified by the patient's lethargy and ABG data (i.e., corrected hypoxemia and substantial hypercapnia). Therefore, it is indicated that the patient receive a low concentration of oxygen via a high-flow oxygen-delivery system, an air entrainment mask at 30% oxygen.

A nasal cannula is a low-flow oxygen-delivery device. It is inappropriate here because the patient is hypoventilating. Under ideal conditions, a nasal cannula will deliver about 32% oxygen at 3 L/min. In the situation described here, the nasal cannula would provide an $FIO_2$ greater than 0.32 because the patient has a lower minute ventilation. For low-flow oxygen-delivery devices, the $FIO_2$ is inversely related to the patient's minute ventilation.

(1:742), (16:375, 1124).

## IIIB2d

120. C. Independent lung ventilation (ILV) has been proved clinically beneficial in treating (1) massive hemoptysis, (2) bronchopleural fistula, and (3) severe unilateral pneumonia or lung infection. The use of ILV is generally reserved for patients with whom conventional measures have proved fruitless.

(1:829).

## IIIE1a

121. A. If a patient is to undergo a biopsy during bronchoscopy, a number of evaluations need to be performed to determine the degree of risk for bleeding complications. Among the evaluations performed are:

- activated partial thromboplastin time (APTT)
- prothrombin time (PT)
- determination of liver disease
- history of malabsorption/malnutrition (associated anemias)
- complete clinical history
- determination of active bleeding during physical exam
- history of hemoptysis
- use of anticoagulants
- history of thromboembolism
- history of disseminated intravascular coagulapathy (DIC)

A detailed history directed toward the identification of bleeding disorders is paramount before a lung biopsy is performed during bronchoscopy.

(10:376), (15:629–630).

## IIIC6b

122. C. Based on the relationship between the $P_{plateau}$ and PIP, this patient likely needs to receive endotracheal suctioning. The PIP contains both elastic (compliance) and nonelastic (resistance) components of the work of breathing.

The difference between the PIP and the $P_{plateau}$ represents the pressure generated to overcome the airway resistance in the patient-ventilator system. The $P_{plateau}$ signifies the pressure residing in the lungs at the end of inspiration. This pressure is keeping the lungs inflated under no airflow conditions.

So, when the $P_{plateau}$ increases and the PIP increases but the PIP-$P_{plateau}$ difference remains constant, the patient's lungs are getting stiffer and compliance decreases. The converse is also true.

When the $P_{plateau}$ remains constant and the PIP increases, more pressure is generated to deliver volume to the lungs. Therefore, airway resistance has increased.

The patient in this problem experienced a progressive widening of the PIP-$P_{plateau}$ gradient (Table 5-10).

**Table 5-10**

| Time | PIP-$P_{plateau}$ |
|------|-------------------|
| 19:00 | 10 cm $H_2O$ |
| 20:00 | 14 cm $H_2O$ |
| 21:00 | 28 cm $H_2O$ |

Because the $P_{plateau}$ remained relatively constant (20 cm $H_2O$, 21 cm $H_2O$, and 22 cm $H_2O$) over the three-hour period and because the PIP rose significantly (30 cm $H_2O$, 35 cm $H_2O$, and 50 cm $H_2O$) during the same time, the patient experienced an increase in airway resistance. An increase in airway resistance can be caused by retained secretions or bronchospasm.

If the endotracheal tube were in the right mainstem bronchus, both the $P_{plateau}$ and PIP would be significantly elevated.

(1:937–938), (9:285–287), (10:257–259).

## IIIA2c

123. C. The volume-pressure tracing shown in this question indicates the patient is experiencing overdistention. Overdistention has occurred because the patient's lung capacity has been exceeded. Therefore, the application of more pressure to the patient's lung produces little to no further increase in volume. Essentially, a volume limit has been achieved.

A sudden decrease in the dynamic compliance along the terminal portion of inspiration signifies the point where the volume limit has been achieved. The decreased dynamic compliance at this point accounts for the characteristic appearance of this curve. The loop takes on a beak-like shape as end-inspiration approaches. This shape is described as "beaking."

Overdistension can cause volutrauma as most of the volume enters normal alveoli and creates over inflation. When overdistension occurs during pressure-targeted ventilation, the situation can be corrected by decreasing the pressure setting. The presence of overdistention can be corrected in volume-targeted ventilation by decreasing the volume setting.

In the situation presented with this question, the 70-kg asthmatic is receiving too high a tidal volume. Asthmatics experience overdistension because of air trapping associated with the pathophysiology of their condition. Consequently, if an asthmatic requires mechanical ventilation stemming from a irreversible acute episode, the tidal volume delivered should range from 8 to 10 cc/kg of ideal body weight. The patient presented in this problem is receiving a tidal volume of 12 cc/kg (850 cc ÷ 70 kg = 12 cc/kg). Therefore, to correct the overdistension experienced by the patient as demonstrated by the volume-pressure graphic, the tidal volume needs to be reduced.

The volume-pressure tracing shown in Figure 5-28 indicates the appearance of the graphic after the tidal volume was reduced to 700 cc. Also, notice the lower PIP.

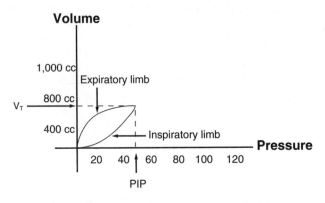

**Figure 5-28:** Volume-pressure loop after tidal volume has been reduced resulting in elimination of overdistention.

(10:236–237), (15:717)

## IIIA1l

124. A. The Fick equation can be used to determine the C.O.:

$$C.O. = \frac{\dot{V}_{O_2}}{CaO_2 - C\bar{v}O_2}$$

where

$C.O.$ = cardiac output (L/min.)
$\dot{V}_{O_2}$ = oxygen consumption (ml/min.)
$CaO_2 - C\bar{v}O_2$ = arterial-venous oxygen content difference (vol%)

Calculate the C.O. knowing that the $\dot{V}_{O_2}$ is 245 ml/min. and that the $CaO_2 - C\bar{v}O_2$ equals 6.0 vol%, or 6 ml $O_2$/100 ml plasma.

$$
\begin{aligned}
C.O. &= \frac{245 \text{ ml/min.}}{6 \text{ ml/100 ml}} \\
&= \frac{245 \text{ ml/minute}}{0.06} \\
&= 4,083 \text{ ml/min. or } 4.08 \text{ L/min.}
\end{aligned}
$$

If the arterial–venous oxygen content ($CaO_2 - C\bar{v}O_2$) is known, and if the oxygen consumption ($\dot{V}_{O_2}$) is also known, the C.O. can be calculated according to the Fick equation.

(1:225–226, 930), (9:298).

## IIIC7b

125. D. Endotracheal suctioning has the potential for a number of complications, including hypoxemia, dysrhythmias, hypotension, and lung collapse. If the suction catheter is too large for the ET tube, it might increase the incidence of some of these complications. For adults and older children the diameter of the suction catheter should not be more than one-half to two-thirds the inner diameter of the ET tube. The original suction catheter used (16 Fr) was too large. A 12 Fr catheter is a more appropriate size.

When suctioning neonates, the guideline that the suction catheter should be no larger than one-half to two-thirds of the internal diameter of the ET tube does not apply. The internal diameter of a neonatal ET tube is rather small. Therefore, using a suction catheter one-half to two-thirds that size would require the suction catheter to be extremely small. Such a small suction catheter would render suctioning difficult. Consequently, the largest possible suction catheter that can easily fit down the neonatal ET tube should be used.

(1:618), (13:182), (16:604).

## IIIA1m(3)

126. D. It would be appropriate at this time to simply monitor and evaluate the patient's response to the CPAP of 10 cm $H_2O$. Furthermore, the actions listed (other than D) are inappropriate. Lowering the CPAP level would be premature because it was just begun. Actually, the CPAP seemed to have reduced the C.O. significantly (i.e., from 13 L/min. to 6 L/ min.). The C.O. of 13

L/min. was likely a response to the patient's cardiopulmonary status. He was extremely hypoxemic ($PaO_2$ 45 torr). Both the heart rate and C.O. increase in the presence of hypoxemia. Fortunately, the person's youth is responsible for his tremendous cardiopulmonary reserve.

The C.I. while on CPAP is normal. Therefore, a volume expander is not indicated. The elimination of hypoxemia has diminished the hypoxic stimulus that was stimulating the heart to work harder. Additionally, the CPAP of 10 cm $H_2O$ might have elevated the mean intrathoracic pressure somewhat and reduced the venous return, contributing to the decreased C.O. and a normalization of the C.I. The formula for the C.I. is as follows:

$$C.I. = \frac{C.O.}{BSA}$$

The patient's arterial $PO_2$ of 80 torr on a CPAP of 10 cm $H_2O$ is acceptable, especially in light of the 7.42 pH. Based on the oxyhemoglobin dissociation curve, these data reflect an arterial oxygen saturation ($SaO_2$) of about 95%. Therefore, it is unnecessary to consider raising the $FiO_2$.

Last, the patient's ABG and acid-base status are essentially normal. Sedating this patient is contraindicated because he is maintaining a sufficient cardiopulmonary status. This patient's work of breathing has already been significantly reduced since the CPAP was initiated. Furthermore, sedation could likely induce ventilatory failure. Again, at this time it is appropriate to monitor this patient and evaluate his response to therapy.

(1:783), (9:309, 314–315), (15:724–728).

## IIIC6a

127. D. When an oral endotracheal tube either migrates or is inserted into the right mainstem bronchus, the right lung receives the entire mechanically delivered tidal volume while the left lung receives essentially no ventilation. Auscultatory findings of this condition reveal diminished or no breath sounds on the left side. Breath sounds on the right side can be heard, of course, because all the volume is being delivered to the right lung. Inspection generally demonstrates little or no chest wall movement on the left side because the left lung is virtually deprived of ventilation. The right lung will receive ventilation. Because of the disparity between the tidal volumes of the two lungs, asymmetrical chest wall movement tends to occur.

(15:834–835).

## IIIC7a

128. A. A number of complications can arise from endotracheal suctioning. One of them, bradycardia, is caused by the vagal-vagal reflex. When the suction catheter impinges upon the carina, the vagal-vagal reflex is stimulated. The consequence is generally bradycardia and a fall in blood pressure.

The patient in this problem experienced a decrease in heart rate from 80 beats/min. to 60 beats/min., or a fall of 20 beats/min. This drop in heart rate can be significant enough to compromise myocardial oxygenation, potentially causing a lethal dysrhythmia. The prudent action to take at this time is to terminate suctioning immediately and hyperoxygenate and hyperinflate the patient.

(1:619–620).

## IIIC5

129. C. Positive expiratory pressure (PEP) mask therapy is one type of therapy indicated for the mobilization of retained secretions in cystic fibrosis and chronic bronchitis patients. PEP mask therapy is a bronchial hygiene technique that can serve as an effective alternative to CPT to mobilize secretions. The patient places the mask tightly, but comfortably, over her mouth and nose. The patient is then instructed to relax and breathe deeply from the diaphragm. Exhalation is intended to be active, but not forced, by using a PEP of 10 to 20 cm $H_2O$. The patient takes 10 to 20 breaths through the mask, and then the mask is removed and the patient coughs to expectorate sputum. This treatment modality may be more cost-effective and provide more patient compliance than CPT.

(Malmeister, M., Fink, J., Hoffman, G., and Fifer, L., "Positive-Expiratory-Pressure Mask Therapy: Theoretical and Practical Considerations and a Review of the Literature," November 1991, *Respiratory Care, 36* (11), pp. 1218–1229), (AARC Clinical Practice Guidelines, "Use of Positive Airway Pressure Adjunct to Bronchial Hygiene Therapy," May 1993, *Respiratory Care, 38* (5), pp. 516–521).

## IIIA1m(2)

130. D. The end-tidal carbon dioxide tension ($PetCO_2$) is measured via capnography. Capnography is the measurement of carbon dioxide in exhaled gas. Ordinarily, gas is sampled from an adaptor located between the ventilator circuitry and the ET tube. The sample is analyzed either via infrared analysis or mass spectrometry.

Under normal and stable cardiovascular conditions, the $PetCO_2$ reflects the alveolar $CO_2$ tension ($PACO_2$), which in turn represents the arterial $CO_2$ tension ($PaCO_2$). The usual difference between the $PaCO_2$ and the $P_{ET}CO_2$ is less than 3 to 5 torr. This gradient widens as a result of the influence of a number of factors.

The $P_{ET}CO_2$ values are reported as either a partial pressure (normal range: 35 to 43 torr) or a percentage (normal range: 4.6% to 5.6%).

Capnography can provide for single-breath monitoring (tracing below), where Phase I represents the onset of exhalation (i.e., air from the anatomic dead space leaves the lungs). Note that Phase I gas is devoid of $CO_2$. The tracing begins an upward deflection in Phase II when $CO_2$ from the alveoli begins to mix with the remnant anatomic dead space gas. Phase III provides the actual $P_{ET}CO_2$ measurement as gas from the alveoli is exclusively exhaled.

Capnography can also be performed continuously at either a slow or fast speed, as represented in the following tracing (Figure 5-29, A–B).

The slow-speed tracing shows that five breaths were analyzed and that the end-tidal $CO_2$ value reached a level of about 5.3%. The fast-speed tracing illustrates the components of a single breath. Line a–b (upward deflection) is exhalation as measured $CO_2$ levels rise. Line b–c is the alveolar gas plateau. Line c–d (downward deflection) reflects inspiration as measured $CO_2$ levels decrease with fresh gas entering the lungs. Point C is the $P_{ET}CO_2$.

(1:363–365), (9:290), (10:101–102).

### IIIA1h

131. C. The formula that needs to be used to solve this problem is as follows:

*Current Values*      *Desired Values*

$$[(V_T - V_D) \times f]PaCO_2 = [(V_T - V_D) \times f]PaCo_2$$

where

    $V_T$ = tidal volume (cc)
    $V_D$ = dead space volume (cc)
     f = ventilatory rate (breaths/min.)
 $PaCO_2$ = arterial $CO_2$ tension (torr)

Because

$$V_T = V_D + V_A$$

where $V_A$ equals the alveolar volume (cc) and because

$$V_A = V_T - V_D$$

Multiplying $f \times V_A$ to obtain the alveolar ventilation ($\dot{V}_A$) can substitute for $V_T - V_D$ in the first formula

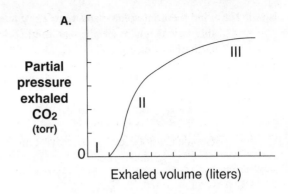

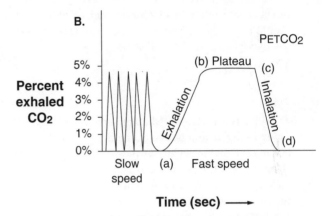

**Figure 5-29:** (A) Single-breath exhaled carbon dioxide tracing; exhaled carbon dioxide ($CO_2$) measurements begin to appear during Phase II and continue through Phase III. No exhaled $CO_2$ detected during Phase I. Phase I represents anatomic dead space. (B) Slow- and fast-speed capnograph tracings: slow-speed tracing analyzing end-tidal $CO_2$ during 5 normal breaths. Fast-speed tracing illustrates components of a single breath; Line a–b signifies exhalation, Line b–c is alveolar gas plateau, Line c–d indicates inspiration, and Point c represents the end-tidal $CO_2$ tension ($P_{ET}CO_2$).

presented here. Alternatively, the following equation can also be used:

$$\dot{V}_A \times PaCO_2 = \dot{V}_A \times PaCO_2$$

STEP 1:    Insert the values given in the problem and solve for the desired alveolar ventilation ($\dot{V}_A$).

$$[(800 \text{ cc} - 150 \text{ cc})10 \text{ bpm}]60 \text{ torr} = (\dot{V}_A)50 \text{ torr}$$

$$\frac{(6,500 \text{ cc/min.}) \, 60 \text{ torr}}{50 \text{ torr}} = \dot{V}_A$$

$$\frac{390,000 \text{ cc/min.}}{50} = \dot{V}_A$$

$$7,800 \text{ cc/min.} = \dot{V}_A$$

STEP 2:    Find the tidal volume and ventilatory rate that would render an alveolar ventilation ($\dot{V}_A$) of 7,800 cc/min.

Choice A: (750 cc − 150 cc)14 bpm = 8,400 cc/min.
Choice B: (800 cc − 150 cc)14 bpm = 9,100 cc/min.
Choice C: (800 cc − 150 cc)12 bpm = 7,800 cc/min.
Choice D: (850 cc − 150 cc)10 bpm = 7,000 cc/min.

An alveolar ventilation of 7,800 cc/min. or 7.80 L/min. would be provided by a tidal volume of 800 cc and a ventilatory rate of 12 breaths/min.

(10:250–251), (17:35–38).

## IIIB2c

132.  D. APRV is a mode somewhat similar to PC-IRV. APRV achieves ventilation by increasing the FRC and lowering the PIP and mean airway pressure. Compared with controlled continuous mechanical ventilation and PCV, APRV is associated with lowering PIP. It can produce an inverse ratio that might improve gas distribution in patients who have severely diminished lung compliance by decreasing physiologic dead-space ventilation and improving arterial oxygenation. The expiratory time of pressure release has to remain less than two seconds or else a decreased arterial $PO_2$ might be observed.

(East, T., "The Magic Bullets in the War on ARDS: Aggressive Therapy for Oxygen Failure," June 1993, *Respiratory Care, 38* (6), p. 692), (Lefebvre, D., and Stock, C., "Airway Pressure Release Ventilation, *Problems in Respiratory Care, 2* (1), pp. 61–68) (15:961–962).

## IIIA1b

133.  D. Air has a lower $PCO_2$ than arterial blood does. Therefore, the $CO_2$ will move from the blood to the gas bubble, lowering the $PaCO_2$. Room air has a $PO_2$ of about 150 mm Hg. This patient's $PaO_2$ should be greater than 250 mm Hg based on an $FIO_2$ of 0.40. This gradient will also lead to a net movement of oxygen from the blood to the air bubbles, lowering the $PaO_2$. There is likely to be a pH change that would be toward the alkalotic range because of the decreased $PaCO_2$.

(3:311), (4:27, 28).

## IIIA2a(4)

134.  B. A normal capnogram has the characteristic contour and features shown in Figure 5-30.

The shape of the capnogram changes with various clinical conditions. The specific changes in shape reflect certain clinical situations. Changes in the shape

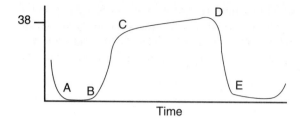

A-B:    Exhalation of $CO_2$—free gas from dead space.
B-C:    Combination of dead space and alveolar gas.
C-D:    Exhalation of mostly alveolar gas (alveolar plateau).
D:      "End-tidal": point—$CO_2$ exhalation at maximum point.
D-E:    Inhalation of $CO_2$—free gas.

**Figure 5-30:**   Normal, fast-speed $CO_2$ waveform highlighting tracing components.

of the capnogram can be used to detect (1) hyperventilation, (2) hypoventilation, (3) increased dead space ventilation, (4) changes in cardiac output, (5) recovery from a neuromuscular blocking agent, and (6) carbon dioxide retention.

The shape of the capnogram in the question can be interpreted as any of the following clinical conditions:

- cardiac arrest with continued alveolar ventilation
- hypotensive episode (e.g., hemorrhage)
- pulmonary embolism
- cardiopulmonary bypass

(1:366, 933), (4:296–300), (10:100–103).

## IIIC7a

135.  C. The patient is experiencing sinus bradycardia. This dysrhythmia is characterized by a heart rate of fewer than 60 beats/min. The RRT would likely cause no harm to the patient when applying suction because the suction catheter is withdrawn in approximately 10 seconds. This dysrhythmia is not uncommon; it sometimes develops in response to increased vagus nerve tone caused by the impingement of the suction catheter against the carina. Once the suction catheter is withdrawn, the patient must be hyperoxygenated and closely observed. Sinus bradycardia is frequently a transient occurrence associated with the suction procedure.

(1:326), (9:203), (16:858).

## IIIE1i

136.  A. To ascertain proper ET tube placement, the RRT must auscultate both sides of the chest wall along the mid-axillary lines. The sound of distinct air move-

ment indicates the likelihood of a properly placed ET tube. Additionally, auscultating over the epigastric region and perceiving no airflow sounds help substantiate that the ET tube has not been inserted into the esophagus.

Using capnometry to measure the end-tidal carbon dioxide tension ($P_{ET}CO_2$) lends evidence to determining the placement of an ET tube. For example, if the ET tube is situated in the trachea, the capnograph will render a reading of approximately 5.6% to 6.0%. On the other hand, if the ET tube has been inserted into the esophagus, a reading near 0% for the end-tidal $CO_2$ will be indicated. Ultimately, to definitively confirm that the ET tube is situated in the trachea appropriately, a portable chest radiograph must be performed.

(1:598, 606), (9:165–166).

## IIIE1e

137. B. A number of medications can be administered to relieve the anxiety of a patient who is about to experience bronchoscopy. Meperidine (Demerol) is a synthetic analgesic with morphine-like activity. It alleviates moderate to severe pain via action through the central nervous system.

Naloxone reverses ventilatory depression caused by narcotics. Lidocaine (1% to 4%) is used as a topical anesthetic during bronchoscopy. It is also given I.V. for its antidysrhythmic activity. Succinylcholine is a depolarizing neuromuscular blocking agent. Its use in conjunction with bronchoscopy is unwarranted because it would produce flaccid paralysis and require mechanical ventilation.

(1:623), (10:380) (15:630–632).

## IIIA2a(1)

138. B. Positive end-expiratory pressure (PEEP) has numerous physiologic effects. A number of them depend on the level of PEEP applied to the lungs as well as lung compliance. The intent of PEEP is usually to increase the arterial $PO_2$ by increasing the FRC and decreasing intrapulmonary shunting. In the process, however, it might have a variety of influences, including (1) a decreasing C.O., (2) a decreasing venous return, (3) an increasing intracranial pressure, and (4) an increasing pulmonary vascular resistance.

Lung compliance will change with the application of PEEP. PEEP improves lung compliance as long as alveoli are recruited. When additional PEEP is administered beyond the point of alveolar recruitment, lung compliance will decrease and the arterial $PO_2$ will fall. The sigmoid compliance curve shifts to the left, and alveoli become overdistended. The C.O. falls further, and the arterial $PO_2$ decreases. Ordinarily, the arterial

$PCO_2$ does not change, but with excessive PEEP it increases. Similarly, the work of breathing increases with excessive PEEP.

(1:880, 914), (9:316, 353), (10:267).

## IIIB1a

139. D. The decision to perform a tracheotomy or continue with ET intubation is not a clear one. Much controversy has centered on this dilemma. The duration of intubation has increased in recent years. Certain references adhere to a policy of " . . . if on the third day of intubation there is a reasonable chance for the patient not to need an artificial airway for an additional 72 hours, leave the endotracheal tube in place." If it is determined that the patient will definitely need an artificial airway, then a tracheotomy should be performed. This "guideline" is very much based on the patient's medical condition, however. The RRT should be cautious in forming absolute statements relative to this clinical question. Studies attempting to answer this question have shown that an absolute criterion cannot be established regarding when to perform a tracheotomy on an intubated patient.

(1:601), (16:599, 601).

## IIIB2c

140. B. Pressure control ventilation (PCV) is a volume-variable mode of ventilatory support. Inspiration is time initiated. During inspiration, a pre-established pressure is rapidly developed and maintained throughout inspiration. An adjusted inspiratory flow delivered by the ventilator is responsible for maintaining the pressure. At a preset time, inspiration ends (i.e., time cycled).

PCV appears to be most beneficial when applied to patients who have severe ARDS. It is generally implemented in conjunction with low control pressure, high flow rates, and inverse ratios. It is a primary indication for patients with ARDS when conventional ventilation and PEEP do not seem to be effective. PCV permits the clinician to use reduced PIP (recommending beginning with pressures one-half the PIP used with conventional ventilation) and PEEP settings while increasing mean airway pressure, which often improves oxygenation. The benefits of PCV are a potential reduction in the risk of barotrauma and improved oxygenation.

(1:837, 850, 875), (10:198–199).

## IIID1b

141. A. The ECG presented shows the occurrence of premature ventricular contractions (PVCs). A succession of PVCs can lead to the development of ventricular tachycardia or ventricular fibrillation. For some reason,

the ventricle begins to contract before the signal from the pacemaker (sinoatrial node) reaches the ventricle. The stroke volume and cardiac output are jeopardized when PVCs take place because the ventricle contracts before it has had sufficient time to fill. Furthermore, the strength of contraction of the PVC is suboptimal because the myocardial fibers are not adequately stretched before a PVC. Both of these circumstances compromise the stroke volume and cardiac output.

(1:330–331), (9:204–205).

### IIIA1f

142. D. Left-ventricular preload is defined as the amount of ventricular stretch occurring immediately prior to systole. This stretch is directly related to the amount of fluid within the ventricle and is inversely related to the elastic properties of the ventricle. Recall that as a muscle is stretched, the amount of tension that it can develop will increase. If the muscle is stretched too far, however, the amount of tension that it can develop will fall. The graph in Figure 5-31 illustrates this principle.

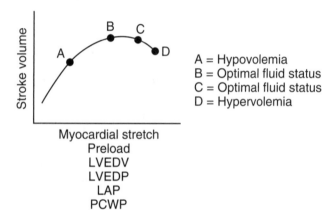

| | A = Hypovolemia |
| B = Optimal fluid status |
| C = Optimal fluid status |
| D = Hypervolemia |

Myocardial stretch
Preload
LVEDV
LVEDP
LAP
PCWP

**Figure 5-31:** Relationship between stroke volume and pulmonary capillary wedge pressure (PCWP). Point A fluids needed to optimize C.O. (hypovolemia and decreased stroke volume), Points B and C optimal fluid balance and optimal PCWP, and Point D hypervolemia and decreased stroke volume. *X* axis might also represent myocardial stretch, preload, LVEDV, LVEDP, and LAP.

This figure illustrates the relationship among left ventricular end-diastolic volume (LVEDV), left ventricular end-diastolic pressure (LVEDP), left atrial pressure (LAP), pulmonary capillary wedge pressure (PCWP), and stroke volume. The most clinically accessible pressure reading is the PCWP, and this reading is what is used to approximate the LVEDV and to gauge fluid administration in the patient. A patient who has the characteristics of stroke volume and PCWP shown at Point A would require more fluids to optimize his C.O. A patient at or between Points B and C would have an optimal fluid balance and PCWP. Finally, Point D

shows diminishing stroke volumes and represents hypervolemia. Diuretics are indicated for this stroke volume and PCWP combination.

(1:946–950), (9:354–358), (10:126–127).

### IIIB4a

143. C. This patient's $PaO_2$ of 120 mm Hg is more than adequate. In fact, it should be reduced because it is at least 20 mm Hg greater than the upper limit of normal.

In flail chest, it might be useful to further stabilize the chest wall, which can be achieved via PEEP or CPAP. A patient with flail chest does not necessarily have oxygenation problems. This patient has no lung parenchymal problem that can be helped by PEEP. If a pneumothorax is diagnosed, chest tubes should be used to evacuate air from the intrapleural space. In most instances of flail chest, mechanical ventilatory support is not needed. The presence of associated lung contusions, aspiration of gastric contents, and other injuries, however, dictates the course of treatment.

(1:550), (9:76, 260, 262), (10:135) (15:1077–1080).

### IIIB4b

144. C. Pressure-support ventilation (PSV) is a volume-variable mode of mechanical ventilation. It is a pressure-initiated mode. The patient generates an inspiratory effort that activates the ventilator. In response to the patient's effort, a rapid inspiratory flow develops through the system to rapidly attain and maintain a preset pressure. When the inspiratory flow rate falls to about 25% of its initial flow rate, inspiration terminates (i.e., flow cycled). The pressure-support level is adjusted by the RRT. The patient establishes his own inspiratory time, peak inspiratory flow, tidal volume, and ventilatory rate.

PSV is useful in assisting the patient's spontaneous breathing through an ET tube. It will overcome the resistance of the ventilator circuit and ET tube as well as any demand-valve ventilation systems that might be present. PSV also enables the patient to gradually build muscle strength during the weaning process without added work of the mechanical system.

PSV significantly reduces the work of breathing imposed on the respiratory system by demand-flow systems, ET tubes, and ventilatory circuitry. Therefore, PSV can be used in conjunction with SIMV to lessen the work of breathing. When these two ventilatory modes are used together, both PSV and SIMV function independently. In the process, PSV enables the patient to increase muscle strength during the weaning process.

(1:864, 910), (10:85, 199, 214), (15:960).

**IIIE1i**

145. B. When patients who are sedated or who have a reduced level of consciousness receive endotracheal intubation via the oral route, an assistant can help with the placement of the endotracheal tube by pressing the patient's larynx near the cricoid cartilage gently with two fingers.

This technique is called the Sellick maneuver and also helps prevent gastric contents from being aspirated because this technique causes the esophagus to be compressed.

(16:589–590).

**IIIB4a**

146. B. This patient has experienced carbon monoxide poisoning evidenced by a carboxyhemoglobin (COHb) level of 45%. Carbon monoxide interferes with oxygen transport by avidly binding to hemoglobin with an affinity of 210 times greater than oxygen. Despite the magnitude of hemoglobin's affinity for oxygen, oxygen continues to dissolve adequately in plasma as the arterial $PO_2$. In fact, it is the latter vehicle of oxygen transport that prevents the peripheral chemoreceptors (carotid and aortic bodies) from sending hyperventilatory signals to the medulla, helping make carbon monoxide such a lethal gas.

What is warranted in many cases of carbon-monoxide poisoning is a high concentration of oxygen to reduce the half-life of carbon monoxide bound to hemoglobin. In the situation presented here, the patient obviously has an adequate ventilatory drive because the arterial $PCO_2$ is 25 mm Hg and the ventilatory rate is 20 breaths/min. Therefore, intubation and mechanical ventilation would be premature interventions at this time.

The oxygen-delivery system capable of providing the highest $FiO_2$ should be used. Mask CPAP with 100% oxygen can certainly be the first choice because the patient has a sufficient spontaneous ventilatory status. Ideally, this patient would benefit from hyperbaric oxygenation at 2 to 3 ATA (atmospheres absolute) with a high oxygen concentration to reduce the half-life of carbon monoxide in the blood more quickly.

(1:229, 764–765), (9:126–127), (15:109, 328, 1107, 1109) (16:396, 1092).

**IIIC3a**

147. B. A simple oxygen mask is designed to accommodate a source flow of 5 to 10 L/min. Exceeding the flow limit of a device might cause inadequate humidification of the source gas. When the upper respiratory tract dehydrates, it is not uncommon for patients to complain of upper airway drying, irritation, and nonproductive coughing. An additional factor in this situation might be the water level in the humidifier. If it is

low, even more dry gas will be delivered to the patient's airway.

In this case, the RRT should ensure a proper water level in the humidifier, lower the oxygen flow rate, and monitor the patient. At the same time, the RRT must evaluate the patient's ventilatory status (tidal volume, ventilatory rate, and ventilatory pattern) to ensure that this patient meets the criteria for a low-flow oxygen-delivery device (simple mask). If this patient has a high minute ventilation ($V_T \times f = \dot{V}_E$), the $FiO_2$ delivered by the simple mask, even with the flow rate reduced, will be lower than the patient needs. For a low-flow oxygen-delivery system, as the minute ventilation increases, the $FiO_2$ decreases. The converse is also true. Additionally, the RRT needs to check the physician's orders for this patient's oxygen because the order might be inappropriate.

(1:663–664), (5:94), (13:104, 108, 119), (15:794–795).

**IIIA1i**

148. B. Positive pressure is being maintained in the continuous-flow IMV system throughout the ventilatory cycle. PEEP has been applied to this system; therefore the 12 cm $H_2O$ pressure registering on the pressure manometer on exhalation is expected and is not a problem. It is inappropriate for the pressure gauge to indicate 3 cm $H_2O$ pressure during spontaneous inspiration, however. The problem can be rectified by increasing the flow rate of the gas flowing through the IMV system.

Consequently, when this type of system is being set up, consideration must be given to the patient's inspiratory flow demands. Continuous-flow IMV systems should incorporate the use of a 3- to 5-liter gas reservoir bag. The gas flow rate should be at least four times the patient's own spontaneous minute ventilation (i.e., approximately ranging between 60 to 90 L/min.).

(1:861–863), (10:329–330), (15:1038–1039).

**IIIE1c**

149. C. Transtracheal aspiration is a specimen collection technique whereby a needle is inserted into the trachea through the cricothyroid membrane. Before the cricothyroid membrane is invaded, the skin area must be liberally anesthetized with local anesthetic. Once the trachea has been penetrated, a catheter is passed through the needle. The catheter can then be advanced into the lower respiratory tract. A syringe attached to the distal end of the catheter is used to aspirate and collect the specimen. This technique is useful for obtaining specimens that are not contaminated by passing through the upper airway.

(15:625), (16:1061).

**IIIC5**

150. C. The best schedule would be to give the albuterol therapy, followed by postural drainage and chest per-

cussion, at 7 A.M., 11 A.M., 3 P.M., and 7 P.M. The Atrovent could then be given at 9 A.M., 1 P.M., 5 P.M., and 9 P.M. to ensure that the patient was receiving a bronchodilator every two hours from 7 A.M. to 9 P.M. Albuterol is a preferential beta-two bronchodilator, whereas Atrovent is a cholenergic blocking agent. Both could safely be given at the same time, however, if desired.

(1:702), (16:1028, 1031).

## IIIA2a(2)

151. C. The following characteristics of a patient's cough are important to identify:

- dry or loose
- productive or nonproductive
- acute or chronic
- prevalence of occurrence (i.e., day or night)

A dry, non-productive cough is often associated with pulmonary fibrosis or congestive heart failure. On the other hand, a loose, productive cough tends to occur with bronchitis or asthma.

(1:298–299).

## IIIA1h

152. C. The mode of ventilation and associated settings causing the least elevation in the patient's mean intrathoracic pressure is IMV delivering a ventilatory rate of 6 breaths/min., along with 5 cm $H_2O$ PEEP and a tidal volume setting based on 15 cc/kg.

The number of positive pressure breaths is limited to six per minute. In between this mandatory positive pressure ventilatory rate, the patient is able to breathe spontaneously. A higher mandatory ventilation rate would enable fewer spontaneous breaths, thereby resulting in a comparatively higher mean intrathoracic pressure. Even with the addition of 5 cm $H_2O$ PEEP, a mandatory rate of 6 breaths/min. does not produce as high a mean intrathoracic pressure as does the SIMV mode at 10 breaths/min. Note that both the IMV and SIMV modes used 15 cc/kg for the tidal volume setting, and both employed a PEEP of 5 cm $H_2O$. Therefore, the difference between these two modes was the mandatory rate.

Adding pressure support to the SIMV (rate of 10 breaths/min.; 5 cm $H_2O$ PEEP; 15 cc/kg) causes a greater elevation of the mean intrathoracic pressure during the spontaneous breaths taken by the patient. Consequently, this additional mode of ventilation causes a larger elevation of the mean intrathoracic pressure than SIMV alone.

The controlled mechanical ventilation at a rate of 12 breaths/min. and 5 cm $H_2O$ of PEEP also would produce a higher mean intrathoracic pressure.

(1:861–863, 874), (15:957–960), (16:616).

## IIIA1e

153. A. The airway resistance in a patient–ventilator system can be approximated when the ventilator is operating with a square waveflow pattern. The following steps illustrate the method of calculation of the airway resistance.

STEP 1: Determine the pressure that was generated to overcome the airway resistance ($P_{Raw}$).

$$PIP - \text{plateau pressure} = P_{Raw}$$

$$50 \text{ cm } H_2O - 25 \text{ cm } H_2O = 25 \text{ cm } H_2O.$$

STEP 2: Convert the peak inspiratory flow rate of 60 L/min. to L/sec.

$$\frac{60 \text{ L/min.}}{60 \text{ sec./min.}} = 1 \text{ L/sec.}$$

STEP 3: Calculate the airway resistance by using the formula $R_{aw} = \dfrac{P_{Raw}}{\dot{V}}$.

$$\frac{25 \text{ cm } H_2O}{1 \text{ L/sec.}} = 25 \text{ cm } H_2O/\text{L/sec.}$$

(1:202, 938), (10:258), (15:89, 457–458).

## IIIA1d

154. B. The C.O. is the product of the stroke volume (ml/beat) and the heart rate (beats/min.). Note the following equation:

$$\text{stroke volume} \times \text{heart rate} = \text{C.O.}$$

$$60 \text{ ml/beat} \times 100 \text{ beats/min.} = 6,000 \text{ ml/min.}$$

Changing ml/min. to L/min., the C.O. becomes

$$\frac{6,000 \text{ ml/min.}}{1,000 \text{ ml/liter}} = 6.0 \text{ L/min.}$$

In addition to being designated as C.O., the C.O. can also be symbolized as $\dot{Q}_T$. The $\dot{Q}$ represents perfusion in units of volume per time (e.g., L/min.). The subscript "T" indicates the total C.O. The $\dot{Q}_T$ has two components: $\dot{Q}_S$ and $\dot{Q}_C$. These are related as follows:

$$\dot{Q}_T = \dot{Q}_S + \dot{Q}_C$$

where

$\dot{Q}_T$ = total C.O. (L/min.)

$\dot{Q}_S$ = shunted C.O. (L/min.)

$\dot{Q}_C$ = C.O. participating in gas exchange (L/min.)

(1:949), (9:276, 309), (10:118, 136).

## IIIA1m(2)

155. D. The Enghoff modification of the Bohr equation is used to calculate the mean exhaled carbon dioxide tension ($P\bar{E}CO_2$). The equation is as follows:

$$\frac{V_D}{V_T} = \frac{PaCO_2 - P\bar{E}CO_2}{PaCO_2}$$

STEP 1:  Convert the body weight expressed in kilograms (kg) to pounds (lbs).

$$(75 \text{ kg})(2.2 \text{ lbs/kg}) = 165 \text{ lbs.}$$

STEP 2:  Use the guideline stating that 1 lb of IBW is approximately equivalent to 1 cc of anatomic dead space.

165 lbs of IBW $\simeq$ 165 cc of anatomic dead space

STEP 3:  Employ the dead space-tidal volume ($V_D/V_T$) equation and solve for the $P\bar{E}CO_2$.

$$\frac{V_D}{V_T} = \frac{PaCO_2 - P\bar{E}CO_2}{PaCO_2}$$

$$\frac{165 \text{ cc}}{520 \text{ cc}} = \frac{44 \text{ torr} - P\bar{E}CO_2}{44 \text{ torr}}$$

$$(0.32)(44 \text{ torr}) = 44 \text{ torr} - P\bar{E}CO_2$$

$$P\bar{E}CO_2 = 44 \text{ torr} - 14 \text{ torr}$$

$$= 30 \text{ torr}$$

To actually conduct a $V_D/V_T$ measurement, the RRT must perform simultaneous exhaled gas and ABG sampling. For spontaneously breathing patients, a 40-liter collection balloon is usually used, whereas a 5-liter sample generally is sufficient for mechanically ventilated patients. From the Bohr equation, one can see that the degree of alveolar $CO_2$ dilution in the exhaled gas (as indicated by the $P\bar{E}CO_2$) will increase as the amount of dead space increases. As dead space increases, the $P\bar{E}CO_2$ decreases.

(1:212), (9:290–292), (15:489).

## IIIE2e

156. A. The duration of exercise is patient dependent. Most patients will begin with a short session and increase exercise time as tolerated, however. Frequency should be established at a minimum of three sessions per week. Intensity and mode of exercise is largely determined by the patient's symptoms and tolerance.

(1:1094–1096), (15:1144–1146).

## IIIA1l

157. A. The C.O. is a function of the volume of blood pumped by the heart to the systemic circulation (stroke volume) multiplied by the frequency of cardiac contraction (heart rate). In general, the venous return (ml/min.) is effectively equal to the C.O. This statement is true because the circulatory system is essentially a closed system.

(1:949), (9:276, 309), (10:118, 136).

## IIIE1i

158. A. A straight route from the mouth to the glottis should be achieved. The head and neck should be extended and raised to a plane above shoulder level. This position is called the *sniffing position*. Note the two diagrams that follow (Figure 5-32). Diagram A illustrates the correct head and neck position, whereas Diagram B demonstrates an incorrect position.

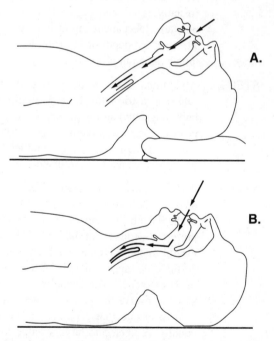

**Figure 5-32:** (A) Correct head and neck position, and (B) incorrect head and neck position.

(1:595), (16:561, 589).

## IIIA1m(1)

159. A. The $C(a-\bar{v})O_2$ represents the amount of oxygen extracted by the tissues from the arterial blood. The normal $C(a-\bar{v})O_2$ ranges from 4.0 vol% to 6.0 vol%. When the $C(a-\bar{v})O_2$ is below 4.0 vol%, the cause might be (1) septic shock, (2) increased cardiac output, (3) anemia, and (4) an increased hemoglobin-oxygen affinity (left shift of the oxyhemoglobin dissociation curve). Values greater than 6.0 vol% can result from a decreased cardiac output, increasing oxygen consumption, and a decreased hemoglobin-oxygen affinity (right shift of the oxyhemoglobin dissociation curve).

(1:223–225), (9:299–300).

## IIIB1e

160. D. To ensure proper placement of an ET tube, the RRT should perform the following steps:

STEP 1: Auscultate both sides of the patient's chest to ensure that a right or left mainstem bronchi intubation has not occurred.

STEP 2: Note the position of the ET tube at the teeth. This information must be noted and written on the patient's flow sheet, because migration of the tube might occur following tape changes and so on. If the tube migrates too far into the patient's airway, a mainstem bronchus intubation (usually right) can occur. If it migrates outward, the patient might be extubated. The average depth of insertion for an ET tube in an adult is approximately 23 cm.

STEP 3: Abdominal auscultation is important to rule out gastric intubation. A gurgling or bubbling sound during the application of a positive pressure breath would indicate that the patient's esophagus, rather than upper airway, has been intubated.

STEP 4: A chest X-ray is an important recommendation to definitively confirm the location of the ET tube in the patient's trachea. The preferred depth of intubation would have the tip of the ET tube at the level of the aortic knob, approximately in the middle of the trachea. Additionally, the RRT should observe the patient's chest excursion to ensure that each side is moving equally. A fiberoptic laryngoscope might obviate the need for chest X-rays by directly visualization of the carina. Finally, a $CO_2$ detector can be used to ensure that the end-tidal $CO_2$ $PetCO_2$ rises and falls with ventilation.

(1:598, 606), (9:165–166), (15:833–834).

## IIIA1l

161. B. The C.O. varies considerably among the normal population because of differences in body size. Therefore, C.O. is not a reliable indicator of cardiovascular function. Instead, the C.I., which is the C.O. divided by the person's BSA, offers measurement that is more useful when comparing the cardiac status of one person to another. The C.I. is obtained by dividing the C.O. by the BSA, expressed in square meters $(m^2)$. The equation is as follows:

$$C.I. = \frac{C.O.}{BSA} = liters/min./m^2$$

STEP 1: Calculate the C.O by multiplying the stoke volume (ml/beat) by the heart rate (beats/ min.).

$$C.O. = stroke\ volume \times heart\ rate$$
$$= 65\ ml/beat \times 82\ beats/min.$$
$$= 5,330\ ml/min.$$

STEP 2: Convert the C.O. to L/min.

$$C.O. = \frac{5,330\ ml/min.}{1,000\ ml/liter}$$
$$= 5.33\ L/min.$$

STEP 3: Obtain the BSA from the Dubois body surface chart (Figure 5-33). By extending a straightedge through 6-ft. 6-in. and 210 pounds, the BSA is 2.31 $m^2$.

STEP 4: Calculate the C.I.

$$C.I. = \frac{5.33\ L/min.}{2.31\ m^2}$$
$$= 2.31\ L/min./m^2$$

The normal C.I. range is 2.50 to 4.00 L/min./$m^2$. This person has a lower-than-normal C.I.

(1:783), (9:309, 314–315), (15:76, 530, 921).

## IIIA1m(a)

162. B. The shunt equation enables the calculation of the percent shunt. For example,

$$\frac{\dot{Q}_S}{\dot{Q}_T} = \frac{C\dot{c}O_2 - CaO_2}{C\dot{c}O_2 - C\bar{v}O_2}$$

where

$\dot{Q}_S$ = shunt cardiac output (L/min.)
$\dot{Q}_T$ = cardiac output (L/min.)
$C\dot{c}O_2$ = end-pulmonary capillary $O_2$ content (vol%)

## Dubois Body Surface Chart

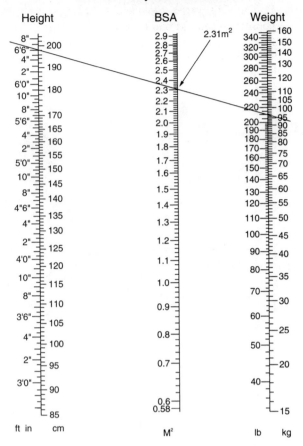

| Height | BSA | Weight |
|---|---|---|

**Figure 5-33:** Dubois body surface chart with straight line connecting height (6-ft. 6-in.) and weight (210 pounds) showing a BSA of 2.31 m² (arrow).

$CaO_2$ = total arterial $O_2$ content (vol%)

$C\bar{v}O_2$ = total mixed venous $O_2$ content (vol%)

Insert the given values into the equation.

$$\frac{\dot{Q}_S}{\dot{Q}_T} = \frac{24.78 \text{ vol\%} - 24.36 \text{ vol\%}}{24.78 \text{ vol\%} - 20.86 \text{ vol\%}}$$

$$= \frac{0.42 \text{ vol\%}}{3.92 \text{ vol\%}} \times 100$$

$$= (0.1071)(100)$$

$$= 10.71\%, \text{ or } 0.1071$$

(1:225–226, 930), (9:323–324).

### IIIA1l

163. C. A relatively simple method employed to differentiate between a diffusion defect and the presence of right-to-left shunting (capillary shunting) is calculating the $P(A\text{-}a)O_2$ following the administration of 100% oxygen. If a diffusion defect is present, an $FIO_2$ of 1.0 will cause the $P(A\text{-}a)O_2$ to decrease (narrow). Conversely, the administration of 100% oxygen causes

the $P(A\text{-}a)O_2$ to increase (widen) when capillary shunting is present. The degree of shunting can be grossly estimated from the $P(A\text{-}a)O_2$ value while 100% oxygen is breathed. For example, every 10 to 15 torr $P(A\text{-}a)O_2$ approximates a 1.0% shunt. Therefore, if the patient's $P(A\text{-}a)O_2$ were 200 torr, about a 13% to 20% shunt would be present.

$$\frac{200 \text{ torr}}{15 \text{ torr}} \cong 13\% \quad \text{and} \quad \frac{200 \text{ torr}}{10 \text{ torr}} \cong 20\%$$

(1:217, 234–235, 821, 929), (10:21, 181, 274).

### IIIC5

164. A. This patient has developed a lung infection as evidenced by the changed characteristics of the sputum and the cough. The sputum transformed from mucoid (clear and thin) to purulent (yellowish-green), and the patient's cough became more frequent.

The utility of CPT as an effective therapeutic technique for the mobilization of secretions is controversial. Its efficacy toward accomplishing that goal appears to vary from patient to patient. It appears as if CPT is not helping this patient much. Therefore, a combination of therapies might be more efficacious. Adding a heated aerosol treatment and a bronchodilator to the regimen might help mobilize this patient's secretions. Incentive spirometry is not intended to mobilize secretions. Rather, its main therapeutic goal is to prevent and/or reverse atelectasis.

(1:811–812), (16:516, 969).

### IIIC5

165. C. One of the guidelines governing the use of incentive spirometry states that when a patient's postoperative inspiratory capacity (IC) is at least 80% of the preoperative level, daily therapeutic evaluations can be terminated. Therapeutic assessments can then be performed on a less frequent basis—perhaps every three days. In the case illustrated here, the patient's postoperative IC is only 66% of the preoperative level; that is,

$$\frac{2.0 \text{ L (IC on 4th postop day)}}{3.0 \text{ L (preop IC)}} \times 100 = 66\%$$

The appropriate recommendation at this time is to maintain the incentive spirometry to continue establishing therapeutic goals for the patient and perform daily therapeutic evaluations. PEP mask therapy is not indicated here because the mobilization of secretions was not stated to be problematic.

(1:774, 777), (16:523, 530).

166. C. Positive expiratory pressure (PEP) mask therapy is a positive airway pressure adjunct to bronchial hygiene therapy. The patient exhales against a fixed orifice resistor, thereby establishing a positive expiratory pressure. The fixed orifice resistors available can develop a pressure of 10 to 20 cm $H_2O$. This therapeutic modality helps "splint" the airways open during exhalation. It simultaneously affords air the opportunity to help move secretions to larger airways.

(AARC Clinical Practice Guideline, May 1993, *Use of Positive Airway Pressure Adjuncts to Bronchial Hygiene Therapy, 38* (5), pp. 516–519).

## IIIA1h

167. A. Bronchospasm and the accumulation of tracheobronchial secretions increase the PIP by increasing the pressure needed to overcome airway resistance ($P_{Raw}$). The pressure needed to overcome airway resistance ($P_{Raw}$) when a volume of gas is delivered from a mechanical ventilator to a patient is represented by the pressure difference between the peak inspiratory pressure (PIP) and the plateau (static) pressure. The following pressure manometers illustrate the two conditions referred to in this question. Manometer A (Figure 5-34) represents the original pressure conditions encountered by the RRT.

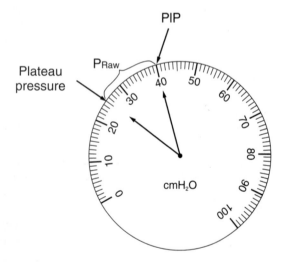

**Figure 5-34:** PIP 40 cm $H_2O$, plateau pressure 25 cm $H_2O$, $P_{Raw}$ 15 cm $H_2O$.

A) PIP: 40 cm $H_2O$
plateau pressure: 25 cm $H_2O$
$P_{Raw}$: 15 cm $H_2O$

Manometer B (Figure 5-35) demonstrates the pressure readings when the RRT observed the changes while performing ventilator rounds.

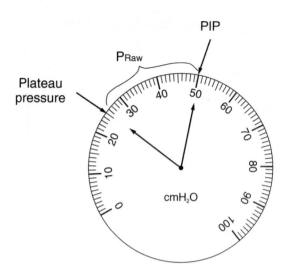

**Figure 5-35:** PIP 50 cm $H_2O$, plateau pressure 25 cm $H_2O$, $P_{Raw}$ 25 cm $H_2O$.

B) PIP: 50 cm $H_2O$
plateau pressure: 25 cm $H_2O$
$P_{Raw}$: 25 cm $H_2O$

The plateau pressure has not changed in this situation, signifying that the lung compliance has not decreased. If the lung compliance had decreased, the plateau pressure would indicate a reading higher than 25 cm $H_2O$. Therefore, because the PIP–plateau pressure gradient increased (widened), the cause for the higher PIP can be attributed to an increased airway resistance. Both mucous plugging (retained secretions) and bronchospasm result in an increased airway resistance. Consequently, in the face of either of these conditions, the pressure generated to overcome airway resistance ($P_{Raw}$) will increase.

(1:937), (10:256–257), (15:642–644), (17:98).

## IIIB2c

168. C. PSV is a pressure-limited, flow-cycled form of ventilatory support. The preset pressure augments the level of the patient's inspiratory efforts. The patient controls the tidal volume, ventilatory rate, inspiratory time, and flow. The actual tidal volume achieved by a patient during PSV is determined by the patient's effort and the pressure-support level set.

PSV is purported to decrease the imposed work of breathing (WOB). The imposed WOB is generally caused by the ET tube and the ventilator circuitry. The patient here has an ET tube with a small internal diameter (6.5 mm). This situation, along with the fact that the patient is recovering from her pulmonary condition and possesses a reliable ventilatory drive, makes her a suitable candidate for PSV.

(1:864, 877), (10:85, 199, 214), (15:960, 1085).

## IIIA1e

169. B. After seven days of incentive spirometry and daily therapeutic evaluations, the patient has achieved an inspiratory capacity (IC) that is more than 80% of the preoperative level. For example,

Preoperative IC: 3.6 liters
IC on 7th postoperative day: 3.0 liters

$$\frac{3.0 \text{ L}}{3.6 \text{ L}} \times 100 = 83\%$$

The recommendation is that when a patient's postoperative IC is at least 80% of the preoperative measurement, the daily therapeutic evaluations can be terminated. The patient will still be expected to continue incentive spirometry treatments and establish and work toward achieving personal therapeutic goals. Therapeutic assessments performed by the RRT can occur on a less frequent basis.

(1:774, 777), (16:523, 530).

## IIIC4

170. B. A helium–oxygen mixture is less dense than an air–oxygen mixture. Therefore, if an oxygen flow meter is used to deliver a helium–oxygen mixture, correction factors must be used to determine the flow rate setting. For example, if a 70–30 helium–oxygen mixture is being administered with an oxygen flow meter, the RRT must divide the desired flow rate by the factor 1.6:

$$\frac{12 \text{ L/min.}}{1.6} = 7.5 \text{ L/min.}$$

Therefore, setting a flow rate of 7.5 L/min. on the oxygen flow meter will result in a helium–oxygen gas flow rate of 12 L/min. If an 80–20 helium–oxygen mixture is being used, the correction factor is 1.8.

(1:717, 768), (16:339, 340, 396).

## IIIB1a

171. C. A fenestrated tracheotomy tube has three components: (1) outer cannula, (2) inner cannula, and (3) decannulation cannula. The outer cannula is inserted through the stoma and has an elliptically shaped opening (fenestration) on its shoulder or curved surface. Through this opening, the patient is allowed to breathe through his upper airway. Generally, when only the outer cannula is in place, the cuff is also deflated to permit a larger flow of air to pass across the vocal cords and through the upper airway. The decannulation cannula caps the outer cannula, thereby forcing the patient to breathe entirely through his upper airway.

When the inner cannula is inserted, it fits inside the outer cannula and directs much of the patient's ex-

haled volume through the tube, assuming that the cuff is deflated. If the cuff is inflated and the inner cannula is in place, all of the air breathed by the patient passes through the tube. Positive pressure mechanical ventilation can be accommodated via the inner cannula with the cuff inflated.

(1:614), (5:247), (13:173–174), (15:829).

## IIIC3a

172. A. Advantages of a closed-suction catheter system include a reduced loss of $F_IO_2$, decreased possibility of suction-induced hypoxia and cardiac dysrhythmias, reduced risk of contamination, and reduced loss of PEEP. Despite these advantages, elevating the $F_IO_2$ to 1.00 before suctioning is still advocated because volume and oxygen are removed from the lungs when suction is applied.

(Trach Care(R) product information, Ballard Medical Products), (Steri-Cath D.L. Closed Ventilation Suction System, product information Concord/Portex), (1:618).

## IIIC7a

173. B. The patient in this situation is experiencing about 20 premature ventricular contractions (PVCs) per minute. The number of PVCs is estimated from this six-second (30 large horizontal blocks) ECG strip. The six-second ECG tracing represents one-tenth of a minute's electrophysiologic activity. Therefore, multiplying the two PVCs that appear on this strip by 10 provides an estimate of the number of PVCs occurring each minute (i.e., 2 PVCs × 10 = 20 PVCs).

The PVCs appearing on the six-second tracing might represent a relatively random occurrence. Consequently, a longer time interval for this tracing should be observed to obtain a more precise count. An isolated PVC is considered to be innocuous. When PVCs become numerous and frequent, however, they can be a harbinger of a serious dysrhythmia (i.e., ventricular tachycardia). Therefore, in this situation, removing the suction catheter immediately is appropriate because the myocardium might become more irritable if suctioning continued as more lung volume and oxygen were evacuated. Adequate pre- and postsuctioning oxygenation are essential to prevent precipitous arterial desaturation. The cardiac tracing shown here, along with the two PVCs, is a normal sinus rhythm at a rate of approximately 80 beats/min. Note the tracing in Figure 5-36 on page 330.

(1:330–331), (9:204–205), (16:864).

## IIIB1a

174. B. The amount of pressure placed into the cuff of a tracheostomy or ET tube is critical from two standpoints.

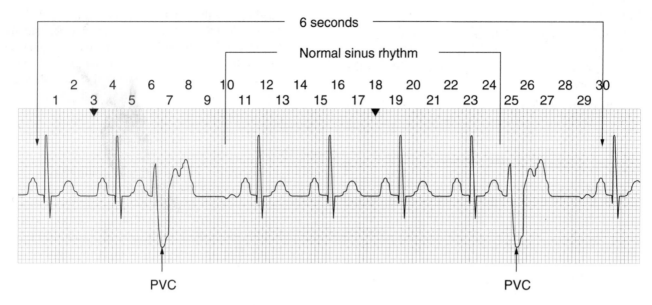

**Figure 5-36:** Lead II ECG tracing showing two PVCs (arrows) and a normal sinus rhythm at 80 beats/min.

First, an adequate seal within the airway is essential for proper ventilation, especially during positive pressure mechanical ventilation. Second, extreme care must be taken to ensure that excess pressure does not develop inside the cuff. High intracuff pressures can interfere with arterial and venous blood flow through the vessels in the tracheal wall in contact with the tube's cuff.

Arterial blood flow through the trachea is around 30 mm Hg, or 42 cm $H_2O$. Venous outflow pressure is about 18 mm Hg, or 24 cm $H_2O$. Therefore, an intracuff pressure range of 20 to 25 mm Hg (27 to 33 cm $H_2O$) is acceptable. If less pressure can be generated within the cuff and still afford an effective seal, however, then larger volumes of air should not be injected into the cuff. Table 5-11 outlines the approximate circulatory pressures that exist in the trachea.

**Table 5-11** Tracheal Circulatory Pressures

| Arterial | | Venous | |
|---|---|---|---|
| mm Hg | cm $H_2O$ | mm Hg | cm $H_2O$ |
| 30 | 42 | 18 | 24 |

In the situation presented here, an intracuff pressure of 42 cm $H_2O$ or 30 mm Hg is too high because it could impede tracheal capillary blood flow, causing tracheal necrosis. The appropriate action to take is to release some of the volume from the cuff to reduce the intracuff pressure to an acceptable level. That range again is 20 to 25 mm Hg, or 27 to 33 cm $H_2O$.

(1:609–610), (5:248–249), (15:836).

**IIIC4**

175. D. A helium-oxygen (He–$O_2$) gas mixture is less dense than an air–oxygen (air–$O_2$) mixture. When oxygen is therapeutically administered, a pressure-compensated oxygen flow meter is customarily used. When a He–$O_2$ gas mixture is administered to a patient who has COPD or upper airway obstruction, a helium–oxygen flow meter might not be readily available. Therefore, an oxygen flow meter can be used to deliver this therapeutic gas mixture. In such circumstances, the flow rate indicated on the oxygen flow meter will be less than the actual flow rate of the 80–20 He–$O_2$.

To obtain the actual flow rate of the 80–20 He–$O_2$, one has to multiply the flow rate setting on the oxygen flow meter by the factor 1.8. For example, if a patient is receiving an 80–20 He–$O_2$ gas mixture via an oxygen flow meter set at 8 L/min., the actual flow rate received by the patient is 14.4 L/min.

$$\left( \begin{array}{c} \text{oxygen flow meter} \\ \text{setting} \end{array} \right)(1.8) = \left( \begin{array}{c} \text{actual 80-20,} \\ \text{He-}O_2 \text{ flow rate} \end{array} \right)$$

$$(8 \text{ L/min.})(1.8) = 14.4 \text{ L/min.}$$

Alternatively, the following formula can be used:

$$\left( \begin{array}{c} \text{oxygen flow} \\ \text{meter setting} \end{array} \right)\left( \frac{\text{density of } O_2}{\begin{array}{c}\text{density of 80-20,}\\ \text{He-}O_2 \text{ mixture}\end{array}} \right) = \left( \begin{array}{c} \text{actual 80-20,} \\ \text{He-}O_2 \text{ flow rate} \end{array} \right)$$

$$(8 \text{ L/min.})\left( \frac{\sqrt{1.43}}{\sqrt{0.43}} \right) =$$

$$(8 \text{ L/min.})\left(\frac{1.196}{0.656}\right) =$$

$$(8 \text{ L/min.})(1.8) = 14.4 \text{ L/min.}$$

If a 70–30 He–$O_2$ gas mixture is administered via an oxygen flow meter, the multiplication factor is 1.6. Table 5-12 indicates the difference among the densities for oxygen, air, and helium.

**Table 5-12** Gas Density Comparison

| Gas | Density (grams/liter) |
|---|---|
| oxygen (O2) | 1.430 |
| air | 1.293 |
| helium (He) | 0.176 |

(1:717, 768), (13:59–60), (15:887–888).

## IIID1a

176. C. Pupillary size and reactivity are indices of cerebral oxygenation. In the course of CPR, this assessment should be performed periodically. The assessment is accomplished by opening one of the victim's eyelids and observing the pupil's response to light. Table 5-13 outlines the evaluation of pupillary response.

**Table 5-13** Assessment of Cerebral Oxygenation

| Pupillary Size and Reactivity | Cerebral Oxygenation |
|---|---|
| • Constricted and responsive to light adequate | adequate |
| • Dilated and responsive to light | inadequate |
| • Fixed and dilated (15–30 minutes) | irreversible brain death likely |

(1:630–631), (16:562–563).

## IIIA1a

177. B. The following four variables can be control variables: (1) pressure, (2) volume, (3) flow, and (4) time. Therefore, a ventilator can be either a pressure controller, volume controller, flow controller, or time controller. The variable that is the control variable is unaffected by lung compliance and/or airway resistance changes. The other variables will vary with changes in lung compliance and airway resistance.

If a ventilator is a flow controller and the patient's airway resistance (Raw) increases, the peak inspiratory pressure will also increase and the flow will remain constant. This relationship is based on the following formula:

$$Raw = \frac{P}{\dot{V}} \quad [\textbf{Remember, flow } (\dot{V}) \textbf{ is constant.}]$$

Rearranging the formula to solve for the constant $\dot{V}$,

$$\dot{V} = \frac{P}{R_{aw}}, \quad \text{or} \quad k = \frac{P}{R_{aw}}$$

Because the airway resistance and the pressure (P) are directly proportional in the formula, the pressure will increase proportionately when Raw increases. Conversely, when Raw decreases, the P will decrease proportionately.

(1:836–840), (5:368–371), (10:75–76), (13:368–372).

## IIID1b

178. A. When medications (epinephrine, lidocaine, atropine, and $NaHCO_3$) are endotracheally administered, they should be given at 2.0 to 2.5 times their recommended I.V. dose. They should also be diluted in 10 ml of normal saline or distilled water. This form of medication administration might adversely affect the arterial $PO_2$. A catheter should be attached to the syringe and its tip passed down the ET tube beyond the ET tube's tip. Once in that location, the medication should be rapidly sprayed to create an aerosol and to quicken reabsorption. Chest compressions should be stopped but resumed immediately after the medication is instilled.

("Guidelines 2000 Cardiopulmonary Resuscitation and Emergency Cardiovascular Care," I-113).

## IIIC1a

179. A. If a patient cycles on a positive pressure breathing device by exerting a negative 2 cm $H_2O$ pressure, as indicated on the pressure manometer, the patient is assuming some of the WOB (i.e., initiating inspiration). Actually, the patient need not exert an inspiratory effort of greater than −3 cm $H_2O$ to initiate inspiration. If the patient "pulls" a more negative inspiratory pressure, the sensitivity control should be adjusted. In this instance, no change needs to be instituted because −2 cm $H_2O$ is not considered exertional for the patient.

(1:781), (15:846).

## Situational Sets
## IIIA1h

180. B. The static pressure refers to the pressure that is responsible for maintaining lung inflation after a volume

change has occurred in the lungs. Other expressions that are synonymous with the static pressure include alveolar distending pressure and plateau pressure. The value for static pressure is used in the denominator of the formula for pulmonary (lung) compliance:

$$C_L = \frac{\Delta V}{\Delta P}$$

where

$C_L$ = pulmonary compliance (L/cm $H_2O$)
$\Delta V$ = changes in volume, generally the tidal volume (liters)
$\Delta P$ = change in pressure; static pressure − PEEP (cm $H_2O$)

STEP 1: Convert the tidal volume ($V_T$) to liters.

$$V_T = \frac{850 \text{ ml}}{1,000 \text{ ml/liter}}$$

$$= 0.85 \text{ liter}$$

STEP 2: Rearrange the aforementioned formula to solve for the static pressure.

$$\Delta P = \frac{\Delta V}{C_L} = \text{static pressure}$$

$$= \frac{0.85 \text{ L}}{0.07 \text{ L/cm } H_2O}$$

$$= 12 \text{ cm } H_2O$$

A static pressure of 12 cm $H_2O$ represents the pressure needed to sustain alveolar inflation at end inspiration after the ventilator delivered the tidal volume of 850 cc. Recall that the static pressure does not reflect any pressure generated to overcome airway resistance. As the name implies, static pressure refers to the pressure in the lungs under static conditions (i.e., no flow conditions). In this problem, the compressible volume was not taken into account.

(1:937), (10:256), (15:13, 84, 643–644).

## IIIA1h

181. C. The peak inspiratory pressure (PIP) is the pressure generated in the patient–ventilator system during the process of delivering a mechanical breath during inspiration. The PIP incorporates pressure generated to overcome airway resistance as well as the static pressure. In other words, the PIP includes both the static and dynamic components involved in accomplishing the WOB. Because the PIP is the sum of the static pressure and the pressure generated to overcome airway resistance, the following formula can be applied:

$$PIP = P_{static} + P_{Raw}$$

where

PIP = peak inspiratory pressure (cm $H_2O$)
$P_{static}$ = static pressure (cm $H_2O$)
$P_{Raw}$ = pressure generated to overcome airway resistance (cm $H_2O$)

STEP 1: Convert the peak inspiratory flow rate ($\dot{V}$) to L/sec.

$$\dot{V} = \frac{60 \text{ L/min.}}{60 \text{ sec./min.}}$$

$$= 1 \text{ L/sec.}$$

STEP 2: Calculate the pressure generated to overcome airway resistance ($P_{Raw}$) by rearranging the equation used to solve for airway resistance ($R_{aw}$).

$$R_{aw} = \frac{\Delta P}{\dot{V}} \quad \text{or} \quad R_{aw} = \frac{P_{Raw}}{\dot{V}}$$

where

$R_{aw}$ = airway resistance (cm $H_2O$/L/sec.)
$\Delta P$ = pressure generated to overcome airway resistance, also called transairway pressure or $P_{resistance}$ (cm $H_2O$)
$\dot{V}$ = flow rate (L/sec.)

Therefore,

$$P_{Raw} = \dot{V} \times R_{aw}$$

$$= (1 \text{ L/sec.})(12 \text{ cm } H_2O/\text{L/sec.})$$

$$= 12 \text{ cm } H_2O$$

STEP 3: Solve for the PIP.

$$PIP = P_{static} + P_{Raw}$$

$$= 12 \text{ cm } H_2O + 12 \text{ cm } H_2O$$

$$= 24 \text{ cm } H_2O$$

(1:937–938), (10:256–257), (15:17, 89, 643–644).

## IIIA1e

182. C. The flow-time waveform shows the flow during exhalation remaining below the baseline and being interrupted by the inspiratory flow. Essentially, exhalation is prevented from completing. The expiratory gas flow must be allowed to return to baseline before inspiration begins. The consequence of inspiration beginning before exhalation is completed is auto-PEEP, or occult PEEP. Auto-PEEP often goes undetected and can have deleterious effects on the patient's hemodynamics and pulmonary mechanics.

(1:917, 951), (10:152–154, 245–246).

**IIIA1e**

183.  C. The flow-time tracing shown in Figure 5-37 on page 333 demonstrates how the expiratory flow should return to baseline, thereby eliminating auto-PEEP.

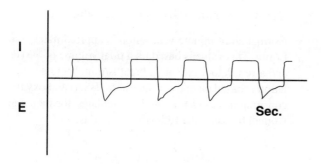

**Figure 5-37**

A number of techniques are available to correct the problems of auto-PEEP. The following list outlines some of the methods:

- endotracheal suctioning
- bronchodilatation
- a larger I.D. endotracheal tube
- shortening inspiratory time in relation to the total cycle time
- increasing the peak inspiratory flow rate
- increasing the tidal volume and decreasing the ventilatory rate

(1:917), (10:155–156).

**IIIA1f**

184.  A. The formula for calculating the mean arterial pressure for either the systemic or pulmonary circulation is as follows:

$$MAP = \frac{2(DP) + SP}{3}$$

where

MAP = mean arterial pressure (mm Hg)
DP = diastolic pressure (mm Hg)
SP = systolic pressure (mm Hg)

Therefore, in reference to the pulmonary circulation, this formula becomes:

$$\overline{PAP} = \frac{2(PAd) + PAs}{3}$$

where

$\overline{PAP}$ = mean pulmonary artery pressure (mm Hg)
PAd = pulmonary artery diastolic pressure (mm Hg)
PAs = pulmonary artery systolic pressure (mm Hg)

$$\overline{PAP} = \frac{2(20 \text{ mm Hg}) + 40 \text{ mm Hg}}{3}$$

$$= 26.7 \text{ mm Hg}$$

(1:943, 949), (9:336), (10:136).

**IIIA1l**

185.  C. To calculate the pulmonary vascular resistance, use the following equation:

$$PVR = \frac{\overline{PAP} - PCWP}{C.O.}$$

where

PVR = pulmonary vascular resistance (mm Hg/L/min. or dynes-sec./cm$^5$)
$\overline{PAP}$ = mean pulmonary artery pressure (mm Hg)
C.O. = cardiac output (L/min.)

Therefore,

$$PVR = \frac{26.7 \text{ mm Hg} - 12.0 \text{ mm Hg}}{3.5 \text{ L/min.}}$$

$$= 4.2 \text{ mm Hg/L/min.}$$

After multiplying the PVR expressed in mm Hg/L/min. by 79.9, the units become dynes-sec./cm$^5$. Normal PVR is 1.5 to 3.0 mm Hg/L/min., or 150 to 250 dynes-sec./cm$^5$. Therefore, the PVR is higher than normal in this case.

(1:949), (10:119), (15:530).

**IIIA1m(3)**

186.  B. This patient has an increased pulmonary vascular resistance caused by pulmonary hypertension, perhaps resulting from the hypercapnia and acidemia. Fluid overload, or hypervolemia, is not a problem in this case because the PCWP is normal. Hypervolemia, high-pressure pulmonary edema, and mitral valve stenosis are associated with a higher than normal PCWP.

Another indicator of an increased pulmonary vascular resistance is the elevated central venous pressure (CVP). Normally, the CVP is 5 to 15 cm $H_2O$, or 4 to 12 mm Hg. In this case, the CVP is high (17 mm Hg) because of the increased afterload imposed on the right ventricle by the pulmonary vasoconstriction.

(1:946–948), (10:119, 126), (15:530–533).

**IIIB1a**

187.  D. This patient is experiencing impending ventilatory failure from ventilatory muscle fatigue and paralysis. The cause of the decreased ventilatory muscle function is Guillain–Barré syndrome. Guillain–Barré syndrome is a polyneuritis generally affecting peripheral

motor and sensory neurons. The neurons experience a self-limiting and usually reversible demyelination. The specific etiology is unknown. This neuromuscular disease frequently follows a viral illness, however, and sometimes develops after vaccination for the swine flu. This condition ordinarily begins with peripheral muscle weakness and paralysis and can progress to the muscles of ventilation, causing ventilatory failure. The lungs are not diseased because the pathophysiology of this condition affects the neurons and weakens muscle activity.

The treatment for Guillain–Barré is generally mechanical ventilation to treat the acute ventilatory failure (acute respiratory acidosis). The prognosis is often good, but any sequelae depends on the extent of the demyelination that occurred. Mechanical ventilation is often required for 6 to 8 weeks.

(1:545), (10:235), (15:306, 1065).

## IIIB2c

188. C. Again, this patient is in impending ventilatory failure because of ventilatory muscle weakness and paralysis. Therefore, any form of mechanical ventilation that relies either solely or heavily on the patient's own spontaneous breathing efforts to cycle on inspiration or to generate an adequate tidal volume is inappropriate. Because this patient is at great risk for experiencing complete ventilatory muscle paralysis, the mode of ventilation selected must provide her complete ventilatory needs at this time.

Therefore, the assist-control mode at a controlled rate of 8 to 10 breaths/min. will deliver sufficient ventilation during this time of ventilatory muscle weakness and paralysis. If complete ventilatory muscle paralysis ensues, the patient's ventilatory needs will continue to be provided. On the other hand, if the disease process begins to reverse, the patient will have the opportunity to "trigger" the ventilator with her own spontaneous efforts, at which time the controlled rate would be altered according to ABG data and overall patient assessment.

Modes such as IMV or SIMV would be acceptable only if the mandatory rates were sufficient enough to render her ventilatory needs. Otherwise, these modes at low rates would impose a greater work of breathing on this patient and would contribute to her ventilatory failure. The pressure-support mode would be acceptable here if a backup mode were available in the event that the patient became apneic. Last, there would be no need to sedate this patient because it is unlikely that she would "fight" the ventilator. The nature of her clinical pathophysiology is having a paralyzing effect.

(1:545), (10:235, 299–300), (15:955–962).

## IIIB2c

189. A. Appropriate ventilator settings for this patient would include the following:

1. minute ventilation ($\dot{V}_E$) of 6.0 L/min.
2. tidal volume ($V_T$) of 700 cc
3. ventilatory rate (f) of 8 to 10 breaths/min.

Normal adult minute ventilation is approximately 6.0 L/min. This value is based on a tidal volume of 500 cc and a ventilatory rate of 12 breaths/min. Minute ventilation is based on body surface area (BSA) and oxygen consumption ($\dot{V}O_2$). It can be calculated for men and women by using the following formulas:

$$(\textbf{Men})\ \dot{V}_E = 4.0 \times BSA$$

$$(\textbf{Women})\ \dot{V}_E = 3.5 \times BSA$$

STEP 1: Use the Dubois body surface chart to obtain this patient's BSA (Figure 5-38).

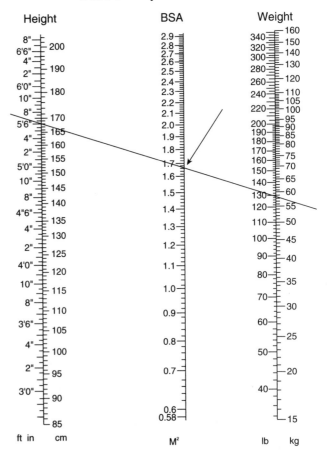

## Dubois Body Surface Chart

**Figure 5-38:** Dubois body surface chart with straight line connecting height (5ft. 6in.) and weight (130 pounds) showing a BSA of 1.66 m² (arrow).

This patient's BSA is 1.66 m² (arrow on chart), based on her height of 5-ft. 6-in. and her weight of 130 pounds.

STEP 2: Use the female version of the $\dot{V}_E$ formula.

$$\dot{V}_E = 3.5 \times 1.66 \text{ m}^2$$

$$= 5.81 \text{ L/min. (round off to 6.0 L/min.)}.$$

STEP 3: Calculate this patient's IBW, which will be used to determine the tidal volume setting.

(Men) IBW (lbs) = 106 + [6 × (height in inches − 60)]

(Women) IBW (lbs) = 105 + [5 × (height in inches − 60)]

Therefore,

IBW (lbs) = 105 + [5 × (66 inches − 60)]

$$= 105 + (5 \times 6)$$

$$= 105 + 30$$

$$= 135 \text{ lbs}$$

STEP 4: Convert the IBW of 135 lbs to kilograms (kg).

$$kg = \frac{135 \text{ lbs}}{2.2 \text{ lbs/kg}}$$

$$= 61 \text{ kg (IBW)}$$

STEP 5: The tidal volume setting is ordinarily based on the guideline of 10 to 15 cc/kg of IBW. Therefore, the tidal volume setting will be within the range of 610 to 915 cc.

(61 kg)(10 cc/kg) = 610 cc

(61 kg)(15 cc/kg) = 915 cc

STEP 6: Determine the ventilatory rate by using the following formula. A $V_T$ of 700 cc, or 0.7 liter, will be delivered.

$$f = \frac{\dot{V}_E}{V_T}$$

$$= \frac{6.0 \text{ L/min.}}{0.7 \text{ L/breath}}$$

$$= 8.57 \text{ breaths/min.}$$

(1:949), (9:309, 311), (10:119, 136), (15:966–968).

**IB9c**

190. D. The following steps outline the method whereby the patient's alveolar ventilation ($\dot{V}_A$) can be calculated:

STEP 1: Convert 90 kg to lbs by using the conversion factor of 1 kg equals 2.2 lbs.

$$lbs = 90 \text{ kg} \times 2.2 \text{ lbs/kg}$$

$$= 198 \text{ lbs}$$

STEP 2: Estimate the amount of anatomic dead space. *Guideline:* There is one cubic centimeter (cc) of anatomic dead space ($V_D$) per pound (lb) of IBW. Therefore, 198 lb × 1 cc/lb of IBW 5 198 cc ($V_D$)

STEP 3: Calculate the alveolar volume ($V_A$).

$$V_A = V_T - V_D$$

$$= 800 \text{ cc} - 198 \text{ cc}$$

$$= 602 \text{ cc/breath}$$

STEP 4: Calculate the alveolar ventilation ($\dot{V}_A$).

$$\dot{V}_A = (V_A)(\text{ventilatory rate})$$

$$= (602 \text{ cc/breath})(15 \text{ breaths/min.})$$

$$= 9,030 \text{ cc/min., or } 9.03 \text{ L/min.}$$

(1:211–213), (17:289).

**IIIB4a**

191. C. The pH is within the normal range (7.35 to 7.45). Therefore, no intervention is indicated to alter the pH. Likewise, the $PaCO_2$ value lies within normal limits ($PaCO_2$ 35 to 45 mm Hg). Consequently, no corrective measures are required for this parameter either. The $PaO_2$ value, however, is low. The $FiO_2$ of 0.60 is already in the high range. Applying PEEP might serve to increase the $PaO_2$. Because no cardiovascular problem is mentioned in this situation, it can be assumed that the application of PEEP would not be contraindicated.

The patient should be monitored for any of the adverse effects of PEEP, however: (1) decreased venous return, (2) decreased C.O., and (3) decreased lung compliance (causing increases in the arterial $PCO_2$).

(1:880, 939), (10:672).

**IB9b**

192. D. The tidal volume delivered by the Siemens Servo 900C is not directly set on the ventilator. It is a function of the preset minute ventilation and the ventilatory rate setting. Use the following steps to calculate the tidal volume delivered by the ventilator in this situation.

STEP 1: Convert minute ventilation ($\dot{V}_E$) expressed in L/min. to cc/min.

$$6 \text{ L/min.} \times 1,000 \text{ cc/liter} = 6,000 \text{ cc/min.}$$

STEP 2: Calculate the tidal volume ($V_T$).

$$V_T = \frac{\dot{V}_E}{\text{ventilatory rate}}$$

$$= \frac{6,000 \text{ cc/min.}}{10 \text{ breaths/min.}}$$

$$= 600 \text{ cc/breath}$$

(5:478), (13:518–519).

## IIIA1h

193. B. On the 900C, the inspiratory time is based on the two settings; that is, the inspiratory time percent (20%, 25%, 33%, 50%, 67%, and 80%) and the inspiratory pause percent (0%, 5%, 10%, 20%, and 30%). Calculate the patient's inspiratory time ($T_I$) according to the following steps:

STEP 1: Determine the total ventilatory cycle time (TCT).

$$TCT = \frac{\text{time conversion factor}}{\text{ventilatory rate}}$$

$$= \frac{60 \text{ sec./min.}}{10 \text{ breaths/min.}}$$

$$= 6 \text{ sec./breath}$$

STEP 2: Calculate the inspiratory time by multiplying the TCT by the sum of the $T_{I\%}$ and the inspiratory pause time percent.

$$T_I = TCT(T_{I\%} + \text{inspiratory pause time\%})$$

$$= (6 \text{ sec./breath})\left(\frac{33}{100} + 0\right)$$

$$= 1.98 \text{ sec.}$$

(5:477–478), (13:516–521).

## IIIA1h

194. C. Calculate the expiratory time ($T_E$) by subtracting the $T_I$ from the TCT.

$$T_E = TCT - T_I$$

$$= 6.0 \text{ sec.} - 1.98 \text{ sec.}$$

$$= 4.02 \text{ sec.}$$

The inspiratory:expiratory (I:E) ratio can be obtained by dividing both the inspiratory time ($T_I$) and the expiratory time ($T_E$) by the sum of the $T_{I\%}$ and the inspiratory pause time percent, multiplied by the TCT. In the question here, the I:E ratio would be determined as follows:

$$\text{I:E} = \frac{1.98 \text{ sec.}}{1.98 \text{ sec.}} : \frac{4.02 \text{ sec.}}{1.98 \text{ sec.}}$$

$$= 1:2$$

(1:860), (10:205–206).

## IIIA1e

195. B. When a mechanical ventilator delivers a tidal volume to a patient, a portion of the delivered volume remains in the ventilator tubing at end inspiration. This volume is called the *compressed,* or *lost,* volume. To calculate the actual tidal volume or actual minute ventilation received by the patient, the compressed or lost volume in the ventilator tubing must be obtained. To perform this calculation, however, the compliance or compressibility factor of the ventilator circuit must be known.

To derive the tubing compressibility factor, a low tidal volume must be set, the high-pressure limit must be dialed to its maximum, and the patient Y connector must be occluded when the ventilator cycles on. Once the machine cycles on to inspiration, the Y connector should be occluded and the PIP should be noted. The procedure for calculating the tubing compliance factor is outlined as follows.

STEP 1: Determine the tidal volume delivered by the Siemens Servo 900C.

$$V_T = \frac{\dot{V}_E}{f}$$

where

$V_T$ = tidal volume (cc)
$\dot{V}_E$ = minute ventilation (L/min.)
$f$ = ventilatory rate (breaths/min.)

$$V_T = \frac{2 \text{ L/min.}}{12 \text{ breaths/min.}}$$

$$= 0.167 \text{ L/breath, or } 167 \text{ cc/breath}$$

STEP 2: Calculate the tubing compliance factor by using the following formula:

$$C_T = \frac{V_T}{PIP - PEEP}$$

where

$C_T$ = tubing compliance (cc/cm $H_2O$)
$V_T$ = tidal volume (cc)
PIP = peak inspiratory pressure (cm $H_2O$)
PEEP = positive end-expiratory pressure (cm $H_2O$)

$$C_T = \frac{167 \text{ cc}}{50 \text{ cm } H_2O - 5 \text{ cm } H_2O}$$

$$= 3.71 \text{ cc/cm } H_2O$$

This value indicates that for each cm $H_2O$ pressure generated during inspiration, 3.71 cc of volume are compressed (lost) in the ventilator tubing.

(1:937–938), (9:285), (10:256).

## IIIA1h

196. B.

STEP 1: Determine the delivered tidal volume by using the following formula:

$$V_T = \frac{\dot{V}_E}{f}$$

$$= \frac{8 \text{ L/min.}}{12 \text{ breaths/min.}}$$

$$= 0.667 \text{ L/breath or}$$
$$667 \text{ cc/breath}$$

STEP 2: Determine the volume compressed (lost) in the tubing by solving for $V_{lost}$.

$$C_T = \frac{V_{lost}}{PIP - PEEP}$$

After rearranging the formula,

$$V_{lost} = (C_T)(PIP - PEEP)$$

$$= (3.71 \text{ cc/cm } H_2O)(35 \text{ cm } H_2O - 5 \text{ cm } H_2O)$$

$$= (3.71 \text{ cc/cm } H_2O)(30 \text{ cm } H_2O)$$

$$= 111.3 \text{ cc}$$

STEP 3: Calculate this patient's actual tidal volume.

$$V_T = \text{ventilator volume} - \text{compressed volume}$$

$$= 667 \text{ cc} - 111 \text{ cc}$$

$$= 556 \text{ cc}$$

(1:937–938), (9:285), (10:256).

## IIIA1e

197. D. This patient's IBW was given in pounds; therefore, we must convert it to kg.

$$kg = \frac{85 \text{ lbs}}{2.2 \text{ lbs/kg}}$$

$$= 39.5 \text{ kg}$$

If we know the patient's IBW in kilograms, we can determine the tidal volume recommended by the physician (12 cc/kg):

$$V_T = (12 \text{ cc/kg})(39.5 \text{ kg})$$

$$= 474 \text{ cc}$$

At this time, the ventilator is delivering a tidal volume of 667 cc. This volume is too large and must be reduced in order to comply with the physician's order. The new tidal volume must be sufficient enough to deliver the 474 cc plus the 111 cc compressed in the ventilator tubing. Consequently, the tidal volume sought must be equal to 585 cc (474 cc plus 111 cc). The target tidal volume can be achieved by either increasing the ventilatory rate or decreasing the minute ventilation. The SIMV rate does not influence the tidal volume.

Consider the ventilatory rate first. The change in the ventilatory rate can be calculated as follows:

$$f = \frac{\dot{V}_E}{V_T}$$

$$= \frac{10,000 \text{ cc/min.}}{585 \text{ cc/breath}}$$

$$= 17 \text{ breaths/min.}$$

This ventilatory rate is not available among the choices presented. Therefore, manipulation of the ventilatory rate can be excluded as a means of achieving the target tidal volume in this problem. Keep in mind, however, that the combination of a 10 L/min. $\dot{V}_E$ and a 17 breath/min. ventilatory rate would render a tidal volume of approximately 585 cc. Besides, the physician has not indicated any desire to change the ventilatory rate.

As we switch our attention to the possibility of decreasing the minute ventilation, the following formula can be used:

$$\dot{V}_E = (V_T)(f)$$

$$= (585 \text{ cc/breath})(12 \text{ breaths/min.})$$

$$\approx 7,000 \text{ cc/min. or } 7 \text{ L/min.}$$

Decreasing the minute ventilation from 10 L/min. to 7 L/min. will provide a tidal volume of 585 cc at a ventilatory rate of 12 breaths/min.

Be aware that a slight decrease in the compressed volume will occur as a result of the smaller tidal volume now delivered. The reduced tidal volume will generate a lower PIP. The compressible volume can be recalculated based on the new PIP if it is necessary to be that precise.

(1:909), (10:251).

## IIIB2c

198. B. The primary concerns for a patient who has massive cerebral hemorrhage are to provide an adequate alveolar ventilation and to reduce the intracranial pressure (ICP). The ICP can be lowered by increasing cerebral vascular resistance (vasoconstriction) and still providing adequate cerebral blood flow.

The patient's inablity to maintain an adequate spontaneous minute ventilation requires him to be mechanically ventilated. A $V_T$ of 270 cc and a ventilatory rate of 7 breaths/min. is not sufficient to meet his metabolic demands. It is important to precisely control the $PaCO_2$ because an increased $PaCO_2$ causes cerebral vasodilatation, thereby increasing the intracranial pressure. Controlled ventilation is indicated.

Maintaining an arterial $PCO_2$ of between 20 to 25 torr generally causes adequate cerebral vasoconstriction yet provides sufficient cerebral blood flow for brain perfusion. It is believed that the reduction of cerebral blood flow is maximized at an arterial $PCO_2$ around 20 torr. At this arterial $PCO_2$, evidence indicates that the vasoconstriction effect is counterbalanced by the vasodilatation caused by cerebral hypoxia.

(10:147–148), (15:1095–1102).

## IIIB2c

199. A. Intracranial pressure (ICP) can be monitored continuously via a subarachnoid bolt, a Scott cannula placed in the lateral ventricle, or a Richmond subdural screw. Hypoxia and hypercapnia produce cerebral vasodilatation, increasing cerebral blood volume and increasing the ICP. An increased ICP, in turn, will reduce cerebral perfusion pressure and cause a decrease in cerebral blood flow. Therefore, it is necessary to control the ICP while continuing to maintain cerebral blood flow above critically low levels to avoid cerebral infarction.

From a ventilatory standpoint, the arterial $PO_2$ and $PCO_2$ can be manipulated to influence the ICP. Maintaining a satisfactory arterial $PO_2$ to reduce cerebral vasodilation is one important measure. Another useful intervention is to iatrogenically induce a respiratory alkalosis. The patient should be hyperventilated to an arterial $PCO_2$ level of 20 to 25 torr. This level of hypocapnia results in maximum cerebral vasoconstriction.

High PIP should be avoided whenever possible because high PIP tends to increase the ICP. Patient coughing and gagging should be minimized because both of these activities temporarily increase the ICP.

PEEP should not be employed unless absolutely necessary because it increases the ICP.

(10:147–148), (15:1095–1102).

## IIIB2c

200. B. In cases of increased intracranial pressure, the $PaCO_2$ should be maintained in a range of 20 to 25 mm Hg.

(10:147–148), (15:1095–1102).

## IB2b

201. B. A number of conditions can cause a unilateral reduction in chest-wall excursion. These conditions include atelectasis, pneumothorax, pleural effusion, and consolidation. Dull percussion notes are caused by atelectasis, underlying neoplasms, pleural effusion, and consolidation. Increased resonance is perceived in lung regions experiencing hyperinflation. Diminished breaths sounds via auscultation result from atelectasis, consolidation, hyperaeration, and pleural effusion. Atelectasis in the region of the left lower lobe would cause the intrapleural pressure in that area to become more subatmospheric, thereby causing the left hemidiaphragm to rise. Alveolar collapse will show up as an increased density on a chest roentgenogram. The decreased lucency will present as a radiopaque area. The findings of this physical chest assessment and chest radiography are consistent with left lower-lobe atelectasis.

(1:309), (9:71–74, 261–262), (15:436–443).

## IIIC1a

202. D. Patients who have thoracic or abdominal surgery often find it difficult to breathe deeply because of pain caused by the incision. The lack of deep breathing prevents complete lung expansion as well as periodic sighing. The consequence is atelectasis. To overcome the potential problem of post-operative atelectasis, it is imperative to have preoperative instructions given to the patient on how to perform either IPPB or incentive spirometry (IS), both of which are indicated as a prophylaxis to atelectasis or as a therapeutic modality to treat that condition.

There are different protocols used to determine which deep-breathing technique (IPPB or IS) should be used. One such protocol is based on the comparison of the patient's pre- and postoperative inspiratory capacity (IC). Table 5-14 outlines this protocol.

(1:309), (9:71–74, 261–262), (15:436–443).

## IA1h

203. D. Persistent pulmonary hypertension of the newborn (PPHN) ordinarily occurs in term or post-term infants. Characteristically, their cyanosis is more severe than the

**Table 5-14** Postoperative Thoracotomy/Laparotomy
Deep-Breathing Protocol

| Pre- to Postoperative IC | Deep Breathing Technique |
|---|---|
| > 50% | IPPB |
| 50% to 80% | IS |
| > 80% | Monitor patient for pulmonary complications |

radiographic presentation of their lung problem. The cyanosis is caused by the right-to-left shunting occurring across the foramen ovale and/or the ductus arteriosus.

The muscular pulmonary arterioles of the newborn constrict in resonse to the severe hypoxemia, hypercapnia, and acidemia. Consequently, the resulting pulmonary vasoconstriction causes much of the C.O. to be shunted right to left through the foramen ovale and/or the ductus arteriosus.

Clinical manifestations of PPHN include cyanosis and respiratory distress. A significant disparity existing between pre- and postductal $PaO_2$s is deemed diagnostic. Postductal blood (umbilical artery catheter sample) contains more venous blood and therefore will reflect a lower oxygen value than the preductal (radial artery) sample.

The oxygenation data given in this question (radial artery: $PO_2$ 45 torr; UAC: $PO_2$ 28 torr) reflect a significant pre- and postductal $PaO_2$ disparity. In the presence of significant right-to-left shunting, however, pre- and postductal $PaO_2$s can be equal.

(1:1034), (16:940–943).

**IIIA1b**

204. B. The common method of treatment of PPHN is hyperventilation via mechanical ventilation. The intent of the hyperventilation is to lower the arterial $PCO_2$ to an approximate range of 20 to 25 torr, and to relieve the acidemia.

The hypercapnia and associated acidemia contribute to pulmonary vasoconstriction and pulmonary hypertension. Another factor that is frequently involved in the development of these two pathophysiologic conditions is hypoxemia. The hyperventilation producing the low arterial $PCO_2$ and increased pH eliminates two of the three factors that produce pulmonary vasoconstriction and pulmonary hypertension. Frequently, the pulmonary vasoconstriction and pulmonary hypertension are ameliorated by mechanical ventilation, as evidenced by an improved arterial $PO_2$. The treatment of PPHN includes the administration of an increased

$FiO_2$, in addition to the mechanical hyperventilation. The intent of the elevated $FiO_2$ is to produce both bronchodilatation and vasodilatation.

To reiterate, the therapeutic approach to PPHN includes mechanical hyperventilation to decrease the arterial $PCO_2$ and elevate the pH. Additionally, a high $FiO_2$ is administered to eliminate the hypoxemia. Overall, improvement of these ABG and acid-base measurements promotes pulmonary vasodilatation and relieves the pulmonary hypertension.

However, not all neonates respond favorably to the hyperventilation and oxygenation. The patient in this question represents such a situation. Despite receiving a high $FiO_2$, a high PIP, and a high ventilatory rate, severe hypoxemia persists. The risk of barotrauma at this point should be obvious.

An action worthy of consideration at this time is I.V. administration of the vasodilator tolazoline (Priscoline). Tolazoline is an alpha adrenergic antagonist with a histamine-like action. However, varying degrees of success have been met with the use of tolazoline. Therefore, its use should be considered in light of its potential side effects, which include pulmonary hemorrhage, hypotension, thrombocytopenia, and GI bleeding. More recently, some PPHN patients who fail to respond to conventional treatment undergo extracorporeal membrane oxygenation (ECMO).

(1:1034), (16:940–943).

**IA1b**

205. C. Epiglottitis is generally caused by the bacterium *Hemophilus influenzae* type B. The inflammation (obstruction) occurs above the glottis. Specifically, the structures affected by this disease are the epiglottis, the arytenoid cartilages, and the aryepiglottic folds. These three anatomical structures comprise the laryngeal inlet.

The age group usually afflicted with this infectious process ranges from two to six years. Clinical manifestations include (1) high fever; (2) hoarseness; (3) a brassy, barking cough; (4) inspiratory and expiratory stridor; (5) sore throat; (6) dysphagia; (7) muffled voice; (8) drooling; and (9) dyspnea. Patients who have this disease commonly lean forward and assume the sniffing position.

Lateral neck roentgenograms indicate an enlarged epiglottis. Specifically, the epiglottis appears broad and thick. This appearance is often described as the thumb sign because the epiglottis resembles the shape of an adult's thumb. Other radiographic findings include thickening of the aryepiglottic folds and ballooning of the hypopharynx. The lateral neck X-ray often distinguishes croup from epiglottitis. Characteristically, croup reveals subglottic narrowing. The following diagram illustrates the anatomic location of the inflammatory process associated with epiglottitis (Figure 5-39).

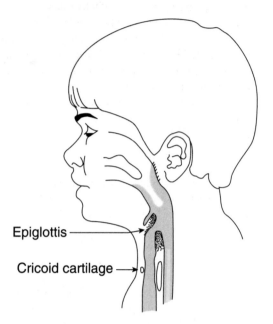

**Figure 5-39:** Epiglottitis: note the swollen supraglottic region.

Again, the epiglottitis is characterized by a swollen epiglottis and laryngeal inlet and therefore is supraglottic.

Laryngotracheobronchitis, or croup, is the inflammation of the airway below the vocal cords. It is shown in Figure 5-40 to be the region of the cricoid cartilage in the larynx.

(1:1039–1040), (16:597, 983–984).

### IIIB1a

206. A. Quite often, epiglottitis is a respiratory emergency warranting the immediate establishment of a patent airway because of the acute and rapid nature of this upper airway obstruction. Therefore, ET intubation is attempted. In some instances, the route of ET intubation might be blocked, requiring a tracheostomy to be performed. Direct laryngoscopy or the use of a tongue depressor to visualize the larynx is contraindicated in epiglottitis because of the potential risk of producing a complete airway obstruction. Again, the artificial airway preferred is an ET tube. If an ET tube cannot be inserted, however, a tracheostomy must be performed.

(1:1039–1040), (16:597, 983–984).

### IA1f(4)

207. A. To calculate this patient's airway resistance, one needs to determine the pressure that was generated to overcome the airway resistance during the inspiratory phase of ventilation. This pressure, designated as $P_{Raw}$, is the difference between the PIP and the static pressure ($P_{static}$). This relationship is expressed as follows:

$$P_{Raw} = PIP - P_{static}$$

Table 5-15 shows the PIP–$P_{static}$ gradient, or the $P_{Raw}$ ($\Delta P$), for each ventilator check.

**Table 5-15** Data from Ventilator Check

| Time | PIP | $P_{static}$ | $P_{Raw}$ (PIP − $P_{static}$, or $\Delta P$) |
|---|---|---|---|
| 4:10 P.M. | 36 cm $H_2O$ | 24 cm $H_2O$ | 12 cm $H_2O$ |
| 5:15 P.M. | 38 cm $H_2O$ | 26 cm $H_2O$ | 12 cm $H_2O$ |
| 6:05 P.M. | 41 cm $H_2O$ | 29 cm $H_2O$ | 12 cm $H_2O$ |
| 7:15 P.M. | 42 cm $H_2O$ | 30 cm $H_2O$ | 12 cm $H_2O$ |
| 8:10 P.M. | 45 cm $H_2O$ | 33 cm $H_2O$ | 12 cm $H_2O$ |

The difference between the PIP and $P_{static}$ has remained constant at 12 cm $H_2O$ pressure over the four-hour period discussed here. Because the peak inspiratory flow rate and the $P_{Raw}$ have remained constant from 4:10 P.M. to 8:10 P.M., the airway resistance ($R_{aw}$) has not changed. If the formula for airway resistance is applied to each ventilator check made, it can be seen that the airway resistance has remained constant.

$$R_{aw} = \frac{PIP - P_{static}}{\dot{V}}$$

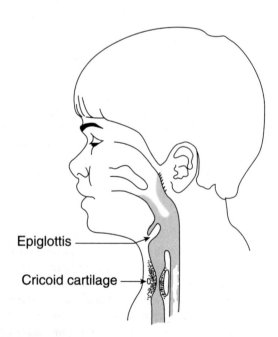

**Figure 5-40:** Laryngotracheobronchitis: note the subglottic inflammation in the cricoid cartilage region.

Table 5-16 shows the calculated airway resistance for each ventilator check made. The peak inspiratory flow has been converted to L/sec. (50 L/min. = 0.833 L/sec.).

**Table 5-16** Calculator $R_{aw}$ for Ventilator Checks

| Time | $P_{RAW}$ or $\Delta P$ (cm H$_2$O) | $\dot{V}$ (L/sec.) | $R_{AW}$ (cm H$_2$O/L/sec.) |
|------|------|------|------|
| 4:10 P.M. | 12 | 0.833 | 14.4 |
| 5:15 P.M. | 12 | 0.833 | 14.4 |
| 6:05 P.M. | 12 | 0.833 | 14.4 |
| 7:15 P.M. | 12 | 0.833 | 14.4 |
| 8:10 P.M. | 12 | 0.833 | 14.4 |

(1:937–938), (10:256–257), (15:89).

**IIIC6a**

208. B. When the PIP and the static pressure both increase to the same extent over time, a decrease in the effective static compliance is taking place. It has been demonstrated from the data in the previous question that the airway resistance remained constant over the four-hour period. Therefore, the only other component responsible for the changes in the PIP and the static pressure is the effective static compliance. The equation used for solving for the effective static compliance follows:

$$C_{static} = \frac{\Delta V}{\Delta P} = \frac{V_T}{P_{static} - PEEP}$$

Table 5-17 illustrates the effective static compliance values for each of the ventilator checks given in this problem. The $C_{static}$ column shows the progressive decrease in the compliance value. The tidal volume of 1,000 cc has been converted to 1 liter.

**Table 5-17** $C_{static}$ for Ventilator Checks

| Time | Volume (liter) | $P_{static}$ − PEEP (cm H$_2$O) | $C_{static}$ (L/cm H$_2$O) |
|------|------|------|------|
| 4:10 P.M. | 1 | 19 | 0.053 |
| 5:15 P.M. | 1 | 21 | 0.048 |
| 6:05 P.M. | 1 | 24 | 0.042 |
| 7:15 P.M. | 1 | 25 | 0.040 |
| 8:10 P.M. | 1 | 28 | 0.036 |

The effective static compliance generally reflects the lung–chest-wall compliance because the compliance of the tubing and the ventilator system are ordinarily constant. Furthermore, when the chest wall is normal, the chest-wall compliance is assumed to be constant.

Therefore, changes in the static pressure under these circumstances infer changes in the status of the lungs.

Clinical conditions that are associated with a decreased lung compliance (decreased effective static compliance) include atelectasis, pneumothorax, pleural effusion, and slippage of an ET tube into the right mainstem bronchus. Likewise, right mainstem bronchus intubation widens the static pressure–PIP gradient because more pressure is encountered by depositing all the $V_T$ into one lung. In these conditions, the same tidal volume is being deposited into a smaller "container," the result of which is an increased static pressure and PIP. In most instances, right mainstem bronchus intubation would not occur gradually, so it can be ruled out as a likely cause of the decrease in static compliance. Airway resistance problems (e.g., increased tracheobronchial secretions) are identified by a widened PIP–$P_{static}$ gradient.

(1:937–938), (10:256–257), (15:89).

**IIIC5**

209. Some patients who have severe COPD are susceptible to small airway collapse because of generating high intrapleural pressures during coughing. Directed cough is a voluntary effort made by the patient with the intention of duplicating the characteristics of an effective spontaneous cough. When this maneuver is performed, intrapleural pressure might become supra-atmospheric. Consequently, some patients who have severe COPD experience small airway collapse when their intrapleural pressures become supra-atmospheric (positive). Therefore, these patients require a modified, directed cough technique. Such modifications include (1) forced expiratory technique (FET), (2) active cycle breathing, and (3) autogenic drainage.

Splinting is considered a modified, directed cough procedure but is used for post-surgical patients experiencing abdominal or thoracic pain while they cough.

Postural drainage with percussion and vibration is sometimes effective in moving secretions from peripheral airways to central airways, but it is not a coughing procedure. Coughing must accompany postural drainage with percussion and vibration for this bronchial hygiene procedure to be effective.

(1:803-807).

**IIIC5**

210. B. Because the elderly, arthritic grandmother of the 10-year-old cystic fibrosis patient cannot comply with the child's bronchial hygiene regimen of postural drainage with percussion and vibration, an alternative form of bronchial hygiene therapy must be instituted. The alternative therapy must not require the involvement of the patient's grandmother. The patient must become her own caregiver.

Suitable forms of bronchial hygiene therapy the patient can self-administer include PEP therapy, flutter therapy, or intrapulmonary percussive ventilation. A mechanical percussor would still require the patient's grandmother to perform the therapy on her granddaughter. Therefore, this form of therapy is inadvisable.

Forced expiratory technique is a modification of the normal directed cough. No evidence was given implying that the patient required modification of the directed cough technique.

(1:803, 810-811).

## IIIC2

211.  A. The effectiveness of a small volume nebulizer is less technique-dependent compared to a metered-dose inhaler or a dry powder inhaler. The optimal breathing pattern associated with a small volume nebulizer includes having the patient breathe slowly through the mouth at a normal tidal volume. Deep breathing and breathholding while using a small volume nebulizer does not appreciably improve drug deposition.

(1:696).

## IIIB3

212.  D. The cough mechanism has four components: the irritation phase, the inspiration phase, the compression phase, and the expulsion phase. A number of factors can adversely influence each of these phases and hinder the patient's ability to cough up pulmonary secretions. For example, general anesthesia, narcotic-analgesics (morphine), and central nervous system depression interfere with the irritation phase. Post-surgical pain from abdominal or thoracic surgery and obesity can prevent the patient from inspiring a large enough tidal volume to produce an effective cough. Abdominal muscle weakness and soreness and a tracheal airway impair the compression phase by prohibiting the pressure within the lungs to rise sufficiently. Again, abdominal muscle weakness and soreness prevent the abdominal musculature from vigorously contracting and producing a rapid expulsion of air.

(1:792-794).

## IIIC2

213.  B. When using a metered-dose inhaler (MDI), the patient must be instructed to open his mouth widely with the MDI outlet pointing toward the mouth. The MDI should be positioned a distance of about two fingers away from the mouth. After the patient exhales normally, he needs to begin inspiring slowly, at which

time the actuator is depressed. Inspiration then continues to total lung capacity. When total lung capacity is achieved, a 10-second breathhold takes place.

(1:689).

## IIIB3

214.  C. Patients who have neuromuscular disease, e.g., myasthenia gravis and Guillain-Barré syndrome, generally cannot generate a vigorous cough because of their inability to produce a forceful expulsion of air. When their neuromuscular disease affects their abdominal and thoracic musculature, this problem arises.

These patients often benefit from manually assisted coughing. After the patient takes a deep breath or receives a large manual breath (bag-mask), external chest wall or epigastric compression is coordinated with a forced exhalation. If the patient is unable to inspire an adequate deep breath, a breath is administered via a manual resuscitator.

PEP therapy, flutter therapy, and intrapulmonary percussive ventilation require functional abdominal musculature to be effective forms of bronchial hygiene therapy. Actually, an effective cough is necessary for most bronchial hygiene techniques to be successful.

(1:807-811).

## IIIC2

215.  C. A dry powder inhaler (DPI) is activated by the patient's inspiratory effort. The patient must develop a rapid inspiratory flow rate (exceeding 40 L/min.) to create aerosol particles capable of entering the lungs. If the patient is unable to generate such a high inspiratory flow rate, the device cannot be used and another mode of drug delivery (a metered-dose inhaler or small-volume nebulizer) must be ordered.

To optimally use a DPI, the patient must be instructed to exhale slowly to functional residual capacity (FRC), place the DPI mouthpiece between his lips, and create a seal. Then, the patient needs to inhale deeply and forcefully. Breathholding with a DPI is unnecessary.

(1:691-693).

## IIIC8a

216.  B. Draining the condensate from the breathing circuit provides only a temporary solution to the problem of "rain-out" in the ventilator tubing. Using a heated-wire breathing circuit and setting the temperatures of the humidifier and the heated-wire circuit appropriately

will correct the condensation problem. The temperature of the humidifier should be set at 33°C ± 2°C, and the heated-wire circuit temperature should be set at 37°C. The temperature of the heated-wire circuit being higher than the humidifier increases the capacity of the flowing gas to hold moisture. Therefore, little to no condensate forms in the tubing.

Note that as the temperature of the heated-wire circuit is raised above that of the humidifier, the relative humidity of the gas in the inspiratory limb of the breathing circuit is less than the relative humidity at the humidifier. Remember the formula for relative humidity:

$$\% \text{ relative humidity} = \frac{\text{content}}{\text{capacity}} \times 100$$

(1:671), (9:114-115).

## IIIC8c

217. D. If a patient is receiving assist or assist-control mechanical ventilation and develops a respiratory alkalosis that persists despite ventilator setting adjustments, mechanical dead space can be added. In the situation presented in this question, the patient's respiratory alkalosis continued although the mandatory rate (and later, the tidal volume) were reduced.

Various lengths of large-bore (22 mm) tubing added between the endotracheal tube adapter and the Y connector of the breathing circuit constitute mechanical dead space.

Another alternative to solve this problem of persistent respiratory alkalosis is to change the mode of mechanical ventilation, e.g., IMV, SMV, or pressure support. These modes would enable the patient to breathe without a mandatory breath with every inspiration.

Sedating the patient to control the patient's breathing would also correct this respiratory acid-base disturbance problem.

(10:235, 251, 434).

## IIIC4

218. B. Helium-oxygen (heliox) gas mixtures are available in two concentrations: 80-20 (80% helium; 20% oxygen) and 70-30 (70% helium; 30% oxygen). These specialty gas mixtures are available in compressed gas cylinders color coded brown and green.

Because helium diffuses so readily, heliox mixtures should be administered via a nonrebreathing mask (which is essentially a closed system). Alternatively,

heliox can be given by way of a small-volume reservoir device, e.g., a simple mask.

For patients who have an endotracheal tube inserted, an intermittent positive-pressure delivery device is often used.

If an oxygen flowmeter is used, it will register a flow rate lower than the actual flow rate because heliox is less dense than both 100% $O_2$ and oxygen enriched air.

(1:768), (16:887-888).

## IIIC4

219. A. Although heliox mixtures are commercially available in compressed gas cylinders, the contents of the cylinders might be unmixed. What might occur is a layering effect in the cylinder with the helium (density: 0.43 g/L) accumulating near the top of the tank and the oxygen (density: 1.43 g/L) settling lower in the cylinder. The concentration of the oxygen flowing from the cylinder must be analyzed to determine the oxygen concentration delivered by the cylinder. Otherwise, the patient might develop hypoxemia and aggravate the current condition.

In such a situation as described in this question, the patient appears to be experiencing hypoxemia because inadequate oxygen is being delivered. At this time, the patient should be given 100% oxygen via a nonrebreathing mask to relieve the likely hypoxemia and respiratory distress. The physician must also be notified of this situation.

(1:719, 768), (16:887-888).

## IIIB3

220. D. Patients who undergo thoracic or abdominal surgery do not breathe deeply because of the incisional pain. Consequently, their ability to generate an effective cough is greatly compromised. The tendency is for these patients is to retain secretions if bronchial hygiene and lung expansion measures are not instituted.

This patient is demonstrating an inability to clear secretions as supported by the presence of inspiratory and expiratory crackles. These adventitious breath sounds are caused by the build-up of secretions. The fact that these abnormal lung sounds sometimes disappear when the patient generates an effective cough indicates that their origin is retained secretions.

What this patient needs is a combination of therapeutic modalities. Incentive spirometry is intended to help the patient breathe deeply. The aerosol therapy is intended to help liquify the secretions to facilitate their removal. The postural drainage is administered to mobilize secretions from peripheral airways to the central airways. Splinting is taught to help this patient generate a more effective cough to then remove the secretions from the central airways.

(1:772-774, 793-799, 803).

## IIIC6b

221. D. A fenestrated tracheostomy tube is designed to help patients wean from a tracheostomy tube. Before the actual weaning takes place, the patient needs to meet certain criteria. The patient needs to demonstrate a desire to have the tracheal airway removed. The patient's upper airway reflexes must be intact.

Once the patient meets these and other mechanical and physiologic requirements, the patient can begin weaning from the tracheostomy tube.

Before the tracheostomy tube cuff is deflated, the patient's upper airway must be suctioned to prevent the aspiration of secretions. Once the cuff is deflated, suctioning of the trachea and oropharynx might be necessary again. The inner cannula is then removed, and the tracheostomy tube opening is covered with a decannulation cannula (plug). The patient can then breathe air around the deflated cuff and through the outer cannula and out the fenestration, thereby through the upper airway.

(1:614-615).

## IIIC8b

222. C. The volume lost through chest tubes when the same tidal volume is being delivered can be estimated by subtracting the measured exhaled tidal volume after chest tube insertion from the measured exhaled tidal volume before chest tube insertion.

In the problem presented, the patient's ventilator is set to deliver a tidal volume of 450 ml. Before the pneumothorax, the measured exhaled tidal volume was 400 ml. After the chest tubes were inserted, the measured exhaled tidal volume was 250 ml.

Therefore, 150 ml of gas is being lost through the chest tubes, e.g.,

$$400 \text{ ml} - 250 \text{ ml} = 150 \text{ ml}$$

(1:488).

# REFERENCES

1. Scanlan, C., Spearman, C., and Sheldon, R., *Egan's Fundamentals of Respiratory Care*, 7th ed., Mosby-Year Book, Inc., St. Louis, MO, 1999.

2. Kacmarek, R., Mack, C., and Dimas, S., *The Essentials of Respiratory Care*, 3rd ed., Mosby-Year Book, Inc., St. Louis, MO, 1990.

3. Shapiro B., Peruzzi, W., and Kozlowska-Templin, R., *Clinical Applications of Blood Gases*, 5th ed., Mosby-Year Book, Inc., St. Louis, MO, 1994.

4. Malley, W., *Clinical Blood Gases: Application and Noninvasive Alternatives*, W.B. Saunders Co., Philadelphia, PA, 1990.

5. White, G., *Equipment Theory for Respiratory Care*, 3rd ed., Delmar, Albany, NY, 1999.

6. Ruppel, G., *Manual of Pulmonary Function Testing*, 7th ed., Mosby-Year Book, Inc., St. Louis, MO, 1998.

7. Barnes, T., *Core Textbook of Respiratory Care Practice*, 2nd ed., Mosby-Year Book, Inc., St. Louis, MO, 1994.

8. Rau, J., *Respiratory Care Pharmacology*, 5th ed., Mosby-Year Book, Inc., St. Louis, MO, 1998.

9. Wilkins, R., Sheldon, R., and Krider, S., *Clinical Assessment in Respiratory Care*, 4th ed., Mosby-Year Book, Inc., St. Louis, MO, 2000.

10. Pilbeam, S., *Mechanical Ventilation: Physiological and Clinical Applications*, 3rd ed., Mosby-Year Book, Inc., St. Louis, MO, 1998.

11. Madama, V., *Pulmonary Function Testing and Cardiopulmonary Stress Testing*, 2nd ed., Delmar, Albany, NY, 1998.

12. Koff, P., Eitzman, D., and New, J., *Neonatal and Pediatric Respiratory Care*, 2nd ed., Mosby-Year Book, Inc., St. Louis, MO, 1993.

13. Branson, R., Hess, D., and Chatburn, R., *Respiratory Care Equipment*, J.B. Lippincott, Co., Philadelphia, PA, 1995.

14. Darovic, G., *Hemodynamic Monitoring: Invasive and Noninvasive Clinical Application*, 2nd ed., W.B. Saunders Company, Philadelphia, PA, 1995.

15. Pierson, D, and Kacmarek, R., *Foundations of Respiratory Care*, Churchill Livingston, Inc., New York, NY, 1992.

16. Burton, et al., *Respiratory Care: A Guide to Clinical Practice*, 4th ed., Lippincott-Raven Publishers, Philadelphia, PA, 1997.

17. Wojciechowski, W., *Respiratory Care Sciences: An Integrated Approach*, 3rd ed., Delmar, Albany, NY, 2000.

18. Aloan, C., *Respiratory Care of the Newborn and Child*, 2nd ed., Lippincott-Raven Publishers, Philadelphia, PA, 1997.

19. Dantzker, D., MacIntyre, N., and Bakow, E., *Comprehensive Respiratory Care*, W.B. Saunders Company, Philadelphia, PA, 1998.

20. Farzan, S., and Farzan, D., *A Concise Handbook of Respiratory Diseases*, 4th ed., Appleton & Lange, Stamford, CT, 1997.

**PURPOSE:**  The posttest contained here represents your final phase in preparing for the Written Registry Examination. The content of the posttest parallels that which you will encounter on the Written Registry Examination offered by the National Board for Respiratory Care (NBRC). The posttest contains 100 test items that match the Written Registry Examination Matrix. The content areas included on the posttest are as follows:

- Clinical Data (17 items)
- Equipment (20 items)
- Therapeutic Procedures (63 items)

Remember to allow yourself two (uninterrupted) hours for the posttest and use the answer sheet located on the next page. Score the posttest soon after you complete it. Begin reviewing the posttest analyses and references and the NBRC matrix designations as soon as you have a reasonable block of time available.

# Posttest Answer Sheet

**DIRECTIONS:**     Darken the space under the selected answer.

|  | A | B | C | D |  |  | A | B | C | D |
|---|---|---|---|---|---|---|---|---|---|---|
| 1. | ❑ | ❑ | ❑ | ❑ |  | 25. | ❑ | ❑ | ❑ | ❑ |
| 2. | ❑ | ❑ | ❑ | ❑ |  | 26. | ❑ | ❑ | ❑ | ❑ |
| 3. | ❑ | ❑ | ❑ | ❑ |  | 27. | ❑ | ❑ | ❑ | ❑ |
| 4. | ❑ | ❑ | ❑ | ❑ |  | 28. | ❑ | ❑ | ❑ | ❑ |
| 5. | ❑ | ❑ | ❑ | ❑ |  | 29. | ❑ | ❑ | ❑ | ❑ |
| 6. | ❑ | ❑ | ❑ | ❑ |  | 30. | ❑ | ❑ | ❑ | ❑ |
| 7. | ❑ | ❑ | ❑ | ❑ |  | 31. | ❑ | ❑ | ❑ | ❑ |
| 8. | ❑ | ❑ | ❑ | ❑ |  | 32. | ❑ | ❑ | ❑ | ❑ |
| 9. | ❑ | ❑ | ❑ | ❑ |  | 33. | ❑ | ❑ | ❑ | ❑ |
| 10. | ❑ | ❑ | ❑ | ❑ |  | 34. | ❑ | ❑ | ❑ | ❑ |
| 11. | ❑ | ❑ | ❑ | ❑ |  | 35. | ❑ | ❑ | ❑ | ❑ |
| 12. | ❑ | ❑ | ❑ | ❑ |  | 36. | ❑ | ❑ | ❑ | ❑ |
| 13. | ❑ | ❑ | ❑ | ❑ |  | 37. | ❑ | ❑ | ❑ | ❑ |
| 14. | ❑ | ❑ | ❑ | ❑ |  | 38. | ❑ | ❑ | ❑ | ❑ |
| 15. | ❑ | ❑ | ❑ | ❑ |  | 39. | ❑ | ❑ | ❑ | ❑ |
| 16. | ❑ | ❑ | ❑ | ❑ |  | 40. | ❑ | ❑ | ❑ | ❑ |
| 17. | ❑ | ❑ | ❑ | ❑ |  | 41. | ❑ | ❑ | ❑ | ❑ |
| 18. | ❑ | ❑ | ❑ | ❑ |  | 42. | ❑ | ❑ | ❑ | ❑ |
| 19. | ❑ | ❑ | ❑ | ❑ |  | 43. | ❑ | ❑ | ❑ | ❑ |
| 20. | ❑ | ❑ | ❑ | ❑ |  | 44. | ❑ | ❑ | ❑ | ❑ |
| 21. | ❑ | ❑ | ❑ | ❑ |  | 45. | ❑ | ❑ | ❑ | ❑ |
| 22. | ❑ | ❑ | ❑ | ❑ |  | 46. | ❑ | ❑ | ❑ | ❑ |
| 23. | ❑ | ❑ | ❑ | ❑ |  | 47. | ❑ | ❑ | ❑ | ❑ |
| 24. | ❑ | ❑ | ❑ | ❑ |  | 48. | ❑ | ❑ | ❑ | ❑ |

|       | A | B | C | D |       |       | A | B | C | D |
|-------|---|---|---|---|-------|-------|---|---|---|---|
| 49.   | ❏ | ❏ | ❏ | ❏ |       | 75.   | ❏ | ❏ | ❏ | ❏ |
| 50.   | ❏ | ❏ | ❏ | ❏ |       | 76.   | ❏ | ❏ | ❏ | ❏ |
| 51.   | ❏ | ❏ | ❏ | ❏ |       | 77.   | ❏ | ❏ | ❏ | ❏ |
| 52.   | ❏ | ❏ | ❏ | ❏ |       | 78.   | ❏ | ❏ | ❏ | ❏ |
| 53.   | ❏ | ❏ | ❏ | ❏ |       | 79.   | ❏ | ❏ | ❏ | ❏ |
| 54.   | ❏ | ❏ | ❏ | ❏ |       | 80.   | ❏ | ❏ | ❏ | ❏ |
| 55.   | ❏ | ❏ | ❏ | ❏ |       | 81.   | ❏ | ❏ | ❏ | ❏ |
| 56.   | ❏ | ❏ | ❏ | ❏ |       | 82.   | ❏ | ❏ | ❏ | ❏ |
| 57.   | ❏ | ❏ | ❏ | ❏ |       | 83.   | ❏ | ❏ | ❏ | ❏ |
| 58.   | ❏ | ❏ | ❏ | ❏ |       | 84.   | ❏ | ❏ | ❏ | ❏ |
| 59.   | ❏ | ❏ | ❏ | ❏ |       | 85.   | ❏ | ❏ | ❏ | ❏ |
| 60.   | ❏ | ❏ | ❏ | ❏ |       | 86.   | ❏ | ❏ | ❏ | ❏ |
| 61.   | ❏ | ❏ | ❏ | ❏ |       | 87.   | ❏ | ❏ | ❏ | ❏ |
| 62.   | ❏ | ❏ | ❏ | ❏ |       | 88.   | ❏ | ❏ | ❏ | ❏ |
| 63.   | ❏ | ❏ | ❏ | ❏ |       | 89.   | ❏ | ❏ | ❏ | ❏ |
| 64.   | ❏ | ❏ | ❏ | ❏ |       | 90.   | ❏ | ❏ | ❏ | ❏ |
| 65.   | ❏ | ❏ | ❏ | ❏ |       | 91.   | ❏ | ❏ | ❏ | ❏ |
| 66.   | ❏ | ❏ | ❏ | ❏ |       | 92.   | ❏ | ❏ | ❏ | ❏ |
| 67.   | ❏ | ❏ | ❏ | ❏ |       | 93.   | ❏ | ❏ | ❏ | ❏ |
| 68.   | ❏ | ❏ | ❏ | ❏ |       | 94.   | ❏ | ❏ | ❏ | ❏ |
| 69.   | ❏ | ❏ | ❏ | ❏ |       | 95.   | ❏ | ❏ | ❏ | ❏ |
| 70.   | ❏ | ❏ | ❏ | ❏ |       | 96.   | ❏ | ❏ | ❏ | ❏ |
| 71.   | ❏ | ❏ | ❏ | ❏ |       | 97.   | ❏ | ❏ | ❏ | ❏ |
| 72.   | ❏ | ❏ | ❏ | ❏ |       | 98.   | ❏ | ❏ | ❏ | ❏ |
| 73.   | ❏ | ❏ | ❏ | ❏ |       | 99.   | ❏ | ❏ | ❏ | ❏ |
| 74.   | ❏ | ❏ | ❏ | ❏ |       | 100.  | ❏ | ❏ | ❏ | ❏ |

# Posttest Assessment

**DIRECTIONS:** Each of the questions or incomplete statements below is followed by four suggested answers or completions. Select the one that is best in each case and then blacken the corresponding space on the answer sheet found in the front of this chapter. Good luck.

1. An RRT working in the adult, surgical ICU has been performing ventilator rounds and has charted the ventilator data in Table 6-1 from a postoperative laparotomy patient who is receiving mechanical ventilatory support via a microprocessor ventilator.

**Table 6-1** Ventilator Data

| Time | Peak Inspiratory Pressure | Static Pressure |
|------|---------------------------|-----------------|
| 3:00 P.M. | 30 cm H$_2$O | 19 cm H$_2$O |
| 4:00 P.M. | 33 cm H$_2$O | 18 cm H$_2$O |
| 5:15 P.M. | 35 cm H$_2$O | 20 cm H$_2$O |
| 6:10 P.M. | 37 cm H$_2$O | 19 cm H$_2$O |
| 7:05 P.M. | 42 cm H$_2$O | 19 cm H$_2$O |

The patient has the following ventilator settings:

tidal volume: 900 cc
F$_I$O$_2$: 0.40
mode: synchronized intermittent mandatory ventilation (SIMV)
ventilatory rate: 6 breaths/min.

What intervention should be implemented at this time?

A. endotracheal suctioning
B. pilot balloon cuff inflation
C. insertion of chest tubes
D. reduction of the high pressure limit

2. Which of the following recommendations should *not* be included in the respiratory care plan of a COPD patient who has cor pulmonale and is being treated at home?

  I. flutter therapy
 II. mask CPAP
III. chest physiotherapy
IV. metered-dose inhaler

A. II only
B. IV only
C. I, II only
D. III, IV only

3. While monitoring a patient who has a pulmonary artery catheter in place, the RRT observes the following tracing (Figure 6-1).

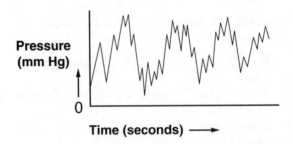

**Pressure (mm Hg)**

**Time (seconds)** ⟶

**Figure 6-1:** Pulmonary artery catheter tracing.

How should she interpret this situation?

A. This represents a normal right ventricular tracing.
B. The transducer has been relocated above the phlebostatic axis.
C. The catheter has coiled in the right atrium.
D. The catheter is stuck in the wedge position.

4. During cardiopulmonary resuscitation, a patient continues to display ventricular fibrillation on the cardiac monitor despite having been defibrillated twice. The physician is considering defibrillating the patient for a third time and asks the RRT assisting in the resuscitation to recommend an appropriate energy level for the defibrillation. What energy level should the RRT recommend at this time?

A. 200 joules
B. 275 joules
C. 330 joules
D. 360 joules

5. The RRT is auscultating the apical region of a patient's thorax. As the patient breathes, the RRT hears high-pitched sounds having an expiratory component equal to or slightly longer than the inspiratory component. How should the RRT describe these findings in the patient's chart?

A. bronchovesicular
B. crackles
C. bronchial
D. rhonchi

6. While administering 3.0 ml of 10% Mucomyst in 2.0 ml of normal saline via a small volume nebulizer, the RRT hears bilateral wheezing upon auscultating the

patient's chest. The patient also complains of dyspnea. What action should the RRT take at this time?

A. Change the concentration of Mycomyst to 20%.
B. Stop the treatment to allow the patient to rest.
C. Administer 0.3 ml of albuterol.
D. Install 3 to 5 ml of normal saline into the patient's airway and perform nasotracheal suctioning immediately.

7. What is(are) the purpose(s) for assessing pupillary response during emergency situations?

I. It establishes a baseline for determining future changes.
II. It allows for the early detection of epidural hematoma.
III. It establishes a measure of the higher cerebral functions.
IV. It is an indicator of hypoxia or drug overdose.

A. II, III only
B. I only
C. I, II, IV only
D. I, III, IV only

8. A patient who is receiving an $F_IO_2$ of 0.40 via mask CPAP has the following arterial blood gas data:

$PaO_2$ 85 torr
$PaCO_2$ 40 torr
pH 7.44
$HCO_3^-$ 26 mEq/L
B.E.: 2 mEq/L

Calculate this patient's $P(A-a)O_2$. Assume a normal respiratory quotient and standard atmospheric pressure.

A. 297 torr
B. 206 torr
C. 154 torr
D. 98 torr

9. The RRT is attempting to measure the exhaled tidal volume of a patient receiving continuous-flow intermittent mandatory ventilation (H-valve assembly). She notices the dial on the Wright Respirometer is spinning continually, preventing her from obtaining a reading. What is the cause of this situation?

A. She has the exhalation port of the Wright Respirometer attached to the ventilator circuit.
B. She has the Wright Respirometer attached to the exhalation limb of the ventilator tubing.
C. She has the Wright Respirometer attached to patient's ET tube.
D. She has the Wright Respirometer attached to the ventilator outlet.

10. The RRT is attaching electrodes to a patient for a sleep study. Where should the electromyographic leads be located?

A. over the outer canthi of the eyes
B. on the chin
C. on the chest just above the nipple line
D. on both sides of the neck

11. A patient who has a pulmonary artery catheter inserted has the following arterial and mixed venous blood gas data:

| Arterial | Mixed Venous |
|---|---|
| $SaO_2$ 95% | $S\bar{v}O_2$ 70% |
| $PaO_2$ 100 torr | $P\bar{v}O_2$ 40 torr |
| $PaCO_2$ 45 torr | $P\bar{v}CO_2$ 46 torr |
| pH 7.40 | pH 7.36 |
| $HCO_3^-$ 24 mEq/L | $HCO_3^-$ 24 mEq/L |
| B.E. 0 mEq/L | B.E. 0 mEq/L |

The patient also has a [Hb] of 15 g%.

Calculate this patient's $C(a-\bar{v})O_2$.

A. 4.5 vol%
B. 5.2 vol%
C. 5.9 vol%
D. 6.3 vol%

12. The appropriate continuous positive airway pressure (CPAP) level needed to treat obstructive sleep apnea is determined by adjusting the CPAP level until:

I. The oxygen saturation is maintained above 90% for 30 minutes.
II. Snoring is eliminated.
III. The apnea episodes stop.
IV. The patient's ventilatory efforts become rhythmic.

A. I, II, III only
B. II, III only
C. I, IV only
D. I, II, III, IV

13. Which of the following clinical signs are included in the Apgar score for clinically evaluating a neonate?

I. heart rate
II. ventilatory rate
III. color
IV. reflex irritability
V. muscle tone

A. I, II, III, IV, V
B. I, II, III only
C. II, IV, V only
D. I, III, IV, V only

14. The RRT is about to perform ET suctioning on a COPD patient receiving 30% $O_2$ via a Briggs adaptor. How should the patient be preoxygenated before the suction procedure?

   A. The patient should receive two manual ventilations with room air.
   B. The patient should be bagged at the $FiO_2$ he is receiving.
   C. The patient should be bagged at an $FiO_2$ of 0.40.
   D. The patient should have two manual breaths delivered at an $FiO_2$ of 0.80.

15. A 34-year-old, 110-pound female diabetic patient enters the emergency department displaying Kussmaul's breathing. Room air ABG data indicate the following:

   PO$_2$ 110 torr
   PCO$_2$ 10 torr
   pH 7.22
   HCO$_3^-$ 4 mEq/liter
   B.E. $-20$ mEq/liter

   She also has the following vital signs:

   blood pressure: 133/96 torr
   heart rate: 143 beats/min.
   ventilatory rate: 51 breaths/min.
   body temperature: 98.6°F

   Which of the following laboratory data would be appropriate to obtain on this patient?

   A. electrolytes
   B. cardiac enzymes
   C. liver enzymes
   D. complete blood count

16. The RRT is preparing to calibrate a blood gas analyzer. The compressed gas tanks containing the calibration gases have the following oxygen and carbon dioxide gas mixtures:

   | Cylinder A | Cylinder B |
   |------------|------------|
   | 5.0% $CO_2$ | 10.0% $CO_2$ |
   | 12.0% $O_2$ | 0.0% $O_2$ |

   Calculate the high $O_2$ and $CO_2$ partial pressure values. Assume one atmosphere of pressure.

   A. PO$_2$ 149.73 torr; PCO$_2$ 71.30 torr
   B. PO$_2$ 91.20 torr; PCO$_2$ 38.00 torr
   C. PO$_2$ 85.56 torr; PCO$_2$ 71.30 torr
   D. PO$_2$ 71.30 torr; PCO$_2$ 35.65 torr

17. The RRT obtained the following hemodynamic data from a 70-kg patient in the ICU:

   pulmonary artery systolic pressure: 25 mm Hg
   pulmonary artery diastolic pressure: 7 mm Hg
   mean pulmonary artery pressure: 14 mm Hg
   pulmonary capillary wedge pressure: 27 mm Hg
   cardiac output: 5.5 L/min

   Which of the following interpretations of this hemodynamic data is most appropriate?

   A. The patient has left ventricular dysfunction.
   B. The patient is experiencing volume overload.
   C. The patient has pulmonary hypertension.
   D. The data are erroneous.

18. A patient's blood analysis reveals the following data:

   hemoglobin concentration: 19 g/dl
   red blood cell count: $6.5 \times 10^6/mm^3$

   Which of the following descriptions match these blood data?

   I. anemia
   II. polycythemia
   III. erythrocytopenia
   IV. hemocytopenia

   A. I, IV only
   B. II only
   C. II, III only
   D. III only

19. What should the RRT consider doing if positive expiratory pressure (PEP) therapy at 25 cm $H_2O$ for 30 minutes does *not* increase sputum production in a patient who produces more than 30 ml of sputum a day without PEP therapy?

   A. increasing the PEP to 30 cm $H_2O$
   B. increasing the PEP therapy frequency to every hour while the patient is awake
   C. discontinuing PEP therapy
   D. increasing the duration of PEP therapy to 30 minutes

20. An infant is being mechanically ventilated via a pressure-limited, time-cycled ventilator displaying a descending ramp pressure waveform. Given the following data, calculate the mean airway pressure.

   ventilator rate: 50 breaths/min.
   peak inspiratory flow: 10 L/min.
   PIP: 27 cm $H_2O$
   $FiO_2$: 0.60
   PEEP: 5 cm $H_2O$
   inspiratory time: 0.4 second
   expiratory time: 0.8 second

   A. 5.0 cm $H_2O$
   B. 6.7 cm $H_2O$

C. 8.6 cm H$_2$O

D. 12.3 cm H$_2$O

21. The RRT has been asked to administer a 70% helium–30% oxygen gas mixture to a 3-year-old boy who has epiglottitis. The only flow meter that the RRT could find is an oxygen flow meter. What flow rate setting on the oxygen flow meter will deliver 15 L/min. of the prescribed gas mixture?

A. 12.0 L/min.

B. 9.5 L/min.

C. 7.0 L/min.

D. 6.5 L/min.

22. A flow-directed pulmonary artery catheter has been inserted in a patient in the coronary care unit. A portion of this patient's hemodynamic profile is presented as follows:

pulmonary artery systolic pressure: 55 mm Hg
pulmonary artery diastolic pressure: 35 mm Hg
pulmonary capillary wedge pressure: 25 mm Hg
cardiac output: 10 liters/min
arterial-mixed venous O$_2$ content difference: 2.5 vol%
oxygen consumption: 250 ml/min

How should the RRT interpret this hemodynamic data?

A. The patient has hypervolemia.

B. The patient is experiencing left ventricular failure.

C. The patient exhibits systemic hypertension.

D. The data are erroneous.

23. During cardiopulmonary resuscitation (CPR) of an intubated neonatal patient, the manual resuscitator fails. At the bedside is a gas-powered resuscitator. What should the RRT do at this time?

A. Use the gas-powered resuscitator because *nothing* else is available.

B. Use the gas-powered resuscitator because it will provide an adequate volume.

C. Use it because it will provide an adequate F$_I$O$_2$.

D. Do *not* use it because it should *not* be used with infants or children.

24. A patient is receiving a 5-ml bronchodilator solution via continuous nebulization from a small-volume nebulizer. The RRT notes that the treatment is extremely brief. What can she do to prolong the treatment to enhance particle deposition?

A. Have the patient breathe more slowly.

B. Instruct the patient to breath-hold at peak inspiration.

C. Switch to intermittent nebulization.

D. Add more medication to the nebulizer.

25. Which of the following diseases are ordinarily associated with digital clubbing?

I. asthma

II. cystic fibrosis

III. bronchiolitis

IV. congenital cardiac anomalies

V. epiglottitis

A. I, III only

B. II, IV only

C. II, III, IV, V only

D. II, IV, V only

26. The RRT has set up a transcutaneous P$_O_2$ monitor on an adult patient. Using the following data, which PaO$_2$ and PtcO$_2$ values are likely to belong to this patient? Assume a normal fluid balance.

stroke volume: 45 ml/beat
heart rate: 50 beats/min.
body surface area: 2.25 m$^2$

A. PaO$_2$ 95 torr; PtcO$_2$ 95 torr

B. PaO$_2$ 90 torr; PtcO$_2$ 60 torr

C. PaO$_2$ 60 torr; PtcO$_2$ 90 torr

D. The PaO$_2$ and PtcO$_2$ values will fluctuate.

27. What is(are) the expected advantage(s) of using the method illustrated in Figure 6-2 for patient extubation and/or discontinuance from mechanical ventilation?

I. It increases the mechanical dead space, thereby challenging the patient to breathe spontaneously.

II. The reservoir tubing serves to maintain a consistent F$_I$O$_2$.

III. The system provides continous distending airway pressure as the patient breathes without mechanical assistance.

IV. It allows for fluctuations in the F$_I$O$_2$ and challenges the peripheral chemoreceptors.

A. I, IV only

B. I, II only

C. II, III only

D. II only

28. The RRT is working with a 72-hour postoperative thoracotomy patient. Auscultation of the chest indicates diminished, bilateral, basilar breath sounds. The chest roentgenogram reveals bilateral basilar infiltrates. What should the RRT do at this time?

A. Intubate the patient and perform ET suctioning.

B. Administer an aerosolized $\beta_2$ agonist.

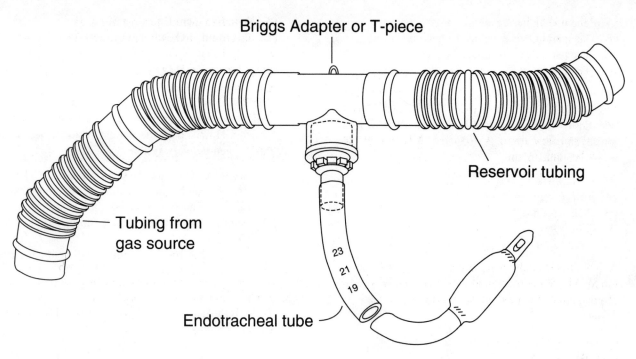

Briggs Adapter or T-piece

Reservoir tubing

Tubing from gas source

23
21
19

Endotracheal tube

**Figure 6-2:** Briggs adaptor setup.

C. Administer aerosol therapy, chest percussion, postural drainage, and incentive spirometry.

D. Place the patient on an air entrainment mask at an $F_{IO_2}$ of 0.30.

29. Following a cardiopulmonary arrest, a patient is intubated and given 100% oxygen via a manual resuscitator. The patient is *not* responding as expected. The RRT suggests the use of capnometry to evaluate the ET tube location. Which of the following statements is true regarding capnometry in this situation?

A. Capnometry *cannot* replace auscultation in determining ET tube location.

B. End-tidal air contains approximately 6.0% $CO_2$, whereas nonend-tidal gas has less than 0.5% $CO_2$.

C. If the ET tube is malplaced, measured expired $CO_2$ levels rise rapidly.

D. Capnometry can ascertain right mainstem bronchus intubation.

30. Which of the following factors affect the end-tidal $CO_2$ measurements obtained via capnography?

I. cardiac output
II. ventilation–perfusion ratio
III. alveolar ventilation
IV. fraction of inspired oxygen

A. I, II, III, IV
B. II, III only

C. I, II, III only
D. I, II, IV only

31. The RRT notices an intensive care unit (ICU) patient experiencing premature ventricular contractions. What antiarrhythmic medication is appropriate to use?

A. propranolol
B. digitalis
C. adenosine
D. lidocaine

32. Which factor(s) is(are) commonly used for assessing a patient's perfusion state?

I. sensorium
II. capillary refill
III. $Q_S/Q_T$
IV. $V_D/V_T$

A. I, II, III, IV
B. I only
C. I, II only
D. I, IV only

33. The RRT has just completed administering 10% Mucomyst via a small-volume nebulizer to a patient. Upon auscultation, the RRT hears bilateral wheezing. At the same time, the patient complains of dyspnea. Which of the following interpretations of the patient's condition should the RRT report to the physician?

A. The patient has developed bronchospasm.
B. The patient has developed a pneumothorax.
C. The patient has aspirated the medication.
D. The patient needs to receive 20% Mucomyst.

34. Given the following data, calculate this patient's C.O.

blood pressure: 135/88 mm Hg
pulse: 88 beats/min.
stroke volume: 67 ml
cardiac index (C.I.): 3.64 L/min./m²

A. 6.10 L/min.
B. 5.89 L/min.
C. 5.76 L/min.
D. 3.20 L/min.

35. What is wrong with the following diagram (Figure 6-3)?

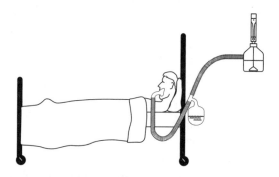

**Figure 6-3:** Patient who is receiving aerosol therapy.

A. The water collection trap is misplaced.
B. An oxygen blender should be used.
C. The water level in the humidifier is low.
D. A reservoir bag is lacking.

36. A hemodynamically monitored patient in the ICU has the following cardiovascular data:

pulmonary artery systolic pressure: 20 mm Hg
pulmonary artery diastolic pressure: 5 mm Hg
pulmonary capillary wedge pressure: 3 mm Hg
arterial-mixed venous $O_2$ content difference: 8.0 vol%
body temperature: 37°C

Which of the following conditions is likely causing these hemodynamic data?

A. left ventricular failure
B. pulmonary hypertension
C. hypovolemia
D. mitral regurgitation

37. Assuming that a patient is receiving PSV to overcome the imposed work of breathing, at what pressure-support level would it generally be acceptable to extubate the patient?

A. less than 2 cm $H_2O$
B. 3 to 7 cm $H_2O$
C. 8 to 12 cm $H_2O$
D. 13 to 15 cm $H_2O$

38. The RRT has been informed that a home-care patient will be receiving transtracheal oxygen via a SCOOP-1 catheter. How should the patient be instructed about this oxygen-delivery system?

I. that she can increase the $O_2$ flow rate up to 5 L/min.
II. that she can begin immediately receiving oxygen once the transtracheal procedure is performed
III. that the transtracheal catheter might require daily cleaning
IV. that the transtracheal catheter will not be inserted until the stent is removed

A. I, III, IV only
B. I, II only
C. III, IV only
D. II, III only

39. A tracheostomy patient is receiving 40% oxygen via a trach mask using an unheated large-reservoir, air-entrainment nebulizer filled with sterile distilled water. ABGs at this time reveal the following:

$PO_2$ 80 torr
$PCO_2$ 40 torr
pH 7.40

Upon suctioning the patient, the RRT notes that the patient's secretions are thick and tenacious. Which of the following equipment changes would be most appropriate?

A. Replace the nebulizer with an ultrasonic nebulizer filled with 0.45% NaCl, using a 50% Venturi for oxygen mixing.
B. Replace the trach mask with a Briggs adaptor to increase the inspired humidity and oxygen concentration.
C. Use a heated pneumatic jet nebulizer operating at 40% oxygen.
D. Increase to 0.50 the $FIO_2$ delivered by the unheated pneumatic nebulizer.

40. The RRT suspects that air is leaking into the intrapleural space, which has been draining via a three-bottle pleural drainage system (Figure 6-4 on page 355).

How can he determine the source of the air leak?

A. Momentarily clamp the chest drainage tube.
B. Briefly clamp the tubing that connects the suction-control bottle and the water seal bottle.

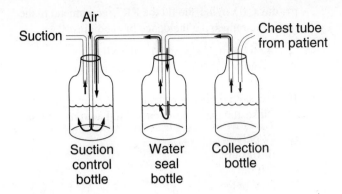

**Figure 6-4:** Three-bottle pleural drainage system.

C. Increase the source vacuum and observe the bubbling.

D. Turn off the source vacuum and observe the water level rise in the water seal bottle.

41. What is the significance of a low left ventricular, end-diastolic pressure obtained via pulmonary artery catheterization?

   A. an increased left ventricular preload
   B. an increased left ventricular afterload
   C. a decreased left ventricular preload
   D. an increased left ventricular stroke volume

42. A galvanic cell oxygen analyzer is being used in-line to measure the oxygen concentration delivered to a mechanically ventilated patient. How will the analyzed $O_2$ concentration be affected if the sensor is located on the inspiratory limb near the patient Y connector?

   A. The measured $O_2\%$ will be less than the actual $O_2$ concentration.
   B. The measured $O_2\%$ will be greater than the actual $O_2$ concentration.
   C. The measured $O_2\%$ will *not* be influenced at all.
   D. The measured $O_2\%$ will fluctuate above and below the actual $O_2$ concentration.

43. The RRT is about to perform ET suctioning on an adult patient and notices that the suction-pressure gauge indicates $-10$ mm Hg. What action should she take at this time?

   A. Proceed with the ET suctioning procedure.
   B. Adjust the suction pressure until the gauge indicates $-120$ mm Hg.
   C. Adjust the suction pressure until the manometer reads $-80$ mm Hg.
   D. Report the situation to the maintenance department for repair.

44. Which of the following statements are true regarding subjective data elicited from a patient?

   I. Subjective data are less accurate than objective data.
   II. Subjective data are usually gathered during the "Review of Systems" portion of the history and physical.
   III. The existence of subjective data are evident to the skilled and sensitive observer.
   IV. Subjective data are called *symptoms*.
   V. Subjective data refer to feelings, sensations, and perceptions.

   A. I, II only
   B. I, III, V only
   C. II, III only
   D. II, IV, V only

45. A 110-pound female patient suspected of having myasthenia gravis has been monitored by the RRT for the past four hours. The patient's forced vital capacity (FVC) and maximum inspiratory pressure (MIP) are shown in Table 6-2.

**Table 6-2** FVC and MIP Data

| Time | Ventilatory Measurement | Valve |
|------|------------------------|-------|
| 5:20 P.M. | FVC | 3.5 liters |
|  | MIP | −50 cm $H_2O$ |
| 6:30 P.M. | FVC | 2.5 liters |
|  | MIP | −40 cm $H_2O$ |
| 7:15 P.M. | FVC | 1.5 liters |
|  | MIP | −30 cm $H_2O$ |
| 8:25 P.M. | FVC | 0.5 liter |
|  | MIP | −20 cm $H_2O$ |

The FVC and MIP obtained at 8:25 P.M. are the most recent data. What should the RRT recommend at this time?

   A. administration of an aerosol mask delivering 40% oxygen
   B. administration of a nasal cannula set at 4 L/min.
   C. insertion of a pulmonary artery catheter
   D. intubation and mechanical ventilation

46. Which corrective action(s) is(are) effective in reducing auto-PEEP?

   I. establishing a low tidal volume
   II. shortening the inspiratory time
   III. reducing the ventilatory rate
   IV. using the largest internal diameter ET tube possible

   A. II, III only
   B. I, IV only

C. I only

D. I, II, III, IV

47. Which continuous-flow IMV system depicts the appropriate position for the one-way valve (Figures 6-5 A–D)?

48. Which of the following types of patients are likely to benefit from the use of a small-volume nebulizer as opposed to a metered-dose inhaler (MDI)?

I. a patient having an asthmatic episode

II. a patient who has severe COPD

III. an asymptomatic asthmatic patient

IV. a mild COPD patient who also has reversible airways disease

A. II, IV only

B. I, III, IV only

C. III, IV only

D. I, II only

49. An asthmatic patient has just been prescribed beclomethasone for home use via an MDI at two puffs per day QID. What should the RRT recommend to the patient to reduce the incidence of candidiasis?

I. Avoid using a spacer with the MDI.

II. Avoid breath holding for more than one second at end inspiration.

III. Exhale rapidly after the drug has been inhaled.

IV. Rinse and gargle after each MDI administration.

A. IV only

B. II, III only

C. I, II only

D. I, IV only

50. A 38-year-old Caucasian female enters the emergency department displaying the following signs and symptoms: (1) chills and fever, (2) cough, (3) increased white blood cell (WBC) count, and (4) pleuritic pain. The patient also complains of coughing up copious amounts of purulent, foul-smelling, foul-tasting, blood-tinged sputum. Sputum cultures indicate anaerobes and mixed flora. The patient also claims that she has not experienced any weight loss, anorexia, or dyspnea. Amphoric breath sounds can be heard upon aus-

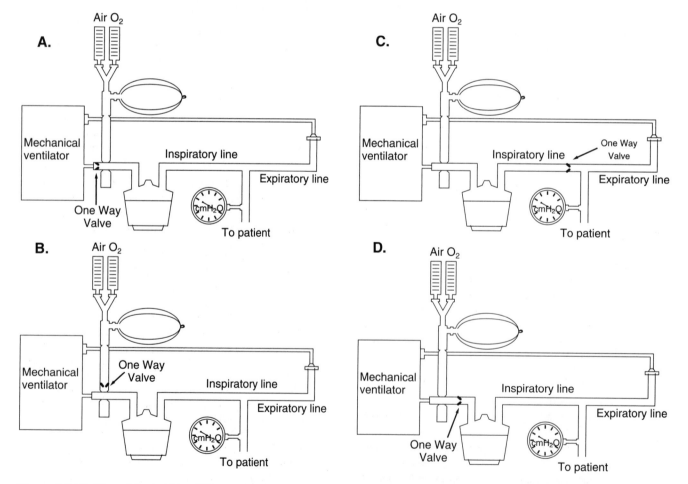

**Figure 6-5 (A–D):** *Adapted from Pilbeam*, Mechanical Ventilation: Physiological and Clinical Applications, *2nd ed.* © *1992, Mosby-Year Book, Inc.*

culation of the right anterior upper chest. Movement of the right upper chest is slightly reduced. The percussion note in that region is dull. Which clinical condition is the probable diagnosis?

A. pulmonary neoplasm
B. lung abscess
C. pleural effusion
D. bronchiectasis

51. When transporting a ventilator patient by fixed-wing aircraft, it is imperative for the RRT to consider that:

   I. as altitude increases, trapped gas will decrease.
   II. as altitude increases, trapped gas will increase.
   III. the $FIO_2$ decreases with increased altitude.
   IV. the ventilator preset volume must be doubled for every 5,000-foot increase in altitude.
   V. the $PaO_2$ decreases with increased altitude.

A. II, III, IV only
B. I, III only
C. II, V only
D. II, III, V only

52. How can right ventricular infarction distort the normal pulmonary artery catheter waveforms?

A. The right atrial, right ventricular, and pulmonary artery pressures might all be higher.
B. The right ventricular pressure and pulmonary artery pressure can be reduced to a level resembling the right atrial pressure.
C. Right atrial pressure can rise to the level of the right ventricular pressure.
D. Right atrial pressure might rise, and right ventricular pressure might fall.

53. Which of the following hemodynamic measurements can be obtained from a four-lumen pulmonary artery catheter having thermodilution capability?

   I. C.O.
   II. mean pulmonary artery pressure ($\overline{PAP}$)
   III. central venous pressure (CVP)
   IV. pulmonary capillary wedge pressure (PCWP)

A. I, II, III, IV
B. I, II, III only
C. II, IV only
D. I, III, IV only

54. An RRT is called to the home of a patient who is being mechanically ventilated with a pneumatically powered ventilator. The problem, as stated by the patient's family, began when the compressed gas cylinders "ran dry" and the nurse connected the ventilator to a liquid oxygen system. The family members indicated that the patient suddenly became distressed and required ven-

tilation with a manual resuscitator. The most likely explanation for causing this overall problem is that:

A. the ventilator was *not* properly attached to the liquid oxygen source outlet.
B. the liquid oxygen system is *not* capable of operating the pneumatically powered ventilator.
C. the ventilator's controls were *not* appropriately adjusted when connected to the liquid oxygen system.
D. the liquid oxygen system vaporizer coils became "frozen" as a result of the demands of the ventilator.

55. A severe ARDS patient is receiving pressure-control ventilation (PCV). The physician wants a pressure-control level to deliver a tidal volume of approximately 600 cc. The patient is generating a PIP of 20 cm $H_2O$ and has an exhaled tidal volume of 400 cc. What adjustment should be made to deliver the requested tidal volume?

A. Increase the PIP.
B. Decrease the ventilatory rate.
C. Institute 10 cm $H_2O$ of positive end-expiratory pressure (PEEP).
D. Increase the expiratory time.

56. Which of the following physiologic measurements might improve when inverse-ratio ventilation is changed from 2:1 to 3:1?

A. oxygenation
B. acid-base balance
C. alveolar ventilation
D. end-tidal $PCO_2$

57. The RRT is about to have a patient perform a maximum expiratory pressure maneuver. From what level of lung volume should the patient be instructed to begin the maneuver?

A. total lung capacity
B. end-tidal inspiration
C. functional residual capacity
D. residual volume

58. During CPR, RRT observes the cardiac monitor displaying the electrocardiogram shown in Figure 6-6 on page 358.

What should he recommend in this situation?

A. defibrillation
B. cardioversion
C. ET instillation of lidocaine
D. I.V. administration of atropine

59. A COPD patient who has excessive secretions is being mechanically ventilated. Humidification is being

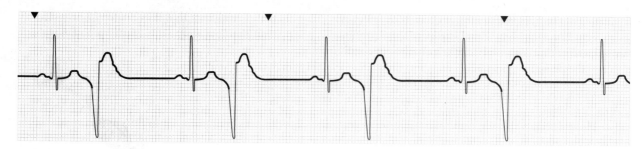

**Figure 6-6:** Lead II ECG tracing.

provided by a heat-moisture exchanger. What precautions need to be taken as a result of using this type of humidifier?

A. Periodic culture and sensitivity testing must be performed on the humidifier to prevent the colonization of bacteria.
B. Close monitoring of patient secretions must occur to prevent obstruction of the tubing.
C. Frequent observation of the inspiratory limb must be maintained to note any degree of circuit melting.
D. Constant temperature monitoring of the inspiratory limb of the ventilator circuit must be maintained to avoid high gas temperatures.

60. The RRT is preparing to insert an arterial line in a patient. Before starting the procedure, he obtained a positive modified Allen's test from the patient's left hand. What should he do at this time?

A. Perform a modified Allen's test on the right hand.
B. Perform another modified Allen's test on the left hand.
C. Cannulate the radial artery of the right hand.
D. Cannulate the radial artery of the left hand.

61. A patient is receiving an $FIO_2$ of 0.40 via an all-purpose nebulizer operating at a source flow rate of 10 L/min. The patient's arterial $PO_2$ has decreased from 75 torr to 60 torr. The patient's peak inspiratory flow rate is 50 L/min. What recommendation should the RRT make to improve this patient's oxygenation status?

A. Increase the $FIO_2$ to 0.60.
B. Increase the source flow rate to 12 L/min.
C. Set-up tandem nebulizers at an $FIO_2$ of 0.40 at 10 L/min.
D. Institute mask CPAP at 5 cm $H_2O$ with an $FIO_2$ of 0.60.

62. As the RRT views a series of chest X-rays, she notes the margins of the pulmonary vessels have become progressively blurred to the point of being indistinct. This observation has been made in the presence of cardiomegaly. Which interpretation would be appropriate?

A. The patient is experiencing right ventricular failure.
B. The patient is developing a lobar pneumonia.
C. The patient is developing more severe pulmonary edema.
D. The patient is progressively developing a pneumothorax.

63. Which of the following ECGs (Figures 6-7 a–d) often require(s) defibrillation?

A. II, III only
B. II only
C. I, III only
D. II, III, IV only

64. A 1-minute old infant has the following characteristics:

- heart rate: 85 beats/min.
- respiratory effort: irregular, weak, gasping
- muscle tone: some flexion of extremities
- reflex irritability: frown when stimulated
- skin color: acrocyanosis

What is the infant's 1-minute Apgar score?

A. 10
B. 7
C. 5
D. 2

65. Which factor(s) can influence where the pulmonary artery catheter tip will become located during insertion?

I. venous return
II. diuresis
III. high PEEP levels
IV. shunt fraction

A. I, II, III only
B. I only
C. II, III, IV only
D. III only

66. An ICU patient with a bronchopleural fistula is being mechanically ventilated with a microprocessor ventilator in the volume-control mode. There is approximately a 500-ml leak through the right chest tube. On

**A.**

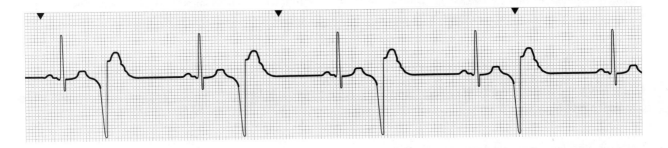

**B.**

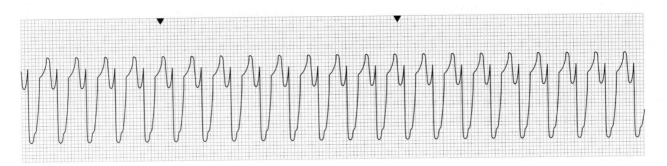

**C.**

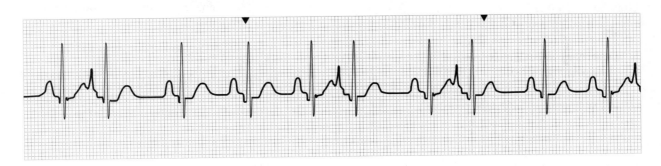

**D.**

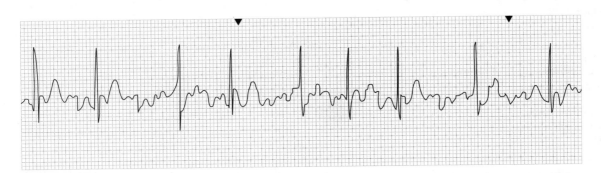

**Figure 6-7 A–D**

rounds, a physician asks the RRT to institute independent lung ventilation and to monitor the effect of the patient's response to this change. What will be the most appropriate measurement to monitor?

A. expired $CO_2$
B. flow rate of the air leak
C. transcutaneous $PO_2$ and $PCO_2$
D. difference between inspiratory and expiratory tidal volumes

67. Determine the dead space–tidal volume ratio for a patient who has a dissolved arterial carbon dioxide tension of 40 torr and a mean exhaled carbon dioxide tension of 28 torr.

A. 1.3
B. 0.7
C. 0.5
D. 0.3

68. A 61-year-old postmyocardial infarction victim has a pulmonary artery catheter in place and exhibits the following hemodynamic data:

heart rate: 105 beats/min.
blood pressure: 90/60 mm Hg
mean pulmonary artery pressure: 32 mm Hg
mean left atrial pressure: 8 mm Hg
C.O.: 3.5 L/min.

Which hemodynamic measurement is likely to be decreased?

A. pulmonary vascular resistance
B. stroke volume
C. pulmonary capillary wedge pressure
D. left ventricular end-diastolic pressure

69. To which circuit must the RRT switch the defibrillator to assure appropriate application of cardioversion for a patient who is displaying atrial fibrillation?

A. central
B. auxiliary
C. synchronized
D. unsynchronized

70. All of the following types of hemoglobin can be measured by a co-oximeter EXCEPT:

A. deoxyhemoglobin
B. methemoglobin
C. sulfhemoglobin
D. carboxyhemoglobin

71. Chest physiotherapy (CPT) has been ordered for a patient who has developed right middle-lobe atelectasis following bypass surgery. A chest tube has been inserted in the third intercostal space along the anterior axillary line on the right side. What should the RRT do in this situation?

A. Avoid placing the patient in the Trendelenburg position.
B. Avoid percussing over the chest tube.
C. The physician should be notified that CPT is contraindicated for this patient.
D. The patient should be instructed *not* to cough.

72. A physician performing endotracheal intubation is assisted by an RRT who is monitoring a capnograph during the procedure. Throughout the intubation procedure, the RRT notices that the capnograph maintains a readout of 0.0% $CO_2$. What interpretation can be made?

A. The ET tube has been inserted into the right mainstem bronchus.
B. The ET tube has been inserted into the esophagus.
C. The patient has been appropriately intubated.
D. The cuff on the ET tube needs to be inflated.

73. A meconium-stained infant has been receiving positive pressure ventilation (PPV) with 100% oxygen via a bag-valve-mask device for approximately two minutes. Her heart rate initially was 80 beats/min. and is now 55 beats/min. Which of the following actions should be taken *first*?

A. Begin external cardiac compressions and continue PPV.
B. Intubate and continue PPV.
C. Administer epinephrine and continue PPV.
D. Continue PPV and monitor the heart rate.

74. A 25-year-old female is brought into the emergency department by paramedics following a severe motor vehicle accident. She is suffering from multiple, deep lacerations and a closed head injury. An ABG is performed and an oxygen saturation is established with a co-oximeter. What additional measurement is necessary to determine the patient's oxygen content?

A. white blood count
B. platelet count
C. cardiac output
D. hemoglobin concentration

75. While performing therapeutic evaluations on patients who are receiving respiratory therapy, the RRT notes that a tracheotomized, severe COPD patient who is re-

ceiving continuous aerosol therapy with a trach collar via a heated, large-volume jet nebulizer operating at 30% oxygen appears to be choking. Gurgling sounds from the patient during inspiration and exhalation are audible with the unaided ear. Pulse oximetry indicates a saturation of 80%. Following aggressive ET suctioning, the gurgling sounds disappear, and the patient *no* longer appears distressed. Upon auscultation of the chest, coarse crackles are perceived during inspiration and exhalation. The arterial saturation is now 96%. What should the RRT recommend for this patient?

A. Maintain the trach collar and institute humidity therapy by using a heated, passover humidifier at 30% $O_2$.
B. Maintain the same apparatus, but increase the $FIO_2$ to 0.40.
C. Change to a T piece with *no* reservoir tubing, but continue with the heated, large-volume nebulizer at 30% $O_2$.
D. Institute a Briggs adaptor with 100 cc of reservoir tubing via a heated, large-volume nebulizer at 40% $O_2$.

76. Which of the following situations concerning blood gas analyzer electrodes can cause data trending?

I. air bubbles in contact with the electrode membrane
II. protein contamination of the electrode
III. an aging electrode
IV. contamination of calibration standards

A. II, III only
B. III, IV only
C. I, IV only
D. I, II only

77. A 59-year-old, 75-kg patient had a myocardial infarction. During CPR, the RRT is asked to recommend an initial dose of $NaHCO_3$ for I.V. administration. What initial dose should he recommend?

A. 37.5 mEq
B. 55.5 mEq
C. 75.0 mEq
D. 150 mEq

78. Upon entering the adult ICU to perform ventilator rounds, the RRT notes that a 160-pound, severe COPD patient who is receiving mechanical ventilation triggers the high pressure alarm on each inspiration. The clinician also hears a gurgling sound coming from the patient. Upon auscultation of the chest, early inspiratory crackles are perceived bilaterally. While inspecting the tubing, he sees that the patient has a heat–moisture ex-

changer (HME) located at the Y adaptor. The ventilator settings include the following:

mode: SIMV
$V_T$: 750 cc
high-pressure limit: 50 cm $H_2O$
low-pressure limit: 5 cm $H_2O$
spontaneous rate: 12 breaths/min.
mechanical rate: 6 breaths/min.
$FIO_2$: 0.35
PEEP: 5 cm $H_2O$

After ET suctioning is performed, the gurgling ceases and the adventitious breath sounds noted earlier disappear. The high pressure alarm continues to sound on each inspiration, however. What should the RRT do at this time?

A. Suggest that the patient receive Pavulon and institute controlled mechanical ventilation.
B. Increase the high-pressure limit to 70 cm $H_2O$.
C. Decrease the tidal volume to 600 cc.
D. Remove the HME and add a cascade humidifier.

79. Upon reviewing the chart of a postmyocardial infarction patient, the RRT finds reference to a pleural effusion described as follows: "Thoracentesis rendered thin, clear fluid. Microscopic examination of the fluid revealed very few cells, while those present were predominantly lymphocytes. *No* microorganisms were cultured. Lab results also indicated 1.5% protein concentration and a specific gravity of 1.00. The effusion did *not* clot upon standing." What is the likely nature of this pleural effusion?

A. hemothorax
B. transudate
C. empyema
D. exudate

80. Calculate the percent shunt of a patient who is receiving controlled mechanical ventilation with an $FIO_2$ of 0.60 and a Swan–Ganz catheter in place.

GIVEN:

$P_B$ 760 torr
body temperature 37°C
$P_{H_2O}$ 47 torr
$PaO_2$ 150 torr
$PaCO_2$ 40 torr
pH 7.35 (arterial)
[Hb] 15 g%
$SaO_2$ 100%
$P\bar{v}O_2$ 30 torr
$P\bar{v}CO_2$ 45 torr

pH 7.32 (venous)
$S\overline{v}O_2$ 75%
respiratory quotient 1.0

A. 11.72%
B. 10.53%
C. 9.29%
D. 7.46%

81. The RRT notices that a sudden increase in ventilating pressures is required to deliver the same tidal volume. She immediately auscultates the patient's chest and determines that breath sounds are decreased over the right lower lobe and that the percussion note is hyper-resonant. A chest X-ray reveals a large pneumothorax in the right lower lobe. What should the RRT recommend to the physician at this time?

A. decreasing the tidal volume
B. inserting a chest tube on the right side of the chest
C. performing a thoracocentesis on the left side of the chest
D. obtaining an arterial blood sample to determine the severity of the problem

82. The RRT notices that the ventilator pressure gauge on a volume ventilator is indicating $-10$ cm $H_2O$ during each spontaneous breath generated by the patient. The patient is receiving demand-flow IMV. Which of the following conditions might be responsible for this situation?

I. The gas flow rate in the IMV circuitry is less than the patient's inspiratory needs.
II. The one-way valve in this system is sticking.
III. The humidifier water level in the ventilator circuit is low.
IV. The ventilator's sensitivity control is turned off.

A. I, II, IV only
B. II, III only
C. I, II only
D. I, III, IV only

83. The RRT enters the room of a patient who is receiving oxygen via a simple mask and notices the flow meter is set at 4 L/min. What should the RRT do in this situation?

A. Reduce the flow rate to 2 L/min.
B. Replace the device with an air-entrainment mask at 50% oxygen.
C. Increase the flow rate to 6 L/min. and then check the physician's orders.
D. Check the water level in the reservoir.

84. An RRT is asked to assist in the performance of a pulmonary stress test for a patient who is being evaluated for respiratory impairment. The patient is being evaluated based on the American Medical Association's *Guides to the Evaluation of Permanent Impairment.* The results of the study show an FVC of 68%, an $FEV_1$ of 72%, and a $VO_2$ max of 23 ml/kg/min. These findings best reflect what level of pulmonary impairment?

A. *no* impairment
B. mild impairment
C. moderate impairment
D. severe impairment

85. The RRT is about to connect a patient to a Siemens Servo 900C ventilator set in the pressure-control mode with inverse-ratio ventilation. This ventilator has waveform monitoring capabilities. How should she establish the appropriate ventilatory rate?

A. Set the inspiratory time percent to 33%.
B. Set the ventilatory rate to coincide with the inspiratory time percent.
C. Set each inspiration to begin just before the terminal flow reaches zero.
D. Set the ventilatory rate in accordance with the inspiratory time until a 2:1 inspiratory:expiratory (I:E) ratio is achieved.

86. A 33-week-old neonate who is receiving 2 cm $H_2O$ of continuous-flow, nasotracheal continuous positive airway pressure (CPAP) on an $FiO_2$ of 0.30 displays the following ABG and acid-base values:

$PO_2$ 80 torr
$PCO_2$ 41 torr
pH 7.39
$HCO_3^-$ 24 mEq/liter
B.E. 0 mEq/liter

What should the RRT do at this time?

A. Extubate the patient.
B. Increase the CPAP to 4 cm $H_2O$.
C. Increase the $FiO_2$ to 0.40.
D. Decrease the $FiO_2$ to 0.25.

87. An endotracheally intubated patient is breathing gas delivered by the device shown in Figure 6-8 on page 363.

The RRT observes a mist exiting from the opening of the reservoir tubing when the patient exhales. When the patient inhales, however, the RRT notices the mist disappears from the entire length of the reservoir tubing. What should he do at this time?

A. Add another 50 cc of reservoir tubing.
B. Increase the $FiO_2$.
C. Increase the flow rate of the source gas.
D. Switch to a tracheostomy collar.

88. A pressure transducer used to measure the central venous pressure (CVP) is about to be calibrated. At which

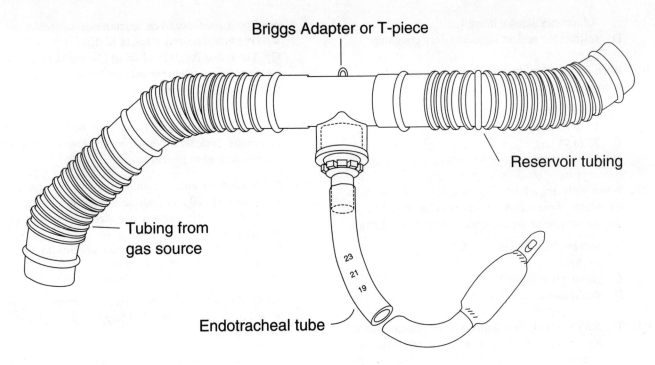

**Figure 6-8:** Briggs adaptor setup.

of the following levels should the pressure transducer be placed?

A. height of the sternum
B. height of the spine
C. mid-axillary
D. lower than the patient's chest

89. The device illustrated in Figure 6-9 was added to the exhalation limb of a mechanical ventilator circuit.

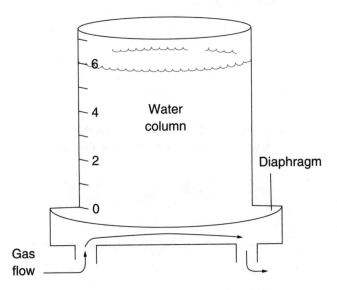

**Figure 6-9:** Device added to exhalation limb of the mechanical ventilator circuit.

The pressure-time tracing in Figure 6-10 was obtained after the device shown in Figure 6-9 was added.

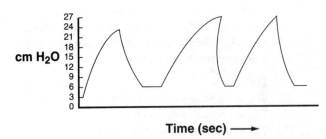

**Figure 6-10:** Pressure-time tracing after the device is added to the exhalation limb of the mechanical ventilator circuit.

The device added to the mechanical ventilator circuit is called a:

A. flow resistor
B. resistive resistor
C. reverse Venturi resistor
D. threshold resistor

90. A patient who has an intracranial pressure of 15 mm Hg has been prescribed CPT for the left lower lobe. What recommendation should the RRT make in this situation?

A. Administer IPPB therapy.
B. Modify postural drainage positions.

C. Administer aerosol therapy.

D. Instruct the patient regarding deep coughing.

91. What is the normal systolic pressure range for the right ventricle?

    A. 5 to 10 torr
    B. 15 to 25 torr
    C. 35 to 45 torr
    D. 50 to 60 torr

92. When analyzing a fetal blood sample with a co-oximeter, which of the following values is most likely to be altered because of the presence of fetal hemoglobin?

    A. reduced hemoglobin
    B. oxyhemoglobin
    C. carboxyhemoglobin
    D. methemoglobin

93. The RRT is checking a liquid oxygen system used by a home care patient. The system weighs 60 pounds and is delivering a liter flow of 3 L/min. How long will this system operate?

    A. 86 hours
    B. 114 hours
    C. 180 hours
    D. 216 hours

94. The RRT notices *no* condensation in the recyclable circuitry of a ventilator to which is attached a heated cascade humidifier. Which of the following situations might account for this condition?

    I. The cascade's heating element has malfunctioned.
    II. The humidifier was *not* turned on.
    III. The temperature was set too low.
    IV. The temperature was set too high.

    A. II, IV only
    B. I, III only
    C. I, II, III only
    D. I, IV only

95. When initiating pressure-control inverse-ratio ventilation (PC-IRV), which of the following considerations is *most* important?

A. The patient should be sedated and paralyzed.
B. The initial I:E ratio should be 4:1.
C. The initial PEEP level should be the same as that used during conventional ventilation of the patient.
D. The initial $F_IO_2$ should be 0.40.

96. Which of the following actions might be helpful when suctioning thick secretions from the lower airway of an intubated adult patient?

    A. Suction the airway continuously for 20 seconds.
    B. Instill 3 to 10 ml of normal saline.
    C. Use a suction catheter one size smaller than the ET tube.
    D. Lower the negative pressure applied to −150 mm Hg.

97. An 850-kg status asthmaticus patient is receiving controlled mechanical ventilatory support. The ventilator settings include the following:

    tidal volume: 800 cc
    ventilatory rate: 12 breaths/min.
    flow rate: 40 L/min.
    $F_IO_2$: 0.50
    I:E: 1:2
    pressure limit: 60 cm $H_2O$

    The RRT notices the patient grimacing and tossing in bed. At the same time, the high pressure alarm sounds with each inspiration, and the pressure manometer is frequently dropping to −12 cm $H_2O$ before and between breaths. The RRT performs aggressive ET suctioning and confirms *no* obstruction in the patient-ventilator system. The high pressure alarm continues to sound, however. What should the RRT recommend at this time?

    A. Recommend lowering the peak inspiratory flow rate.
    B. Suggest that the patient receive sedation.
    C. Recommend administering in-line albuterol.
    D. Suggest lowering the $F_IO_2$.

98. If a monitored CCU patient displayed the ECG shown in Figure 6-11, what course of action should be taken?

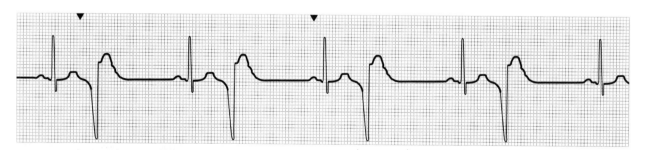

**Figure 6-11:** Lead II ECG tracing.

A. Do *nothing* at this time, but closely monitor the patient.
B. Defibrillate the patient.
C. Administer isoproterenol to increase the heart rate.
D. Administer calcium chloride to increase the force of myocardial contractility.

99. A 70-kg postoperative patient who is receiving volume-cycled ventilation in the control mode at an $F_{I}O_2$ of 0.60 displays the following ABG data:

PO$_2$ 90 mm Hg
PCO$_2$ 28 mm Hg
pH 7.46

Other ventilator settings include the following:

tidal volume: 600 ml
ventilatory rate: 12 breaths/min.

Which action would be most appropriate?

A. decreasing the $F_{I}O_2$
B. decreasing $V_T$
C. increasing the ventilatory rate
D. adding mechanical dead space

100. An infant in an incubator is receiving ribavirin via a SPAG-2 unit. The distal end of the aerosol-delivery tubing from the SPAG-2 unit is emitting particles into the incubator through one of its sleeves. What should the RRT do at this time?

A. Open one of the other incubator sleeves to allow the infant's exhaled $CO_2$ to vent from the enclosure.
B. Attach the distal end of the aerosol-delivery tubing to an oxyhood placed inside the incubator.
C. Place a filter on the distal end of the aerosol-delivery tubing to filter the large particles.
D. Increase the SPAG-2 unit's pressure setting to 50 psig to increase particle output.

# POSTTEST MATRIX CATEGORIES

1. IIIA1e
2. IC4
3. IIB1q(1)
4. IIID1b
5. IIIA2a(2)
6. IIIC5
7. IIID1a
8. IIIA1m(1)
9. IIB1i(3)
10. IIIE1g
11. IIIA1m(1)
12. IIIE1g
13. IA1h
14. IIIB4c
15. IIIA1g
16. IIB3a
17. IC2c
18. IA1c
19. IIIC5
20. IIIA1h
21. IIIC4
22. IC2c
23. IIA1d
24. IIIC2
25. IB1a

26. IIIA1b
27. IIIC3a
28. IIIC5
29. IIIB1e
30. IIIA1m(2)
31. IIID1b
32. IB6a
33. IIIA2a(1)
34. IIIA1l
35. IIB1c
36. IC2a
37. IIIB1c
38. IIIE2b
39. IIIA1c
40. IIB2r
41. IC2c
42. IIB2h(5)
43. IIIC7c
44. IIIA2a(1)
45. IB10d
46. IIIB4a
47. IIB1i(3)
48. IIIC2
49. IIIE2f
50. IA1b

51. IIID3
52. IIIA1f
53. IIA1q(1)
54. IIB2h(2)
55. IIIB2c
56. IIIB4b
57. IB9d
58. IIID1b
59. IIIB1b
60. IIIE1k
61. IIIC3a
62. IB7e
63. IIID1b
64. IA1h
65. IIB1q(1)
66. IIIB2d
67. IC1c
68. IIIA1m(3)
69. IIIE1h
70. IIA1h(4)
71. IIIC5
72. IIIE1i
73. IIID1c
74. IIIA1g
75. IIIC3a

76. IIB1h(4)
77. IIID1b
78. IIIC6a
79. IA1c
80. IIIA1m(1)
81. IIIE1j
82. IIB1e(1)
83. IIIC3a
84. IIIE1e
85. IIIA1h
86. IIIB1c
87. IIB2a(2)
88. IIB1q(1)
89. IIA1i(2)
90. IIIC5
91. IA1g(2)
92. IIIA1b
93. IIIE2a
94. IIB1b
95. IIIB4b
96. IIIC7d
97. IIIE1l
98. IIIA1d
99. IIB2e(1)
100. IIB2s

# Chapter 6 Posttest: Entry-Level Examination Matrix Scoring Form

| Content Area | Posttest Item Number | Posttest Content Area Score | |
|---|---|---|---|
| **I. Clinical Data** | | | |
| A. Review patient records; recommend diagnostic procedures. | 13,18,50,64,79,91 | $\dfrac{}{6} \times 100 = $ _____ % | |
| B. Collect and evaluate additional clinical information. | 25,32,45,57,62 | $\dfrac{}{5} \times 100 = $ _____ % | $\dfrac{}{17} \times 100 = $ _____ % |
| C. Perform procedures, interpret results, and assist in care plan. | 2,17,22,36,41,67 | $\dfrac{}{6} \times 100 = $ _____ % | |
| **II. Equipment** | | | |
| A. Select, obtain, and assure cleanliness. | 23,53,70,89 | $\dfrac{}{4} \times 100 = $ _____ % | $\dfrac{}{20} \times 100 = $ _____ % |
| B. Assemble, check for proper function, identify and/or correct malfunctions, and perform quality control. | 3,9,16,35,40,42, 47,54,65,76,82,87, 88,94,99,100 | $\dfrac{}{16} \times 100 = $ _____ % | |
| **III. Therapeutic Procedures** | | | |
| A. Evaluate, monitor, and record patient's response. | 1,5,8,11,15,20,26, 30,33,34,39,44,52,68, 74,80,85,92,98 | $\dfrac{}{19} \times 100 = $ _____ % | |
| B. Maintain airway, remove secretions, and assure ventilation and tissue oxygenation. | 14,29,37,46,55,56, 59,66,86,95 | $\dfrac{}{10} \times 100 = $ _____ % | $\dfrac{}{63} \times 100 = $ _____ % |
| C. Modify therapy/make recommendations based on patient's response. | 6,19,21,24,27,28, 43,48,61,71,75, 78,83,90,96 | $\dfrac{}{15} \times 100 = $ _____ % | |
| D. Perform emergency procedures. | 4,7,31,51,58,63,73,77 | $\dfrac{}{8} \times 100 = $ _____ % | |
| E. Assist physician and conduct pulmonary rehabilitation/home care. | 10,12,38,49,60,69, 72,81,84,93,97 | $\dfrac{}{11} \times 100 = $ _____ % | |

# NBRC Written Registry Examination for Advanced Respiratory Therapists (RRTs) Content Outline

*This content outline is reprinted with permission of the copyright holder, the National Board For Respiratory Care, Inc., 8310 Nieman Rd, Lenexa, KS 66214. All rights reserved. Effective December 1999.*

## I. Select, Review, Obtain, and Interpret Data

**SETTING:** In any patient care setting, the advanced respiratory care therapist reviews existing clinical data and collects or recommends obtaining additional pertinent clinical data. The therapist evaluates all data to determine the appropriateness of the prescribed respiratory care plan, and participates in the development of the respiratory care plan.

| | RECALL | APPLICATION | ANALYSIS |
|---|---|---|---|
| | 3 | 3 | 11 |
| **A. Review patient records and recommend diagnostic procedures.** | 1* | 1 | 3 |
| 1. Review existing data in patient's record: | | | |
| a. patient history [e.g., present illness, admission notes, respiratory care orders, progress notes] | X** | | |
| b. physical examination [e.g., vital signs, physical findings] | X | | |
| c. lab data [e.g., CBC, chemistries/electrolytes, coagulation studies, Gram stain, culture and sensitivities, urinalysis] | X | X | |
| d. pulmonary function and blood gas results | X | X | |
| e. radiological studies [e.g., X-rays of chest/upper airway, CT, MRI] | X | X | |
| f. monitoring data | | | |
| (1) fluid balance (intake and output) | | | |
| (2) pulmonary mechanics [e.g., maximum inspiratory pressure (MIP), vital capacity] | X | X | |
| (3) respiratory monitoring [e.g., rate, tidal volume, minute volume, I:E, inspiratory and expiratory pressures; flow, volume and pressure waveforms] | X | X | |
| (4) lung compliance, airway resistance, work of breathing | X | X | |

| | RECALL | APPLICATION | ANALYSIS |
|---|---|---|---|
| (5) noninvasive monitoring [e.g., capnography, pulse oximetry, transcutaneous $O_2/CO_2$] | | X | X |
| g. results of cardivascular monitoring | | | |
| (1) ECG, blood pressure, heart rate | | X | X |
| (2) hemodynamic monitoring [e.g., central venous pressure, cardiac output, pulmonary capillary wedge pressure, pulmonary artery pressures, mixed venous $O_2$, $C(a-\bar{v})O_2$, shunt studies ($\dot{Q}s/\dot{Q}t$)] | | X | X |
| h. maternal and perinatal/neonatal history and data [e.g., Apgar scores, gestational age, L/S ration, pre/post-ductal oxygenation studies] | | X | |
| i. other diagnostic studies [e.g., EEG, intracranial pressure monitoring, metabolic studies ($\dot{V}O_2$, $\dot{V}CO_2$, nutritional assessment), ventilation/perfusion scan, pulmonary angiography, sleep studies, other ultrasonography] | | | |
| 2. Recommend the following procedures to obtain additional data: | | | |
| a. CBC, electrolytes, other blood chemistries | | | |
| b. X-ray of chest and upper airway, CT scan, bronchoscopy, ventilation/perfusion lung scan, barium swallow | | X | X |
| c. Gram stain, culture and sensitivities | | X | X |
| d. Spirometry before and/or after bronchodilator, maximum voluntary ventilation, diffusing capacity, functional residual capacity, flow-volume loops, body plethysmography, nitrogen washout distribution test, total lung capacity, $CO_2$ response curve, closing volume, airway resistance, bronchoprovocation, maximum inspiratory pressure (MIP), maximum expiratory pressure (MEP) | | X | X |
| e. blood gas analysis, insertion of arterial, umbilical and/or central venous, pulmonary artery monitoring lines | | X | X |
| f. lung compliance, airway resistance, lung mechanics, work of breathing | | X | X |

*The number in each column is the number of items in that content area and cognitive level contained in each examination. For example, in category I.A., one item will be asked at the recall level, one item at the application level, and three items at the analysis level. The items could be asked relative to any tasks listed (1–2) under category I.A.

**Note: An "X" denotes the examination does NOT contain items for the given task at the cognitive level indicated in the respective column (Recall, Application, Analysis).

| | RECALL | APPLICATION | ANALYSIS |
|---|---|---|---|
| g. ECG, echocardiography, pulse oximetry, transcutaneous $O_2/CO_2$ monitoring | X | X | |
| h. $V_D/V_T$, $\dot{Q}s/\dot{Q}t$, cardiac output, cardiopulmonary stress testing | | | |
| **B. Collect and evaluate clinical information.** | **1** | **1** | **5** |
| 1. Assess patient's overall cardiopulmonary status by *inspection* to determine: | | | |
|   a. general appearance, muscle wasting, venous distention, peripheral edema, diaphoresis, digital clubbing, cyanosis, capillary refill | X | X | |
|   b. chest configuration, evidence of diaphragmatic movement, breathing pattern, accesory muscle activity, asymmetrical chest movement, intercostal and/or sternal retractions, nasal flaring, character of cough, amount and character of sputum | X | X | |
|   c. transillumination of chest, Apgar score, gestational age | X | X | |
| 2. Assess patient's overall cardiopulmonary status by *palpation* to determine: | | | |
|   a. heart rate, rhythm, force | X | X | |
|   b. asymmetrical chest movements, tactile fremitus, crepitus, tenderness, secretions in the airway, tracheal deviation, endotracheal tube placement | X | X | |
| 3. Assess patient's overall cardiopulmonary status by *percussion* to determine diaphragmatic excursion and areas of altered resonance | X | X | |
| 4. Assess patient's overall cardiopulmonary status by *auscultation* to determine presence of: | | | |
|   a. breath sounds [e.g., normal, bilateral, increased, decreased, absent, unequal, rhonchi or crackles (râles), wheezing, stridor, friction rub] | X | X | |
|   b. heart sounds, dysrhythmias, murmurs, bruits | X | X | |
|   c. blood pressure | X | X | |
| 5. Assess patient's learning needs [e.g., age and language appropriateness, education level, prior disease and medication knowledge] | X | X | |
| 6. Interview patient to determine: | | | |
|   a. level of consciousness, orientation to time, place and person, emotional state, ability to cooperate | X | X | |
|   b. presence of dyspnea and/or orthopnea, work of breathing, sputum | | | |

| | RECALL | APPLICATION | ANALYSIS |
|---|---|---|---|
| production, exercise tolerance and activities of daily living | X | X | |
|   c. physical environment, social support systems, nutritional status | X | X | |
| 7. Review chest X-ray to determine: | | | |
|   a. presence of, or changes in, pheumothorax or subcutaneous emphysema, other extra-pulmonary air, consolidation and/or atelectasis, pulmonary infiltrates | X | X | |
|   b. presence and postion of foreign bodies | X | X | |
|   c. position of endotracheal or tracheostomy tube, evidence of endotracheal or tracheostomy tube cuff hyperinflation | X | X | |
|   d. position of chest tube(s), nasogastric and/or feeding tube, pulmonary artery catheter (Swan-Ganz), pacemaker, CVP, and other catheters | X | | |
|   e. position of, or changes in, hemidiaphragms, hyperinflation, pleural fluid, pulmonary edema, mediastinal shift, patency and size of major airways | X | X | |
| 8. Review lateral neck X-ray to determine: | | | |
|   a. presence of epiglottitis and subglottic edema | X | X | |
|   b. presence or position of foreign bodies | X | X | |
|   c. airway narrowing | X | X | |
| 9. Perform bedside procedures to determine: | | | |
|   a. ECG, pulse oximetry, transcutaneous $O_2/CO_2$ monitoring, capnography, mass spectrometry | X | X | |
|   b. tidal volume, minute volume, I:E | X | X | |
|   c. blood gas analysis, $P(A-a)O_2$, alveolar ventilation, $V_D/V_T$, $\dot{Q}s/\dot{Q}t$, mixed venous sampling | X | X | |
|   d. peak flow, maximum inspiratory pressure, maximum expiratory pressure, forced vital capacity, timed forced expiratory volumes [e.g., $FEV_1$], lung compliance, lung mechanics | X | X | |
|   e. cardiac output, pulmonary capillary wedge pressure, central venous pressure, pulmonary artery pressures, fluid balance (intake and output) | | | |
|   f. pulmonary vascular resistance and systemic vascular resistance | | | |
|   g. apnea monitoring, sleep studies, respiratory impedance plethysmography | X | X | |
|   h. tracheal tube cuff pressure, volume | X | X | |

| | RECALL | APPLICATION | ANALYSIS |
|---|:---:|:---:|:---:|
| 10. Interpret results of bedside procedures to determine: | | | |
| a. ECG, pulse oximetry, transcutaneous $O_2/CO_2$ monitoring, capnography, mass spectrometry | X | X | |
| b. tidal volume, minute volume, I:E | X | X | |
| c. blood gas analysis, P(A-a)$O_2$, alveolar ventilation, $V_D/V_T$, Qs/Qt, mixed venous sampling | X | X | |
| d. peak flow, maximum inspiratory pressure, maximum expiratory pressure, forced vital capacity, timed forced expiratory volumes [e.g., $FEV_1$], lung compliance, lung mechanics | X | X | |
| e. cardiac output, pulmonary capillary wedge pressure, central venous pressure, pulmonary artery pressures, fluid balance (intake and output) | | | |
| f. pulmonary vascular resistance and systematic vascular resistance | | | |
| g. apnea monitoring, sleep studies, respiratory impedance plethysmography | X | X | |
| h. tracheal tube cuff pressure, volume | X | X | |
| **C. Perform procedures and interpret results, determine appropriateness of and participate in developing and recommending modifications to respiratory care plan.** | 1 | 1 | 3 |
| 1. Perform and/or measure the following: | | | |
| a. spirometry before and/or after bronchodilator, maximum voluntary ventilation, diffusing capacity, functional residual capacity, flow-volume loops, body plethysmography, nitrogen washout distribution test, total lung capacity, $CO_2$ response curve, closing volume, airway resistance | X | X | |
| b. ECG, pulse oximetry, transcutaneous $O_2/CO_2$ monitoring | X | X | |
| c. $V_D/V_T$, Qs/Qt, mixed venous sampling, C(a-$\bar{v}$)$O_2$, cardiac output, pulmonary capillary wedge pressure, central venous pressure, pulmonary artery pressures, cardiopulmonary stress testing | | | |
| d. fluid balance (intake and output) | | | |

| | RECALL | APPLICATION | ANALYSIS |
|---|:---:|:---:|:---:|
| e. arterial sampling and blood gas analysis, co-oximetry, P(A-a)$O_2$ | X | X | |
| f. sleep studies, metabolic studies [e.g., indirect calorimetry] | | | |
| g. ventilator flow, volume, and pressure waveforms, lung compliance | X | X | |
| 2. Interpret results of the following: | | | |
| a. spirometry before aad/or after bronchodilator, maximum voluntary ventilation, diffusing capacity, functional residual capacity, flow-volume loops, body plethysmography, nitrogen washout distribution test, total lung capacity, $CO_2$ response curve, closing volume, airway resistance, bronchoprovocation | X | X | |
| b. ECG, pulse oximetry, transcutaneous $O_2/CO_2$ monitoring | X | X | |
| c. $V_D/V_T$, Qs/Qt, mixed venous sampling, C(a-$\bar{v}$) $O_2$, cardiac output, pulmonary capillary wedge pressure, central venous pressure, pulmonary artery pressures, cardiopulmonary stress testing | | | |
| d. fluid balance (intake and output) | | | |
| e. arterial sampling and blood gas analysis, co-oximetry, P(A-a)$O_2$ | X | X | |
| f. peripheral venipuncture or insertion of intravenous line | | | |
| g. sleep studies, metabolic studies [e.g., indirect calorimetry] | | | |
| h. insertion of arterial and umbilical monitoring lines | | | |
| i. ventilator flow, volume, and pressure waveforms, lung compliance | X | X | |
| 3. Determine the appropriateness of the prescribed respiratory care plan and recommend modifications where indicated: | | | |
| a. perform respiratory care quality assurance | X | X | |
| b. develop quality improvement program | X | X | |
| c. review interdisciplinary patient and family care plan | X | X | |
| 4. Participate in development of respiratory care plan [e.g., case management, develop and apply protocols, disease management education] | X | X | |

| | RECALL | APPLICATION | ANALYSIS |
|---|---|---|---|
| **II. Select, Assemble, and Check Equipment for Proper Function, Operation, and Cleanliness**<br><br>**SETTING:** In any patient care setting, the advanced respiratory therapist selects, assembles, and assures cleanliness of all equipment used in providing respiratory care. The therapist checks all equipment and corrects malfunctions. | 3 | 4 | 13 |
| **A. Select and obtain equipment and assure equipment cleanliness.** | 1 | 2 | 5 |
| 1. Select and obtain equipment appropriate to the respiratory care plan: | | | |
| a. oxygen administration devices | | | |
| (1) nasal cannula, mask, reservior mask (partial rebreathing, nonrebreathing), face tents, transtracheal oxygen catheter, oxygen conserving cannulas | X | X | |
| (2) air-entrainment devices, tracheostomy collar and T-piece, oxygen hoods and tents | X | X | |
| (3) CPAP devices | X | X | |
| b. humidifiers [e.g., bubble, passover, cascade, wick, heat moisture exchanger] | X | X | |
| c. aerosol generators [e.g., pneumatic nebulizer, ultrasonic nebulizer] | X | X | |
| d. resuscitation devices [e.g, manual resuscitator (bag-valve), pneumatic (demand-valve), mouth-to-valve mask resuscitator] | X | X | |
| e. ventilators | | | |
| (1) pneumatic, electric, microprocessor, fluidic | X | X | |
| (2) high frequency | | | |
| (3) noninvasive positive pressure | X | X | |
| f. artificial airways | | | |
| (1) oro- and nasopharyngeal airways | X | X | |
| (2) oral, nasal and double-lumen endotracheal tubes | X | X | |
| (3) tracheostomy tubes and buttons | X | X | |

| | RECALL | APPLICATION | ANALYSIS |
|---|---|---|---|
| (4) intubation equipment [e.g., laryngoscope and blades, exhaled $CO_2$ detection devices] | X | X | |
| (5) other airways [e.g., laryngeal mask airway (LMA), Esophageal Tracheal Combitube® (ETC)] | | | |
| g. suctioning devices [e.g., suction catheters, specimen collectors, oropharyngeal suction devices] | X | X | |
| h. gas delivery, metering and clinical analyzing devices | | | |
| (1) regulators, redcing valves, connectors and flowmeters, air/oxygen blenders, pulse-dose systems | X | X | |
| (2) oxygen concentrators, air compressors, liquid oxygen systems | X | X | |
| (3) gas cylinders, bulk systems and manifolds | X | X | |
| (4) capnograph, blood gas analyzer and sampling devices, co-oximeter, transcutaneous $O_2/CO_2$ monitor, pulse oximeter | X | X | |
| (5) CO, He, $O_2$ and specialty gas analyzers | X | X | |
| i. patient breathing circuits | | | |
| (1) IPPB, continuous mechanical ventilation | X | X | |
| (2) CPAP, PEEP valve assembly | X | X | |
| (3) H-valve assembly | | | X |
| j. environmental devices | | | |
| (1) incubators, radiant warmers | | | |
| (2) aerosol (mist) tents | X | X | |
| (3) scavenging systems | | X | X |
| k. positive expiratory pressure device (PEP) | | | |
| l. Flutter® mucous clearance device | | | X |
| m. other therapeutic gases [e.g., $O_2/CO_2$, $He/O_2$] | | | |
| n. manometers and gauges | | | |
| (1) manometers—water, mercury and aneroid, inspiratory/expiratory pressure meters, cuff pressure manometers | X | X | |
| (2) pressure transducers | X | X | |
| o. respirometers [e.g., flow-sensing devices (pneumotachometer), volume displacement] | X | X | |

| | RECALL | APPLICATION | ANALYSIS |
|---|---|---|---|
| p. electrocardiography devices [e.g., ECG oscilloscope monitors, ECG machines (12-lead), Holter monitors] | X | X | |
| q. hemodynamic monitoring devices | | | |
| (1) central venous catheters, pulmonary artery catheters [e.g., Swan-Ganz], cardiac output, continuous $S\bar{v}O_2$ monitors | | | |
| (2) arterial catheters | | | |
| r. vacuum systems [e.g., pumps, regulators, collection bottles, pleural drainage devices] | X | X | |
| s. metered dose inhalers (MDI), MDI spacers | X | X | |
| t. Small Particle Aerosol Generators (SPAG) | X | X | |
| u. bronchoscopes | X | X | |
| 2. Assure selected equipment cleanliness [e.g., select or determine appropriate agent and technique for disinfection and/or sterilization, perform procedures for disinfection and/or sterilization, monitor effectiveness of sterilization procedures] | X | X | |
| **B. Assemble and check equipment function, identify and correct equipment malfunctions, and perform quality control.** | **2** | **2** | **8** |
| 1. Assemble, check for proper function, and identify malfunctions of equipment: | | | |
| a. oxygen administration devices | | | |
| (1) nasal cannula, mask, reservoir mask (partial rebreathing, nonrebreathing), face tents, transtracheal oxygen catheter, oxygen conserving cannulas | X | X | |
| (2) air-entrainment devices, tracheostomy collar and T-piece, oxygen hoods and tents | X | X | |
| (3) CPAP devices | X | X | |
| b. humidifiers [e.g., bubble, passover, cascade, wick, heat moisture exchanger] | X | X | |
| c. aerosol generators [e.g., pneumatic nebulizer, ultrasonic nebulizer] | X | X | |
| d. resuscitation devices [e.g., manual resuscitator (bag-valve), pneumatic (demand-valve), mouth-to-valve mask resuscitator] | X | X | |
| e. ventilators | | | |
| (1) pneumatic, electric, microprocessor, fluidic | X | X | |
| (2) high frequency | | | |
| (3) noninvasive positive pressure | X | X | |

| | RECALL | APPLICATION | ANALYSIS |
|---|---|---|---|
| f. artificial airways | | | |
| (1) oro- and nasopharyngeal airways | X | X | |
| (2) oral, nasal and double-lumen endotracheal tubes | X | X | |
| (3) tracheostomy tubes and buttons | X | X | |
| (4) intubation equipment [e.g., laryngoscope and blades, exhaled $CO_2$ detection devices] | X | X | |
| g. suctioning devices [e.g., suction catheters, speciment collectors, oropharyngeal suction devices] | X | X | |
| h. gas delivery, metering and clinical analyzing devices | | | |
| (1) regulators, reducing valves, connectors and flowmeters, air/oxygen blenders, pulse-dose systems | X | X | |
| (2) oxygen concentrators, air compressors, liquid oxygen systems | X | X | |
| (3) gas cylinders, bulk, systems and manifolds | X | X | |
| (4) capnograph, blood gas analyzer and sampling devices, co-oximeter, transcutaneous $O_2/CO_2$ monitor, pulse oximeter | X | X | |
| (5) CO, He, $O_2$ and specialty gas analyzers | X | X | |
| i. patient breathing circuits | | | |
| (1) IPPB, continuous mechanical ventilation | X | X | |
| (2) CPAP, PEEP valve assembly | X | X | |
| (3) H-valve assembly | | X | X |
| j. environmental devices | | | |
| (1) incubators, radiant warmers | | | |
| (2) aerosol (mist) tents | X | X | |
| k. positive expiratory pressure (PEP) device | | | |
| l. Flutter® mucous clearance device | | | X |
| m. other therapeutic gases [e.g., $O_2/CO_2$, $He/O_2$] | | | |
| n. manometers and gauges | | | |
| (1) manometers—water, mercury and aneroid, inspiratory/expiratory pressure meters, cuff pressure manometers | X | X | |
| (2) pressure transducers | | | |
| o. respirometers [e.g., flow-sensing devices (pneumotachometer), volume displacement] | X | X | |
| p. electrocardiography devices [e.g., ECG oscilloscope monitors, ECG machines (12-lead), Holter monitors] | X | X | |

| | RECALL | APPLICATION | ANALYSIS |
|---|---|---|---|
| q. hemodynamic monitoring devices | | | |
| (1) central venous catheters, pulmonary artery catheters [e.g., Swan-Ganz], cardiac output, continuous $\bar{s}vO_2$ monitors | | | |
| (2) arterial catheters | | | |
| r. vacuum systems [e.g., pumps, regulators, collection bottles, pleural drainage devices] | X | X | |
| s. bronchoscopes | | | X |
| 2. Take action to correct malfunctions of equipment: | | | |
| a. oxygen administration devices | | | |
| (1) nasal cannula, mask, reservoir mask (partial rebreathing, nonrebreathing), face tents, transtracheal oxygen catheter, oxygen conserving cannulas | X | X | |
| (2) air-entrainment devices, tracheostomy collar and T-piece, oxygen hoods and tents | X | X | |
| (3) CPAP devices | X | X | |
| b. humidifiers [e.g., bubble, passover, cascade, wick, heat moisture exchanger] | X | X | |
| c. aerosol generators [e.g., pneumatic nebulizer, ultrasonic nebulizer] | X | X | |
| d. resuscitation devices [e.g., manual resuscitator (bag-valve), pneumatic (demand-valve), mouth-to-valve mask resuscitator] | X | X | |
| e. ventilators | | | |
| (1) pneumatic, electric, microprocessor, fluidic | X | X | |
| (2) high frequency | | | |
| (3) noninvasive positive pressure | X | X | |
| f. artificial airways | | | |
| (1) oro- and nasopharyngeal airways | X | X | |
| (2) oral, nasal and double-lumen endotracheal tubes | X | X | |
| (3) tracheostomy tubes and buttons | X | X | |
| (4) intubation equipment [e.g., laryngoscope and blades, exhaled $CO_2$ detection devices] | X | X | |
| g. suctioning devices [e.g., suction catheters, specimen collectors, oropharyngeal suction devices] | X | X | |
| h. gas delivery, metering and clinical analyzing devices | | | |
| (1) regulators, reducing valves, connectors and flowmeters, air/oxygen blenders, pulse-dose systems | X | X | |
| (2) oxygen concentrators, air compressors, liquid oxygen systems | X | X | |

| | RECALL | APPLICATION | ANALYSIS |
|---|---|---|---|
| (3) gas cylinders, bulk systems and manifolds | X | X | |
| (4) capnograph, blood gas analyzer and sampling devices, co-oximeter, transcutaneous $O_2/CO_2$ monitor, pulse oximeter | X | X | |
| (5) CO, He, $O_2$ and specialty gas analyzers | | | |
| i. patient breathing circuits | | | |
| (1) IPPB, continuous mechanical ventilation | X | X | |
| (2) CPAP, PEEP valve assembly | X | X | |
| (3) H-valve assembly | | | X |
| j. environmental devices | | | |
| (1) incubators, radiant warmers | | | X |
| (2) aerosol (mist) tents | X | X | |
| k. positive expiratory pressure (PEP) device | | | |
| l. Flutter® mucous clearance device | | | X |
| m. other therapeutic gases [e.g., $O_2/CO_2$, $He/O_2$] | | | |
| n. manometers and gauges | | | |
| (1) manometers—water, mercury and aneroid, inspiratory/expiratory pressure meters, cuff pressure manometers | X | X | |
| (2) pressure transducers | | | |
| o. respirometers [e.g., flow-sensing devices (pneumotachometer), volume displacement] | X | X | |
| p. electrocardiography devices [e.g., ECG oscilloscope monitors, ECG machines (12-lead), Holter monitors] | | | |
| q. hemodynamic monitoring devices | | | |
| (1) central venous catheters, pulmonary artery catheters [e.g., Swan-Ganz], cardiac output, continuous $S\bar{v}O_2$ monitors | | | |
| (2) arterial catheters | | | |
| r. vacuum systems [e.g., pumps, regulators, collection bottles, pleural drainage devices] | X | X | |
| s. Small Particle Aerosol Generators (SPAG) | | X | X |
| t. bronchoscopes | | | X |
| 3. Perform quality control procedures for: | | | |
| a. blood gas analyzers and sampling devices, co-oximeters | X | X | |
| b. pulmonary function equipment, ventilator volume/flow/pressure calibration | X | X | |
| c. gas metering devices | X | X | |
| d. noninvasive monitors [e.g., transcutaneous] | | | |

| | RECALL | APPLICATION | ANALYSIS |
|---|---|---|---|

## III. Initiate, Conduct, and Modify Prescribed Therapeutic Procedures

**SETTING:** In any patient care setting, the RRT evaluates, monitors, and records the patient's response to care. The therapist maintains patient records and communicates with other healthcare team members. The therapist initiates, conducts, and modifies prescribed therapeutic procedures to achieve the desired objectives. The therapist provides care in emergency settings, assists the physician, and conducts pulmonary rehabilitation and homecare.

| | RECALL | APPLICATION | ANALYSIS |
|---|---|---|---|
| III. Initiate, Conduct, and Modify Prescribed Therapeutic Procedures | 6 | 8 | 49 |
| **A. Evaluate, monitor, and record patient's response to respiratory care.** | 2 | 3 | 13 |
| 1. Evaluate and monitor patient's response to respiratory care: | | | |
| a. recommend and review chest X-ray | X | X | |
| b. perform arterial puncture, capillary blood gas sampling, and venipuncture; obtaion blood from arterial or pulmonary artery lines; perform transcutaneous $O_2/CO_2$, pulse oximetry, co-oximetry, and capnography monitoring | X | X | |
| c. observe changes in sputum production and consistency, note patient's subjective response to therapy and mechanical ventilation | X | X | |
| d. measure and record vital signs, monitor cardiac rhythm, evaluate fluid balance (intake and output) | X | X | |
| e. perform spirometry/determine vital capacity, measure lung compliance and airway resistance, interpret ventilator flow, volume, and pressure waveforms, measure peak flow | X | X | |
| f. determine and record central venous pressure, pulmonary artery pressures, pulmonary capillary wedge pressure and/or cardiac output | | | |

| | RECALL | APPLICATION | ANALYSIS |
|---|---|---|---|
| g. recommend measurement of electrolytes, hemoglobin, CBC and/or chemistries | | | |
| h. monitor mean airway pressure, adjust and check alarm systems, measure tidal volume, respiratory rate, airway pressures, I:E, and maximum inspiratory pressure (MIP) | X | X | |
| i. measure $FIO_2$ and/or liter flow | X | X | |
| j. monitor endotracheal or tracheostomy tube cuff pressure | X | X | |
| k. auscultate chest and interpret changes in breath sounds | X | X | |
| l. perform hemodynamic calculations [e.g., shunt studies ($\dot{Q}s/\dot{Q}t$), cardiac output, cardiac index, pulmonary vascular resistance and systemic vascular resistance, stroke volume] | | | |
| m. interpret hemodynamic calculations: | | | |
| (1) calculate and interpret $P(A-a)O_2$, $C(a-\bar{v})O_2$, $\dot{Q}s/\dot{Q}t$ | | | |
| (2) exhaled $CO_2$ monitoring, $V_D/V_T$ | | | |
| (3) cardiac output, cardiac index, pulmonary vascular resistance and systemic vascular resistance, stroke volume | | | |
| 2. Maintain records and communication: | | | |
| a. record therapy and results using conventional terminology as required in the healthcare setting and/or by regulatory agencies by noting and interpreting: | | | |
| (1) patient's response to therapy including the effects of therapy, adverse reactions, patient's subjective and attitudinal response to therapy | X | X | |
| (2) auscultatory findings, cough and sputum production and characteristics | X | X | |
| (3) vital signs [e.g., heart rate, respiratory rate, blood pressure, body temperature] | X | X | |
| (4) pulse oximetry, heart rhythm, capnography | X | X | |
| b. verify computations and note erroneous data | X | X | |

| | RECALL | APPLICATION | ANALYSIS |
|---|---|---|---|
| c. apply computer technology to patient management [e.g., ventilator waveform analysis, electronic charting, patient care algorithms] | | X | X |
| d. communicate results of therapy and alter therapy per protocol(s) | | X | X |
| **B. Conduct therapeutic procedures to maintain a patent airway, achieve adequate ventilation and oxygenation, and remove bronchopulmonary secretions.** | 1 | 1 | 10 |
| 1. Maintain a patent airway including the care of artificial airways: | | | |
| a. insert oro- and nasopharyngeal airway, select endotracheal or tracheostomy tube, perform endotracheal intubation, change tracheostomy tube, maintain proper cuff inflation, position of endotracheal or tracheostomy tube | | X | X |
| b. maintain adequate humidification | | X | X |
| c. extubate the patient | | X | X |
| d. properly position patient | | X | X |
| e. identify endotracheal tube placement by available means | | X | X |
| 2. Achieve adequate spontaneous and artificial ventilation: | | | |
| a. initiate and adjust IPPB therapy | | X | X |
| b. initiate and select appropriate settings for high frequency ventilation | | | |
| c. initiate and adjust ventilator modes (e.g., A/C, SIMV, pressure support ventilation (PSV), pressure control ventilation (PCV)] | | X | X |
| d. initiate and adjust independent (differential) lung ventilation | | | |
| 3. Remove bronchopulmonary secretions by instructing and encouraging bronchopulmonary hygiene techniques (e.g., coughing techniques, autogenic drainage, positive expiratory pressure device (PEP), intrapulmonary percussive ventilation (IPV), Flutter®, High Frequency Chest Wall Oscillation (HFCWO)] | | X | X |
| 4. Achieve adequate arterial and tissue oxygenation: | | | |
| a. initiate and adjust CPAP, PEEP, and noninvasive positive pressure | | X | X |
| b. initiate and adjust combinations of ventilatory techniques [e.g., SIMV, PEEP, PS, PCV] | | X | X |

| | RECALL | APPLICATION | ANALYSIS |
|---|---|---|---|
| c. position patient to minimize hypoxemia, administer oxygen (on or off ventilator), prevent procedure-associated hypoxemia [e.g., oxygenate before and after suctioning and equipment changes] | | X | X |
| **C. Make necessary modifications in therapeutic procedures based on patient response.** | 0 | 1 | 10 |
| 1. Modify IPPB: | | | |
| a. adjust sensitivity, flow, volume, pressure, $FiO_2$ | | X | X |
| b. adjust expiratory retard | | X | X |
| c. change patient—machine interface [e.g., mouthpiece, mask] | | X | X |
| 2. Modify patient breathing pattern during aerosol therapy | | X | X |
| 3. Modify oxygen therapy: | | | |
| a. change mode of administration, adjust flow, and $FiO_2$ | | X | X |
| b. set up an $O_2$ concentrator or liquid $O_2$ system | | X | X |
| 4. Modify specialty gas [e.g., $He/O_2$, $O_2/CO_2$] therapy [e.g., change mode of administration, adjust flow, adjust gas concentration] | | X | |
| 5. Modify bronchial hygiene therapy [e.g., alter position of patient, alter duration of treatment and techniques, coordinate sequence of therapies, alter equipment used and PEP therapy] | | X | X |
| 6. Modify artificial airway management: | | | |
| a. alter endotracheal or tracheostomy tube position, change endotracheal or tracheostomy tube | | X | X |
| b. initiate suctioning | | X | X |
| c. inflate and deflate the cuff | | X | X |
| 7. Modify suctioning: | | | |
| a. alter frequency and duration of suctioning | | X | X |
| b. change size and type of catheter | | X | X |
| c. alter negative pressure | | X | X |
| d. instill irrigating solutions | | X | X |
| 8. Modify mechanical ventilation: | | | |
| a. change patient breathing circuitry, change type of ventilator | | X | X |
| b. measure volume loss through chest tube(s) | | X | |
| c. change mechanical dead space | | X | X |

| | RECALL | APPLICATION | ANALYSIS |
|---|---|---|---|
| **D. Initiate, conduct, or modify respiratory care techniques in an emergency setting.** | 1 | 1 | 10 |
| 1. Treat cardiopulmonary collapse according to: | | | |
|   a. BCLS | X | X | |
|   b. ACLS | X | X | |
|   c. PALS | X | X | |
|   d. NRP | X | X | |
| 2. Treat tension pneumothorax | | | |
| 3. Participate in land/air patient transport | | | |
| **E. Assist physician, initiate, and conduct pulmonary rehabilitation.** | 2 | 2 | 6 |
| 1. Act as an assistant to the physician performing special procedures including: | | | |
|   a. bronchoscopy | X | X | |
|   b. thoracentesis | X | X | |
|   c. transtracheal aspiration | | | |
|   d. tracheostomy | X | X | |
|   e. cardiopulmonary stress testing | | | |
|   f. percutaneous needle biopsies of the lung | | | |
|   g. sleep studies | | | |
|   h. cardioversion | X | X | |
|   i. intubation | X | X | |
|   j. insertion of chest tubes | | | |
|   k. insertion of lines for invasive monitoring [e.g., central venous pressure, pulmonary artery catheters, Swan-Ganz, arterial lines] | | | |
|   l. conscious sedation | | | |
| 2. Initiate and conuct pulmonary rehabilitation and home care within the prescription: | | | |
|   a. monitor and maintain home respiratory care equipment, maintain apnea monitors | | | |
|   b. explain planned therapy and goals to patient in understandable terms to achieve optimal therapeutic outcome, counsel patient and family concerning smoking cessation, disease management | X | X | |
|   c. assure safety and infection control | X | X | |
|   d. modify respiratory care procedures for use in the home | X | X | |
|   e. implement and monitor graded exercise program | | | |
|   f. conduct patient education and disease management programs | X | X | |
| **TOTALS** | 12 | 15 | 73 |

# Posttest Answers and Analyses

**NOTE:** The references listed after each analysis are numbered and keyed to the reference list located at the end of this section. The first number indicates the text. The second number indicates the page where information about the questions can be found. For example, (1:114, 187) means that on pages 114 and 187 of reference 1, information about the question will be found. Frequently, it will be necessary to read beyond the page number indicated to obtain complete information. Therefore, reference to the question will be found either on the page indicated or on subsequent pages.

## IIIA1e

1.  A. Over a four-hour period, the RRT has indicated that the peak inspiratory pressure (PIP) has risen from 30 cm $H_2O$ to 42 cm $H_2O$ while the static or plateau pressure remained essentially constant. The PIP has two components: a static component and a dynamic component. When an inspiratory hold or pause is initiated at the time the PIP is achieved, the static pressure is obtained. The static pressure represents the pressure that is necessary to maintain lung inflation at the tidal volume (900 cc) set on the ventilator. Changes in the static pressure indicate changes in the lung–chest wall (or total) compliance.

    Assuming that the chest wall is normal (constant), the static pressure will reflect changes in lung compliance specifically. For example, if the plateau (static) pressure increases, pulmonary compliance has decreased (i.e., the lungs have become stiffer). On the other hand, a decrease in the plateau pressure reflects an increased lung compliance.

    In this problem, the plateau pressure has remained the same but the PIP has increased—indicating that airway resistance, or the nonelastic component of the work of breathing (WOB), has increased. From the choices presented, the only item that would correct an airway resistance problem is ET suctioning.

    (1:937), (10:257–258, (15:643–644).

## IC4

2.  A. Continuous positive airway pressure (CPAP) would be contraindicated for a patient who has COPD and cor pulmonale. This patient has pulmonary hypertension and a failing right ventricle.

    The elevated mean-intrathoracic pressure from the CPAP device could aggravate the pulmonary hypertension. At the same time, CPAP might impose a greater afterload on the right ventricle, causing this chamber to work harder.

    CPAP is contraindicated for patients who are hemodynamically unstable.

    (1:783), (10:268, 271).

## IIB1q(1)

3.  C. The situation illustrated on the tracing, represented by exaggerated oscillations, can occur under the following conditions: catheter coiling in either the right atrium or right ventricle or catheter positioning near the pulmonic valve exposed to turbulent flow.

    (14:303-307).

## IIID1b

4.  D. According to the American Heart Association, adults should receive an initial energy of 200 joules for defibrillation. If a second defibrillation is indicated, the energy level should range between 200 and 300 joules. For third and subsequent defibrillations, the energy level must be raised to 360 joules.

    For children and infants, the recommendations state 2 joules/kg for the initial and second shocks and 4 joules/kg for the third and subsequent defibrillations.

    (1:657), (16:814).

## IIIA2a(2)

5.  C. Bronchial or tracheal breath sounds are described as high-pitched sounds with an expiratory component equal to or slightly longer than the inspiratory component. Bronchovesicular breath sounds are not as loud as bronchial breath sounds and are slightly lower in pitch. Bronchovesicular breath sounds tend to have equal inspiratory and expiratory components. Crackles refer to adventitious sounds characterized by discontinuous abnormal lung sounds. Rhonchi are low-pitched continuous sounds. Wheezes are high-pitched continuous sounds.

    (1:313-314), (9:81-82).

## IIIC5

6.  C. Mucomyst (acetylcysteine) is a mucolytic agent often used to treat the problem of copious, viscous pulmonary secretions. Patients who sometimes benefit from the administration of either 10% or 20% Mucomyst are those who have COPD, bronchiectasis, or acute tracheobronchitis.

Mucomyst can cause bronchospasm in certain patients. When this happens, the RRT needs to administer a beta adrenergic bronchodilator (e.g., albuterol) immediately. In fact, if the RRT anticipates the likelihood of bronchospasm associated with Mucomyst administration, she should give the patient a beta adrenergic bronchodilator before the Mucomyst treatment. Alternatively, the bronchodilator can be placed in the small-volume nebulizer with the mucolytic agent, having both nebulized concurrently.

(1:574, 579-580), (16:475).

## IIID1a

7. C. Pupillary reflexes are part of every neurological examination and part of the initial assessment in emergency situations. The information obtained will establish a baseline for comparison with future examinations. Among the factors that can affect pupil size and reaction time are hypoxia, trauma, increased intracranial pressure, intracranial bleeding, and drug reactions.

(15:1095–1100).

## IIIA1m(1)

8. C. This patient's P(A-a)O$_2$ can be calculated as follows:

STEP 1:   Calculate the P$_A$O$_2$ using the alveolar air equation.

$$P_AO_2 = F_IO_2(P_B - P_{H_2O}) - PaCO_2\left(F_IO_2 + \frac{1 - F_IO_2}{R}\right)$$

$$= 0.4 (760\ torr - 47\ torr) - 40\ torr\left(0.4 + \frac{1 - 0.4}{0.8}\right)$$

$$= 239\ torr$$

STEP 2:   Calculate the P(A-a)O$_2$.

$$P(A\text{-}a)O_2 = PaO_2 - PaO_2$$

$$= 239\ torr - 85\ torr$$

$$= 154\ torr$$

(1:217, 235, 929), (9:125, 294), (16:256).

## IIB1i(3)

9. B. When using a Wright Respirometer to measure the exhaled tidal volume of a patient who is receiving continuous-flow IMV through an H-valve assembly (Figure 6-12), the RRT must attach the device to the patient's ET tube and maintain the IMV system disconnected from the patient's ET tube. Otherwise, the dial on the respirometer will be prone to the effects of both the continuous gas flow and the flow from the ventilator during mandatory breath delivery. If the respirometer is attached to the exhalation port of the ventilator circuit, the dial will continually spin (caused

by the continuous gas flow). If the device is connected along the inspiratory limb, it will be influenced by the continuous IMV flow and the ventilator's mandatory breaths.

The diagram in Figure 6-12 illustrates how the H-valve IMV system connects to the ventilator circuitry.

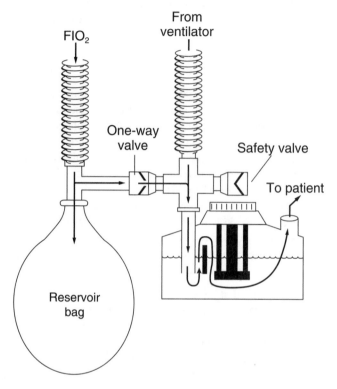

**Figure 6-12:** H-valve IMV assembly added to a mechanical ventilator circuit.

(1:861–862), (10:329–331).

## IIIE1g

10. B. When polysomnography is performed, a number of recordings are obtained to determine when the patient is asleep and to identify when the different stages of sleep are occurring. The two general sleep stages are nonrapid eye movement (nonREM) and rapid eye movement (REM).

To ascertain the specific stage of sleep during polysomnography, the following tracings need to be recorded: (1) an electroencephalogram (EEG), (2) an electrooculogram (EOG), and (3) an electromyogram (EMG). The EEG is obtained from two leads placed on the top of the patient's head. The EOG waveforms are derived from electrodes located over the outer canthi of the eyes. The EMG tracing is generated from leads attached to the patient's chin.

(1:557–559), (9:410–414), (15:579–582).

**IIIA1m(1)**

11. B. The following steps are used to calculate the $C(a\text{-}\bar{v})O_2$:

STEP 1: Determine the arterial oxygen content ($CaO_2$).

$$CaO_2 = (PaO_2)(0.003 \text{ vol\%/torr}) +$$
$$(1.34 \text{ ml } O_2/g \text{ Hb})(SaO_2)([Hb])$$
$$= (100 \text{ torr})(0.003 \text{ vol\%/torr}) +$$
$$(1.34 \text{ ml } O_2/g \text{ Hb})(0.95)(15 \text{ g Hb}/100 \text{ ml})$$
$$= 0.3 \text{ vol\%} + 19.1 \text{ vol\%}$$
$$= 19.4 \text{ vol\%}$$

STEP 2: Calculate the mixed venous oxygen content ($C\bar{v}O_2$).

$$C\bar{v}O_2 = (P\bar{v}O_2)(0.003 \text{ vol\%/torr}) +$$
$$(1.34 \text{ ml } O_2/g \text{ Hb})(S\bar{v}O_2)([Hb])$$
$$= (46 \text{ torr})(0.003 \text{ vol\%/torr}) +$$
$$(1.34 \text{ ml } O_2/g \text{ Hb})(0.70)(15 \text{ g Hb}/100 \text{ ml})$$
$$= 0.14 \text{ vol\%} + 14.1 \text{ vol\%}$$
$$= 14.2 \text{ vol\%}$$

STEP 3: Obtain the $C(a\text{-}\bar{v})O_2$ by subtracting the $C\bar{v}O_2$ from the $CaO_2$.

$$C(a-\bar{v})O_2 = CaO_2 - C\bar{v}O_2$$
$$= 19.4 \text{ vol\%} - 14.2 \text{ vol\%}$$
$$= 5.2 \text{ vol\%}$$

A $C(a\text{-}\bar{v})O_2$ of 5.0 vol% is normal. According to the Fick equation,

$$\dot{Q}_T = \frac{\dot{V}O_2}{C(a-\bar{v})O_2}, \text{ or } \dot{V}O_2 = \dot{Q}_T \times C(a-\bar{v})O_2$$

If the tissue oxygen consumption remains constant, the $C(a\text{-}\bar{v})O_2$ will decrease as the cardiac output increases. On the other hand, if the $\dot{V}O_2$ remains constant, the $C(a\text{-}\bar{v})O_2$ will increase as the cardiac output decreases.

(1:226-227), (9:125-126), (16:256).

**IIIE1g**

12. B. The level of CPAP appropriate for the treatment of obstructive sleep apnea is determined by polysomnography. After an initial sleep study has revealed that sleep apnea is present and that CPAP is indicated, a follow-up sleep study is performed to determine the therapeutic CPAP level. Once the sleep apnea syndrome has been reconfirmed during a non-CPAP sleep trial, a nasal CPAP of 5 cm $H_2O$ is applied. If necessary, the CPAP level is raised in increments of about 2 cm $H_2O$ until the patient stops snoring and the obstructive apnea episodes are eliminated. If the patient demonstrates oxygen desaturation below 85%, oxygen is supplied to the CPAP system until a saturation of 90% is achieved. Oxygen saturation is *not* a criterion for determining the appropriate CPAP level in this clinical condition. It is simply addressed by administering oxygen therapy along with the CPAP if the patient exhibits desaturation below 85%.

(1:557–559), (9:410–414), (15:579–582).

**IA1h**

13. D. The purpose of the Apgar score is to clinically evaluate the cardiopulmonary status of a newborn. The Apgar score is composed of the following clinical signs: (1) heart rate, (2) respiratory (ventilatory) effort, (3) muscle tone, (4) reflex irritability, and (5) color. Ventilatory rate is *not* one of the clinical signs included; ventilatory effort is. The Apgar scale is shown in Table 6-3.

The Apgar score is based on a scale of 0 to 10. Apgar score ranges and their corresponding clinical interventions are listed in Table 6-4 on page 380. Apgar scores

**Table 6-3** Apgar Scale

| Sign | Score | | |
| --- | --- | --- | --- |
| | 0 | 1 | 2 |
| Heart rate | Absent | < 100 bpm | > 100 bpm |
| Ventilatory effort | Absent | Weak, irregular | Good, crying |
| Muscle tone | Flaccid, limp | Some flexion of extremities | Active, well flexed |
| Reflex irritability | No response | Grimace | Cough, sneeze |
| Color | Peripheral and central cyanosis | Peripheral cyanosis | Completely pink |

should be determined at one and five minutes after birth.

**Table 6-4** Clinical Application of Apgar Score

| Apgar Score | Clinical Intervention |
| --- | --- |
| 7–10 | Resuscitative measures are not needed |
| 4–6 | Mild to moderate asphyxia, suctioning and oxygenation indicated; ventilation considered |
| 0–3 | Cardiopulmonary resuscitation indicated |

(1:1002), (9:215), (18:43–44).

**IIIB4c**

14. C. Chronic obstructive pulmonary disease (COPD) patients characteristically have maldistribution of ventilation throughout their tracheobronchial tree. This nonuniform distribution of inspired gas results in many areas of the lung possessing low ventilation–perfusion ratios, or perfusion in excess of ventilation (venous admixture or shunt effect units).

Nitrogen, an inert and relatively insoluble gas, functions as a filler gas—thereby maintaining lung volume. When increased oxygen is administered, oxygen replaces (washes out) nitrogen molecules. The oxygen that replaces the nitrogen in situations where the patient's lungs have nonuniform ventilation and many alveolar units with perfusion in excess of ventilation is rapidly absorbed by the blood. The result is alveolar collapse, or absorption atelectasis.

The general guideline of hyperoxygenating a patient with 100% $O_2$ before performing ET suctioning should be abandoned whenever the patient has chronic obstructive airflow. Nonetheless, hyperoxygenation should still be performed to help reduce the risk of hypoxemia developing during the procedure. The degree of hyperoxygenation for a COPD patient should be no more than 0.10 $FIO_2$ greater than what the patient is receiving. In this case, the patient is receiving an $FIO_2$ of 0.30; therefore, the hyperoxygenated $FIO_2$ should not be greater than 0.40.

(1:619), (16:606).

**IIIA1g**

15. A. ABG and acid-base data indicate a severe metabolic acidosis associated with a low arterial $PCO_2$ and an above-normal arterial $PO_2$. The patient has hyperventilated because of peripheral chemoreceptor (carotid and aortic bodies) stimulation caused by the acute increase of $H^+$ ions in the arterial blood. The cause of this metabolic problem is the patient's diabetes. The cells of the body require glucose for fuel during aero-

bic respiration. Insulin is essential for the transport of glucose into the cells. When a diabetic patient's insulin blood level is low, not enough glucose can enter the cells. The cells then respire via an alternate pathway, whereby free fatty acids in circulation are metabolized by the liver. The metabolic by-products of this alternate metabolic route are ketones. Therefore, the acidosis produced is termed *diabetic ketoacidosis*. The diabetic ketoacidosis experienced by this patient cannot be compensated for by hyperventilation. This type of metabolic acidosis is characterized by an accumulation of nonvolatile acids (ketoacids) that cannot be excreted by the lungs; rather, they can only be excreted via the kidneys.

Treating diabetic ketoacidosis with I.V. fluids, insulin, and electrolytes is customary. Therefore, electrolytes must be measured to ascertain the electrolyte imbalance. Generally, $HCO_3^-$ administration is withheld unless the arterial pH is less than 7.10. When the patient's acidemia is corrected, hyperventilation will eventually diminish and normal ventilation will be reestablished.

The arterial $PO_2$ is above normal because of the increased minute ventilation and the low arterial $PCO_2$. Hyperventilation in situations as this can result in inordinately high room air arterial $PO_2$s. Kussmaul's breathing is associated with diabetic ketoacidosis. It is characterized by deep and rapid ventilatory efforts.

(1:275), (4:115, 236, 251), (9:131), (15:291, 675).

**IIB3a**

16. C. The calculation for the high $O_2$ and $CO_2$ gas tension of the calibration gas cylinders for a blood gas analyzer are shown as follows:

***High $O_2$ Calibration (torr)***

STEP 1: Correct the measured barometric pressure (from barometer reading) for the presence of water vapor at 37°C.

$$\left(\begin{array}{c} one \\ atmosphere \end{array}\right) - \left(\begin{array}{c} P_{H_2O} \\ at\ 37°C \end{array}\right) = \left(\begin{array}{c} corrected \\ barometric\ pressure \end{array}\right)$$

760 torr − 47 torr = 713 torr

STEP 2: Convert the gas percentage to its decimal equivalent ($F_{gas}$).

$$F_{gas} = \frac{\%\ gas}{100}$$

$$= \frac{12.0\%\ O_2}{100}$$

$$= 0.12$$

STEP 3: Calculate the partial pressure value of the high $O_2$ gas ($P_{gas}$).

$$P_{gas} = \text{(corrected barometric pressure)} \times (F_{gas})$$

$$= 713 \text{ torr} \times 0.12 \ F_IO_2$$

$$= 85.56 \text{ torr}$$

### High CO₂ Calibration (torr)

STEP 1:  Correct the measured barometric pressure.

$$PB_{corrected} = 760 \text{ torr} - 47 \text{ torr}$$

$$= 713 \text{ torr}$$

STEP 2:  Determine the $FCO_2$.

$$FCO_2 = \frac{10.0\% \ CO_2}{100}$$

$$= 0.10$$

STEP 3:  Calculate the high $PCO_2$ value.

$$PCO_2 = 713 \text{ torr} \times 0.10 \ FCO_2$$

$$= 71.30 \text{ torr}$$

(6:309), (15:11), (17:261–263).

## IC2c

17.  D. According to the hemodynamic data presented, the patient has a PCWP greater than the PAd and the PAs pressures. Ordinarily, the PCWP is somewhat lower than the PAd pressure. Furthermore, if the PCWP exceeded the PAs pressure, blood would flow theoretically from the left ventricle to the right ventricle—a situation we all know is impossible.

Because these data are incompatible with normal physiology, they are erroneous. New measurements must be obtained.

(1:943-949), (9:338-350, 356-358).

## IA1c

18.  B. The blood data presented in the question indicate that the patient has an increased hemoglobin concentration (19 g/dl or 19 g%) and an increased red blood cell concentration (6.5 × 10⁶/mm³). The term *polycythemia* describes this condition. *Anemia* refers to hemoglobin concentrations less than 12 g%. The suffix *-penia* means decrease from normal or deficiency. Therefore, the terms *erythrocytopenia* and *hemocy-*

*topenia* would refer to conditions of low red blood cell concentrations and low blood cell concentrations, respectively.

Table 6-5 shows normal ranges for some red blood cell values in the blood.

(9:103, 115), (16:178).

## IIIC5

19.  C. One purpose of PEP therapy is to increase sputum production in patients who already have excessive sputum production (i.e., cystic fibrosis and chronic bronchitis patients). If PEP therapy does not accomplish this objective, it should be discontinued.

(American Association for Respiratory Care Clinical Practice Guideline [May, 1993], "Use of Positive Airway Pressure Adjuncts to Bronchial Hygiene," *Respiratory Care, 38* (5), pp. 516–519).

## IIIA1h

20.  C. The formula to use is as follows:

$$\overline{P}_{aw} = K(PIP - PEEP)(T_I/TCT) + PEEP$$

where

$\overline{P}_{aw}$ = mean airway pressure (cm $H_2O$)
$K^*$ = waveform constant
$PIP$ = peak inspiratory pressure (cm $H_2O$)
$PEEP$ = positive end-expiratory pressure (cm $H_2O$)
$T_I$ = inspiratory time (seconds)
$TCT$ = total cycle time (seconds)

*K equals 0.5 for ascending or descending ramp pressure waveforms. For square or rectangular pressure waveforms, K equals 1.0.

STEP 1:  Determine the total cycle time (TCT).

$$T_I + T_E = TCT$$

$$0.4 \text{ sec.} + 0.8 \text{ sec.} = 1.2 \text{ sec.}$$

STEP 2:  Insert the known values into the mean airway pressure ($\overline{P}_{aw}$) equation.

$$\overline{P}_{aw} = K(PIP - PEEP)(T_I/TCT) + PEEP$$

$$= 0.5(27 \text{ cm } H_2O - 5 \text{ cm } H_2O)(0.4 \ \cancel{\text{sec.}}/1.2 \ \cancel{\text{sec.}}) +$$

$$5 \text{ cm } H_2O$$

**Table 6-5** Normal Ranges for Red Blood Cell Values in Blood

|  | Red Blood Cell (RBC) or Erythrocyte Count | Hemoglobin Concentration | Hematocrit |
|---|---|---|---|
| Male | 4.6–6.2 × 10⁶/mm³ | 13.5–16.5 g% | 40%–54% |
| Female | 4.2–5.5 × 10⁶/mm³ | 12.0–15.0 g% | 38%–47% |

$= 0.5(22 \text{ cm H}_2\text{O})(0.33) + 5 \text{ cm H}_2\text{O}$

$= 3.6 \text{ cm H}_2\text{O} + 5 \text{ cm H}_2\text{O}$

$= 8.6 \text{ cm H}_2\text{O}$

(1:888), (9:287), (10:265).

## IC2c

21. B. By dividing the prescribed 70–30 heliox flow rate by the 1.6 conversion factor, the actual oxygen flow meter setting can be determined. For example,

$$\frac{\text{required 70-30 heliox flow rate}}{\text{conversion factor}} = \text{oxygen flow meter setting}$$

$$\frac{15 \text{ L/min.}}{1.6} = 9.375 \text{ L/min.}$$

Setting the oxygen flow meter at 9.5 L/min. will supply about 15 L/min. of 70–30 heliox to the patient. The conversion factors for 80–20 heliox and 60–40 heliox are 1.8 and 1.4, respectively.

(1:768), (13:59–60), (16:357–358).

## IC2c

22. A. Whenever the pulmonary capillary wedge pressure (PCWP) is elevated, such as, greater than 15 mm Hg, one of two conditions is likely the cause. They are either left ventricular failure or hypervolemia. Left ventricular failure is frequently caused by myocardial infarction or mitral regurgitation.

Left ventricular failure can be differentiated from hypervolemia if the cardiac output and $C(a-\bar{v})O_2$ are known. In this case, the cardiac output (10 liters/min.) is elevated. Such a situation is impossible for a patient who has left ventricular failure because the left heart is an inadequate pump. Left ventricular failure generally produces a lower-than-normal cardiac output.

Although the $C(a-\bar{v})O_2$ is less than normal, the increased cardiac output is assuring a normal tissue oxygen consumption ($VO_2$). This situation can be verified by the Fick equation, which states that

$$\dot{Q}_T = \frac{\dot{V}o_2}{C(a - \bar{v})O_2}, \text{ or } \dot{V}o_2 = \dot{Q}_T \times C(a - \bar{v})O_2$$

Therefore,

$(10 \text{ liters/min.})(2.5 \text{ vol\%}/100) = 250 \text{ ml/min.}$

The problem here is hypervolemia.

(1:943–949), (9:347–353).

## IIA1d

23. D. Disadvantages of using gas-powered resuscitation devices include variable delivered volumes, potentially high pressure, and high flow rates; the latter two can contribute to the incidence of barotrauma and massive gastric insufflation.

(5:235–237), (13:201–202).

## IIIC2

24. C. Continuous nebulization occurs during both inspiration and exhalation. Therefore, medication is wasted while the patient exhales because he does not derive any benefit from its nebulization during that phase of the ventilatory cycle. Instituting intermittent nebulization, whereby the patient controls the flow of the nebulizing gas to the nebulizer during inspiration only, will prolong the treatment and provide the patient with more medication. The patient's breathing pattern during continuous nebulization has no influence on the length of the treatment (e.g., breathing slowly and performing an inspiratory hold at end-inspiration will have no bearing on duration). Such a breathing pattern will prolong treatment time if nebulization occurs only during inspiration (not during exhalation or during the inspiratory pause).

(1:694), (15:807–808).

## IB1a

25. B. Digital clubbing refers to the painless enlargement of the terminal phalanges of the fingers and toes that develops over years from a variety of pulmonary and nonpulmonary disorders. Digital clubbing is manifested as an alteration of the angle between the nail and the adjacent skin to 180° or more. The normal angle is 160°. Cardiac anomalies that produce cyanosis cause digital clubbing (e.g., coarctation of the aorta [preductal], tricuspid atresia, tetralogy of Fallot, truncus arteriosus, anomalous venous return, and transposition of the great vessels). Pulmonary disorders that usually cause digital clubbing include cystic fibrosis, bronchiectasis, interstitial fibrosis, bronchogenic carcinoma, and chronic bronchitis.

(1:317–318), (15:438, 672–673), (18:250–264).

## IIIA1b

26. B. Only neonates can have a perfect correlation between the $PtcO_2$ and the $PaO_2$. A neonate's skin is more conducive to the diffusion of oxygen; hence, the correlation between the $PtcO_2$ and $PaO_2$ can be 1 to 1. The quality of an adult's skin differs; consequently, the correlation between these two measurements depends on the patient's perfusion status (cardiac output) and fluid balance. A decreased cardiac output (hypoperfu-

sion) causes peripheral vasoconstriction and reduces capillary blood flow. Therefore, under such conditions the $PtcO_2$ falls below the $PaO_2$.

The patient in this question had a cardiac output of 2,250 ml/min. or 2.25 liters/min. (i.e., 45 ml/beat × 50 beats/min). Judgment concerning the correlation between the $PaO_2$ and $PtcO_2$ cannot be made solely on the cardiac output because the cardiac output varies with body size. The cardiac index (C.I.) relates the cardiac output to body surface area (BSA) as follows:

$$C.I. = \frac{C.O.}{BSA}$$

The normal range for the C.I. is 2.5 to 4.0 liters/min./m². Based on the data given here, this patient's cardiac index is

$$C.I. = \frac{2.25 \text{ liters/min.}}{2.25 \text{ m}^2}$$
$$= 1 \text{ liter/min./m}^2$$

This C.I. is well below the lower limit of normal for this measurement. Therefore, this patient is experiencing low perfusion.

The $PtcO_2$ falls below the $PaO_2$ as perfusion decreases. Hence, a $PaO_2$ of 90 torr and a $PtcO_2$ of 60 torr are consistent with such a physiologic situation.

(1:353-356), (9:227, 309-310), (10:102,104).

## IIIC3a

27. D. The T-piece or Briggs adapter enables trial periods of spontaneous ventilation. It acts as a weaning technique before the decision to extubate the patient and discontinue mechanical ventilatory support. The reservoir tubing serves to maintain a constant $FIO_2$. A flow meter setting of at least 10 L/min. and reservoir tubing of 120 cc can generally maintain an $FIO_2$ of 0.50 without much difficulty.

Another advantage of this system is that it is easily adaptable to reinstituting mechanical ventilatory support if the patient requires it. The system is free from all the effects of positive airway pressure, however. During these trials, the patient might experience hypoventilation, atelectasis, and increased intrapulmonary shunting. Consequently, an $FIO_2$ greater than that set on the mechanical ventilator should be provided by this mode of gas delivery. Other forms of weaning from mechanical ventilation include intermittent mandatory ventilation (IMV) and inspiratory pressure support ventilation.

(1:755, 976–977), (10:331–332), (15:1032).

## IIIC5

28. C. This patient is having difficulty deep breathing because of the pain associated with the recent thoracotomy. During the postoperative period, this patient should have been receiving aerosol therapy along with incentive spirometry and coughing instructions (splinting of the incision). CPT would also be a reasonable adjunct at this time.

Based on the situation presented in this question, the patient appears to have retained secretions, as evidenced by auscultation and chest X-ray findings. Therefore, the patient's condition warrants the implementation of therapeutic modalities directed toward bronchopulmonary hygiene. In this case, aerosol therapy followed by CPT (postural drainage and percussion), along with incentive spirometry should enhance the mobilization of secretions.

(1:799, 812–813), (15:790, 802–803, 844).

## IIIB1e

29. B. Capnometry can be used instead of observation and auscultation to determine whether an ET tube has been inserted into the trachea. A properly located ET tube results in measured end-tidal $CO_2$ levels of about 6.0%, which will vary, of course, with the phase of ventilation. A malplaced ET tube results in low or absent end-tidal $CO_2$ measurements because esophageal intubation leads to the stomach. Caution must be applied to the interpretation of a low end-tidal $CO_2$ reading, because in cardiac arrest situations, low perfusion might account for the low $PetCO_2$ readings and not a malplaced ET tube. Similarly, a large $V_D/V_T$ ratio, as in pulmonary embolism, can produce low $PetCO_2$ values.

("Guidelines 2000 Cardiopulmonary Resuscitation and Emergency Cardiovascular Care," page I–101), (15:500–501, 834–835).

## IIIA1m(2)

30. C. Capnography is a noninvasive method for the continuous measurement of the end-tidal carbon dioxide tension ($PetCO_2$) via infrared or mass spectrometry. The utility of measuring the ($PetCO_2$) is that under normal and stable cardiovascular conditions, it reflects the alveolar $CO_2$ tension and in turn the arterial $CO_2$ tension. The usual difference between the arterial $PCO_2$ and the $PetCO_2$ is less than 3 to 5 torr. This gradient widens as a result of the influence of a number of factors.

For example, a low C.O. causes less metabolically produced $CO_2$ to be delivered to the pulmonary circulation for gas exchange, thereby causing the arterial $PCO_2$ to become much greater than the $P_{ET}CO_2$. Ventilation-perfusion ($\dot{V}_A/\dot{Q}_C$) imbalances, likewise, produce an increased disparity between these two measurements. Similarly, an alveolar ventilation that is out of phase with the level of carbon dioxide production ($\dot{V}CO_2$) widens the arterial $PCO_2$-$P_{ET}CO_2$ gradient.

Some infants experience an increased arterial $PCO_2$ as a result of the added dead space of the $CO_2$ sensor. Tachypneic infants might breathe too rapidly for an accurate measurement to be made. Aside from being independent of tissue perfusion and displaying waveforms reflecting cardiopulmonary conditions, capnography is associated with a variety of technical difficulties.

(1:364–366, 933), (9:290), (10:101–102).

## IIID1b

31. D. Lidocaine (Xylocaine) is an antiarrhythmic medication administered I.V. to treat premature ventricular contractions (PVCs) and in some situations to control tachycardia. Digitalis is a cardiac glycoside that increases the strength of myocardial contraction (positive inotropism). It is useful for the treatment of congestive heart failure, certain atrial dysrhythmias, and ventricular tachycardia. Adenosine is indicated for the treatment of supraventricular tachycardia. Verapamil is a calcium channel blocker used to treat supraventricular tachycardia.

(14:405, 422–423, 692), (16:850, 853, 1032, 1135).

32. C. When one evaluates the cardiovascular system, the blood pressure is measured, the heart rate (pulse) is taken, and the peripheral perfusion status is determined. The perfusion status is assessed by (1) observing the patient's skin color (e.g., pink, ashen, and cyanosis), (2) noting skin texture or turgor, (3) checking capillary refill, (4) noting the patient's sensorium (level of consciousness), (5) measuring or observing the extent of urine output, (6) perceiving skin temperature, and (7) palpating peripheral pulses.

(1:302–305), (9:52–53, 58–65), (15:431–433).

## IIIA2a(1)

33. A. Mucomyst, or n-acetylcysteine, is a mucolytic agent and is available for nebulization in 10% and 20% concentrations. Conditions such as acute tracheobronchitis, COPD, and tuberculosis indicate its use.

Mucus consists of polypeptide and carbohydrate chains interlinked, creating highly viscous material. Mucomyst splits the sulfur-sulfur (disulfide) bonds, making mucus less viscous and more easily removed.

Mucomyst sometimes irritates the lining of the airways, however, causing bronchospasm. This side effect is more prevalent with asthmatics.

The bilateral wheezing heard by the RRT and the dyspnea expressed by the asthmatic patient in this question indicates the likelihood of bronchospasm. If Mucomyst must be given to an asthmatic, strong consideration should be given to nebulizing it concomitantly with a bronchodilator.

(1:579-580), (15:189), (16:442, 444).

## IIIA1l

34. B. The C.O. is a product of the stroke volume and the heart rate. It can be calculated according to the following steps:

STEP 1: Convert the stroke volume (SV) to liters.

$$SV = \frac{67 \text{ ml}}{1{,}000 \text{ ml/liter}}$$

$$= 0.067 \text{ liter}$$

STEP 2: Calculate the C.O.

$$C.O. = SV \times HR$$
$$= 0.067 \text{ L/beat} \times 88 \text{ beats/min.}$$
$$= 5.90 \text{ L/min.}$$

(1:949), (9:308), (10:118–119), (15:76, 530).

## IIB1c

35. A. A water-collection trap must be incorporated in all aerosol-delivery systems to help control the amount of condensation developing in the tubing system. Increased levels of condensate in the inspiratory line reduce the efficiency of the air-entrainment port of the nebulizer because back pressure can reduce the velocity of the source gas flow, causing less room air to be entrained. In order to function properly, the water-collection trap must be situated along the most gravity-dependent portion of the aerosol tubing. This location assures drainage of the condensate into the trap.

(1:671).

## IC2c

36. C. The PCWP has a normal range of 5 to 15 mm Hg. The most frequent cause of a decreased PCWP is hypovolemia. A $C(a-\bar{v})O_2$ greater than 5 vol%, combined with a normal body temperature, reflects a decreased cardiac output. The decreased cardiac output and the decreased PCWP indicate the patient has hypovolemia.

The minimally normal PAs and PAd are not consistent with left ventricular failure, hypervolemia, or mitral regurgitation. All the pulmonary artery pressures (PAs, PAd, PAP, and PCWP) become elevated when any of these conditions is present.

(1:943-949), (9:347-353).

37. B. Pressure support ventilation (PSV) can be applied in three clinical situations: (1) PSV can be used to help overcome the imposed WOB created by the resistance to airflow through the ET tube, as well as that developed by breathing through the ventilator circuit; (2) PSV can be used in conjunction with IMV and SIMV, reducing some of the workload placed on the muscles of ventilation; and (3) PSV can sometimes be used as a stand alone mode of ventilation referred to as maximum pressure support, or $PS_{max}$.

When PSV is used solely to overcome the imposed WOB, pressure-support levels of less than 20 cm $H_2O$ are usually used. When the pressure-support level is lowered to about 3 to 7 cm $H_2O$, extubation can generally be performed. When PSV is used with SIMV to facilitate the weaning process, the amount of pressure support to provide a tidal volume of 10 to 12 ml/kg is applied. PSV used in this manner requires the SIMV breaths to be gradually decreased to accomplish weaning. As a stand alone form of ventilation, the same tidal volume (i.e., 10 to 12 ml/kg) is sought. In this instance, however, backup controlled ventilation should be available should the patient fatigue or become apneic.

(1:864–877, 980), (10:85, 199, 214), (15:960–961).

38. C. Transtracheal oxygen therapy improves patient compliance (24 hours/day) as well as improves the cosmetic aspect of oxygen therapy. Following the transtracheal procedure, a stenting device is inserted for about one week. After that time, the stenting device is removed, and an operational SCOOP-1 catheter is inserted. The SCOOP-1 catheter remains in place for about 5 to 7 weeks to allow for epithelialization. Once the tract has epithelialized, the patient can remove the catheter for periodic cleaning.

SCOOP-1 catheters are used for patients who require 2 L/min. or less of oxygen. The SCOOP-2 transtracheal catheter provides for flow rates greater than 2 L/min. Generally, the transtracheal catheter cleaning protocol varies from two times per day to daily cleaning with the catheter in position. Removal of the catheter is usually performed every few weeks.

(13:72–73), (15:1166–1169).

39. C. A heated pneumatic nebulizer is capable of delivering 100% body humidity (44 mg $H_2O$/liter) plus a mist of moderate density. This setup can be useful in mobilizing secretions. The patient's $PaO_2$ here on 40% oxygen is 80 torr, which is adequate. One would probably not wish to increase or decrease the patient's $FiO_2$, however.

An unheated pneumatic jet nebulizer has a total water output of generally less than 44 mg $H_2O$/liter and would be of little value in adding water to the mucous blanket. Ultrasonic nebulizers and room humidifiers are rarely used in most hospitals today and would make the use of supplemental oxygen more difficult.

(1:693–694).

40. A. If an air leak is present in a three-bottle pleural drainage system, it will be leaking into the intrapleural space or into the drainage system. To differentiate between these two sources of air leaks, the RRT should momentarily clamp the chest drainage tube and observe the suction-control bottle at the same time. If the suction-control bottle continues to bubble, the leak is not associated with the drainage system; instead the problem is an air leak into the intrapleural space around the chest tube. In this situation, the physician must be summoned immediately.

(1:487–488), (9:264–268), (15:1092–1094).

41. C. Ideally, the left ventricular end-diastolic pressure (LVEDP) represents the volume of blood that is in the left ventricle immediately before systole. In other words, it reflects the left ventricular preload. The LVEDP also signifies the compliance of the left ventricle. Therefore, when the LVEDP is low, the pulmonary capillary wedge pressure (PCWP) is also generally low. The RRT must be aware that there are times when the PCWP does not accurately reflect left-ventricular preload, however. For example, when aortic regurgitation is present, the PCWP is less than the LVEDP. When the PAC balloon tip is in either Zone 1 or 2 or when mitral valve regurgitation is present, the PCWP is greater than the LVEDP. In myocardial hypertrophy, the PCWP equals the LVEDP.

(1:948–949), (9:357), (15:530–532).

42. A. If the sensor of either a galvanic cell or polarographic oxygen analyzer is located along the ventilator tubing at a point after the gas had been humidified, the measured $O_2$% will be less than the actual $O_2$ concentration. Because most of these types of oxygen analyzers are calibrated with dry gas, their sensors must be situated in gas circuits before the humidification devices. The formula that can be used to compare dry gas and saturated gas oxygen analysis is shown as follows:

$$\text{analyzed } O_2\% = \frac{P_B - P_{H_2O}}{P_B} FiO_2 \times 100$$

where

$P_B$ = barometric pressure (torr)
$P_{H_2O}$ = partial pressure of water vapor (torr)
$F_IO_2$ = fraction of inspired oxygen

(1:339), (6:263).

## IIIC7c

43. A. There is a degree of discrepancy among clinicians as to what ranges of negative pressure are appropriate for ET suctioning of adult, pediatric, and neonatal patients. Some clinicians advocate using $-120$ mm Hg to $-150$ mm Hg for adults, $-80$ mm Hg to $-120$ mm Hg for pediatric patients, and $-60$ mm Hg to $-80$ mm Hg for neonates. Others recommend $-100$ mm Hg to $-120$ mm Hg for adults, $-80$ mm Hg to $-100$ mm Hg for children, and $-60$ mm Hg to $-80$ mm Hg for infants. Still others suggest applying $-80$ mm Hg to $-120$ mm Hg for adults, $-60$ to $-80$ mm Hg for children, and $-40$ to $-60$ mm Hg for newborns.

Obviously, these proposed suction-pressure settings are only guidelines. Ultimately, the nature of the tracheobronchial secretions will dictate the pressure used. In this situation, $-110$ mm Hg for an adult patient is a suitable subatmospheric pressure to use during ET suctioning.

(1:616), (18:400).

## IIIA2a(1)

44. D. Subjective data or responses are not directly measurable. They can be explained by the patient, however. They consist of perceptions, feelings, pain, or discomfort. Nausea, dizziness, confusion, and distrust are examples of subjective data that might affect the patient's response to therapy. Although the subjective data or symptoms might not be directly evident, their presence can be inferred by observation of the patient's body language, facial expressions, tone of voice, and other outward signs. These perceptions are often discovered in the Review of Systems.

(1:300), (9:15–16, 17).

## IB10d

45. D. Myasthenia gravis is an autoimmune neuromuscular disease that generally afflicts women in their 20s to 40s and men in their 50s to 60s. Antibodies are formed against the acetylcholine receptors at the myoneural junction, thereby preventing the normal binding between the neurotransmitter acetylcholine and the receptors on the postsynaptic membrane. The consequence of this condition is a generalized weakness often starting with the muscles innervated by the cranial nerves, as well as the peripheral muscles. The paralysis can spread centrally and affect the muscles of ventilation, causing ventilatory failure.

It is important to frequently monitor the ventilatory mechanics of such patients to determine the need to intervene before the patient develops acute ventilatory failure. The point at which intervention should occur is established by the guideline, which states that spontaneous ventilation cannot be maintained when the FVC is less than 10 to 15 ml/kg and the MIP is less than $-20$ to $-25$ cm $H_2O$.

The patient presented here deteriorated over a four-hour period in terms of both of these ventilatory measurements. The FVC diminished from 3.5 liters, or 70 ml/kg, to 0.5 liter, or 10 ml/kg. These values are based on the following calculations:

STEP 1: $\dfrac{110 \text{ lbs (patient weight)}}{2.2 \text{ lbs/kg}} = 50 \text{ kg}$

STEP 2: 3.5 liters = 3,500 ml

STEP 3: $\dfrac{3,500 \text{ ml}}{50 \text{ kg}} = 70 \text{ ml/kg (5:20 P.M. FVC value)}$

STEP 4: 0.5 liter = 500 ml

STEP 5: $\dfrac{500 \text{ ml}}{50 \text{ kg}} = 10 \text{ ml/kg (8:25 P.M. FVC value)}$

Likewise, the MIP decreased in four hours from $-50$ cm $H_2O$ to $-20$ cm $H_2O$. This patient is experiencing impending ventilatory failure and requires ET intubation and mechanical ventilation.

(1:543–544), (15:230, 1066).

## IIIB4a

46. D. Auto-PEEP (inadvertent or undetectable PEEP) usually develops when insufficient time is provided for exhalation. Under such circumstances, the next breath begins before the previous breath is completed. The result is incomplete emptying of the lungs (in other words, air trapping or auto-PEEP).

Auto-PEEP can be reduced by a number of ways: (1) employing low-compliance ventilator tubing, (2) inserting a large-caliber ET tube, (3) increasing the inspiratory flow rate, (4) shortening the inspiratory time, (5) prolonging the expiratory time, (6) establishing a lower tidal volume, (7) setting a reduced ventilatory rate, and (8) instituting extrinsic PEEP.

(1:828, 880, 917, 951–953), (15:901–907), (9:286–287), (10:152, 153–154, 245–246).

## IIB1i(3)

47. B. The continuous-flow IMV system enables the spontaneously breathing patient to intersperse spontaneous breaths between mandatory positive pressure breaths delivered by the ventilator. A one-way valve positioned between the ventilator circuitry and the contin-

uous-flow (H) system prevents these two gas-delivery mechanisms from interfering with each other.

For example, between positive pressure breaths, the patient can obtain a tidal volume from the continuous-flow system by generating a negative pressure that is sufficient enough to open the one-way valve located at the T connector. When the one-way valve is open, gas flows into the inspiratory limb of the ventilator circuit to the patient's lungs. As soon as the ventilator delivers a mandatory breath, the one-way valve closes and the patient receives a preset tidal volume. With this arrangement, there are times when a spontaneous breath is in the process of being delivered and the mandatory breath cycles on. Under such circumstances, the patient receives a hyperinflated, or stacked, breath.

(1:861–862), (10:329–330), (15:1053).

## IIIC2

48.　D. In most instances when an MDI is available, it is preferred over a small-volume nebulizer. Despite that many patients improperly use MDIs, these devices are efficacious, easy to use, and more cost-effective than small-volume nebulizers. Each patient situation needs to be evaluated as to which device is more appropriate. A patient who is having an asthmatic attack is probably unable to properly use an MDI. Such a patient would have difficulty taking a slow inhalation from FRC to total lung capacity as well as performing a 4- to 10-second breath-hold maneuver. A patient who is suffering from severe COPD would be confronted with similar problems.

(1:688–699), (5:123–126), (15:813–814).

## IIIE2f

49.　A. Some asthmatic patients, especially those who have chronic, severe asthma, require long-term, systemically administered corticosteroids. Glucocorticoids are extremely useful in treating chronic severe asthma because they (1) inhibit phospholipase-A2 and arachidonic acid breakdown, (2) enhance the patient's responsiveness of beta-2 receptors to beta-2 agonists, (3) inhibit the release of certain inflammatory mediators, and (4) suppress IgE binding on cell surfaces.

Long-term use of glucocorticoids generally causes Cushing's syndrome, however. Therefore, these patients should be placed on alternate-day steroid therapy and/or prescribed steroid MDIs as soon as possible to lower the systemic steroid concentration.

Treatment with steroids via MDIs (e.g., beclomethasone [Vanceril], triamcinolone [Azmacort] and flunisolide [AeroBid]) can lead to thrush or oral candidiasis (fungal infection with *Candida albicans*), as a result of changing the normal respiratory flora. To avoid this occurrence, the patient should be instructed to use a spacer and to rinse and gargle his mouth after each MDI administration.

(1:454, 583), (15:185, 681), (16:488–490).

## IA1b

50.　B. The early clinical presentation of lung abscess resembles that of pneumonia: cough, pleuritic pain, leukocytosis (increased white blood cell count), fever, chills, and general malaise. The abscess often produces large amounts of foul-smelling (fetid), foul-tasting, blood-tinged sputum. The sputum produced in bronchiectasis generally is also foul-smelling and blood-tinged; however, it separates into three distinct layers upon settling. Weight loss and anorexia are usually associated with pulmonary neoplasms. Amphoric breath sounds are characteristic of cavitations associated with lung abscesses. Amphoric breath sounds resemble the sound produced as air is blown over the mouth of an empty pop bottle. These sounds occur when the cavitation is large and communicates with a bronchus. Chest wall movement might be normal or slightly reduced on the affected side, and the percussion note is usually dull.

(15:351–352), (16:197, 203, 285).

## IIID3

51.　C. Barometric (atmospheric) pressure decreases with increasing altitude. Likewise, the individual partial pressures that constitute the components of a gas mixture (e.g., atmospheric air) decrease with increasing altitude. The percentages of the constituent gases remain the same, however. This physical principle (Dalton's law of partial pressure) can have a major impact on an infant's oxygenation status. For example, if an infant who is being transported via a fixed-wing aircraft has a borderline arterial $PO_2$ at sea level, he might experience significant arterial desaturation resulting from a relatively small decrease in the alveolar $PO_2$ at an increased altitude. To avoid this potentially catastrophic circumstance, the aircraft can be flown at a lower altitude or the cabin pressure can be increased.

Additionally, Boyle's law plays an important role in aviation physiology. Boyle's law states that the gas pressure is inversely related to the gas volume when the mass and temperature of the gas are constant ($P_1V_1 = P_2V_2$). Consequently, as altitude increases (decreased pressure), the volume of any trapped (loculated) gas will increase. For example, if an infant has an untreated pneumothorax, the volume of air in the intrapleural space will expand at an increased altitude. To circumvent this potential problem, all air that can be reached should be evacuated via chest tubes and oro- or nasogastric tubes.

(16:251, 358).

52. B. Pathophysiologic disorders often distort the normal pulmonary artery catheter waveforms shown in Figure 6-13.

The pressures developed in the right ventricle can be reduced by the presence of necrotic tissue in the right ventricle, caused by a right-ventricular myocardial infarction. These right ventricular and pulmonary artery pressures might be so low that they resemble those in the right atrium, thereby causing the waveforms to appear as indistinguishable.

(1:947), (9:347), (10:122).

## IIIA1q(1)

53. A. The pulmonary artery, or Swan–Ganz, catheter is capable of monitoring (1) the cardiac output (C.O.), (2) the pulmonary artery pressure, (3) the central venous pressure (CVP), and (4) the pulmonary capillary wedge pressure (PCWP).

A number of other hemodynamic measurements can be calculated from the data derived from a Swan–Ganz catheter. These measurements include the cardiac index (C.I.), systemic vascular resistance (SVR), pulmonary vascular resistance (PVR), stroke index (SI), and intrapulmonary shunt fraction ($\dot{Q}_S/\dot{Q}_T$).

(1:946), (9:348), (10:122).

## IIB1h(2)

54. B. Liquid oxygen systems are used in the home for oxygen supplementation. Oxygen in the liquid state can be stored more efficiently and used more cost-effectively than tanks. Liquid systems do have certain drawbacks, however. One is that they operate at pressures below 50 psig (generally at 20 to 22 psig); thus, they are not capable of providing a sufficient pressure source to power ventilators. This patient would be better served with an electrically driven ventilator and with supplemental oxygen bled into the ventilator.

(1:1111, 1114–1115), (5:25), (13:22–24).

## IIB2c

55. A. Pressure-control ventilation (PCV) is a volume-variable mode of mechanical ventilation. During PCV, inspiration is time initiated. During inspiration, a pre-

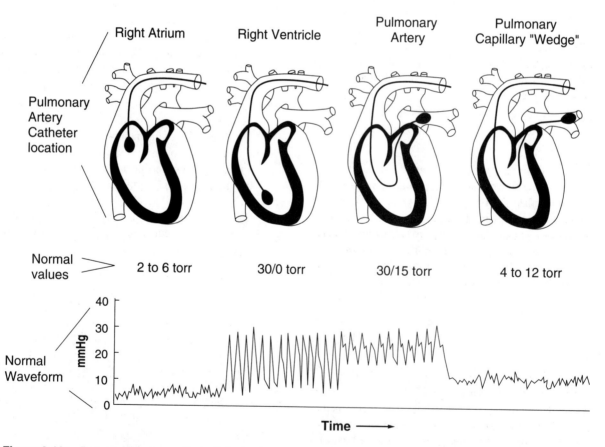

**Figure 6-13:** Pulmonary artery catheter location indicating corresponding normal values and normal waveforms.

set pressure is rapidly achieved and held constant throughout the inspiratory phase. This predetermined pressure is maintained by adjusting the ventilator's peak inspiratory flow rate. Inspiration terminates when a pre-established time elapses. The tidal volume during PCV is affected by the delivered pressure and patient's lung characteristics (i.e., pulmonary compliance and airway resistance). When the patient's lung characteristics are constant, increasing the PIP can accomplish increasing the delivered tidal volume.

(1:837, 875, 878), (10:198–199, 216).

## IIIB4b

56. A. During inverse-ratio ventilation, the inspiratory time equals or exceeds the expiratory time. When a patient has a severe decrease in lung compliance and hypoxemia that does not respond to high levels of $F_1O_2$ and PEEP, inverse-ratio ventilation frequently improves oxygenation. The improved oxygenation is often linked to an increased mean airway pressure. Patients who have ARDS are frequently ventilated with inverse-ratio ventilation for that specific purpose. Inverse-ratio ventilation is generally achieved through PCV and airway-pressure-release ventilation.

(1:518–519, 827, 876), (10:156, 199, 285–286).

## IB9d

57. A. The maximum expiratory pressure (MEP) maneuver is ordinarily performed in the pulmonary function laboratory instead of at the patient's bedside, because this measurement renders little useful information in the critical care setting. Diagnostically, however, it provides information concerning ventilatory muscle function.

To perform an MEP correctly, the patient must be instructed to exhale as forcefully as possible from total lung capacity. The patient forcefully exhales through a mouthpiece connected to a pressure gauge and a one-way valve system that permits the patient to inspire but prevents exhalation. The maneuver usually lasts five seconds.

(1:825), (6:52–53), (10:179–180), (15:555–556).

## IIID1b

58. C. The cardiac dysrhythmia displayed represents premature ventricular contractions (PVCs). PVCs arise in the ventricles and are followed by a compensatory pause. PVCs can range from innocuous in normal persons to life threatening when they cause the cardiac pattern to deteriorate to ventricular tachycardia. Lido-

caine can be administered via the ET tube to depress ventricular electrical activity. Lidocaine is an anti-dysrhythmic medication that can be administered either I.V. or endotracheally.

When lidocaine (actually any medication) is instilled through the ET tube, it is given at 2.0 to 2.5 times the recommended I.V. drug dose. It should also be diluted in 10 ml of either normal saline or distilled water. Cardiac compressions are momentarily terminated to allow the rapid insertion of a catheter projecting beyond the tip of the ET tube so that the lidocaine can be quickly sprayed into the tracheobronchial tree. It is also recommended that two or three rapid insufflations with the manual resuscitator be applied immediately following the instillation of the drug. Cardiac compressions are again withheld at this time.

("Guidelines 2000 Cardiopulmonary Resuscitation and Emergency Cardiovascular Care," pages I–114).

## IIIB1b

59. B. Generally, a condensing humidifier or a heat–moisture exchanger (HME) is not recommended for patients who have excessive secretions. COPD patients frequently produce copious amounts of secretions. Therefore, some other form of humidification is recommended. If an HME must be used, however, it is critical for close observation of the airway status to take place to avoid the disaster of airway obstruction. Other conditions that might contraindicate the use of a condensing humidifier include patients who have low tidal volumes and patients who have large airway leaks.

(1:697, 903), (10:209, 228), (13:123–124, 130).

## IIIE1k

60. D. The modified Allen's test is performed to assess the adequacy of collateral circulation to the hand. Specifically, the modified Allen's test assesses the presence of ulnar circulation. This assessment must be conducted before cannulation of the radial artery is attempted.

A modified Allen's test is performed by (1) instructing the patient to clench his fist while pressure is applied to the radial and ulnar arteries, (2) opening the hand (fist) to note the blanched nature of the palm and hand, and (2) removing the pressure applied to the ulnar artery. When the pressure applied to the ulnar artery is removed, either the hand will return to its normal pink color (positive Allen's test) or it will remain blanched (negative Allen's test). Therefore, a positive Allen's test indicates that the ulnar arterial blood supply to the hand is adequate. In such circumstances, an arterial catheter can be placed in that hand. Other methods for evaluating collateral circulation include using a Doppler flow probe and the finger pulse transducer.

(4:12–14), (9:121).

## IIIC3a

61. C. This patient's peak inspiratory flow rate (50 L/min.) is exceeding the output of the all-purpose nebulizer. The all-purpose nebulizer set at 40% oxygen with a 10 L/min. flow rate is able to provide only 40 L/min. of total flow. This total flow is based on the fact that an $F_IO_2$ of 0.40 has an air:$O_2$ ratio of 3:1.

If the $F_IO_2$ is increased to 0.60, the total flow rate received by the patient will be grossly inadequate. The air:$O_2$ ratio for 60% oxygen is 1:1. Therefore, the patient would receive only 10 L/min. of air and 10 L/min. of oxygen, or a total flow rate of only 20 L/min. This flow rate would be half of what the patient was originally receiving.

Maintaining the setting on the all-purpose nebulizer at 40% oxygen and increasing the source flow rate to 12 L/min. would still render an inadequate flow rate to the patient. The 3:1 air:$O_2$ ratio for 40% oxygen would result in 36 L/min. of air and 12 L/min. of oxygen (48 L/min. delivered flow). That total flow still falls short of the patient's own 50 L/min. inspiratory flow rate.

Instituting 5 cm $H_2O$ of mask CPAP at an $F_IO_2$ of 0.60 might correct this patient's hypoxemia. This level of therapeutic intervention might not be necessary at this time, however. Consider the fact that the initial setup, intended to correct the hypoxemia, was not adjusted properly to meet this patient's inspiratory needs. As long as the patient is not in any immediate danger, an effort should be made to correct the system in place to deliver the proper flow rate.

A tandem arrangement of two all-purpose nebulizers each set to deliver an $F_IO_2$ of 0.40 at 10 to 15 L/min. would provide a total flow rate in excess of the patient's inspiratory demands. Each nebulizer at 10 L/min. would render 40 L/min. The sum flow rate delivered by the two nebulizers in tandem would be 80 L/min. If this apparatus does not ameliorate the patient's hypoxemia, the patient might be evaluated for CPAP.

(15:879, 882–883).

## IB7e

62. C. Pulmonary edema results from either high pulmonary intravascular pressures (high-pressure or cardiogenic pulmonary edema) or a loss of integrity of the pulmonary vasculature (permeability or noncardiogenic pulmonary edema). High-pressure pulmonary edema is generally associated with an enlarged heart, indicating left ventricular failure. As the left ventricle fails, it is unable to maintain a C.O. matching that of the right ventricle. Consequently, the pulmonary vas-

culature becomes engorged with blood and the pulmonary vascular pressures elevate. As pulmonary capillary hydrostatic approaches the level of the oncotic pressure (colloid osmotic pressure), peribronchial cuffing occurs. Peribronchial cuffing represents an apparent thickening of the bronchial walls. This condition is usually best observed in the larger perihilar bronchi.

In the presence of a deteriorating left ventricle and increasing pulmonary intravascular pressures, more vascular fluid enters the pulmonary interstitium, causing the margins of the pulmonary vessels to become obscured. These events, in the presence of cardiomegaly, indicate a worsening of high-pressure (cardiogenic) pulmonary edema. Other radiographic signs of pulmonary edema include interstitial and alveolar infiltrates and Kerley B lines.

(1:508, 512, 513–514, 904), (15:606–607).

## IIID1b

63. B. Ventricular tachycardia is characterized by a ventricular rate of 140 to 300 beats/min. The P waves, which represent atrial contraction (depolarization), are masked by the numerous QRS complexes, which are widened and irregular. Ventricular tachycardia is frequently caused by a myocardial infarction. Treatment of this dysrhythmia usually includes an antidysrhythmic medication (e.g., lidocaine and procainamide). Defibrillation is often used to attempt to convert this dysrhythmia to a normal sinus rhythm. Synchronized cardioversion in ventricular tachycardia might be difficult to achieve because of the form of this dysrhythmia. A patient who displays ventricular tachycardia and is pulseless, unconscious, hypotensive, or in pulmonary edema should receive unsynchronized shocks (defibrillation) to avoid the delay associated with attempts to synchronize.

The first electrocardiogram (ECG) illustrated represents premature ventricular contractions (PVCs). PVCs can develop during a normal sinus rhythm, sinus bradycardia, or sinus tachycardia. PVCs originate in the ventricles. After a PVC occurs, a compensatory pause ensues before a normal P wave develops. Myocardial ischemia and myocardial irritability are believed to influence the onset of PVCs. Frequently occurring PVCs can cause ventricular fibrillation to develop.

The third (Roman numeral III) ECG depicts atrial fibrillation. This dysrhythmia is characterized by an atrial rate of 350 to 450 beats/min. No P waves can be perceived, and an undulating (wavy) baseline appears. Normal QRS complexes appear irregularly depending on conduction time through the atrioventricular node. The C.O. is compromised because the atria do not adequately fill the ventricles. Digitalis and cardioversion are often used to treat atrial fibrillation.

The fourth (Roman numeral IV) abnormal ECG pattern presented reflects premature atrial contractions (PACs). The rate is generally normal or increased. An ectopic focus causes the PACs. The ectopic focus originates in the atria. Factors such as smoking, alcohol ingestion, anxiety, or excitement can trigger this dysrhythmia.

(16:140–143), ("Guidelines 2000 Cardiopulmonary Resuscitation and Emergency Cardiovascular Care," pages I–158 to I–165).

## IA1h

64.  C. An Apgar score is comprised of the ratings of five components used to evaluate newborns at one minute and five minutes after birth. The Apgar scoring criteria are listed in Table 6-6.

Based on the characteristics of this infant, a one-minute Apgar score of 5 was recorded.

The following actions are warranted for the corresponding one-minute Apgar scores:

$\leq$ 2: severely depressed infant requiring immediate resuscitation
3-6: some stimulation and oxygen needed
$\geq$ 7: stable infant requiring monitoring only

(10:215), (18:43–44).

## IIB1q(1)

65.  A. The lungs are divided into three vertical zones based on the relationship among the pulmonary artery pressure (Pa), the alveolar pressure ($P_A$), and the pulmonary venous pressure (Pv), as illustrated Figure 6-14 on page 392. Ordinarily, the pulmonary artery catheter tip "floats" into Zone 3 during insertion because the blood flow to Zone 3 is greater than in Zones 1 or 2. If the catheter tip ends up in Zone 1 or 2, the pulmonary capillary wedge pressure (PCWP) will be greater than the left ventricular end-diastolic pressure (LVEDP).

Certain clinical situations can influence the extent (size) of Zone 3. In other words, certain interventions can reduce the vertical dimension of Zone 3, making insertion of the catheter tip into that zone difficult.

Two such interventions are PEEP and diuretic therapy. High levels of PEEP tend to reduce the area of Zone 3 by increasing the alveolar pressure above the pulmonary venous pressure, lessening the ver-tical flow of blood. Areas in the lung where this situation occurs become Zone 2. Similarly, diuresis reduces fluid volume, and if extensive enough, it can reduce the area of Zone 3 and convert portions of it to Zone 2. Likewise, a decreased venous return can result in a reduced height of the vertical dimension of Zone 3. Therefore, impaired venous return can also influence the placement of a pulmonary artery catheter. Ordinarily, when the pulmonary artery catheter is inserted, its tip enters Zone 3 where the pulmonary artery pressure exceeds the pulmonary venous pressure, which in turn is greater than the alveolar pressure. Therefore, the pulmonary wedge pressure taken in Zone 3 will reflect the left ventricular end-diastolic pressure (LVEDP).

(1:948), (9:350–351), (15:531–533).

## IIIB2d

66.  D. Independent lung ventilation has been used primarily for major bronchopleural leak. Although the actual flow rate through the leak can and should be measured with high-frequency jet ventilation, the least complicated approach to determine optimal ventilator settings for the affected lung during conventional ventilation is to measure the difference between inspiratory and expiratory volumes (as long as no other leak is present).

(1:829), (15:736, 1090–1091).

## IC1c

67.  D. The Enghoff modified Bohr equation is used to determine the dead space–tidal volume ($V_D/V_T$) ratio. When the dissolved arterial carbon dioxide tension ($PaCO_2$) and the mean exhaled carbon dioxide tension ($P_{\overline{E}}CO_2$) are given, the ($V_D/V_T$) can be calculated as follows:

**Table 6-6** APGAR Score

| Category | 0 Points | 1 Point | 2 Points |
|---|---|---|---|
| | | Score | |
| heart rate | absent | < 100 bpm | > 100 bpm |
| respiratory effort | absent | irregular, weak, gasping | crying, rigorous breathing |
| muscle tone | flaccid | some flexion of extremities | active flexion of extremities, good motion, resistance to extension |
| reflex irritability | unresponsive | frowns or grimaces when stimulated | active movement, crying, coughing or sneezing |
| skin color | totally cyanotic, pale, or gray | acrocyanosis, i.e., hands and feet cyanotic with a pink body | completely pink |

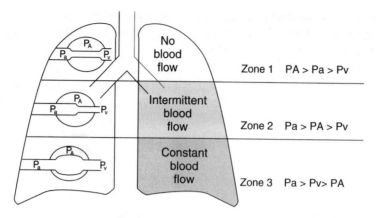

**Figure 6-14:** Pulmonary vascular blood flow zones ($P_A$ = intra-alveolar pressure, $P_a$ = pulmonary arterial pressure, and $P_v$ = pulmonary venous pressure).

$$\frac{V_D}{V_T} = \frac{PaCO_2 - P\overline{E}CO_2}{PaCO_2}$$

$$\frac{V_D}{V_T} = \frac{40 \text{ torr} - 28 \text{ torr}}{40 \text{ torr}}$$

$$\frac{V_D}{V_T} = \frac{12 \text{ torr}}{40 \text{ torr}}$$

$$\frac{V_D}{V_T} = 0.30$$

(1:927, 935), (10:434), (17:25–29).

**IIIA1m(1)**

68. B. The stroke volume can be calculated by rearranging the following formula:

$$C.O. = SV \times HR$$

Solving for the stroke volume, the equation becomes the following

$$SV = \frac{C.O.}{HR}$$

$$= \frac{3.5 \text{ L/min.}}{105 \text{ beats/min.}}$$

$$= 0.033 \text{ L/beat}$$

or

$$= 33 \text{ ml/beat}$$

The normal range for stroke volume is 50 to 80 ml/beat.

The other hemodynamic measurements are not decreased by this condition. A myocardial infarction frequently reduces the left ventricle's ability to contract. Blood will back up in the pulmonary vasculature and influence the given factors as follows. The pulmonary vascular resistance will either increase or remain the same. It depends on how much blood backs into the pulmonary vasculature. The capillary osmotic pressure actually increases a bit because of the fluid that leaves the vasculature and enters the pulmonary interstitium. The PCWP and LVEDP are also elevated. The stroke volume is low because the left ventricle has lost contractile myocardial tissue. Therefore, the amount of blood ejected from that chamber is reduced.

(1:949), (9:313–314), (16:862, 1134).

**IIIE1h**

69. C. Synchronized cardioversion is the delivery of a countershock in phase with the QRS complex (ventricular depolarization) on the ECG pattern. In the synchronized mode, the capacitors discharge when the defibrillator/monitor "seeks" the R wave of the QRS complex. The electric shock is delivered a few milliseconds following the apex of the R wave.

Synchronized cardioversion must only be performed when the tachycardia associated with the dysrhythmia is 150 to 160 beats/min. or less. Otherwise, the defibrillator/monitor might not be capable of discriminating between an R wave and a T wave (ventricular repolarization). Discharge of the shock during a T wave can result in ventricular fibrillation. Therefore, synchronized cardioversion is indicated for dysrhythmias such as supraventricular tachycardia, atrial flutter, and atrial fibrillation because these abnormal ECG patterns generally have discernable R waves and QRS complexes and have a rate of 150 to 160 beats/min. or less.

("Guidelines 2000 Cardiopulmonary Resuscitation and Emergency Cardiovascular Care," pages I–92 to I–93).

**IIA1h(4)**

70. C. Four different wavelengths of light are used in a co-oximeter to obtain the absorbance pattern of the following four types of hemoglobin: (1) deoxyhemoglobin, (2) oxyhemoglobin, (3) methemoglobin, and

(4) carboxyhemoglobin. Sulfhemoglobin cannot be measured by a co-oximeter. The wavelength for sulfhemoglobin is similar to that for methemoglobin, however. Therefore, the absorbance pattern for these two types of hemoglobin will be similar. Consequently, sulfhemoglobin levels in the blood can cause incorrect methemoglobin readings.

(1:348, 358), (9:296), (10:97).

## IIIC5

71. B. The objective of chest physiotherapy (CPT) is the removal of tracheobronchial secretions. Atelectasis can be relieved by the removal of secretions. At the same time, better aeration of the affected lung regions can be accomplished. Drainage of the lower lobes is best accomplished with the patient in the Trendelenburg (head-down) position.

Percussion should be avoided directly over incisions, chest tubes, and catheters. The patient should be placed in an upright position following postural drainage, percussion, and vibration and then encouraged to cough. If coughing occurs while the patient is prone or in the Trendelenburg position, she should immediately be placed in an upright position to avoid the development of excessive intracranial pressure.

(1:801–802), (16:44, 506–507, 509–516, 521).

## IIIE1i

72. B. Capnography is sometimes used during ET intubation to help determine placement of the tube in the trachea. Up to the time the ET tube enters the trachea, the capnograph will display a readout of near 0.0% $CO_2$. Once the tube is inserted into the trachea, however, the display will indicate an abrupt rise in the exhaled $CO_2$ from 0.0% to around 5.6%. This abrupt rise in the $CO_2$ concentration results from the metabolically produced $CO_2$ leaving the lungs through the ET tube. If the ET tube enters the esophagus, the $CO_2$% will remain around 0.0%. Auscultation of the thorax and chest radiography should also be used to confirm ET tube placement.

(1:598), (15:500).

## IIID1c

73. A. If PPV does not maintain a heart rate at 60 beats/min. or higher, external cardiac compressions must be initiated. If the heart rate remains under 80 beats/min. after 30 seconds of compressions and PPV, intubation should be performed and the appropriate medications should be administered. If the heart rate is rising and exceeds 80 beats/min., cardiac compressions must be discontinued and PPV must be maintained.

(1:1015), (18:158-162, 416-426).

## IIIA1g

74. D. The formula for calculating oxygen content is as follows:

$$CaO_2 = Hb \times 1.34 \times \frac{SaO_2}{100} + 0.003 \times PaO_2$$

where

$CaO_2$ = arterial oxygen content (vol%)
  $Hb$ = hemoglobin concentration (g% or g/dl)
$SaO_2$ = arterial oxygen saturation (%)
$PaO_2$ = partial pressure of oxygen in arterial blood (torr)
 1.34 = ml of $O_2$/g of hemoglobin
0.003 = conversion factor (vol%/torr)

The majority of a person's oxygen is carried bound to hemoglobin. In this example, an arterial saturation of 98%, a hemoglobin of 15 g%, and a $PaO_2$ of 100 torr will result in an arterial content of 20 vol% (Figure 6-15). Approximately 98.5% of this oxygen is carried by the hemoglobin, whereas only 1.5% is physically dissolved in the plasma.

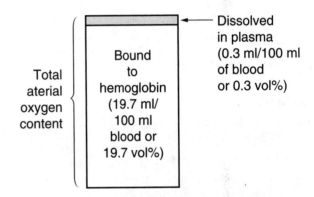

**Figure 6-15:** Comparison of oxygen dissolved in the plasma with oxygen bound to hemoglobin.

Because this patient was involved in a motor vehicle accident and sustained multiple injuries, her hemoglobin is probably quite low. Even if her $PaO_2$ were within acceptable limits, a low hemoglobin concentration would result in an inadequate oxygen content. This situation leads to tissue hypoxia if the C.O. was unable to compensate for the drop in oxygen content. Recall that there are four causes of hypoxia: (a) hypoxemic (low arterial content), (b) anemic (inadequate amounts of functional hemoglobin), (c) circulatory or stagnant (poor C.O.), and (d) histotoxic (cyanide poisoning).

The relationship among the cardiac output ($\dot{Q}_T$), arterial oxygen content ($CaO_2$), and oxgyen delivery ($Do_2$) is summarized by the following equation:

$$oxygen\ delivery = CaO_2 \times \dot{Q}_T$$

As long as the C.O. is able to increase to offset any decrease in the arterial oxygen content, the oxygen delivery will remain constant. If not, inadequate delivery will occur with a resulting lactic acidosis.

Assuming a constant heart rate, C.O. might fall because of decreases in stroke volume. Stroke volume might fall because of a low preload (secondary to bleeding), a high afterload (hypertension and/or a stenosis of semilunar valves), and/or low contractility (poor myocardial performance). Naturally, the heart will beat faster if the stroke volume starts to fall. Especially in the elderly, however, increasing heart rate further exacerbates the problem.

(1:886), (9:293, 296).

## IIIC3a

75. A. The patient in this situation appears to have experienced swelling of retained secretions as a result of the aerosol therapy. The loud gurgling sounds audible during inspiration and exhalation were produced by the secretions in this patient's large airways. This patient was apparently so overwhelmed by them that she began choking.

Once her airways were cleared by the aggressive ET suctioning, her respiratory distress abated and her arterial saturation returned to normal. The fact that coarse crackles were recognized via auscultation indicates that secretion buildup might continue to be a problem. This patient likely does not require particulate water in her airway, however, perhaps leading again to another airway obstruction crisis. Therefore, at this time humidity therapy should be instituted to reduce the amount of water deposited in the airway and still prevent respiratory mucosal drying. This patient should then be more closely monitored.

(15:819–820).

## IIB1h(4)

76. A. Trending, as shown in Figure 6-16, represents a systematic error, which in turn is the repeated movement away from the mean. Trending is the progressive increase or decrease in the deviation from the mean.

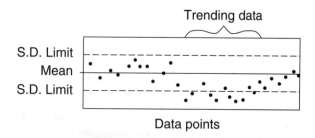

Figure 6-16: Analyzed data demonstrating trending (gradual movement of analyzed results away from the mean).

Conditions related to blood gas analyzer electrodes that can cause trending include (1) protein contamination, (2) electrode aging, and (3) mercury battery aging. Another type of systematic error is shifting. Shifting occurs when there is a sudden shift or change in measurements followed by data plateauing or clustering. Data shifting is illustrated in Figure 6-17.

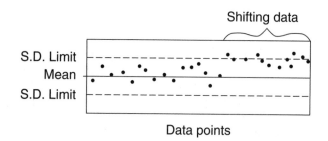

Figure 6-17: Analyzed data illustrating a shift outside the acceptable standard deviation (SD) limit (rapid movement of analyzed results away from the mean).

Conditions that can cause shifting include (1) temperature changes in calibration standards, (2) contamination of calibration standards, and (3) air bubbles under the membrane.

(4:47–49), (13:238).

## IIID1b

77. C. When sodium bicarbonate ($NaHCO_3$) is to be administered during CPR, the initial dose should be 1 mEq/kg. Then, for every 10 minutes thereafter, one-half the initial dose should be given. Therefore, because this patient weighs 75 kg, initially he should receive a dose of 75 mEq followed in 10-minute intervals by doses of 37.5 mEq.

("Guidelines 2000 Cardiopulmonary Resuscitation and Emergency Cardiovascular Care," pages I–133 to I–134).

## IIIC6a

78. D. Although a useful humidification device when indicated, a heat–moisture exchanger (HME) is contraindicated for patients who have excessive secretion production (e.g., COPD and cystic fibrosis patients) and for patients who receive most of their minute ventilation spontaneously. In this situation, the patient needed ET suctioning immediately, indicated by the gurgling and auscultation findings. The problem was not completely rectified, however.

This patient, who has severe COPD, is prone to excessive bronchopulmonary secretion production. Such a condition contraindicates the use of an HME because the secretions increase the resistance through the device as well as pose a threat of complete airway obstruction.

In the problem presented here, the accumulation of mucus in the HME likely elevated the resistance across the hygroscopic material in the device, producing high inspiratory pressures. Therefore, the HME must be replaced by a cascade or wick humidifier, which can generally accommodate high flow rates.

(1:697, 903), (10:209, 228), (13:123–124, 130), (15:798–799).

**IA1c**

79. B. An extremely small volume of fluid resides between the visceral and parietal pleurae, acting as a lubricant as the lungs fill and empty within the thoracic cavity. This fluid results from the transudation of fluid from the pleural capillaries. This movement of fluid is governed by the relationship among the Starling factors, such as capillary hydrostatic pressure and oncotic pressure. In the course of various pathophysiologic processes, abnormal amounts of fluid accumulate in the intrapleural space. The nature of this fluid depends on the pathophysiology present. Two broad classifications of fluid exist: transudate and exudate. Table 6-7 outlines the characteristics of these two categories of intrapleural fluid.

Clinical conditions often associated with a transudative process include congestive heart failure, hypoproteinemia, and fluid overload. Exudates are frequently caused by venous thromboembolism, ARDS, tuberculosis, pneumonia, and pulmonary neoplasm.

In addition to these two general classifications, some pleural effusions are named according to the specific nature of the fluid. For example, frank bleeding into the intrapleural space produces a hemothorax. Pure chyle accumulating in the intrapleural space results in a chylothorax. The end stage of a progressive inflammatory, exudative process often manifests itself as pus in the intrapleural space. The term *empyema,* or *pyothorax,* describes this condition.

(1:478–480), (15:51–53).

**IIIA1m(1)**

80. A.

STEP 1: Use the clinical shunt equation.

$$\frac{\dot{Q}_S}{\dot{Q}_T} = \frac{(P_AO_2 - P_aO_2)0.003 \text{ vol\%/torr}}{(P_AO_2 - P_aO_2)0.003 + (C_aO_2 - C\bar{v}O_2)} \times 100$$

STEP 2: Calculate the arterial $O_2$ content.

$C_aO_2$ = dissolved arterial $O_2$ + combined arterial $O_2$

= (150 torr × 0.003 vol%/torr) +

(1.00 × 15 g% Hb × 1.34)

= 20.55 vol%

STEP 3: Calculate the venous $O_2$ content.

$C\bar{v}O_2$ = dissolved venous $O_2$ + combined venous $O_2$

= (30 torr × 0.003 vol%/torr) +

(0.75 × 15 g% Hb × 1.34)

= 15.17 vol%

STEP 4: Use the alveolar air equation to compute the $P_AO_2$.

$$P_AO_2 = (P_B - P_{H_2O})F_IO_2 - P_ACO_2{}^* \left( F_IO_2 + \frac{1 + F_IO_2}{R} \right)$$

Because R = 1.0,

$$\left( F_IO_2 + \frac{1 - F_IO_2}{R} \right) = \left( 0.6 + \frac{1 - 0.6}{1} \right) = 1.0$$

*The $P_aCO_2$ can substitute for the $P_ACO_2$ in the alveolar air equation because equilibration across the alveolar-capillary membrane is assumed.

Therefore,

$P_AO_2$ = (760 torr − 47 torr)0.6 − 40 torr(1.0) = 388 torr

$$\frac{\dot{Q}_S}{\dot{Q}_T} = \frac{(388 \text{ torr} - 150 \text{ torr})0.003}{(388 \text{ torr} - 150 \text{ torr})0.003 - (20.55 \text{ vol\%} - 15.17 \text{ vol\%})} \times 100$$

$$\frac{\dot{Q}_S}{\dot{Q}_T} = 11.72\%$$

STEP 5: Insert the values into the clinical shunt equation.

**Table 6-7** Intrapleural Fluid Analysis

| Transudate | Exudate |
|---|---|
| • thin | • viscous |
| • clear | • translucent |
| • protein concentration < 3% | • protein concentration > 3% |
| • specific gravity < 1.015 | • specific gravity > 1.015 |
| • does not clot upon standing | • might clot upon standing |
| • very few cells (mainly lymphocytes) | • polymorphonuclear leukocytes (PMNs)/lymphocytes |
| • no microorganisms cultured | • microorganisms might be cultured |

Alternatively, the following classic shunt equation can be used:

$$\frac{\dot{Q}_S}{\dot{Q}_T} = \frac{C\acute{c}O_2 - CaO_2}{C\acute{c}O_2 - C\bar{v}O_2} \times 100$$

where

$\dot{Q}_S$ = that portion of the C.O. that does not exchange with alveolar air (L/min.)

$\dot{Q}_T$ = total C.O. (L/min.)

$C\acute{c}O_2$ = total end-pulmonary capillary oxygen content (vol%)

$CaO_2$ = total arterial oxygen content (vol%)

$C\bar{v}O_2$ = total venous oxygen content (vol%)

(1:930), (9:295), (15:487–488).

### IIIE1j

81. B. Once a pneumothorax on a mechanically ventilated patient is identified, the air must be evacuated from the intrapleural space as soon as possible. The appropriate intervention for a large-volume pneumothorax is to have a tube thoracostomy performed so that the chest tubes can drain the air from the intrapleural space. If the pneumothorax were small, insertion of chest tubes might still be considered in view of the fact that the pa-tient is receiving positive pressure ventilation, which could worsen the situation at any moment. Needle aspiration of a pneumothorax is not uncommon if the volume of air is small and if the patient is spontaneously breathing without the support of positive pressure.

In the situation presented here, chest tubes would be placed along either the mid-axillary or posterior axillary lines between the sixth or seventh interspace on the right side.

(1:145, 482, 487–489).

### IIB1i(3)

82. C. When a patient is receiving IMV, the ventilator's sensitivity control is generally turned off, thereby preventing the ventilator from cycling on when the patient generates a negative pressure to obtain a spontaneous breath. A −10 cm $H_2O$ is definitely too great an effort for a patient. It will certainly increase her WOB greatly. Conditions that can cause this inordinately large negative pressure to be generated include a malfunctioning demand valve and an inadequate gas flow rate in the spontaneous breathing circuit. Figure 6-18 illustrates a demand-flow IMV system.

(1:850, 861–863, 874), (10:164, 197–198, 199, 246, 329).

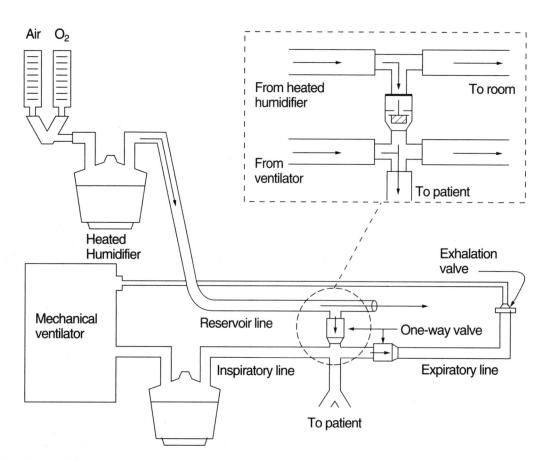

**Figure 6-18:** Demand-flow IMV.

### IIIC3a

83. C. A simple oxygen mask must operate at a minimum flow rate of 6 L/min. to ensure that the patient's expirate is flushed out of the mask. A flow rate of 4 L/min. is too low; it increases the likelihood that the patient will inhale a portion of her own exhaled gas, placing the patient at risk for developing hypercapnia. The RRT needs to increase the flow rate to at least 6 L/min. and then check the physician's order to determine the prescribed flow rate. He then needs to readjust the flow rate if the liter flow was ordered at more than 6 L/min.

(1:749–750), (5:71), (13:73).

### IIIE1e

84. B. Pulmonary stress testing is done for a number of reasons. One reason is to evaluate a subject for disability and impairment. One of the guides for evaluation of respiratory impairment was developed by Engelberg. These guides are published by the American Medical Association as *Guides to the Evaluation of Permanent Impairment.* The range of results are listed in Table 6-8.

When the RRT views the chart and the results noted above, he will see that this patient is in the category of mild impairment.

(Engelberg, A.L., *Guides to the Evaluation of Permanent Impairment,* 3rd ed., American Medical Association, Chicago, 1988, pp. 107–144), (15: 522).

### IIIA1h

85. C. During PC-IRV, a rapid insufflation with a decelerating flow pattern maintains a preset pressure throughout inspiration. The ventilatory rate is established based on the flow pattern. When the expiratory flow is about to reach the baseline, the inspiratory flow is set to cycle on. The ventilatory rate that interrupts the terminal expiratory flow just before it reaches zero becomes the established rate.

Preventing exhalation from going to completion causes auto-PEEP. Hence, PC-IRV is not generally recommended for patients who have dynamic airflow limitation. Patients who have dynamic airflow limitation include those who have COPD or asthma.

(1:518–519, 827, 876), (10:156, 199, 286–287).

### IIIB1c

86. A. Continuous positive airway pressure (CPAP) is generally discontinued when the patient can support his own breathing without fatiguing on a CPAP level of about 2 cm $H_2O$ with an $FIO_2$ of less than 0.40. The ABG and acid-base data here certainly reveal normal acid-base status and sufficient oxygenation:

$PaO_2$ 80 torr
$PaCO_2$ 41 torr
pH 7.39
$HCO_3^-$ 24 mEq/liter

Because the general guidelines for CPAP removal are met in this case, extubation is warranted. The neonate should be placed in an oxyhood with an $FIO_2$ of less than or equal to 0.30 after CPAP removal and extubation.

(10:285), (18:299–300).

### IIB2a(2)

87. C. A Briggs adaptor or a T-piece is used to deliver more precise oxygen concentrations to certain intubated patients. When this device is used, the mist exiting the distal opening of the T-piece must be visible throughout the entire ventilatory cycle. If the mist disappears

**Table 6-8** Classes of Respiratory Impairment

|  | Class 1 | Class 2 | Class 3 | Class 4 |
|---|---|---|---|---|
|  | 0%<br>No Impairment<br>of the Whole Person | 10–25%<br>Mild Impairment<br>of the Whole Person | 30–45%<br>Moderate Impairment<br>of the Whole Person | 50–100%<br>Severe Impairment<br>of the Whole Person |
| FVC | ≥ 80% | 60–79% | 51–59% | ≤ 50% |
|  | and | or | or | or |
| FEV$_1$ | ≥ 80% | 60–79% | 41–59% | ≤ 40% |
|  | and | or | or | or |
| FEV$_1$/FVC | ≥ 70% | 60–69% | 41–59% | ≤ 40% |
|  | and | or | or | or |
| D$_L$CO | ≥ 80% | 60–79% | 41–59% | ≤ 40% |
| or | or | or | or | or |
| $\dot{V}O_2$max | > 25 mL/kg/min. | 20–25 mL/kg/min. | 15–20 mL/kg/min. | < 15 mL/kg/min. |

* Percentages equal percent of predicted. (From Engelberg,[9] with permission)

during inspiration, the likelihood exists that the patient is rebreathing his own exhaled gas and/or the $F_{I}O_2$ received by the patient is less than that intended. To correct this situation, the RRT needs to increase the flow rate of the source gas.

(1:755–756), (13:77–78), (15:885–887).

## IIB1q(1)

88. C. To ensure accurate and consistant readings from a pressure transducer used to measure central venous pressure (CVP) levels (usually from the proximal port on a pulmonary artery catheter), the pressure transducer should be placed even with the patient's mid-axillary level. Although the precise location of the catheter tip is not precisely known, it is assumed to be in the mid-chest position at the junction of the superior vena cava and the right atrium. Any number of methods can be used to estimate this level.

- Place a mark on the patient's lateral chest wall that is midway between the anterior and posterior thorax.
- Measure 10 cm up from the top of the mattress, and place a mark on the patient's chest at that point.
- Place a mark at the mid-axillary level and at the fourth intercostal space.

If the transducer is zeroed at this point and then lowered with respect to the original level, the hydrostatic pressure of the water column in the catheter will falsely elevate the CVP reading. Similarly, raising the transducer's location above the original level will result in a false drop in the patient's CVP reading.

(9:361–363), (14:165–167, 170, 240).

## IIA1i(2)

89. D. The device shown is a water column used to institute PEEP. A water column PEEP device is known as a *threshold resistor*. Ordinarily, threshold resistors are placed in the expiratory limb of a ventilator breathing circuit. The threshold resistor shown here is applying 6 cm $H_2O$ PEEP to the patient's airways at end exhalation. The effect of this device can be perceived by observing the ventilator's pressure-time tracing. Note that the pressure does not return to zero, but rather it returns to 6 cm $H_2O$ at end exhalation. The PIP reaches 24 cm $H_2O$ without the PEEP and 30 cm $H_2O$ with the PEEP applied. Other threshold resistors commonly used to establish PEEP include spring-loaded diaphragms, electromechanical valves, reverse Venturis, and balloon valves.

(13:648–650, 653–654).

## IIIC5

90. B. The normal intracranial pressure is below 10 mm Hg. An intracranial pressure of 15 mm Hg will likely decrease cerebral blood flow. The lung region in this situation, which has been targeted for CPT, ordinarily requires the patient to assume the Trendelenburg position. The left lower lobe has four segments, three of which require the Trendelenburg position for drainage (i.e., posterior basal segment, anteromedial basal segment, and lateral basal segment). The superior basal segment is drained by placing the patient flat on her stomach.

The RRT should recommend to the physician modification of the postural drainage positions because of the elevated intracranial pressure. Positioning the patient head down will aggravate the problem of the increased intracranial pressure. Both IPPB therapy and deep coughing are contraindicated here because both of these therapeutic interventions would further elevate the patient's intracranial pressure. Aerosol therapy might be a useful adjunct to the CPT. It would not necessarily mobilize the secretions from the left lower lobe, however.

(1:799–800).

## IA1g(2)

91. B. The systolic pressure of the right and left ventricles of the heart range approximately 15 to 25 torr and 90 to 140 torr, respectively. The low resistance to blood flow through the pulmonary vasculature, caused by the mechanical phenomena referred to as *recruitment* and *distention*, account for the low right-ventricular pressures.

(1:215).

## IIIA1b

92. C. Fetal hemoglobin is not specifically measured by the co-oximeter. When present in a sample of blood, however, it produces false carboxyhemoglobin results. Many co-oximeters are capable of compensating for the presence of fetal hemoglobin via operator direction.

(1:328), (15:492).

## IIIE2a

93. B. The RRT must consider the weight of a liquid oxygen system, rather than rely on the pressure-gauge reading when calculating the duration of oxygen from a liquid system.

STEP 1: Calculate the volume of gaseous oxygen provided by the liquid system. Use the following formula and incorporate the gas volume–liquid weight factor (344 L/lb):

$$\begin{pmatrix} \text{volume of} \\ \text{gaseous} \\ \text{oxygen} \\ \text{(L)} \end{pmatrix} = \begin{pmatrix} \text{weight of} \\ \text{liquid oxygen} \\ \text{system} \\ \text{(lb)} \end{pmatrix} \times \begin{pmatrix} \text{gas volume-} \\ \text{liquid weight} \\ \text{conversion} \\ \text{factor (L/lb)} \end{pmatrix}$$

$$= 60 \text{ lbs} \times 344 \text{ L/lb}$$

$$= 20,640 \text{ L}$$

STEP 2: Determine the approximate flow duration from this liquid oxygen system.

$$\text{flow duration (min.)} = \frac{\text{volume of gaseous oxygen (L)}}{\text{liter flow (L/min.)}}$$

$$= \frac{20,640 \text{ L}}{3 \text{ L/min.}}$$

$$= 6,880 \text{ min.}$$

STEP 3: Convert minutes to hours.

$$\text{hours} = \frac{\text{min.}}{60 \text{ min./hour}}$$

$$= \frac{6,880 \text{ min.}}{60 \text{ min./hour}}$$

$$= 114 \text{ hours}$$

(1:1115), (5:28), (13:49).

## IIB1b

94. C. If the cascade humidifier has not been turned on or if the heating element inside the cascade has malfunctioned, the air traveling from the ventilator through the tubing and to the patient will not receive humidification. As a result, there will be no condensation accumulating in the ventilator tubing. Likewise, if the cascade temperature was set too low, the inspired gas would be insufficiently humidified. Again, no condensation would be deposited in the tubing. Conversely, if the cascade humidifier was set too high, condensation would develop in the ventilator circuit because the temperature of the gas would decrease in transit from the humidifier to the patient Y.

(5:107–110), (13:111).

## IIIB4b

95. A. Typically, candidates for inverse-ratio ventilation are already receiving conventional, volume-limited, mechanical ventilation. Most patients should be sedated and paralyzed when inverse-ratio ventilation is begun. If the patient is not sedated and paralyzed, the patient might "fight" the ventilator. The most common method of delivering inverse-ratio ventilation is via pressure control. For PC-IRV, the initial pressure-control level should be approximately one-half to two-thirds what is used during conventional volume ventilation of the patient.

Initially, no PEEP should be used if the original PEEP was less than 8 cm $H_2O$. If the original PEEP level was 8 cm $H_2O$ or greater, about one-half of the original PEEP level should be used. The initial $FIO_2$ should be 1.0. The I:E ratio should gradually be reversed, beginning with 1.5:1 or 2:1.

(1:518–519, 827, 876), (10:156, 286–287).

## IIIC7d

96. B. When secretions are extremely thick, it might be necessary to instill 3 to 10 ml of normal saline (in neonatal patients, only a few drops are required) before suctioning. This procedure is an attempt to "thin" secretions, thus facilitating their removal.

(15:836).

## IIIE1l

97. B. The problem in this situation is that the patient is breathing "against" the ventilator. She is generating a high negative pressure ($-12$ cm $H_2O$) on the pressure manometer. The patient might still be in active bronchospasm and refractory to conventional medication for an acute asthmatic episode. Therefore, sedation with fentanyl (Sublimaze) or another suitable sedative might help settle down the patient and enable her to breathe in phase with the ventilator. With the high pressure alarm continuing to sound, she likely requires sedation. Morphine is a frequently used opiate for sedation. Because morphine causes histamine release, however, it probably is best to avoid administering morphine to asthmatic patients. Fentanyl does not cause histamine release.

(10:311, 317).

## IIIA1d

98. A. The patient is displaying premature ventricular contractions (PVCs). Without additional clinical data, it is difficult to assess the hazard these PVCs are posing to the patient. It is reasonable to assume that the patient is not in any imminent danger, however. The presence of PVCs indicates that the myocardium of the ventricles is irritable and more prone to the development of a lethal dysrhythmia. Administration of lidocaine or some other suitable antidysrhythmia medication might be considered to reduce myocardial irritability.

(1:330–331), (9:204–206).

## IIB2e(1)

99. D. A pH of 7.46 and a $PaO_2$ of 80 mm Hg both approximately lie within normal limits, although a pH of 7.46 is 0.01 pH unit above the upper limit of normal. Patients are commonly ventilated in the range of 10 to

15 ml/kg of IBW. The tidal volume here (600 ml) represents 8.6 ml/kg; that is,

$$\frac{600 \text{ ml}}{70 \text{ kg}} = 8.6 \text{ ml/kg}$$

Therefore, the tidal volume is not excessive.

Similarly, a ventilatory rate of 12 breaths/min. is not excessive. This patient's minute ventilation ($V_T \times f = \dot{V}_E$) is 7.2 L/min., which is certainly reasonable. Reducing the tidal volume or ventilatory rate might lower the $PaO_2$ in this situation. Therefore, neither one should be reduced. The best approach here is to add some mechanical dead space to elevate the $PaCO_2$. Because the patient is in the control mode, elevating the $PaCO_2$ in this manner would not be difficult to accomplish. With the added mechanical dead space, however, the arterial $PO_2$ might decrease. If the dead space fails to achieve the therapeutic goal, it will need to be removed.

(1:935), (10:209, 248, 251–252, 434).

**IIB2s**

100. B. The manner in which the medication is now being delivered (directly into the incubator) is inappropriate because the infant is not receiving the full benefit of the aerosolized ribavirin. Much of the drug is settling out in the interior of the incubator and is not being inhaled by the infant. As much of the medication as possible should be delivered to the patient's face. An oxyhood needs to be placed over the infant's head and attached to the distal end of the aerosol-delivery tubing. The infant would then be in a situation to inhale more of the aerosolized ribavirin. Note that Figure 6-19 illustrates a SPAG-2 unit depositing its aerosolized output into an oxyhood.

The SPAG-2 unit is also designed to be connected to a face mask or tent. A number of clinical facilities have incorporated filters into their ventilator circuitry to administer aerosolized ribavirin via the SPAG-2 unit. The pharmaceutical company that manufactures Virazole (ribavirin) strongly discourages this practice because the buildup of crystallized ribavirin in the ventilator system might cause ventilator malfunction.

(1:697–698), (5:159–163), (13:149–152).

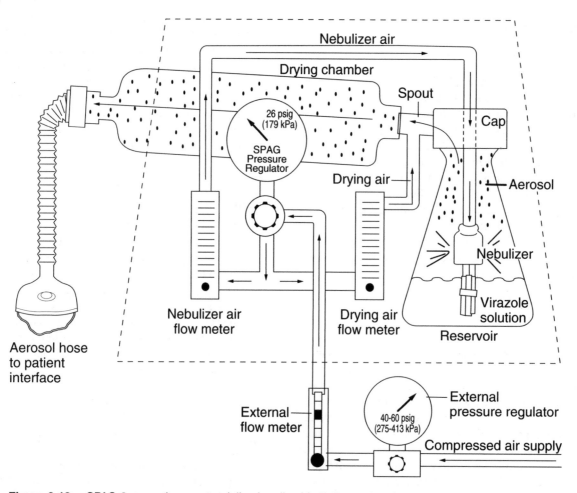

**Figure 6-19:** SPAG-2 aerosol generator delivering ribavirin to the oxyhood.

# REFERENCES

1. Scanlan, C., Spearman, C., and Sheldon, R., *Egan's Fundamentals of Respiratory Care*, 7th ed., Mosby-Year Book, Inc., St. Louis, MO, 1999.

2. Kacmarek, R., Mack, C., and Dimas, S., *The Essentials of Respiratory Care*, 3rd ed., Mosby-Year Book, Inc., St. Louis, MO, 1990.

3. Shapiro B., Peruzzi, W., and Kozlowska-Templin, R., *Clinical Applications of Blood Gases*, 5th ed., Mosby-Year Book, Inc., St. Louis, MO, 1994.

4. Malley, W., *Clinical Blood Gases: Application and Noninvasive Alternatives*, W.B. Saunders Co., Philadelphia, PA, 1990.

5. White, G., *Equipment Theory for Respiratory Care*, 3rd ed., Delmar, Albany, NY, 1999.

6. Ruppel, G., *Manual of Pulmonary Function Testing*, 7th ed., Mosby-Year Book, Inc., St. Louis, MO, 1998.

7. Barnes, T., *Core Textbook of Respiratory Care Practice*, 2nd ed., Mosby-Year Book, Inc., St. Louis, MO, 1994.

8. Rau, J., *Respiratory Care Pharmacology*, 5th ed., Mosby-Year Book, Inc., St. Louis, MO, 1998.

9. Wilkins, R., Sheldon, R., and Krider, S., *Clinical Assessment in Respiratory Care*, 4th ed., Mosby-Year Book, Inc., St. Louis, MO, 2000.

10. Pilbeam, S., *Mechanical Ventilation: Physiological and Clinical Applications*, 3rd ed., Mosby-Year Book, Inc., St. Louis, MO, 1998.

11. Madama, V., *Pulmonary Function Testing and Cardiopulmonary Stress Testing*, 2nd ed., Delmar, Albany, NY, 1998.

12. Koff, P., Eitzman, D., and New, J., *Neonatal and Pediatric Respiratory Care*, 2nd ed., Mosby-Year Book, Inc., St. Louis, MO, 1993.

13. Branson, R., Hess, D., and Chatburn, R., *Respiratory Care Equipment*, J.B. Lippincott, Co., Philadelphia, PA, 1995.

14. Darovic, G., *Hemodynamic Monitoring: Invasive and Noninvasive Clinical Application*, 2nd ed., W.B. Saunders Company, Philadelphia, PA, 1995.

15. Pierson, D., and Kacmarek, R., *Foundations of Respiratory Care*, Churchill Livingston, Inc., New York, NY, 1992.

16. Burton, et al., *Respiratory Care: A Guide to Clinical Practice*, 4th ed., Lippincott-Raven Publishers, Philadelphia, PA, 1997.

17. Wojciechowski, W., *Respiratory Care Sciences: An Integrated Approach*, 3rd ed., Delmar, Albany, NY, 2000.

18. Aloan, C., *Respiratory Care of the Newborn and Child*, 2nd ed., Lippincott-Raven Publishers, Philadelphia, PA, 1997.

19. Dantzker, D., MacIntyre, N., and Bakow, E., *Comprehensive Respiratory Care*, W.B. Saunders Company, Philadelphia, PA, 1998.

20. Farzan, S., and Farzan, D., *A Concise Handbook of Respiratory Diseases*, 4th ed., Appleton & Lange, Stamford, CT, 1997.

# Quick Reference Material—Clinical Data

1. Cylinder Sizes and Correction Factors — 404
2. Atmospheric Pressure Equivalents — 404
3. Causes of Hypoxemia — 404
4. Classification of Hypoxemia — 404
5. Criteria for Instituting Mechanical Ventilation — 404
6. Indications for PEEP — 405
7. Mechanical Ventilation Weaning Criteria — 405
8. Static and Dynamic Compliance Changes (D) — 405
9. Static and Dynamic Compliance Changes (D) and Associated Diagnoses — 405
10. Acid-Base Interpretations — 406
11. Normal Adult Hemodynamic Values — 406
12. Normal Adult Systemic Arterial Pressures — 406
13. Pulmonary Function Interpretations — 406
14. Pulmonary Function Interpretations and Values — 407
15. Blood Gas Analyzer Electrode Accuracy and Calibration Ranges — 407
16. Apgar Scoring Scale — 407

## Cylinder Sizes and Correction Factors

| Cylinder Size | Correction Factor |
|---|---|
| D | 0.16 L/psig |
| E | 0.28 L/psig |
| G | 2.41 L/psig |
| H or K | 3.14 L/psig |

## Atmospheric Pressure Equivalents

760 mm Hg
760 torr
1034 cm $H_2O$
14.7 psig
101.33 kPa

## Causes of Hypoxemia

- Decreased $F_IO_2$ or $P_IO_2$
- A/C membrane diffusion impairment
- Hypoventilation ($\downarrow \dot{V}_A$)
- R–L shunting
- $\dot{V}_A / \dot{V}_C$ mismatching

## Classification of Hypoxemia

| Classification | $PaO_2$ (torr) |
|---|---|
| Mild | 60 to 79 |
| Moderate | 40 to 59 |
| Severe | < 40 |

## Criteria for Instituting Mechanical Ventilation

| Measurement | Normal Value | Critical Value |
|---|---|---|
| • VC | 65 to 75 ml/kg | < 15 ml/kg |
| • $\dot{V}_E$ | 5 to 6 L/min. | > 10 L/min. |
| • f | 12 to 20 breaths/min. | > 35 breaths/min. |
| • $V_T$ | 5 to 7 ml/kg | < 5 ml/kg |
| • MIP (20 sec) | −80 to −100 cm $H_2O$ | > −20 cm $H_2O$ (~ 20 sec.) |
| • $V_D/V_T$ | 0.3 to 0.4 | > 0.6 |
| • $PaCO_2$ | 35 to 45 torr | > 55 torr |
| • pH | 7.35 to 7.45 | < 7.25 |
| • $PaO_2$ | 80 to 100 torr | < 50 torr at 0.50 $F_IO_2$ |
| • P(A-a)$O_2$ | 5 to 10 torr | > 350 torr at 1.00 $F_IO_2$ |

Indications for PEEP

- $PaO_2 < 60$ torr on $FIO_2$ 0.60 to 0.80
- $\dot{Q}_S/\dot{Q}_T > 0.30$
- $P(A\text{-}a)O_2 > 300$ torr on $FIO_2$ 1.0

Mechanical Ventilation Weaning Criteria

| Physiologic Measurement | Acceptable Values |
| --- | --- |
| Spontaneous f | $\leq 25$ breaths/min. |
| Spontaneous $V_T$ | $\geq 3$ ml/kg |
| VC | $\geq 10$ to 15 ml/kg |
| MIP | $\geq -20$ to $-25$ cm $H_2O$ ($\sim 20$ sec.) |
| Spontaneous $\dot{V}_E$ | $< 10$ L/min. |
| $C_T$ on ventilator | $> 30$ ml/cm $H_2O$ |
| $\dot{Q}_S/\dot{Q}_T$ | $< 15\%$ |
| $V_D/V_T$ | $< 0.55$ to 0.60 |
| $PaO_2/FIO_2$ | $> 100$ |
| $P(A\text{-}a)O_2$ on 100% $O_2$ | $< 300$ to 350 torr |
| $PaO_2$ on 100% $O_2$ | $> 300$ torr |
| $PaO_2$ on $< 40\%$ $O_2$ | $\geq 60$ torr |
| $PaO_2/PAO_2$ | $> 0.15$ |

Static and Dynamic Compliance Changes ($\Delta$)

| Condition | $\Delta\,C_{static}$ | $\Delta\,C_{dynamic}$ |
| --- | --- | --- |
| • Increased $R_{aw}$ | No $\Delta$ | Decrease |
| • Decreased $R_{aw}$ | No $\Delta$ | Increase |
| • Increased $C_{Total}$ | Increase | Increase |
| • Decreased $C_{Total}$ | Decrease | Decrease |
| • Increased $R_{aw}$ and decreased $C_{Total}$ | Decrease | Decrease |
| • Decreased $R_{aw}$ and increased $C_{Total}$ | Increase | Increase |
| • Increased $C_{Total}$ and increased $R_{aw}$ | Increase | No $\Delta$ or decrease |
| • Decreased $C_{Total}$ and decreased $R_{aw}$ | Decrease | No $\Delta$ or increase |

Static and Dynamic Compliance Changes ($\Delta$) and Associated Diagnoses

| $\Delta C_{static}$ | $\Delta C_{dynamic}$ | Diagnosis |
| --- | --- | --- |
| Decrease | Decrease | High-pressure (cardiogenic) pulmonary edema |
| Decrease | Decrease | Pneumonia |
| Decrease | Decrease | Adult respiratory distress syndrome (ARDS) |
| Decrease | Decrease | Atelectasis |
| Decrease | Decrease | Pneumothorax |
| No $\Delta$ | Decrease | Bronchospasm |
| No $\Delta$ | Decrease | Retained secretions |

Acid-Base Interpretations

| Acid-Base Abnormality | PaCO$_2$ (mm Hg) | HCO$_3^-$ (mEq/liter) | pH[a] |
|---|---|---|---|
| • uncompensated (acute) respiratory acidosis | > 45 | 22 to 26 | < 7.35 |
| • compensated (chronic) respiratory acidosis | > 45 | > 26 | Just under 7.35 |
| • uncompensated (acute) respiratory alkalosis | < 35 | 22 to 26 | > 7.45 |
| • compensated (chronic) respiratory alkalosis | < 35 | < 22 | Just above 7.45 |
| • uncompensated (acute) metabolic acidosis | 35 to 45 | < 22 | < 7.35 |
| • compensated (chronic) metabolic acidosis | < 35 | < 22 | Just below 7.35 |
| • uncompensated (acute) metabolic alkalosis | 35 to 45 | > 26 | > 7.45 |
| • compensated (chronic) metabolic alkalosis | > 45[b] | > 26 | > 7.45[b] |

[a] Compensatory mechanisms ordinarily do not return the pH value to within normal limits. When compensation has occurred, the pH will generally be just below the lower limit of normal (compensated acidosis) or just above the upper limit of normal (compensated alkalosis), depending on the primary acid-base disturbance.

[b] The PaCO$_2$ rarely exceeds 50 mm Hg during a compensated metabolic alkalosis. Therefore, the pH in this situation will generally be somewhat higher than the upper limit of normal.

Normal Adult Hemodynamic Values

| Physiologic Measurement | Acceptable Range |
|---|---|
| CVP | 0–7 cm H$_2$O (0–5 mm Hg) |
| RA pressure | < 10 mm Hg |
| RV diastolic | 0–8 mm Hg |
| RV systolic | 15–38 mm Hg |
| PA diastolic | 4–15 mm Hg |
| PA systolic | 12–30 mm Hg |
| PA mean | 8–20 mm Hg |
| PCWP mean | 6–12 mm Hg |
| LV diastolic | 4–11 mm Hg |
| LV systolic | 80–140 mm Hg |
| Cardiac output (C.O.) | 4–8 L/min. |
| Stroke volume (SV) | 60–130 ml |
| Cardiac index (CI) | 2.5–4.2 L/min./m$^2$ |
| $\dot{Q}_S/\dot{Q}_T$ | < 5.0% |

Normal Adult Systemic Arterial Pressures

| Measurement | Acceptable Range (mm Hg) |
|---|---|
| Diastolic | 60 to 90 |
| Systolic | 100 to 140 |
| Mean | 70 to 100 |

Pulmonary Function Interpretations

| Measurement | Restriction | Obstruction — Air Trapping | Obstruction — Hyperinflation |
|---|---|---|---|
| TLC | Decreased | Normal | Increased |
| VC | Decreased | Decreased | Normal |
| FRC | Decreased | Increased | Increased |
| RV | Decreased | Increased | Increased |
| RV/TLC | Normal | Increased | Increased |

Pulmonary Function Interpretations and Values

| Measurement | Normal | Restriction | Obstruction | |
| | | | Air Trapping | Hyperinflation |
|---|---|---|---|---|
| TLC (ml) | 6000 | 3600 (60% pred.) | 6000 (100% pred.) | 7500 (125% pred.) |
| VC (ml) | 4800 | 2850 (59% pred.) | 3600 (75% pred.) | 4575 (95% pred.) |
| FRC (ml) | 2400 | 1400 (58% pred.) | 3500 (145% pred.) | 4000 (167% pred.) |
| RV(ml) | 1200 | 750 (63% pred.) | 2400 (200% pred.) | 2925 (243% pred.) |
| RV/TLC (%) | 20% | 20% | 40% | 40% |

Blood Gas Analyzer Electrode Accuracy and Calibration Ranges

| Electrode Accuracy | Calibration |
|---|---|
| pH±0.01 | 6.840 (low) |
| | 7.384 (high) |
| $PCO_2$ ± 2.0% or ± 1 torr at 40 torr | 5.0% $CO_2$ (low) |
| | 10.0% $CO_2$ (high) |
| $PO_2$ ± 3.0% or ± 2.5 torr at 80 torr | 0% $O_2$ (low) |
| | 12% or 20% $O_2$ (high) |

Apgar Scoring Scale

| Sign | Rating | | |
| | 0 | 1 | 2 |
|---|---|---|---|
| Heart rate | Absent | < 100 beats/min. | > 100 beats/min. |
| Ventilatory effort | Absent | Slow, irregular | Good, crying |
| Muscle tone | Limp | Some flexion | Active, motion |
| Reflex irritability | No response | Grimace | Cough or sneeze |
| Color | Central and peripheral cyanosis | Peripheral cyanosis | Completely pink |

# Quick Reference Material— Waveforms and Tracings

1. Spirogram showing lung volumes and capacities     410

2. Normal Lead II ECG tracing showing electrophysiologic events (numbers) and electrocardiographic representation (letters)     410

3. Normal pulmonary artery (Swan–Ganz) catheter pressure tracings during catheter insertion     411

4. Capnography Tracings     412

5. Pressure-time waveforms     415

6. Mean airway pressure     416

7. Flow-time waveforms     416

8. Pressure, volume, and flow waveforms demonstrating controlled mechanical ventilation     417

9. Pressure, volume, and flow waveforms demonstrating SIMV with PSV and PEEP     418

10. Pressure, volume, and flow waveforms showing SIMV with PSV     419

11. Pressure, volume, and flow waveforms depicting pressure control ventilation (PCV)     420

12. Pressure, volume, and flow waveforms depicting assist/control ventilation     421

13. Pressure, volume, and flow waveforms illustrating SIMV     422

14. Pressure-time waveforms representing various modes of mechanical ventilation     423

15. Pressure-volume loop and mechanical ventilator characteristics     424

# 1. Spirogram showing lung volumes and capacities

## LUNG VOLUMES AND CAPACITIES

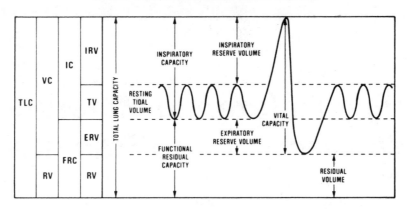

# 2. Normal Lead II ECG tracing showing electrophysiologic events (numbers) and electrocardiographic representation (letters)

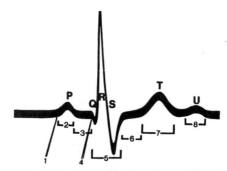

| Sequential electrical events of the cardiac cycle | Electrocardiographic representation |
|---|---|
| 1. Impulse from the sinus node | Not visible |
| 2. Depolarization of the atria | P wave |
| 3. Depolarization of the AV node | Isoelectric |
| 4. Repolarization of the atria | Usually obscured by the QRS complex |
| 5. Depolarization of the ventricles<br>  a. intraventricular septum<br>  b. right and left ventricles | QRS complex<br>  a. initial portion<br>  b. central and terminal portions |
| 6. Activated state of the ventricles immediately after depolarization | ST segment; isoelectric |
| 7. Repolarization of the ventricles | T wave |
| 8. After-potentials following repolarization of the ventricles | U wave |

## 3. Normal pulmonary artery (Swan–Ganz) catheter pressure tracings during catheter insertion

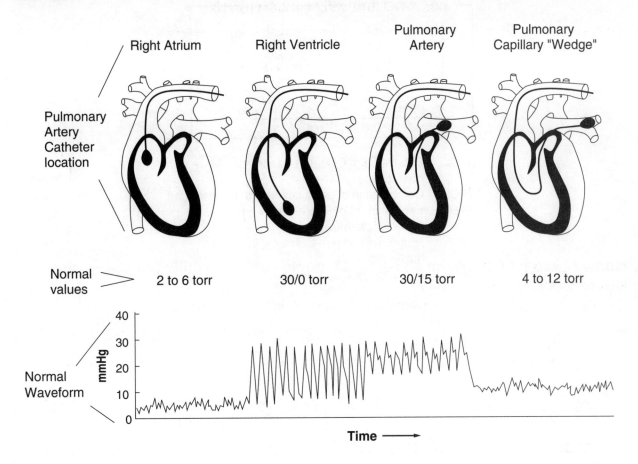

| | Right Atrium | Right Ventricle | Pulmonary Artery | Pulmonary Capillary "Wedge" |
|---|---|---|---|---|
| Pulmonary Artery Catheter location | | | | |
| Normal values | 2 to 6 torr | 30/0 torr | 30/15 torr | 4 to 12 torr |

Normal Waveform

Time ⟶

# 4. Capnography Tracings

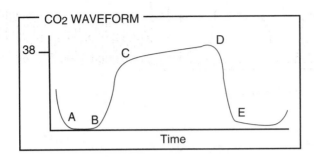

A-B: Exhalation of $CO_2$ free gas from dead space

B-C: Combination of dead space and alveolar gas

C-D: Exhalation of mostly alveolar gas (alveolar plateau)

D: "End-tidal": point—$CO_2$ exhalation at maximum point

D-E: Inhalation of $CO_2$ free gas

(4A) Normal, fast-speed $CO_2$ waveform highlighting tracing components.

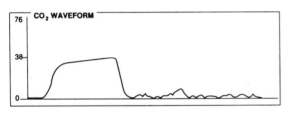
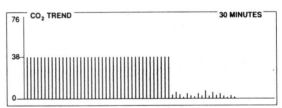

(4B) Abrupt end-tidal $CO_2$ decrease to 0 torr or near 0 torr reflecting the potential loss of ventilation.

## POTENTIAL INTERPRETATIONS:

- esophageal intubation
- ventilator disconnection
- ventilator malfunction
- obstructed or kinked ET tube

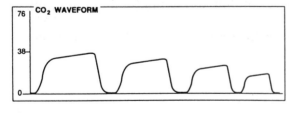
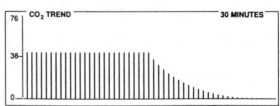

(4C) Exponential decrease in end-tidal $CO_2$ signifying interrupted blood flow.

## POTENTIAL INTERPRETATIONS:

- cardiac arrest with continued alveolar ventilation
- hypotensive episode (hemorrhage)
- pulmonary embolism
- cardiopulmonary bypass

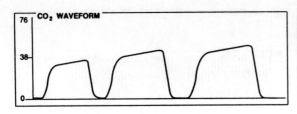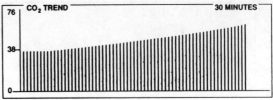

(4D)  Progressively increasing end-tidal $CO_2$.

## POTENTIAL INTERPRETATIONS:

- hypoventilation
- increasing body temperature
- partial airway obstruction
- absorption of $CO_2$ from exogenous source (e.g., laparoscopy)

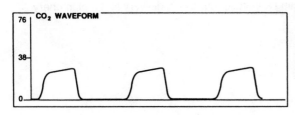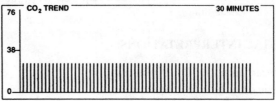

(4E)  Consistently low end-tidal $CO_2$ characterized by a well-defined alveolar plateau indicating a widened P(a-A)$CO_2$ gradient.

## POTENTIAL INTERPRETATIONS:

- hyperventilation
- COPD (pulmonary emphysema, chronic bronchitis)
- asthma
- pulmonary embolism
- hypovolemia

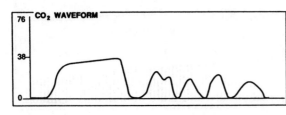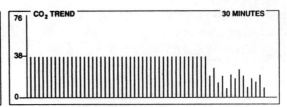

(4F)  Abrupt fall in end-tidal $CO_2$, but not to 0 torr, indicating an incomplete sampling of patient's expirate.

## POTENTIAL INTERPRETATIONS:

- ventilator circuit leak
- partial ventilation circuit disconnection
- retained secretions causing partial airway obstruction
- ET tube in hypopharynx

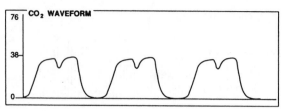 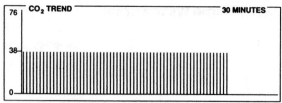

(4G) Alveolar plateau cleft signifying partial recovery from a neuromuscular blockade.

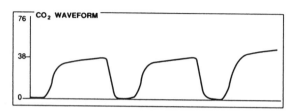 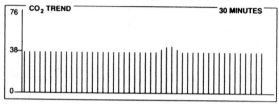

(4H) Abrupt, transient increase in end-tidal $CO_2$ reflecting an acute rise in $CO_2$ delivery to the pulmonary vasculature.

## POTENTIAL INTERPRETATIONS:

- bicarbonate ($HCO_3^-$) administration
- release of limb tourniquet

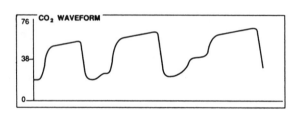 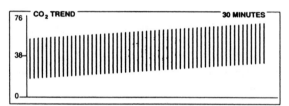

(4I) Abrupt baseline elevation signaling a contaminated sample cell requiring cleaning and recalibration.

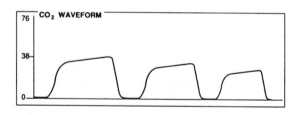 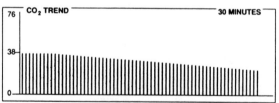

(4J) Progressive drop in end-tidal $CO_2$ suggesting a decreasing $\dot{V}CO_2$ or a decreasing pulmonary perfusion.

## POTENTIAL INTERPRETATIONS:

- hypovolemia
- decreasing cardiac output
- hypoperfusion
- hypothermia

## 5. Pressure-time waveforms

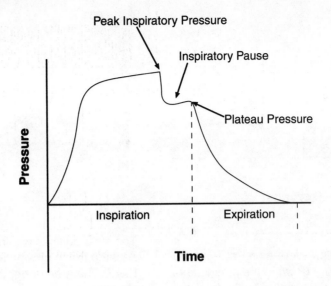

Peak Inspiratory Pressure

Inspiratory Pause

Plateau Pressure

Pressure

Inspiration

Expiration

**Time**

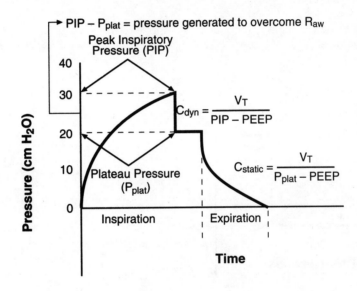

PIP – P_plat = pressure generated to overcome R_aw

Peak Inspiratory Pressure (PIP)

40

30

$C_{dyn} = \dfrac{V_T}{PIP - PEEP}$

20

Plateau Pressure (P_plat)

10

$C_{static} = \dfrac{V_T}{P_{plat} - PEEP}$

0

Pressure (cm H₂O)

Inspiration

Expiration

**Time**

## 6. Mean airway pressure

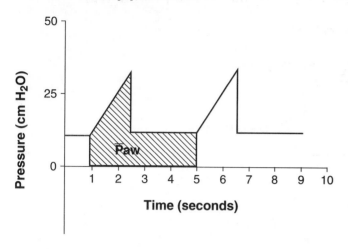

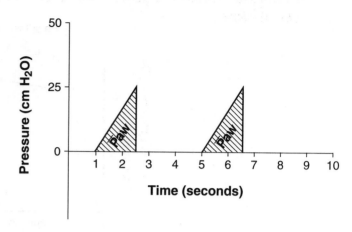

The slashed lines within the pressure-time tracing represent the mean airway pressure ($\bar{P}_{AW}$) in the presence of PEEP. The area under the curve divided by the total cycle time equals the $\bar{P}_{AW}$.

The slashed lines within the pressure-time tracing represent the mean airway pressure ($\bar{P}_{AW}$) in the presence of PEEP. The area under the curve divided by the total cycle time equals the $\bar{P}_{AW}$.

## 7. Flow-time waveforms

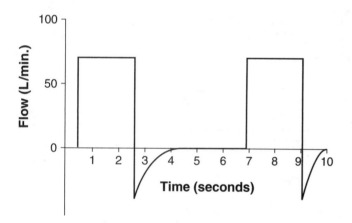

Square flow-time waveform.

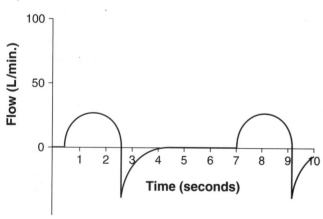

Sinusoidal flow-time waveform.

Decelerating flow-time waveform.

## 8. Pressure, volume, and flow waveforms demonstrating controlled mechanical ventilation

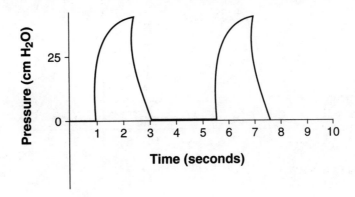

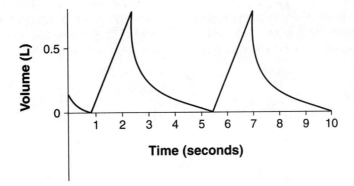

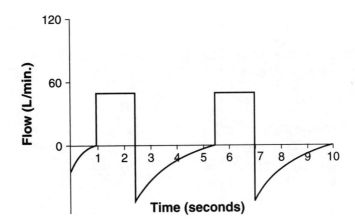

## 9. Pressure, volume, and flow waveforms demonstrating SIMV with PSV and PEEP

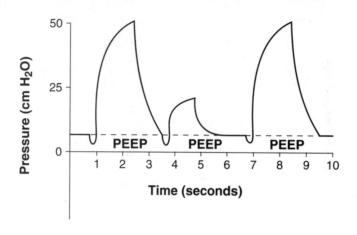

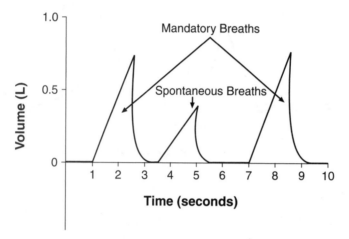

(The spontaneous volume is increased because the breath is pressure supported.)

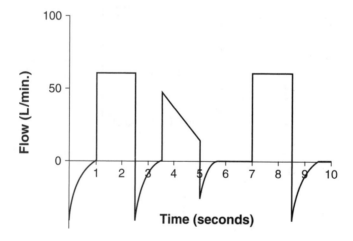

## 10. Pressure, volume, and flow waveforms showing SIMV with PSV

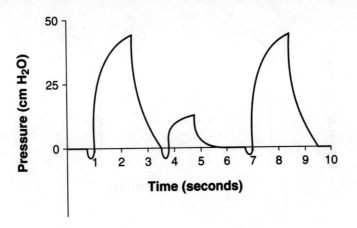

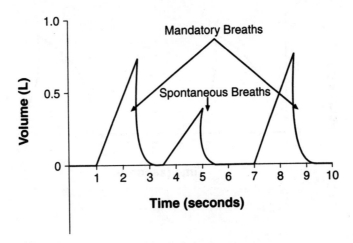

(The spontaneous volume is increased because the breath is pressure supported.)

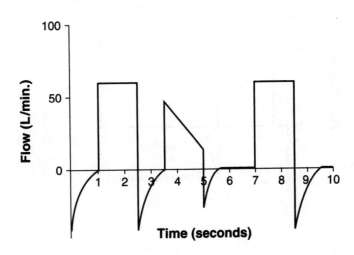

## 11. Pressure, volume, and flow waveforms depicting pressure control ventilation (PCV)

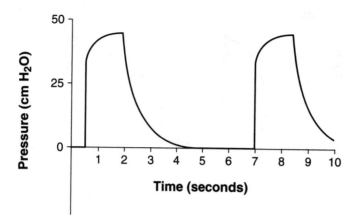

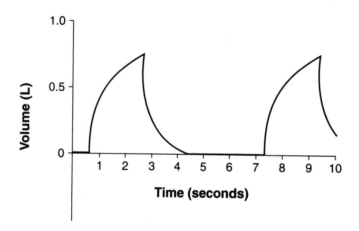

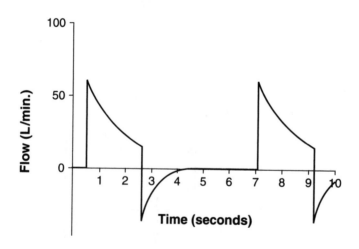

**12. Pressure, volume, and flow waveforms depicting assist/control ventilation**

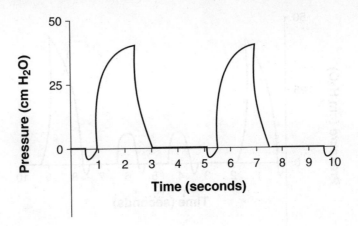

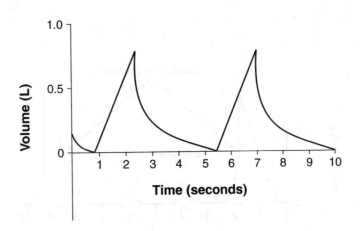

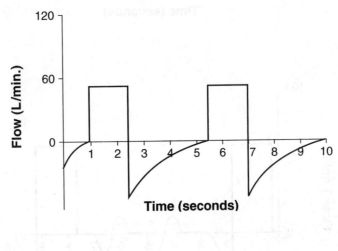

## 13. Pressure, volume, and flow waveforms illustrating SIMV

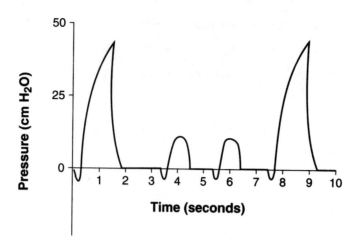

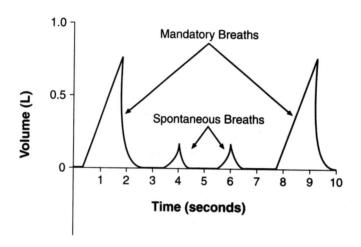

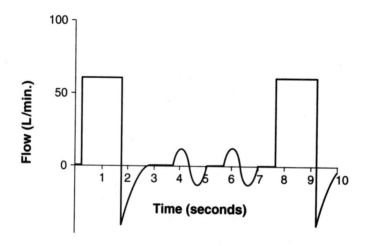

# 14. Pressure-time waveforms representing various modes of mechanical ventilation

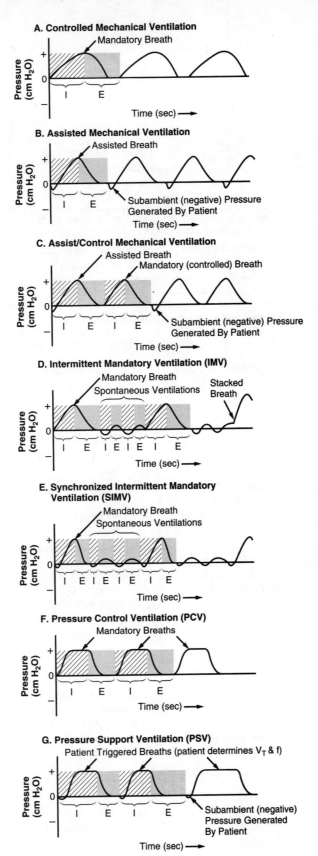

A. Controlled Mechanical Ventilation

Mandatory Breath

Pressure (cm H₂O)

Time (sec) →

B. Assisted Mechanical Ventilation

Assisted Breath

Pressure (cm H₂O)

Subambient (negative) Pressure Generated By Patient

Time (sec) →

C. Assist/Control Mechanical Ventilation

Assisted Breath
Mandatory (controlled) Breath

Pressure (cm H₂O)

Subambient (negative) Pressure Generated By Patient

Time (sec) →

D. Intermittent Mandatory Ventilation (IMV)

Mandatory Breath
Spontaneous Ventilations
Stacked Breath

Pressure (cm H₂O)

Time (sec) →

E. Synchronized Intermittent Mandatory Ventilation (SIMV)

Mandatory Breath
Spontaneous Ventilations

Pressure (cm H₂O)

Time (sec) →

F. Pressure Control Ventilation (PCV)

Mandatory Breaths

Pressure (cm H₂O)

Time (sec) →

G. Pressure Support Ventilation (PSV)

Patient Triggered Breaths (patient determines $V_T$ & f)

Pressure (cm H₂O)

Subambient (negative) Pressure Generated By Patient

Time (sec) →

## 15. Pressure-volume loop

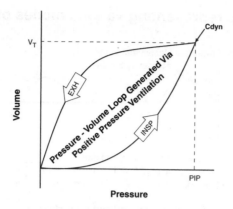

| Mechanical Ventilator Characteristics | | | |
|---|---|---|---|
| | **Constant Flow Ventilator** | **Constant Pressure Ventilator** | **Variable Flow Ventilator** |
| **Modes** | control & SIMV | control & SIMV | control |
| **Variables** | **Independent Variable**<br>• Flow<br><br>**Dependent Variable**<br>• Pressure<br><br>**Limiting Variable**<br>• Volume<br><br>**Triggering Variables**<br>• Time<br>• Pressure<br>• Flow | **Independent Variable**<br>• Pressure<br><br>**Dependent Variables**<br>• Volume<br>• Flow<br><br>**Limiting Variable**<br>• Pressure<br><br>**Triggering Variables**<br>• Time<br>• Pressure<br>• Flow | **Independent Variable**<br>• Volume<br><br>**Dependent Variable**<br>• Pressure<br><br>**Limiting Variable**<br>• Volume<br><br>**Triggering Variables**<br>• Time<br>• Pressure<br>• Flow |
| **Waveform Analysis** | • Pressure-time waveform is affected by airway resistence changes.<br><br>• Flow-time waveform is not affected by compliance and airway resistence changes.<br><br>• Volume-time waveform is not affected by compliance and airway resistence changes. | • Pressure-time waveform is not affected by compliance and airway resistence changes.<br><br>• Flow-time waveform is affected by compliance and airway resistence changes.<br><br>• Volume-time waveform is affected by compliance and airway resistence changes. | • Pressure-time waveform is affected by compliance changes.<br><br>• Flow-time waveform is not affected by airway resistence changes.<br><br>• Volume-time waveform is not affected by compliance and airway resistence changes. |

# Quick Reference Material—
# Physical Examination of the Chest

1. Chronic bronchitis
2. Pulmonary emphysema                                    426
3. Asthma                                                 426
4. Bacterial (lobar) pneumonia                            426
5. Lobar atelectasis                                      426
6. Pneumothorax (unilateral)                              426
7. Pleural effusion (unilateral)                          426

## Physical Examination of the Chest for Some Common Pulmonary Diseases and Conditions[*]

| Disease/Condition | Inspection | Palpation | Percussion | Auscultation |
|---|---|---|---|---|
| Chronic bronchitis | Prolonged exhalation; accessory ventilatory-muscle use and cyanosis in severe form or during acute exacerbation; thoracic excursions might be normal or decreased depending on severity; jugular venous distention with cor pulmonale; slight overweight appearance | Generally normal | Usually unremarkable; hepatomegaly with cor pulmonale | Early inspiratory crackles; expiratory wheezing depending on severity; prolonged exhalation; loud $P_2$ with pulmonary hypertension (cor pulmonale) |
| Pulmonary emphysema | Barrel chest; increased AP chest-wall diameter; kyphosis; accessory ventilatory-muscle use; prolonged exhalation; clavicular lift during inspiration; pursed-lip breathing; prominent anterior chest with elevated ribs; emaciated appearance | Decreased chest-wall expansion; reduced and/or more midline point of maximum impulse; decreased tactile fremitus | Hyperresonance; decreased diaphragmatic excursions | Dimished breath sounds; heart sounds distant; prolonged exhalation |
| Asthma | Accessory ventilatory-muscle use: prolonged exhalation; intracostal and supraclavicular retractions based on severity; increased AP diameter if severe | Frequently normal; decreased chest-wall expansion and decreased tactile fremitus depending on severity | Frequently normal; hyperresonance during acute exacerbation | Prolonged exhalation and expiratory wheezing; inspiratory and expiratory wheezing, or diminished air movement with severity |
| Bacterial (lobar) pneumonia | Accessory ventilatory-muscle use and cyanosis depending on severity; increased ventilatory rate | Reduced thoracic expansion over affected lung area; increased tactile fremitus over consolidated (affected) area | Dull percussion note or decreased resonance over consolidated area | Bronchial breath sounds over consolidated area; if bronchial obstruction is total, breath sounds will be diminished or absent; coarse inspiratory crackles in affected region |
| Lobar atelectasis | Increased ventilatory rate (accessory-muscle use) and shallow breathing; mediastinal and tracheal shift toward affected (atelectatic) region; cyanosis if severe | Decreased tactile fremitus over atelectatic region; reduced chest-wall expansion over affected region | Dull percussion note over atelectatic region | Decreased or absent breath sounds over collapsed region (no air entry); late inspiratory crackles indicate air entry through partial obstruction, inflating atelectatic alveoli |
| Pneumothorax (unilateral) | Tachypnea (ventilatory distress) and cyanosis depending on severity; mediastinal and tracheal deviation away from affected lung, varying with severity | Absent tactile fremitus over affected lung; reduced chest-wall expansion over involved lung | Hyperresonance over affected lung | Absent or diminished breath sounds over affected lung |
| Pleural effusion (unilateral) | Increased ventilatory rate (respiratory distress) and cyanosis varying with severity; mediastinal and tracheal shift away from affected side based on severity (size of effusion) | Absent tactile fremitus over affected area; decreased chest-wall expansion on the affected side | Dull percussion note over affected area | Absent breath sounds over affected region |

[*]The actual clinical manifestations and physical examination findings will vary with the severity of the presentation.